T0400560

Pharmaceutical Perspectives of Cancer Therapeutics

Yi Lu · Ram I. Mahato
Editors

Pharmaceutical Perspectives of Cancer Therapeutics

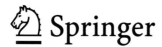 Springer

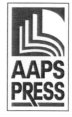

Editors

Yi Lu
Department of Pathology
 & Laboratory Medicine
University of Tennessee
 Health Science Center
19 S. Manassas
Memphis TN 38103
USA
ylu@utmem.edu

Ram I. Mahato
Department of Pharmaceutical Sciences
University of Tennessee
 Health Science Center
19 S. Manassas
Memphis TN 38103
USA
rmahato@utmem.edu

ISBN 978-1-4419-0130-9   e-ISBN 978-1-4419-0131-6
DOI 10.1007/978-1-4419-0131-6
Springer Dordrecht Heidelberg London New York

Library of Congress Control Number: 2009927127

Printed on acid-free paper

Springer is part of Springer Science + Business Media (www.springer.com)

Preface

The goal of our efforts in compiling *Pharmaceutical Perspectives of Cancer Therapeutic* is to produce a comprehensive, yet easy-to-follow review of the principles and current approaches in this ever growing field. With today's broad research perspective and technology expertise, the knowledge in the field of cancer research and drug development has become a challenge not only for students who are eager to learn, but also for seasoned professionals who are willing to update. The complexity of cancer demands a comprehensive and integrated understanding from both cancer biology and pharmaceutical dosage forms and drug delivery, in order to warrant a successful therapeutic regimen. However, no book to date combines together these two aspects, namely the cancer research and the drug design and delivery from an integrated perspective of cancer treatment. Hence, a book that merges the knowledge from these two aspects is greatly desired.

For the purpose of bridging basic research and clinical application, pharmaceutical drug development processes and regulatory issues, drug design and delivery, laboratory and translational experimentation, marketing and postmarketing surveillance, we have invited international experts with a multidisciplinary background, including scientists and clinicians from both academia and industries in their respective fields to contribute to this book. We intend to convey both an introductory understanding and the latest development in the field so that this book can be useful for both novice students and practicing scientists. With a comprehensive and integrated view of cancer therapeutics, we hope that this book will stimulate a deeper understanding and promote interaction in this integrated field for people with diverse expertise and backgrounds, who are working on cancer therapeutics.

We have organized this book to cover a wide variety of topics, including strategies to suppress tumor angiogenesis and metastasis, overcome multidrug resistance in cancer, target telomerase and apoptosis pathways; therapeutic approaches to employ monoclonal antibody and cancer vaccines; introduction of new concepts such as cancer stem cells and new technologies such as nanobiotechnology, RNA interference, microRNA, and cancer cell gene profiling. The use of synthetic carriers, such as lipids, polymers, and peptides for delivery and targeting of small molecules, proteins, and nucleic acids to cancer cells or specific organs *in vivo*, as well as targeted delivery of macromolecular drugs to cancer cells, are described in detail. In addition, the utilization of imaging in cancer therapeutics, development and utilization of HIF-1 knockout animal models in cancer studies, as well as the principles of developing anticancer drugs and designing clinical trials, are also discussed. In summary, this book provides an in-depth review of various aspects of anticancer strategies and drug delivery approaches from different perspectives, including detailed discussion of several clinical trial cases. The book has a wider and more involved focus on cancer therapy with a good balance on diversity. It integrates cancer therapy approaches (both biological- and small compound molecule-based therapy) with drug delivery. By reading this book, not only bench scientists can have an insight for what physicians desire for their clinical use toward cancer treatment, but also physicians will better understand how the approach and drug are developed and therefore will apply the drug more efficiently and accurately in patients. Moreover, this book summarizes current progress and state of the art of cancer therapeutics, while focusing on the novel ideas that are being explored to overcome the existing challenges. We hope that this book will serve as both a refresher and ready reference, as well as an educational tool, to both new entrants and seasoned researchers.

Memphis, Tennessee   Yi Lu and Ram I. Mahato

About the Editors

Yi Lu graduated with B.S. in Biochemistry from Fudan University in Shanghai, China in 1984, and Ph.D. in Biochemistry and Molecular Biology from University of Nebraska Medical Center, Omaha, NE, USA in 1992. He is currently an associate professor at the Departments of Pathology, Medicine, and Pharmaceutical Sciences, University of Tennessee Health Science Center, Memphis, TN, USA. His research interests include tumor angiogenesis and metastasis, gene therapy for prostate cancer and breast cancer, targeted gene expression, and exploration of novel apoptosis-inducing genes. He has written more than 50 publications and holds five patents.

Ram I. Mahato is a full-time associate professor in the Department of Pharmaceutical Sciences at the University of Health Science Center Memphis, TN, USA. He was a research assistant professor at the University of Utah, Salt Lake City, UT, USA senior scientist at GeneMedicine, Inc., The Woodland, TX, USA and postdoctoral fellow at the University of Southern California in Los Angeles, Washington University in St Louis, MO, USA and Kyoto University, Japan. He received his B.S. in Pharmaceutics from China Pharmaceutical University Nanjing, Jiangsu, China in 1989 and Ph.D. in Pharmaceutics and Drug Delivery from the University of Strathclyde, Glasgow, Scotland, UK in 1992. He is an author or co-author of 79 peer-reviewed articles and book chapters. He has also edited/written three books and is a special features editor of *Pharmaceutical Research* and on the editorial board of the *Journal of Drug Targeting*, *Expert Opinion on Drug Delivery*, and *Transplantation and Risk Management*. His research includes delivery and targeting of small molecules, oligonucleotides, siRNA, and genes.

Contents

Contributors

Michael D. Axelson Department of Internal Medicine, Division of Hematology-Oncology, Harold C. Simmons Comprehensive Cancer Center, University of Texas Southwestern Medical Center, Dallas, TX, USA

You Han Bae Department of Pharmaceutics and Pharmaceutical Chemistry, University of Utah, Salt Lake City, UT, USA

Derrick Beech Department of Surgery, Meharry Medical College, Nashville, TN, USA

Reina Bendayan Leslie Dan Faculty of Pharmacy, University of Toronto, Ontario, Canada

Guofeng Cheng Shanghai Research Center for Animal Biotechnology, Shanghai, China

Kun Cheng Department of Pharmaceutical Sciences, University of Missouri-Kansas City, Kansas City, MO, USA

Kyung H. Choi Eppley Institute for Research in Cancer, University of Nebraska Medical Center, Omaha, NE, USA

Michael Danquah Department of Pharmaceutical Sciences, University of Tennessee Health Science Center, Memphis, TN, USA

Divyakant S. Desai Bristol-Myers Squibb, Co., New Brunswick, NJ, USA

Christian Dohmen Pharmaceutical Biology-Biotechnology, Ludwig-Maximilians Universität, München, Germany

Jun Fang BioDynamics Research Laboratory, Kumamoto University, Innoventive Collaborative Organization, Cooperative Research Laboratory, Mashiki, Kumamoto, Japan

David E. Gerber Department of Internal Medicine, Division of Hematology & Oncology, Harold C. Simmons Comprehensive Cancer Center, University of Texas Southwestern Medical Center, Dallas, TX, USA

Célia M.F. Gomes Institute of Biophysics/Biomathematics, IBILI – Faculty of Medicine, Azinhaga de Sta Comba – Celas, Coimbra, Portugal

Weikuan Gu Department of Orthopaedic Surgery, University of Tennessee Health Science Center, Memphis, TN, USA

Hiroshi Harada Department of Radiation Oncology and Image-applied Therapy, Graduate School of Medicine, Kyoto University, Sakyo-ku, Kyoto, Japan

Masahiro Hiraoka Department of Radiation Oncology and Image-applied Therapy, Graduate School of Medicine, Kyoto University, Sakyo-ku, Kyoto, Japan

K.K. Jain Jain PharmaBiotech, Basel, Switzerland

Dineo Khabele Vanderbilt University Medical Center, Ob/Gyn Department, Nashville, TN, USA

Dongin Kim Department of Pharmaceutics and Pharmaceutical Chemistry, University of Utah, Salt Lake City, UT, USA

Maciej S. Lesniak Section of Neurosurgery, Brain Tumor Center, University of Chicago Pritzker School of Medicine, Chicago, IL, USA

Zheng-Rong Lu Department of Pharmaceutics and Pharmaceutical Chemistry, University of Utah, Salt Lake City, UT, USA

Yi Lu Department of Pathology and Laboratory Medicine, University of Tennessee Health Science Center, Memphis, TN, USA

Chikezie O. Madu Department of Pathology and Laboratory Medicine, University of Tennessee Health Science Center, Memphis, TN, USA

Hiroshi Maeda Laboratory of Microbiology and Oncology, Faculty of Pharmaceutical Sciences, Sojo University, Kumamoto, Japan; BioDynamics Research Laboratory, Kumamoto University, Innoventive Collaborative Organization, Cooperative Research Laboratory, Kumamoto, Japan

Ram I. Mahato Department of Pharmaceutical Sciences, University of Tennessee Health Science Center, Memphis, TN, USA

Ajit S. Narang Bristol-Myers Squibb, Co., New Brunswick, NJ, USA

Manfred Ogris Pharmaceutical Biology-Biotechnology, Ludwig-Maximilians Universität, München, Germany

Michel M. Ouellette Eppley Institute for Research in Cancer, University of Nebraska Medical Center, Omaha, NE, USA

Bin Qin Department of Pharmaceutical Sciences, University of Missouri-Kansas City, Kansas City, MO, USA

Jichao Qin Department of Carcinogenesis, University of Texas M.D. Anderson Cancer Center, Science Park-Research Division, Smithville, TX, USA

Arun K. Rishi Karmanos Cancer Institute, Department of Internal Medicine, Wayne State University, John D. Dingell VA Medical Center, Detroit, MI, USA

Tiffany N. Seagroves Department of Pathology and Laboratory Medicine, Center for Cancer Research, University of Tennessee Health Science Center, Memphis, TN, USA

Takahiro Seki Innoventive Collaborative Organization, Kumamoto University, Kumamoto, Japan

Adam Quasar Sugihara Brain Tumor Center, University of Chicago Pritzker School of Medicine, Chicago, IL, USA

Zsuzsanna Tabi Department of Oncology, School of Medicine, Cardiff University, CRW Laboratory, Velindre Hospital, Cardiff, UK

Dean G. Tang Department of Carcinogenesis, University of Texas M.D Anderson Cancer Center, Science Park-Research Division, Smithville, TX, USA; Program in Molecular Carcinogenesis, Graduate School of Biomedical Sciences (GSBS), The University of Texas Health Science Center, Houston, TX, USA

Matthew A. Tyler Brain Tumor Center, University of Chicago Pritzker School of Medicine, Chicago, IL, USA

Ilya V. Ulasov Brain Tumor Center, University of Chicago Pritzker School of Medicine, Chicago, IL, USA

Anagha Vaidya Department of Pharmaceutics and Pharmaceutical Chemistry, University of Utah, Salt Lake City, UT, USA

Anil Wali Karmanos Cancer Institute, Department of Surgery, Wayne State University, John D. Dingell VA Medical Center, Detroit, MI, USA

Ho Lun Wong School of Pharmacy, Temple University, Philadelphia, PA, USA

Xiao Yu Wu Leslie Dan Faculty of Pharmacy, University of Toronto, Ontario, Canada

Hong Yan Department of Carcinogenesis, University of Texas M.D Anderson Cancer Center, Science Park-Research Division, Smithville, TX, USA; Department of Epidemiology, Wuhan University School of Public Health, Wuhan, Hubei, China

Jian Yan Department of Orthopaedic Surgery, University of Tennessee Health Science Center, Memphis, TN, USA

Xinbo Zhang Department of Surgery, Karmanos Cancer Institute, Wayne State University, John D. Dingell VA Medical Center, Detroit, MI, USA

Tumor Microvasculature and Microenvironment: Therapeutic Targets for Inhibition of Tumor Angiogenesis and Metastasis

Chikezie O. Madu and Yi Lu

1 Introduction

The growth of a tumor depends on both the tumor origin and the surrounding environment. Recent developments of therapeutic strategies targeting angiogenesis and other key steps in the metastatic cascade have demonstrated significant improvements on both the inhibition of primary tumor size and the suppression of malignant secondary tumor spreading. In this chapter, we briefly introduce tumor microvasculature and microenvironment, discuss tumor angiogenesis and therapeutic approaches for inhibiting of tumor angiogenesis, and examine the potential therapeutic targets for suppression of tumor progression and metastasis. While this chapter focuses mainly on pharmaceutical approaches for targeting tumor angiogenesis and metastasis, it also mentions other approaches including gene therapy. In addition, the current challenges and future prospects in this field are discussed.

2 Tumor Microvasculature and Microenvironment

2.1 Tumor Microvasculature

Cancer is a general term for malignant diseases characterized by uncontrolled and abnormal cell proliferation. Whereas different types of cancer have specific causes that lead to the abnormality, all types of cancer require a suitable blood supply to facilitate the tumor growth. In a process termed angiogenesis, endothelial cells initially respond to changes in the local environment and migrate toward the growing tumor. The endothelial cells then migrate together forming tubular structures that are ultimately encapsulated by recruiting periendothelial support cells to establish a vascular network that provides

Y. Lu (✉)

Department of Pathology, University of Tennessee Health Science Center, Memphis, TN 38163, USA

e-mail: ylu@utmem.edu

Y. Lu, R.I. Mahato (eds.), *Pharmaceutical Perspectives of Cancer Therapeutics*, DOI 10.1007/978-1-4419-0131-6_1, © Springer Science+Business Media, LLC 2009

1

nutrition and oxygen to the growing tumor [1]. This vascular network is tumor microvasculature.

Solid tumors less than 1–2 mm in diameter in size generally can obtain their nutrition and oxygen needs through diffusion from the existing surrounding microvasculature [2–4]. However, a progressive enlargement of these tumors leads to an increase in demand for nutrients, oxygen, and growth factors, as well as the removal of increasing production of metabolic waste by the cancer cells. An insufficient supply of these requirements necessary for continuous proliferation results in regions of low glucose levels, low pH, low oxygen concentration (hypoxia), and a possible shrinkage and death of these cells. In order to prevent these and prolong its survival, the tumors must develop their own blood supply network, the tumor microvasculature, in order to provide a stable flow of oxygen and nutrients as well as a system of removing waste to guarantee its unremitting growth. Thus, tumor vasculature has naturally emerged as a potential target for cancer therapy.

2.2 Tumor Microenvironment

As the tumor grows, various cytokines and growth factors are released from the cancer cells into the surrounding. Consequently, various types of cells including fibroblasts, endothelial cells, and infiltrating inflammatory cells are recruited to the tumor site where they are reprogrammed to perform new functions, further facilitating tumor growth. This process in turn creates an elevated variety of cytokines released into the local area by these cells. These various types of cells and cytokines at the tumor site together create a tumor microenvironment. Specifically, the tumor microenvironment is the stroma composed of various types of cells and extracellular matrix (ECM) that surround the tumor.

The tumor microenvironment is a diverse and intricate surrounding that is characterized by low pH and nutrient levels, increased interstitial fluid pressure (IFP), and chronic variation of oxygen levels. The abnormality of tumor microenvironment induces alteration of gene expression in local cells. Those altered gene expression, either from the temporary genetic changes or from the buildup of genetic variation over time, provoke tumor cell ability to progression and metastasis. For example, the interaction between the tumor cells and the ECM, which is thought to play a major role in metastasis, can be modified by genetic changes induced by the local tumor environment. Several studies demonstrated that altered gene expression due to low oxygen levels (hypoxia) microenvironment contributes to the increased metastatic ability of tumor cells [5, 6]. Several genes whose expressions are altered in the hypoxic environment have been linked to the steps of metastasis, including growth, angiogenesis, intravasation, extravasation, and survival [5–8]. By using a xenotransplant metastasis model of human melanoma cells, Xu et al. identified a "metastasis/aggressiveness gene expression signature," based on selection of metastatic potential [9]. Not only does this metastasis gene signature correlate well with the expression profile and the aggressiveness of disease from human melanoma patients but also many genes identified in the metastasis gene signature encode secreted and membrane proteins, suggesting the importance of tumor−microenvironment interactions during metastasis. Genetic and molecular properties of the tumor cells have been the center of research for many years. The current focus has been gradually shifted to emphasize more on the interactions between the tumor and its microenvironment (or the ECM) and on the epigenetic and physiological regulation of metastasis [10].

The locally produced cytokines in the microenvironment, together with the immune responses generated, are considered as major factors in determining the progression or regression of a tumor. The pro- and antitumorigenic abilities of cytokines play essential roles in determining whether the tumor would grow or be rejected after the malignant cells interact with immune cells, which trigger further cascades of cytokines, chemokines, and growth factors. A recent review by Sheu et al. [11] has linked the microenvironment-derived cytokines and growth factors to a number of different kinds of human carcinogenesis models. Key factors that contribute to this tumor immune-altering ability include multifunctional cytokines, extracellular matrix mediators, and regulatory cytokines. Also, tumor cells are able to elude immune-system clearance due to the tumor's ability of local immune suppression. Most tumors are immunogenic but often fail to simulate a sufficient immune response. Several mechanisms have been implicated in the ability of the tumor to escape from the host immune surveillance. The tumor microenvironment has recently been revealed as an important component contributing to the dysfunction of dendritic cells, which play a key role in the induction of tumor-specific immune responses [12]. Study has demonstrated that expression of immune-inhibitory B7 molecules was upregulated in the tumor microenvironment, contributing to the immune evasion of tumors [13]. Thus, these inhibitory B7 molecules and their signaling pathways can be targets in new therapeutic approaches for cancer.

Cancer is a heterogeneous disease, whose progression from hyperplasia to malignancy and invasiveness is controlled by multiple mediators produced by the tumor and its stroma (tumor microenvironment), including, but are not limited to, growth factors, cytokines, chemokines, and proteases. The establishment of a tumor vasculature, viability, spreading, and eventual spreading of the tumor cells to secondary organs are all consequences of abnormal expression of these mediators. For example, clinical research indicates that poor patient prognosis in breast cancer is associated with the signaling activation of the ShcA, an adaptor protein that transmits extracellular signals (growth factor, one of such mediators) to downstream of receptor tyrosine kinases [14]. Depending on the microenvironment, tumor cells can either proceed further sequential steps toward malignant progression including initial recruitment of blood vessels or stay at a "tumor dormancy" state and fail to develop to a clinically detectable manifestation of cancer from a microscopic tumor due to lack of angiogenesis [15]. Recent studies have showed that microenvironment stimuli, such as hyaluronan, have critical impact on cancer initiation and progression [16]. Because microenvironment plays such important roles in tumor initiation and progression, the tumor microenvironment including stromal elements has become an attractive therapeutic target for cancer therapy.

3 Angiogenesis

3.1 Physiological Angiogenesis

Physiological angiogenesis occurs when new blood vessels arise from preexisting ones by emerging thin-walled endothelium-tubular structures in the presence or absence of muscular smooth muscle wall and fibrocytes, respectively. It differs from arteriogenesis and lymphangiogenesis and usually takes place during a normal process, such as reproduction, growth and development (embryonic angiogenesis), and wound healing. Physiological angiogenesis is typically focal and self-limited in time [17]. In general, physiological angiogenesis refers to the outgrowth of microvessels that are typically the size of capillary blood vessels in a normal process regulated by an array of balanced angiogenic stimulators (growth factors) and inhibitors.

In a body's natural process like wound healing, an injured tissue initiates the process of physiological angiogenesis by producing and releasing angiogenic growth factors into the wound area. Upon diffusing into the surrounding tissues, these angiogenic growth factors bind to particular receptors on the surface of endothelial cells of adjacent preexisting blood vessels, and consequently activate the endothelial cells. Specific signals are then transduced to the nucleus, which then instigates the production of new substances including enzymes to breakdown the basement membrane that covers the existing blood vessels. The endothelial cells start to proliferate and migrate out through the broken basement membrane of the existing vessels and are recruited toward the damaged tissue. A new blood vessel tube forms when numerous sprouting endothelial cells roll up. Many such individual blood vessel tubes eventually connect to one another, in order to form a new blood vessel network. The final stabilization of the newly formed blood vessel tubes is structurally supported by smooth muscle cells and pericytes [18]. As the vessel extends, the tissue around the vessel is simultaneously remodeled by collagen deposition from ECM and the local replacement of various cells. Once the wound healing process is complete, surplus cells are removed by apoptosis.

3.2 Pathological Angiogenesis

Pathological angiogenesis occurs in both cancer and a variety of nonneoplastic diseases, sometimes collectively dubbed "angiogenesis-dependent diseases;"

These include, but are not limited to, diabetic blindness, age-related macular degeneration, and rheumatoid arthritis. These pathological conditions are characterized by the feeding of diseased tissues with new blood vessels and the destruction of normal tissues. In contrast to physiological angiogenesis, pathological angiogenesis can persist for years and is usually associated with some clinical symptoms. Pathological angiogenesis is an abnormal process of blood vessel formation in which the body loses control and becomes unable to provide a regulated, balanced array of angiogenic stimulators and inhibitors. As a consequence, angiogenesis-dependent diseases can result from either an excessive formation of new blood vessels (i.e., cancer) or an insufficient supply of new blood vessels (i.e., ischemia).

Pathological angiogenesis can lead to various clinical symptoms such as bleeding, vascular leakage, and tissue destruction, and, in more severe states, incapacitation or death —a consequence of angiogenesis-dependent diseases such as cancer and atherosclerosis [17]. In cancer, diseased cells produce aberrant high amounts of angiogenic growth factors, which overpower the regulatory effects of natural angiogenesis inhibitors: consequently, new blood vessels grow rapidly in an uncontrolled manner, and excessive angiogenesis occurs. Pathological angiogenesis is essential for tumors to grow beyond a microscopic dimension size. The new blood vessels provide nutrition and oxygen to the growing tumor, allowing tumor cells to further proliferate and break into the circulation as well as spread to other organs (tumor metastases).

3.3 Angiogenic Switch

Angiogenesis is driven by a delicate balance between different pro- and anti-angiogenesis effector molecules (or so-called angiogenic stimulators and inhibitors) that influence the growth rate of capillaries [19, 20]. The representative angiogenic stimulators include vascular endothelial growth factor (VEGF), basic fibroblast growth factor (bFGF), matrix metalloproteinases (MMP), transforming growth factor beta-1 (TGFß1), epidermal growth factor (EGF), and angiopoietin-1. The representative angiogenic inhibitors include thrombospondin-1 (TSP-1), angiostatin, and endostatin. Normal vessel growth results from balanced and coordinated expression of these opposing factors. A switch from normal to uncontrolled vessel growth can occur by upregulating angiogenic stimulators or downregulating angiogenic inhibitors or a combination of the two [21].

The angiogenic switch, which leads endothelial cells from a quiescent state to active proliferation, occurs when the subtle balance between angiogenic stimulators and inhibitors is altered. While the exact mechanism of the angiogenic switch is still not fully understood, so far, four components have been proposed or identified to play roles in angiogenic switch in tumorigenesis, based on the studies. (1) *Tumor angiogenesis driven by the prevascular tumors*. The diffusion limit determines the radius of a viable prevascular tumor by obtaining nutrition and oxygen from the nearby existing vessels; once beyond that tumor size (usually around 1–2 mm in diameter), the angiogenic switch must be turned on or the tumor undergoes apoptosis or necrosis [3, 4, 22–26]. Nearly 95% of the human cancers are carcinomas that start off as microscopic lesions localized in an epithelial layer devoid of blood vessels and separated by a basement membrane from underlying vasculature of local tissues. The basement membrane serves as a physical barrier to the migratory endothelial cells that are recruited to the tumor from the local neighborhood and form a circle of new microvessels around the tumor. After the rupture of basement membrane by sprouting new vessels, the infiltrated new capillary blood vessels are covered by several layers of tumor cells [27]. (2) *Tumor angiogenesis contributed by circulating endothelial stem cells.* Accumulated laboratory and clinical studies have demonstrated that circulating endothelial progenitor cells derived from stem cells in the postnatal bone marrow can contribute to tumor growth after they are recruited to the vascular bed of certain type of tumors [28–40]. Circulating VEGF may be one of the angiogenic stimulators by which tumors use to recruit circulating endothelial stem cells: VEGF–VEGF receptor signal has been implicated in the mobilization of bone marrow progenitor endothelial cells into the circulation where the endothelial cells are further recruited into the tumor vascular bed [28]. Therefore, both the endothelial cells from the local neighborhood and the bone marrow can convene to the tumor vascular bed to serve as sources of microvascular endothelial cells for tumor angiogenesis, although the ratio of the endothelial cells from these two sources varies for different types of tumors [41–43]. (3) *Tumor angiogenesis contributed by nonendothelial cells.* Besides endothelial cells, tumors may also recruit mast cells, macrophages, and inflammatory cells from the host [44–47]. These nonendothelial cells can release angiogenic stimulators (such as bFGF) and metalloproteinases, which breakdown the basement membrane and further facilitate the effects of angiogenic stimulators, leading to an in situ amplification of tumor angiogenesis [44, 48–50]. In addition, the host stromal cells in the tumor microenvironment can express an elevated level of VEGF to promote amplification of the tumor angiogenesis [51]. (4) *Angiogenic switch in secondary tumors.* In the metastatic process, tumor cells migrate to the target organ and extravasate from the microvessels there. Once the secondary tumor starts to grow around these vessels, the original vessels degenerate due to apoptosis, and a neovascular network subsequently forms around the new tumor by its recruitment of neovascular sprouts from nearby existing vessels. This "vessel cooption" process may represent a transitional or alternative phase in the angiogenic switch [23, 52].

Because tumors are angiogenesis dependent, anti-angiogenic therapy that targets any of these components of the angiogenic switch should serve well for controlling tumor growth and metastasis. For example, circulating VEGF is one of the angiogenic signals by which tumors can recruit endothelial cells from the bone marrow [30, 53, 42, 54]. Therefore, angiogenesis inhibitors targeting

VEGF and other drugs that suppress the release of bone marrow-derived progenitor endothelial cells can be effective in blocking the angiogenic switch and tumor growth.

4 Therapeutic Approaches for Inhibition of Tumor Angiogenesis

4.1 From the Emerging Concept that Tumor Growth Is Angiogenesis-Dependent to Clinical Trials

In early 1970s, Judah Folkman dared to propose a revolutionary concept that blood vessel formation around a tumor was a prerequisite for the growth of the tumor [3]. Best summarized by Folkman, "Once tumor take has occurred, every further increase in tumor cell population must be preceded by an increase in new capillaries that converge upon the tumor" [55]. Based on the observations by him and his colleagues in the 1960s that tumor growth in isolated and perfused organs was significantly constrained without vascularization [56, 57], Folkman hypothesized that tumor growth is angiogenesis-dependent and an anti-angiogenesis approach can be an effective therapy for cancer [3, 58, 59]. By the mid-1980s, a large amount of research data had been gathered in supporting and solidifying the concept that tumor growth is angiogenesis dependent. This concept and the subsequent evidences from biological, pharmacological, and genetic data have provided a scientific basis for the current development and clinical trials of angiogenesis inhibitors.

However, it took many years before the discovery of the first angiogenesis inhibitor. Before 1980, doubts were casted over whether or not such substances ever existed. The development of bioassays for angiogenesis during the 1970s aided in the discovery of angiogenesis inhibitors [60–64]. Incited by the premise that angiogenesis fosters tumor growth and driven by persisted efforts through a continued study over 25 years, the Folkman's group finally identified the first angiogenesis inhibitor, interferon-alpha (IFN-α), in the early 1980s [65, 66] and several additional angiogenesis inhibitors lateron [67–71]. During the same period, more angiogenesis inhibitors were also discovered by several other groups [72–76]. The first clinical trial using angiogenesis inhibitor occurred in 1989 for the treatment of life-threatening hemangiomas (masses of blood capillaries) by IFN-α [77]. In 1992, TNP-470 became the first angiogenesis inhibitor entering clinical trial for cancer patients, and by the mid-1990s, several other anti-angiogenic drugs started entering clinical trials. By 2003, some of these drugs began to receive FDA approval in the United States. At the end of 2007, over 10 angiogenesis inhibitors had been approved by the FDA in the United States [17], and currently there are over 50 anti-angiogenesis-based drugs in clinical trials for cancer worldwide [77]. Among the 67 completed and ongoing/approved clinical trials in the United States which use anti-angiogenesis drugs, the majority (94%) are used for cancer treatment [78]. Bevacizumab (Avastin), a monoclonal antibody against VEGF, came to US market in February 2008, becoming the first anti-angiogenic drug approved to treat breast cancer.

4.2 Category of Angiogenesis Inhibitors

Angiogenesis inhibitors can be grouped by their natures, functions (Sections 4.2.1, 4.2.2, and 4.2.3), or mechanisms of action (Section 4.2.4, 4.2.5, and 4.2.6). These classifications may overlap.

4.2.1 Direct Angiogenesis Inhibitors

These inhibitors directly block vascular endothelial cells from responding to a wide spectrum of angiogenic stimulators, including VEGF, bFGF, PDGF, and others. As a result, the abilities of endothelial cells on proliferation, migration, and survival are suppressed, and angiogenesis is inhibited. This group of angiogenesis inhibitors includes low molecular weight compounds, such as thalidomide and angiostatic steroids; endogenous, naturally occurring proteins, including IFN-α, IL-12, TSP-1, angiostatin, and endostatin; synthetic inhibitors or peptides that are engineered to impede various steps in the angiogenic process, such as inhibitors of metalloproteinases. As demonstrated by animal study in which tumors growing in mice did not develop drug resistance after treatment with this group of inhibitors [79], direct angiogenesis inhibitors are generally less prone to stimulate acquired drug resistance in the host body, probably due to the fact that they target genetically stable endothelial cells rather than unstably mutating tumor cells [80].

4.2.2 Indirect Angiogenesis Inhibitors

Indirect angiogenesis inhibitors generally prevent the expression of or block the activity of a tumor protein that activates angiogenesis. The action is indirect — the effect of the inhibitor is on either blocking or reduction of the expression of an angiogenic product from a tumor, neutralizing the tumor protein itself, or occluding its receptor on endothelial cells. Many of these angiogenic products from the tumor are proteins coded by the oncogenes that promote the angiogenic switch [22, 81–83]. Studies demonstrated that transfection with oncogenes increases output of tumor cell pro-angiogenic factors and/or decreases expression of anti-angiogenic regulators [83–86]. For example, overexpression of bcl-2 oncogene promotes prostate cancer cells to develop larger neovascularized tumors, increased VEGF expression and microvessel density [87]. The pro-angiogenic nature of these oncogenes may be a major component of their tumorigenic activity. Thus, drugs that target these oncogenes, their products, or the receptors of those products should have a two-fold inhibition on tumor growth: one at disruption of angiogenesis as being an indirect angiogenesis inhibitor and another at anti-proliferation of tumor cells or promoting tumor cells' susceptibility to apoptosis by anti-oncogene property. Several novel anticancer drugs have been developed based on their abilities to inhibit the activity of the oncogene or its mediated signal transduction involved in tumor angiogenesis. Examples of this group of drugs include Herceptin, an inhibitor for the HER2 oncogene signal transduction [88], inhibitors of the EGF receptor tyrosine kinase [82, 88, 89], and ras farnesyl transferase inhibitors that block ras signaling pathways which upregulate production of VEGF and downregulate production of TSP-1 [90].

4.2.3 Endogenous Angiogenesis Inhibitors

This group of inhibitors is defined as opposed to synthetic drugs or inhibitors purified from the bacterial organisms. The inhibitors of this group consist of endogenous and natural proteins that exhibit anti-angiogenic activities, including, but are not limited to, TSP-1, angiostatin, endostatin, interferons, tumstatin, arresten, canstatin, and pigment epithelium-derived factor (PEDF) [91]. The endogenous inhibitors can be either direct (endostatin) or indirect (PEDF) angiogenesis inhibitors. The interferons and platelet factor-4 were among the first in this group to be found possessing the abilities to inhibit endothelial cell migration [65, 92], proliferation [93], as well as angiogenesis [94, 95]. The discovery of the existence of endogenous angiogenesis inhibitors has not only suggested the mechanisms for how a tumor may regulate its own growth but also provided us with new strategies to inhibit tumor angiogenesis and control tumor growth. The most known members of this group are endostatin and angiostatin, which have been shown to effectively suppress tumor angiogenesis in both preclinical and clinical studies [77, 96].

4.2.4 Angiogenesis Inhibitors That Block the Signaling Transduction Pathway

This group of inhibitors is categorized based on their abilities to block the angiogenic signaling transduction pathway and cascade. Some of them may overlap with the groups described above. Members of this group include anti-VEGF antibody that interferes with the binding between the VEGF receptor and its ligand VEGF, thus blocking the VEGF-mediated angiogenic transduction signaling. Avastin, a monoclonal antibody against VEGF, is the first of this kind of drug to be approved by the FDA; it has been shown to suppress tumor growth significantly and prolong patient survival in clinical trials [97]. IFN-α is another example of this group that inhibits the production of bFGF and VEGF, the angiogenic growth factors that initiate the angiogenic signaling cascade. In addition, several synthetic drugs that block receptors on endothelial cells are also in clinical trials [97].

4.2.5 Angiogenesis Inhibitors That Prevent ECM Breakdown

This group of inhibitors acts directly against angiogenic products generated by growing endothelial cells that facilitate ECM breakdown, specifically, the matrix metalloproteinases (MMPs). MMPs play essential roles in angiogenesis by enabling endothelial cells to migrate into adjoining tissues through the holes of MMP-digested matrix and proliferate into the new blood vessels. Therefore, drugs that are aimed at MMPs can serve as effective angiogenesis inhibitors. Several clinical trials using synthetic or naturally occurring molecules that inactivate MMPs are currently ongoing [97].

4.2.6 Miscellaneous Angiogenesis Inhibitors

This is a group of drugs whose anti-angiogenesis mechanisms either are vague or do not fit in any group described above. Examples among this group are LBH589, a histone deacetylase inhibitor [98]; CAI, a drug that exerts its anti-endothelial cell growth effect by inhibiting cell's calcium uptake [97]; rhodostomin, a venom disintegrin that exhibits anti-angiogenic effects through blockade of $\alpha_v\beta_3$ integrin, has been reported to successfully suppress solid tumors and prolong survival in mice [99]; and other interesting pharmaceutical drugs that target annexin II [100]. In addition, the anti-angiogenesis drugs and strategies that have antioxidant effects or lead to copper deficiency for cancer chemoprevention are also under investigation [101].

4.3 Anti-angiogenic Therapy and Pharmaceutic Targets

Anti-angiogenic therapy by the pharmaceutic approach refers to the application of particular compounds capable of inhibiting the formation of new blood vessels in the body, in order to fight "angiogenesis-dependent diseases," including cancer. There are presently over 200 biotech, genomics, and pharmaceutical companies either investing in or developing new drugs to target the inhibition of angiogenesis [18]. The majority of these anti-angiogenic drugs that are currently in clinical trials target angiogenic growth factors or their receptors in order to block the angiogenic signaling pathway. A recent review by Folkman has provided a nice overview of the current anti-angiogenic drugs and their status of FDA approval and clinical trial phase [17]. In this chapter, we discuss several targets that can be used to inhibit tumor angiogenesis by pharmaceutical approaches.

4.3.1 VEGF as a Therapeutic Target

Based on the hypothesis initially proposed by Dvorak that tumor angiogenesis is associated with increased microvascular permeability, a protein named as vascular permeability factor (VPF) was identified [102, 103]. The subsequent sequence revealed that VPF is identical to VEGF, a protein independently found by another group and named for its ability to specifically induce angiogenesis [104–106]. VEGF/VPF (also named as VEGF-A later) is a dimeric glycoprotein secreted by cells that promotes tumor-associated angiogenesis [102, 104]. It is an endothelial cell mitogen and motogen [107–109]. The VEGF-A family comprises five isoforms, including polypeptides of 121, 145, 165, 189, and 206 amino acids that are produced by the alternate splicing of a single gene containing eight exons [105, 110–112]. VEGF$_{165}$ is the one most commonly secreted by tumor cells as well as the one most influential in inducing endothelial cells to form new capillaries [113, 114]. Besides VEGF-A, other identified VEGF family members that share structural homologues include VEGF-B, VEGF-C, VEGF-D, and VEGF-E [109, 115]. In this chapter, we will focus on VEGF-A, the most common and well-studied member of the VEGF family.

Signaling of VEGF is initiated via its binding to its receptor. Two high-affinity VEGF receptors, VEGFR1 (Flt-1) [116, 117] and VEGFR2 (Flk-1/KDR or Flk-1) [118, 119], have been identified in endothelial cells. VEGF receptors are tyrosine kinases that share with other growth factor receptors the ability to trans-phosphorylate and, in turn, phosphorylate on specific tyrosine residues of SH2 (Src homology 2) domain-containing signaling molecules [120, 121], thus activating kinase-dependent transcription factors known as STAT (signal transducers and activators of transcription) proteins that are important modulators of cell growth responses induced by VEGF [122]. Studies have shown that it is Flk-1 (not Flt-1), undergoing strong ligand-dependent tyrosine phosphorylation [120, 121], which plays the major role in mediating the mitogenic effect of VEGF in endothelial cells [112]. Several studies showed that VEGF and its cognate receptor Flk-1 play major roles in tumor angiogenesis [123–128]. The importance of VEGF signaling via VEGF/VEGF receptor (VEGF R) in tumor angiogenesis is exemplified in several studies using a dominant-negative Flk-1 receptor [123, 129], neutralization of VEGF by monoclonal antibodies (mAb) [130, 131], and neutralization of Flk-1 mAb [132, 133] or Flk-1 kinase inhibitors [134] all of which were shown to inhibit angiogenesis and tumor growth. Besides VEGF R1 and R2, a third VEGF receptor (VEGF R3 or Flt-4) was identified and is specifically expressed in lymphatic cells [135]. The various members of the VEGF family have overlapping abilities to interact with their receptors. For example, VEGF-A interacts with VEGF R1 and R2, but not R3; VEGF-B only interacts with R1; whereas VEGF-C and VEGF-D interact with both R2 and R3, but not R1 [136].

VEGF (VEGF-A) is the most potent angiogenic factor known and plays a pivotal role in tumor angiogenesis [1, 137–140]. Several strategies have been developed to either directly neutralize VEGF or block VEGF signaling pathway in order to inhibit tumor angiogenesis. These strategies include neutralizing antibody directly to VEGF [23, 141, 130], small interfering RNA [142, 143] or antisense oligonucleotide [78] to VEGF, antibody against VEGF receptor [132, 133, 144], or inhibitor of VEGF receptor kinase [145]. Avastin (Bevacizumab), an mAb directly against VEGF, was the first among those approved by the FDA in

2004 for the clinical trial of treating metastatic colorectal cancer [77]. In addition, downregulation of ligand VEGF gene expression [146] or the depletion of VEGF protein by truncated VEGF receptor [147] is also an effective strategy to inhibit VEGF-mediated tumor angiogenesis.

4.3.2 bFGF as a Therapeutic Target

Another important angiogenic growth factor is basic fibroblast growth factor (bFGF), which is the first angiogenic protein to be isolated and purified from a tumor [148]. bFGF stimulates cell proliferation on both endothelial cells and various stromal cells including fibroblasts, smooth muscle cells, and neurons. bFGF also promotes endothelial cell migration. While there is very low expression of bFGF receptors in endothelium and bFGF lacks a secretion signal sequence [149], bFGF has a high affinity for heparin and heparan sulfate which are abundant in extracellular matrix. Studies showed that bFGF interferes with and prevent adhesion of leukocytes to endothelium, suggesting that tumors may develop a local immunologic escape and tolerance by expressing high levels of bFGF [150–152].

bFGF has been implicated as a vital player in the early stages of tumor progression [153]. The elevated levels of bFGF are associated with advanced disease stages/tumor grades [154–156] and poor diagnosis in cancer patients [157]. Therefore, strategies by targeting bFGF have been developed in order to inhibit angiogenesis. When antibody against bFGF was administered into mice bearing tumors, dramatic reductions in both neovascularization and tumor size were observed [149]. Several substances have been discovered as potent inhibitors of bFGF. Phosphorothioate oligonucleotides have been shown to inhibit bFGF from binding to endothelial cells [158]. Heparin oligosaccharides have been shown to inhibit bFGF-induced neovascularization [159]. Hyaluronan-binding protease, a plasma serine protease with a high affinity to glycosaminoglycans like heparin or hyaluronic acid, was reported to inhibit bFGF-dependent endothelial cell proliferation [160]. Of interest is that certain tumors, such as giant cell bone tumors and angioblastomas, express exclusively or mainly bFGF with no other usual angiogenic factors. When patients with these tumors were treated with interferon-α at low daily doses, bFGF production by tumor cells was inhibited [161, 162].

4.3.3 HIF-1 as a Therapeutic Target

One general characteristic of fast-growing solid tumors is the development of intratumoral hypoxia, whose existence correlates to a more malignant tumor phenotype and worse diagnosis. The tumor cells in hypoxic conditions are inclined to spread and develop multidrug resistance [163], both of which are obstacles in clinical interventions for cancer patients. The characteristics of a hypoxic environment include low oxygen tension, low extracellular pH, high IFP, glucose deficiency, and increased extracellular lactate levels. Adaptation to the hypoxic environment is critical for tumor cells' survival and growth. To prevent cellular damage and avoid cell death, the hypoxic cells in tumors must undergo modification of their gene expression profiles, in order to form new blood vessels to supply oxygen and nutrition. These hypoxic adaptations include the stimulation of genes that control anaerobic metabolism, nitric oxide synthase, and angiogenesis process [44]. The main mediator of this hypoxia response/adaptation is hypoxia-inducible factor-1 (HIF-1) [164, 165].

HIF-1 is a transcriptional activator for a group of genes that are responsible for promoting tumor cell angiogenesis and progression [141]. HIF-1 is composed of an inducible subunit, HIF-1α and a constitutively expressed subunit, HIF-1ß [166]. HIF-1α is a protein of 120 kDa, member of the basic helix-loop-helix superfamily transcription factors, and its expression is very sensitive to oxygen concentration [167, 168]. Under normal oxygen tension, HIF-1α is rapidly degraded by a posttranslational ubiquitination-triggered proteolysis, and this degradation process requires von Hippel Lindau (VHL) protein [169]. However, under low oxygen tensions (hypoxia), HIF-1α becomes stabilized and heterodimerizes with HIF-1ß to form the complex HIF-1, which mediates its nuclear translocation and binds to hypoxic responsive elements (HRE) within the promoter regions of target genes [164, 170]. Hypoxia in the tumor micro-environment is sufficient for activating HIF-1-dependent gene expression [171]. Tumor regional hypoxia and hypoglycaemia are the principal stimulators for the expression of local pro-angiogenic cytokines, especially VEGF [44, 167, 172]. A characteristic of cancer cells, the basal level of the HIF-1α subunit was frequently overexpressed in advanced tumors [173, 174]. HIF-1α is associated with the risk of aggressive behavior and tumor angiogenesis in gastrointestinal stromal tumors [175]. Overexpression of HIF-1α is also observed in many other cancers [176] and associated with increasing expression of VEGF [175]. Upregulation of HIF-1α signaling pathways has been associated with the molecular expression signature of micrometastasis in human breast cancer [174, 177]. HIF-1α is an important transcriptional factor for tumor progression and metastatic potential [178]: activation of HIF-1α stimulates a group of HIF-1α-regulated genes, including VEGF, one of its main downstream effectors that promote cell angiogenesis and tumorigenesis [179].

Many human neoplastic cells, including colon, breast, lung, endometrium gastric, bladder, and prostate, have been recently reported to overexpress HIF-1 and VEGF transcripts. As VEGF is correlated to vascular density, malignant stage of the disease, and poor prognosis [180–184], targeting HIF-1 (the upstream regulator of VEGF) or its pathway has become a strategy for anti-angiogenic cancer therapy. For example, recent research has revealed that drugs capable of pharmacologically inhibiting estrogen-related receptors (ERRs), which interact physically with HIF-1 and are necessary for HIF-1-induced transcription, severely inhibited growth and angiogenesis of human breast tumor xenografts in vivo [185]. Other inhibitors for HIF-1 pathway include camptothecin/topotecan [186], PX-478 [187], YC-1 [188], and deguelin [189]. Some of these drugs are currently in clinical trials.

4.3.4 Other Targets for Angiogenesis Inhibition

Epigenetic steps that stimulate a pro-angiogenic microenvironment for a tumor can also be targeted. One example of such targets is the inducible nitric oxide synthase (iNOS), known to upregulate VEGF expression and thereby promoting tumor angiogenesis. One recent study revealed that several bioactive food components are able to prevent tumor development by suppressing angiogenesis via the iNOS-VEGF pathway [190]. Another recent study has demonstrated that PI3K/Akt pathway plays a significant role in controlling tumor angiogenesis and growth via modulation of HIF-1 and VEGF expression. As evidenced by the frequent mutations of PTEN and dysfunction of PI3K/AKT pathway in human cancer, the key components (PTEN and PI3K/AKT) in this pathway are suitable targets for cancer therapy [191]. Other anti-angiogenesis-based targets and approaches include utilization of natural and synthetic angiogenesis inhibitors such as angiostatin [192], endostatin [192], arresten [193], canstatin [194], and tumstatin [72].

4.4 Gene Therapy and Other Biological Therapeutic Approaches for Anti-angiogenesis

Inhibition of angiogenesis is an effective approach to suppress tumor growth and metastasis. Gene therapy has become the preferred alternative to warranting a continuous supply of an angiogenic inhibitor, due to its prolonged and wide dispensation of the inhibitor as a product of the transgene. Based on the gene delivery system, it can be categorized as nonviral gene therapy or viral gene therapy. The former uses cationic liposome, nanoparticles, and electroporation to deliver the therapeutic transgene, whereas the latter uses various engineered viral vectors including recombinant retroviruses, adenoviruses, and adeno-associated viruses to do so. The therapeutic transgenes include, but are not limited to, expression of angiogenesis inhibitors (such as angiostatin, see below), tumor/metastasis suppressor genes such as maspin [195, 196], and genes that disrupt angiogenic transduction pathway such as dormant negative VEGF receptor [197] or p16 that downregulates expression of angiogenic factors VEGF (see below). Because anti-angiogenic therapy works more effectively on preventing tumor growth than causing regression of established tumors, gene therapy (especially the viral-based gene delivery) offers an ideal strategy for long-term, continuous production of anti-angiogenic agents that may best serve to prevent development of primary or recurrent tumors. With this notion in mind, gene therapy may be best used in conjunction with other standard therapeutic modalities such as surgery, chemotherapy, and radiotherapy.

4.4.1 Gene Therapy Using Angiostatin

Expression of anti-angiogenic genes or angiogenesis inhibitors is a straightforward targeting approach. Angiostatin gene therapy has been proven to effectively suppress tumors and metastases in mice bearing different types of tumors including breast, renal, gliomas, melanoma, Kaposi's sarcoma, squamous cell carcinoma, and leukemia [198–210]. Angiostatin/endostatin released from stably lentiviral transduced bladder carcinoma cells inhibited proliferation of the co-cultured endothelial cells [211]. Viral-mediated gene transfer of angiostatin has been tested in preclinical models for uveal melanomas [212] and ascite tumors [192], both demonstrate a therapeutic efficacy in terms of reduction of tumor size, vascularity, and increase of animal survival.

4.4.2 Gene Therapy Target VEGF

Because VEGF is the major player in tumor angiogenesis [1, 137–140], neutralizing or reducing the effect of VEGF, the ligand that initiates the VEGF-mediated signaling pathway, should effectively suppress tumor growth and metastasis. This goal can be achieved by either depleting functional VEGF protein or directly downregulating VEGF gene expression. Gene therapy-mediated expression of truncated VEGF R2 (flk-1), a competitive inhibitor for VEGF, suppresses neuroblastoma growth in vivo [147]. Viral-mediated expression of tumor suppressor gene *p16* downregulates *VEGF* gene expression in glioma [213] and breast cancer cells [146]. Our group has generated a replication-defective recombinant adenovirus expressing human wild-type p16 under the control of a rous sarcoma virus (RSV) promoter (AdRSVp16) [214]; the inhibitory effects of AdRSVp16 on tumor angiogenesis were examined by both in vitro and in vivo methods using a breast cancer model.

p16 Inhibits VEGF-Mediated Angiogenesis In Vitro

To analyze whether p16 protein has an effect on VEGF-mediated angiogenesis, AdRSVp16 was used to transduce human breast cancer MDA-MB-231 cells; the conditioned medium was collected 72 h later and used for culturing human microvascular endothelial cells (HMEC), cells on the matrigel in order to analyze p16's effect on angiogenesis in vitro. HMEC cells were grown in the conditioned medium from untreated, control virus-treated, or AdRSVp16-treated MDA-MB-231 cells, and the status of the vascular tubular network formation on Matrigel, as an indicator of angiogenic ability of HMEC cells, was examined at 1 h, 6 h, 24 h, respectively. When the HMEC cells grew in conditioned medium isolated from the untreated MDA-MB-231 cells, the cells tended to form tubular structures very quickly on the Matrigel; even at 1 h, the cells started to aggregate together to form a pre-tubular structure (Fig. 1A). The apparent tubular structure was observed at 6 h (Fig. 1B), and the mature tubular network was attained at 24 h (Fig. 1C). These results suggested that there were some growth factors secreted from MDA-MB-231 cells that were able to stimulate angiogenesis of HMEC cells (Fig. 1A–C). In contrast, when HMEC cells grew in conditioned medium isolated from AdRSVp16-treated MDA-MB-231 cells, their abilities to form the tubular network were

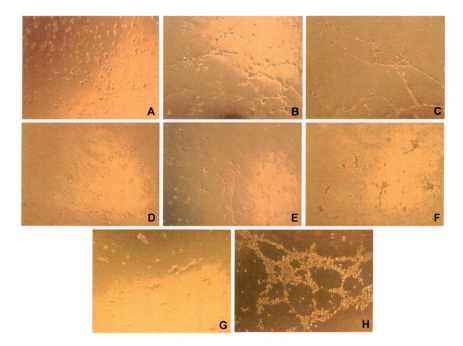

Fig. 1 p16 inhibited HMEC tubular network formation cultured in conditioned medium of MDA-MB-231 cells. HMEC cells were planted onto Matrigel-coated wells in the conditioned medium derived from untreated (**A, B, C**) or AdRSVp16 transduced (**D, E, F**) MDA-MB-231 cells, respectively. The development of the tubular network of HMEC cells was recorded at 1 h (A and D), 6 h (B and E), and 24 h (C and F) after HMEC cell seeding onto the Matrigel. As controls, the images of tubular network of HMEC cells grown in the same conditioned medium derived from untreated MDA-MB-231 cells but containing 1 μg/ml neutralized anti-VEGF antibody (**G**), and in the conditioned medium derived from control virus AdRSV-lacZ transduced MDA-MB-231 cells (**H**) were recorded at 24 h after seeding onto Matrigel

significantly reduced (Fig. 1D–F). Even at 6 h and 24 h time points, where the untreated control groups formed a well-developed tubular network (Fig. 1B and C), the AdRSVp16-treated group had few, if any, visible tubular connections (Fig. 1E and F). These results indicate that p16 effectively inhibited HMEC angiogenesis stimulated by growth factors secreted from MDA-MB-231 cells. When HMEC cells grew in similar conditions as in Fig. 1A–C, but with added neutralizing antibody against VEGF, the cells' abilities to form a tubular network were totally blocked (Fig. 1G), implying that it was VEGF, the downstream effector of HIF-1α-mediated transcription secreted from MDA-MB-231 cells, which played the major role in stimulating HMEC cell angiogenesis. Moreover, this p16-mediated inhibition on the tubular structure was not due to the viral part of AdRSVp16, as the ability to form a tubular network of HMEC cells grown in conditioned medium from control virus (AdRSVlacZ)-treated MDA-MB-231 cells was not reduced, if not somehow increased (Fig.

1H). Taken together, these observations demonstrated that p16 inhibited angiogenesis in an in vitro angiogenic assay, as evidenced by its ability to prevent the
formation of the tubular network in HMEC cells grown on Matrigel in conditioned medium derived from MDA-MB-231 cells (Fig. 2).

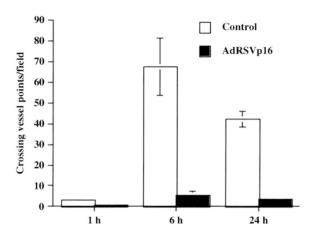

Fig. 2 Quantitation of tubular network formation. The number of tubular connections (i.e.,
crossing vessel points) was counted (five randomly selected fields at each time point), and the
average crossing vessel points per field was presented for a quantitative comparison. The
p values for differences between the control and AdRSVp16 group at 1, 6, and 24 h are all
statistically significant ($p<0.05$). Some error bars are too small to show in this scale

p16 Inhibits VEGF-Mediated Angiogenesis In Vivo

To determine whether p16 inhibits tumor cell-induced angiogenesis, the effect
of p16 on neovascularization of tumor surrounding cells was examined by
dorsal air sac assay [215]. MDA-MB-231 cells were transduced with
AdRSVp16. Forty-eight hours later the cells were harvested and injected into
a chamber that was wrapped with a semipermeable membrane allowing for
diffusion of growth factor, such as VEGF, but not cells. The chamber was
implanted into a dorsal air sac in nude mice, and the newly formed blood vessels
on the undersurface of the chamber were examined 3 days later. As shown in
Fig. 3, PBS-treated mice (as a negative control) did not have any obvious
neovascularization (Fig. 3A). However, the mice injected with MDA-MB-231
cells developed tumor cell-induced neovascularization as evidenced by the
newly formed "zigzagging-shape" small vessels in the air sac fascia (Fig. 3D).
In contrast, mice with AdRSVp16-transduced MDA-MB-231 cells developed
much less newly formed blood vessels (Fig. 3E and F), compared to mice
injected with MDA-MB-231 cells alone (Fig. 3D), or mice injected with control
viral transduced MDA-MB-231 cells (Fig. 3B and C); both of the latter two
induced a more extensive capillary network. When mice were injected with

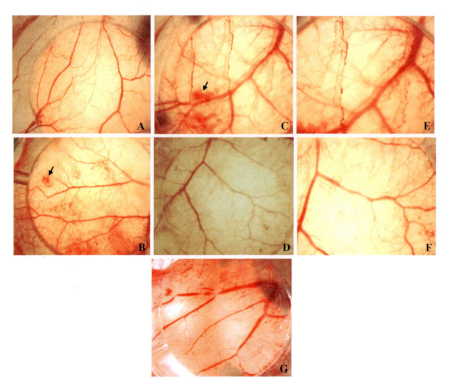

Fig. 3 p16 inhibited tumor-induced neovessel formation in dorsal air sac model. The mouse in the dorsal air sac model [215] was sacrificed on day 3, after chamber implantation, and the implanted chamber was removed from the subcutaneous air fascia, a ring without filters was placed on the same site and then photographed. The newly formed blood vessels were morphologically distinguishable from the preexisting background vessels by their zigzagging characters (see representative *arrows*). Shown are undersurface images of sites from chambers containing PBS only as negative control (**A**), AdRSVlacZ-transduced MDA-MB-231 cells (**B**), MDA-MB-231 cells (**D**), AdRSVp16-transduced MDA-MB-231 cells (**E**), and MDA-MB-231 cells with 1 μg/ml neutralized anti-VEGF antibody (**G**). C and F are the magnified images of B and E, respectively. Original magnifications: A, B, D, E, and G, × 7.5; C and F, × 30

MDA-MB-231 cells along with neutralized anti-VEGF antibody, this tumor-induced angiogenesis disappeared (Fig. 3G). Taken together, these results demonstrate that breast cancer cells can induce neovascularization around the tumor by secreting VEGF to the surrounding environment, and p16 can inhibit this tumor cell-induced neovascularization.

The advantage of using p16 gene therapy is two-fold: first, p16 inhibits tumor angiogenesis by downregulating VEGF gene expression; second, p16 itself is a cyclin D kinase inhibitor that suppresses cell division. Therefore, with the combination of p16's effect on both anti-angiogenesis and anti-proliferation, p16 gene therapy should have significant therapeutic potential in the treatment of cancer patients.

4.4.3 Other Targets and Protein Replacement Therapy for Anti-angiogenesis

PI3K/AKT pathway regulates angiogenesis and several other cell functions including proliferation, transformation, and apoptosis. LY294002, an inhibitor of PI3K, is able to decrease PC-3 prostate cancer cell-induced angiogenesis [191], suggesting that inhibition of PI3K/AKT signaling pathway may be an additional therapeutic approach to inhibit tumor angiogenesis. PTEN, a known inhibitor of PI3K, is frequently found to be mutated or lost in several cancers including prostate cancer. The recent study showed that angiogenesis and tumor growth can be inhibited by restoring wild-type PTEN in PC-3 prostate cancer cells [191]. Furthermore, ectopic PTEN suppressed HIF-1α, VEGF, and PCNA expression in the tumor xenografts. The similar experimental observations were obtained by ectopic expression of AKT-dominant negative mutant [191]. Together, these data suggest that gene therapy targeting PI3K/PTEN/ARK may have efficacy against prostate cancer and other malignant diseases. In fact, a recent study of gene therapy using adenovirus-expressing PTEN effectively inhibited the angiogenesis and invasiveness of PC-3 cells [216].

While most studies on viral-based anti-angiogenesis cancer gene therapy remain in the preclinical stage, the recombinant proteins of some of these targets have entered clinical trials. Among them, angiostatin protein therapy has proved to be very effective when administered systemically to mice bearing a variety of tumors, where a synergistic effect on suppression of metastases has been observed, by combining with endostatin [209, 217, 218], interleukin-12 [219], or chemotherapeutic agents [220, 221]. Recombinant IL-12 is in phase I/II clinical trial [222], and recombinant angiostatin and endostatin have completed phase I/II clinical trials [77, 223], respectively. Endostatin and angiostatin have shown to stabilize the long-term disease and improved quality of life in a small group of patients, with a return of strength, weight, and hair growth − and virtually no toxicity [77]. Angiostatin replacement therapy prevented growth of lung metastases after regression of the primary tumor by radiotherapy [224]. A phase III trial of endostatin was conducted in China for nearly 500 patients with late-stage non-small cell lung cancer. Patients who had endostatin added to their chemotherapy regimen were reported to have increased time to disease progression [77]. In 2005, endostatin was approved for marketing in China. Therapeutic inhibition of vessel formation by gene therapy may be best suited in conjunction with other therapeutic modalities to prevent recurring tumors or micrometastases after surgical removal of primary tumor.

5 Tumor Progression, Metastasis, and Their Therapeutic Targets

5.1 *Angiogenesis as the Prerequisite for Tumor Progression and Metastasis*

Progression from a neoplastic cell to a cancer involves the alteration of many regulatory pathways [225]. Tumors are made up of mixed-cell populations with substantial genetic and phenotypic heterogeneity, which are susceptible to continuous mutations and selections during expansion. During the selection process, some tumor cell populations are eliminated, some are enriched, and some newly mutated populations may rise. The selection can be based on the cells ability to invade and metastasize or on their proliferative advantage in certain or several microenvironments [226, 227]. Accompanying this selection is tumor progression. Metastasis, the spread of tumor cells from a primary site to the distant organs to form secondary tumors, is the optimal phase of tumor progression.

Metastasis is the major cause of death in cancer patients [228]. Metastasis is a complex process including primary tumor growth, invasion through basement membrane and extracellular matrix, dissemination to lymphatic and/or blood circulation, migration to distant organs, vessel cooption, angiogenesis, and colonization in the secondary site [229]. In order to metastasize successfully, a tumor cell must pass through each of the following steps during a metastatic process: it must intravasate into the vasculature from the primary tumor, survive the circulation via blood or lymphatic vessels, reach the microvasculature of the distant organ and extravasate, develop the secondary tumor in situ, and induce angiogenesis in the target organ [230–236]. Involved in both the initiation and the completion of the metastatic cascade cycle, angiogenesis plays an essential role in metastasis.

Two main steps in the metastatic process require angiogenesis: intravasation, the entrance of tumor cells into the blood circulation at the primary tumor site; and extravasation, the exit of tumor cells from the circulation and recolonization at the target organ. By responding to the angiogenic factors from the tumor, the proliferating endothelial cells build up a leaky capillary network around the tumor. Their fragmented basement membranes, due to the effect of tumor-recruited collagenases, allow the tumor cells to penetrate through the capillary and enter into the circulation [237–240]. Once the tumor cells reach the target organ, a reversed process occurs to enable the tumor cells to land successfully in a new environment. By modifying microvessels in the new surrounding such as enhancing vascular permeability and dilation, an angiogenic subpopulation of newly migrated tumor cells start a new cycle of angiogenesis by inducing new vascular sprouts in the secondary organ [241]. However, neovascularization of migrated tumor cells at the secondary site may not always occur immediately. Some metastases may stay in a dormant, undetectable stage for a very long time before angiogenesis occurs [242–244].

Newly transformed neoplastic cells are not generally angiogenic. Angiogenic switch usually occurs during progressive stages of tumorigenesis, such as at the premalignant stage of a spontaneous tumor in transgenic mouse model [1, 245, 246]. Evidences suggest that most presenting patterns of the metastases may be determined by the intensity of angiogenesis in the vascular bed of the primary tumors [247]. For some human malignancy such as cervix cancer, angiogenesis may occur even before the preneoplastic phase, as supported by the evidence that the higher microvessel counts in cervical intraepithelial neoplasia correlates with the later advanced stage of lesions [248]. This explains why for some human tumors when their neovascularizations become detectable, metastases may have already occurred. For the majority of human primary tumors, however, the angiogenic phenotype usually appears after the expression of the malignant phenotype [245]. The tumors can develop and stay locally without neovascularization for a long period before switching to an angiogenic phenotype. For example, the prevascular tumors at the nonangiogenic stage that are found in several metastatic cancers are typically small and slowly growing lesions; they can be dormant for months, even years, without clinical symptoms, and they are rarely metastatic at that stage [248–251]. Likewise, in the animal models, the tumor cells are rarely shed into the circulation before a primary tumor is vascularized, but they do emerge in the circulation following neovascularization of the primary tumor. The number of cells shed from the primary tumor appears to correlate with the density of tumor blood vessels as well as with the number of lung metastases observed later [238, 252]. Therefore, angiogenesis is prerequisite for tumor progression and metastasis.

Accordingly, it is rational and critical to intervene at the key step of the metastatic process, especially angiogenesis, for effective treatment. One of the most promising avenues of cancer research is the development of biologically based therapies to thwart the progression of metastatic disease. However, not all aspects of the metastatic process may be equally clinically applicable; therapies targeting angiogenesis and colonization that involve micrometastatic outgrowth may be the most clinically applicable [229]. In order to recognize a tumor as a whole setting instead of tumor cells alone, therapies targeting components in the tumor environment (e.g., tumor vasculature, hypoxia, cell-ECM) have recently been increasingly developed.

5.2 Therapeutic Targets for Tumor Vasculature

Angiogenesis, the formation of the new vascular network from preexisting vessels to supply the nutrition and oxygen to the growing tumor cells, is required for tumor expansion beyond 1–2 mm in diameter [3, 4, 22–26]. The same neovessel network may also function as a waste transportation pathway to remove the biological end products released from fast-growing tumor cells. It is in the tumor vasculature, the complex of tumor cells and surrounding proliferating endothelial cells, where the individual tumor cell breaks away from an established solid tumor and enters the blood vessel circulation to initiate the metastatic process. There is now evidence to suggest that the blood vessels within a particular solid tumor may actually consist of both endothelial and tumor cells [253]. The mosaic vessels may account for the tumor-cell shedding into the vasculature. Consequently, the growth of resultant metastases requires a similar vascular network for supply of nutrition and oxygen for the growth of the primary tumor [254, 255]. Therefore, targeting tumor vasculature may be an effective approach in suppressing tumor progression and metastasis.

The tumor-associated blood vessels are distinguished different in structure from their normal counterparts of the adjacent tissue; instead of the characterized dichotomous branching in normal vessels, the tumor-associated vessels are dilated, tortuous, often have multiple furcations, and heterogeneous in spatial distribution [59, 66, 146, 256, 257]. In addition, tumor-associated vessels are usually accompanied with a diminished expression of adhesion molecules that facilitate leukocyte-endothelial cell interaction (e.g., ICAM-1, VCAM-1, E-selectin) and an increased expression of CD 44, a cell-surface glycoprotein involved in cell–cell and cell–matrix interactions: overexpression of CD 44 has been linked to the growth and spread of a range of different types of malignancies [148, 258]. The considerably reduced recruitment of leukocytes and natural killer cells, due to decreased expression of adhesion molecules on tumor-associated endothelial cells, may contribute to the escape of tumor vasculature from immune surveillance [55, 258]; on the other hand, the enhanced expression of CD44 may provide growth advantage on the neoplastic cells [180]. Moreover, tumor-associated vessels differ from their normal counterparts in organization and function. Tumor-associated vessels are leaky, and the blood flow is not constant. Whereas the IFP in normal tissues is around 0 mm Hg [259], the IFP in solid tumors is elevated due to vascular hyperpermeability and the lack of functional lymphatic vessels inside tumors. Throughout a tumor, the uniformly high IFP, which drops precipitously in the tumor margin [260], compromises the effective delivery of therapeutic drugs both across the blood vessel wall and interstitum inside tumors. Moreover, the increased fluid flow from the tumor margin into the peri-tumor area by the elevated tumor IFP may facilitate peri-tumor lymphatic hyperplasia and metastasis. In addition, the abnormal microcirculation in tumors, together with lack of oxygen and production of waste, creates ahypoxic and acidic tumor microenvironment which hinders the efficacy of several anticancer treatments, including radiotherapy and chemotherapy. Therefore, the disruption of tumor vasculature will not only destroy tumor cells directly but also help facilitate the drug delivery to the tumor and sensitize other anticancer modalities.

In addition to destroying tumor vasculature directly, an emerging concept to treat cancer is "normalization" of tumor vasculature by restoring the angiogenic balance. As the imbalance of pro- and anti-angiogenic factors contributes to the pathophysiological characteristics of the tumor, reestablishing the balance of pro- and anti-angiogenic factors in the tumors may promote tumor vascular normalization. In fact, several studies have demonstrated that normalization of tumor vasculature and microenvironment can be achieved, albeit transient, by anti-angiogenic treatments either targeting directly on angiogenic (such as VEGF-mediated) signaling pathway by VEGFR2 blockade [261] or indirectly modulating angiogenesisby thalidomide [262]. A synergistic therapeutic effect was observed when cytotoxic therapy was combined with anti-angiogenic treatment during the latter induced "vascular normalization window," when tumors are more susceptible to the chemotherapy agents or radiotherapy [257, 261, 262].

5.3 Therapeutic Target for Tumor Microenvironment – Stroma

A solid tumor, made up of neoplastic cells and nontransformed host stromal cells, is surrounded by ECM. Although not autonomous, the tumor acts as an organ-like entity with the aid of many interdependent cell types, of which the tumor is composed; these cell types contribute to tumor growth and progression. The growth of the tumor and its potential to progress and metastasize is influenced by the tumor microenvironment, or stroma in a succinct term. Stroma consists of ECM, extracellular molecules and various cells including fibroblasts, epithelial cells, adipocytes, smooth muscle cells, immunocytes, glial cells, inflammatory cells, as well as local and recruited endothelial cells. The tumor interacts with its ECM and stromain a dynamic and bidirectional manner. Not only do tumor cells rely on the stroma for proliferation, progression, and metastasis but also tumor cells evolve together with their stroma during tumorigenesis and progression. Examples of bidirectional relationship include the interactions between tumor cells and host endothelial cells, tumor vasculature and host immune cells, and tumor spreading to the regional lymph nodes and lymphangiogenesis. In addition, stromal cells can also affect organ-specific metastasis, as demonstrated by the role of stromal-derived cytokines and growth factors in bone-prone metastasis in certain cancers [263]. However, despite the knowledge of the importance of tumor–stromal interactions in the tumor initiation and progression by the accumulated research evidences, the complex relationship between the tumor cells and the surrounding host cells is still not fully understood.

In addition to their roles in all stages of the tumor progression, especially in the initial stage of tumor development, tumor microenvironment and stromal cells also contribute to the development of tumor drug resistance by altering drug metabolism and hindering drug delivery to the tumor. Recently, there has been increasing attention paid to target the tumor microenvironment, the critical stromal elements, as a cancer therapy approach. One such attempt is to develop drugs that induce apoptosis of stromal cells, disrupt the functions of the stromal cells, or inhibit the factors released by stroma that promote tumor progression and metastasis. It has been shown that bone marrow stromal cells contribute not only to the development of drug resistance but also to the bone metastasis in patients with multiple myeloma. Targeting bone marrow stroma using a proteasome inhibitor leads to significant reduction of bone metastasis [263]. The additional advantage of targeting stroma is that stromal cells, due to their genetic stability, are less likely to develop drug resistance than tumor cells. Drugs targeting endothelial cells in stroma for anti-angiogenesis therapy such as Bevacizumab and Thalidomide have been developed and are currently in clinical trials [17, 263].

The tumor microenvironment and stroma cells can affect tumor progression either positively or negatively. Thus, the interactions between tumor cells and ECM, which can manipulate the malignant behavior of tumor cells in either way, are potential targets for the development of effective therapies. Based on the understanding that alterations in stroma and ECM can trigger and/or promote tumor growth and progression, it is feasible to design strategies that can prevent the tumor development or even revert malignant conversion by manipulating tumor−stromal interactions and reestablishing normal regulation systems. Research work showed that numerous cell functions that are vital for the tumor progression, including growth, differentiation, survival, and migration, could be regulated through physical interactions between cell−cell or cell−ECM. Based on the premise that cancers can be induced by continuous modifications of ECM structure at an experimental system, as demonstrated by the fact that altering mechanical force balance in the ECM, cell and cytoskeletal can induce epithelial tumor progression in vitro [264]. It is reasonable to speculate whether or not cancer can also be reverted to "normal" tissues by remodeling the tumor microenvironment. For instance, certain epithelial cancers can be induced to regain normal tissue morphology after stimulation from the embryonic mesenchyme or exogenous ECM scaffolds, a product derived from epithelial−stromal interactions [264]. The optimal goals of these approaches are to suppress or eradicate tumor metastasis and transform the malignant cancer into a chronic, not life-threatening disease. A better knowledge about the tumor microenvironment would help in developing improved drugs and anticancer strategies.

5.4 Therapeutic Target for Hypoxia and HIF-1

Tumor hypoxia results from a disparity between the demand and the supply of oxygen to the tumor tissue; this consequence occurs when tumor cells are too distant from the vascular supply. By overcoming the hostile hypoxic environment, a tumor induces a new vascular supply to provide oxygen and nutrition − a process called angiogenesis. Accumulated evidences indicate that tumor hypoxia plays an important role in tumor progression and metastasis [5–8]. Studies both in vitro and in vivo demonstrated that hypoxic exposure of tumor cells enhances their metastatic ability [265–269]. Although the mechanism by which hypoxia amplifies the metastatic potential is not fully understood, it is likely that expression of a set of genes, which control processes involved in the metastatic cascade, such as proliferation, angiogenesis, survival, migration, and invasion, is affected by hypoxia. The most and well-studied hypoxia-responsive gene is HIF-1α, which is promptly degraded by proteasomal ubiquitination under normoxic conditions but is stabilized under hypoxic conditions [270]. HIF-1α binds to HIF-1ß, a constitutively repressed subunit [166, 271] to form HIF-1, which acts as a master regulator at the transcription level [164]. HIF-1 drives expression of multiple genes involved in the metastatic process, including the key pro-angiogenic VEGF gene [272], and thus promotes angiogenesis, tumor progression, and metastasis. High levels of HIF-1α have been consistently correlated with tumor progression and poor prognosis in several types of cancers [273], and HIF genes (including HIF-1 and HIF-2) are found to be often upregulated in cancer and their metastases, suggesting that transcription of HIF downstream target genes can promote growth and survival of tumor cells [179].

As interlinked incidents during the process of angiogenesis, the formation of neovasculature is inherently associated with and promoted by the development of tumor hypoxia. Hypoxia is also suggested to affect expression of genes associated with cell–cell and cell–ECM interactions, favoring a metastatic profile by upregulating expression of pro-angiogenic factors and MMPs, as well as downregulating E-cadherin and TIMP1 expression [10]. Furthermore, the tumor resistance to chemotherapy and radiotherapy and a poor prognosis have been associated with hypoxia and high levels of HIF-1α in solid tumor tissues [274]. Therefore, therapies against hypoxia or inhibition of HIF-1 activity may serve as an important component in combination anti-angiogenesis therapies. Flavones extracted from *Portulaca oleracea* are found to have anti-hypoxia effects in the animal study [275]. The anti-angiogenic effects of several novel therapeutic agents that target signal-transduction pathways appear in part due to their ability to reduce HIF-1α levels. Small-molecule inhibitors of HIF-1α are being screened and tested for their efficacy as anticancer agents [164, 276, 277]. Cetuximab, a drug that blocks activation of the epidermal growth factor receptor, decreases HIF-1α protein synthesis through the inhibition of the phosphoinositide-3 kinase (PI3K)/Akt pathway [278].

5.5 Therapeutic Target for Cancer Stem Cells

Tumors consist of heterogeneous populations of cancer cells that constantly divide and grow at a furious pace. The subpopulations of cancer, arisen from rapidly accrued mutations within a tumor, may contribute to the development of drug resistance and thus escape therapy. Other proposed mechanisms responsible for the therapeutic resistance include increased Wnt/beta-catenin and

Notch signaling, amplified checkpoint activation, and upregulated DNA damage repair [279]. Recent work suggests that the cancer stem cells (CSC), a small population of tumor-initiating and self-renewed cancer cells, also contribute to the tumor resistance to chemotherapy and radiotherapy (see Chapter 17 Section 4 for more details). In addition, CSC appears to play a role in angiogenesis; accumulated research work has suggested that CSC is a subpopulation of tumor cells that have metastatic ability [280–282]. Accordingly, therapies targeting molecular mechanisms responsible for CSC-mediated resistance are integrated in the treatment paradigm by anti-angiogenic agents, in order to improve the efficacy of current anti-angiogenesis cancer therapies (for more detailed therapeutical strategies targeting CSC, see Chapter 17).

6 Challenges and Future Prospects

6.1 Unsolved Problems

6.1.1 Resistance to Anti-angiogenesis Therapy

Anti-angiogenic therapy, focused on inhibiting new blood vessel formation, is an effective way to suppress tumor progression. However, one major challenge of this approach is that tumors adapt to and escape from anti-angiogenic therapy. Many angiogenic inhibitors that have been shown to successfully inhibit tumor growth in preclinical models display very poor efficacy on clinical trials [283]. The tumor microenvironment, which modulates the sensitivity of tumors to an anti-angiogenic drug, may be partially responsible for this discrepancy. Even for those anti-angiogenic drugs that show an initial response, the patients may eventually display progression of cancer, indicating that tumors may have developed resistance to anti-angiogenic drugs [284, 285]. In contrast to our great advances in knowledge of the mechanisms of tumor angiogenesis, development of new anti-angiogenic drugs and clinical applications of anti-angiogenic therapies, our current understanding about the process of tumor adaptation to, or mechanism of tumor escape from, angiogenesis inhibition is limited [286]. Accumulated data have started to show that tumors can upregulate angiogenic factors, which mobilize and recruit bone-marrow-derived epithelial cells as well as promote endothelial proliferation in situ as an adaptation/reaction to the anti-angiogenic therapy [22, 287, 288]. Recent studies suggest that CSC and the stromal context may also play important roles in tumor's adaption to anti-angiogenic therapy [280].

Despite our comprehensive understanding on the factors and mechanisms involved in angiogenesis that enable us to develop a variety of angiogenic inhibitors, little is known on the alterations of angiogenic mechanisms under treatment of anti-angiogenic drugs in human cancer. Because of this, investigations are primarily confined to understanding the roles of individual molecules or pathways, instead of providing an integrated view. With the help from analyzing and understanding the functional association between apparently distinct events during angiogenesis and anti-angiogenesis therapy, as well as the identification of the molecular or metabolic features which render tumor cell resistance or sensitivity to anti-angiogenesis therapy, it is possible to design more effective drugs and strategies from an integrated perspective to overcome the tumor resistance to therapy.

6.1.2 Toxicity Associated with Anti-angiogenic Drugs

An obvious side effect of anti-angiogenic therapy is the toxicity to the host body in a long-term treatment, which is usually needed for anti-angiogenic therapy. It not only affects the body's normal process ability such as physiological angiogenesis for wound healing or reproduction but also leads to potential risks like bleeding or clotting disorders and cardiovascular defects [289]. To make matters worse, the toxicity to the host associated with long-term therapy by anti-angiogenic drugs may be delayed and thus hard to detect at the time of drug administration [290]. Despite the fact that therapies aiming at pro-angiogenic growth factors are generally more effective, the direct suppression of the neo-vascularization by targeting endothelial cells appears to have benefits of reduced toxicity and drug-induced resistance [291]. Therefore, selective targeting on the tumor vasculature, especially selective targeting of pathological endothelial cells, has become an important direction in developing the next generation of anti-angiogenic drugs, which are able to specifically block tumor angiogenesis without affecting other physiological angiogenesis process. Recent development of a peptide that binds to specific markers of tumor vasculature and optimization of liposome-based delivery by coupling the peptide with various liposomes conjugated with a chemotherapeutic agent [292–294] may hold hope to the next generation of tumor vasculature-targeting therapeutic agents. In addition, photosensitizers specifically targeting tumor stroma in photodynamic therapy may also help to reach that goal [295].

6.1.3 Lack of Appropriate Animal Models

There are numerous cases in which an anti-angiogenic drug that works very effectively in the animal model fails to deliver the same therapeutic effect in the clinical trial [283]. Multiple factors could be counted for this discrepancy, including the tumor microenvironment's effect on drug sensitivity and tumor adaptation to the drug; the choice of an animal model may be another major cause on the overestimation of the anticancer effect of an anti-angiogenic drug. Due to a very limited number of animal models available that generate clinically relevant, spontaneous tumors, and metastases, most preclinical studies have been done on transplantable tumors (either human tumor xenografts or mouse tumor allografts) that usually grow rapidly as solid, localized tumors in the subcutaneous space. The experimental situation renders the evaluation of drug's anti-angiogenic effects to be mainly focused on the newly formed immature vessels due to rapidly growing nature of the transplantable tumor models; these effects do not necessarily reflect the actual clinical situation. Most of the human solid tumors take a much longer time to develop than mouse transplantable tumors; hence, the human tumors are accompanied by a larger proportion of mature vessels in the tumor mass and therefore become less responsive to anti-angiogenic drugs, which usually work most effectively on newly formed vessels. This may explain why human tumors have a reduced response to the anti-angiogenic drugs than transplantable mouse tumors do. Moreover, those evaluations on the transplanted tumors overlook or are incapable of examining the drug's effects on the distant visceral metastases, the secondary tumors which are the actual cause of cancer deaths. Therefore, clinically relevant animal models which form spontaneous tumors, or orthotopically transplanted tumors which are able to develop secondary lesions by their natural metastatic routes, will be more desirable for preclinical evaluation of anticancer effects of a drug on both primary tumors and metastases.

Besides the above three issues, other remaining obstacles to anti-angiogenic therapy for cancer include high tumor IFP-impaired transport of drugs and vasculogenic mimicry in solid tumors; both are either component of or part of the process in microenvironment and tumor vasculature. Therefore, strategies targeting tumor vasculature and microenvironment have a great potential in developing more effective, new age anticancer drugs.

6.2 Future Directions

The success in cancer therapy, especially on inhibiting tumor angiogenesis and metastasis through targets in tumor microvascular and environment, will rely on the advances on several aspects: further understanding of the biology of malignant tumors and elucidation of mechanisms of pathways that are critical for tumor progression and metastasis, especially on the roles of stroma and CSC in tumor development and malignant progression; identification of the new therapeutic targets and invention of the new generation drugs that are more efficacious and less toxic; exploration and validation of more reliable biomarkers and improvement of imaging technology to better monitor tumor development and evaluation of drugs; and more efficient and beneficial translation of basic research findings into clinical applications. The advance of research tools, such as 3-D culture technology and clinically relevant disease animal models, will greatly facilitate and have significant impacts on laboratory scientists' ability to design and develop better drugs, investigate the mechanism of a drug, and study its effect on tumors as well as on interaction between tumor cell and the microenvironment. Future directions in this field should include, but are not limited to, the following areas.

6.2.1 Establishment of Reliable Biomarkers

Presently, there are at least ten anti-angiogenic therapy-based drugs currently in clinical trials [17]. The biomarkers of angiogenesis are critical in evaluating the efficacy of a new drug and developing an anti-angiogenic therapy. In early clinical studies, the pharmacodynamic effects of drugs observed were important in confirming drug activities. In the long term, however, biomarkers are more desired for the successful evaluation of new drugs and the improved clinical use of FDA-approved drugs, as both evaluations rely heavily on the close surveillance of angiogenesis status and drug activity in patients. Unfortunately, there is no validated biomarker available to date of either angiogenesis or anti-angiogenesis for routine clinical use [296]. The search for biomarkers of angiogenesis and, especially, of clinically successful anti-angiogenic therapy, has therefore become a major challenge in translational and clinical cancer research.

6.2.2 Target Stroma and Cancer Stem Cells

The better understanding of the roles that stroma microenvironment and cancer stem cells (CSC) play in tumor progression and metastasis would facilitate the diagnosis, treatment, and prevention of cancer, as well as translate this information into useful clinical applications. For example, identification of the alterations of the components in the stroma during carcinogenesis would help develop strategies and drugs targeting the stromal cells or specific factors produced by stromal cells that are required for tumor development, progression, and site-specific metastasis. Further characterization of CSC and understanding their roles as well as their interaction with stromal cells in the metastaticprocess would lead to the development of better strategies to identify and eliminate CSC and suppress metastasis.

6.2.3 Combination Therapy

Anti-angiogenic therapy appears to work at much higher efficacy when combined with chemotherapy. Recent clinical trials have revealed that the anti-VEGF mAb Bevacizumab adds to the effect of chemotherapy for the treatment of metastatic non-small cell lung cancer [297]. Other anti-angiogenic therapies that inhibit VEGF receptor tyrosine kinase or combinatively inhibit VEGF and EGF receptors have also been tested in conjunction with chemotherapy [297]. Besides chemotherapy, other therapeutic modalities including gene therapy, immunologic therapy, and radiation therapy, can also be used in conjunction with anti-angiogenic therapy to improve the anticancer therapeutic index.

6.2.4 Novel Therapies

Anti-neovascular Therapy

Partially due to a lack of specific tumor-endothelial markers, the conventional anti-angiogenic inhibitors are designed to target new vessels instead of existing tumor vessels, that is, to inhibit further formation of neovessels rather than to disrupt newly formed angiogenic vessels. As a consequence, tumor growth is stopped but the tumor cells may not be eradicated, so this strategy is essentially a tumor dormancy therapy. In contrast, a novel concept of anti-angiogenic therapy is applying cytotoxic drugs to target and destroy angiogenic, rapid-growing endothelial cells in the tumor vasculature. This is called anti-neovascular therapy (ANET), in which the cytotoxic drugs are efficiently delivered to the neovessels in order to successfully damage the EC cells, thereby possibly leading to a complete cut-off of vital supplies to the tumors. As this strategy causes strong cytotoxicity to the tumor vasculature rather than cytostasis to the tumor alone [298, 299], ANET may eradicate primary tumors and suppress metastasis. With the help of drug delivery system technology and development of angiogenic vasculature-targeting probes, ANET is being tested to deliver the cytotoxic anticancer agents to the angiogenic EC of tumor vasculature [300–302]. ANET may also provide improved therapeutic index when combined with conventional anti-angiogenic therapy.

Targeting Key Transduction Pathway Kinase

The prognosis of cancer patients with metastases remains poor due to the fact that current therapeutic strategies, including some new chemotherapeutic treatment, fail to significantly improve survival. In order to identify the novel therapeutic targets for more effective treatment, some attention has been focused on the better understanding of the molecular mechanisms and signal transduction pathways that contribute to tumor progression and metastasis. For example, new treatment approaches utilizing drugs that specifically target kinase transduction pathways involved in tumor growth have shown some promise either as individual agents or as conjugates combined with conventional chemotherapy [303].

Cancer "Normalization"

An intriguing view in the current field of cancer research is to question the possibility of whether remodeling the tumor microenvironment can reverse the cancer. Based on the hypothesis that cancer is probably a reversible disease, which is a consequence from progressive deregulation of tissue architecture to physical changes in cells, altered mechanical signaling, and eventually to cancer [264], it is possible to "normalize" the cancer by developing a tissue engineering approach in which biologically inspired materials that mimic the embryonic microenvironment can be used to induce and convert cancers into normal tissues.

Discovery of New Drugs by Chemical Genomics

The application of a novel chemical genomics approach on angiogenesis study has led to the discovery of new small molecules and novel targets in angiogenic therapy [304]. Taking advantage of being an inter- and multidisciplinary research engine, chemical genomics utilizes small molecules to dissect the roles of genes and facilitate the discovery of new drugs that are capable of inhibiting angiogenesis. With the help of specific molecular recognition of small molecules with target protein, the mechanism of actions of small molecules may be elucidated; hence, a better drug can be designed based on the structure and activity.

Acknowledgments Some original results are derived from research projects supported by National Institutes of Health grant CA107162 (YL). We thank Andrew Lu for reviewing this manuscript.

References

1. Hanahan D, Folkman J. Patterns and emerging mechanisms of the angiogenic switch during tumorigenesis. *Cell* 1996; **86**: 353–364.
2. Vaupel P, Kallinowski F, Okunieff P. Blood flow, oxygen and nutrient supply, and metabolic microenvironment of human tumors: A review. *Cancer Res* 1989; **49**: 6449–6465.
3. Folkman J. Tumor angiogenesis: Therapeutic implications. *N Engl J Med* 1971; **285**: 1182–1186.
4. Freitas T, Baronzio GF. Tumor hypoxia, reoxygenation and oxygenation strategies: Possible role in photodynamic therapy. *J Photochem Photobiol B Biol* 1991; **11**: 3–30.
5. Chan DA, Giaccia AJ. Hypoxia, gene expression, and metastasis. *Cancer Metastasis Rev* 2007; **26**: 333–339.
6. Rofstad EK. Microenvironment-induced cancer metastasis. *Int J Radiat Biol* 2000; **76**: 589–605.
7. Sullivan R, Graham CH. Hypoxia-driven selection of the metastatic phenotype. *Cancer Metastasis Rev* 2007; **26**: 319–331.
8. Subarsky P, Hill RP. The hypoxic tumour microenvironment and metastatic progression. *Clin Exp Metastasis* 2003; **20**: 237–250.
9. Xu L, Shen SS, Hoshida Y, Subramanian A, Ross K, Brunet JP, Wagner SN, Ramaswamy S, Mesirov JP, Hynes RO. Gene expression changes in an animal melanoma model correlate with aggressiveness of human melanoma metastases. *Mol Cancer Res* 2008; **6**: 760–769.
10. Lunt SJ, Chaudary N, Hill RP. The tumor microenvironment and metastatic disease. *Clin Exp Metastasis* 2008; June 16. [Epub ahead of print], doi:10.1007/s10585-008-9182-2.
11. Sheu BC, Chang WC, Cheng CY, Lin HH, Chang DY, Huang SC. Cytokine regulation networks in the cancer microenvironment. *Front Biosci* 2008; **13**: 6255–6268.
12. Bennaceur K, Chapman J, Brikci-Nigassa L, Sanhadji K, Touraine JL, Portoukalian J. Dendritic cells dysfunction in tumour environment. *Cancer Lett* 2008; June 26. [Epub ahead of print], doi:10.1016/j.canlet.2008.05.017.
13. Zou W, Chen L. Inhibitory B7-family molecules in the tumor microenvironment. *Nat Rev Immunol* 2008; **8**: 467–477.
14. Ursini-Siegel J, Muller WJ. The ShcA adaptor protein is a critical regulator of breast cancer progression. *Cell Cycle* 2008; 7: 1936–1943.

15. Naumov GN, Folkman J, Straume O. Tumor dormancy due to failure of angiogenesis: role of the microenvironment. *Clin Exp Metastasis* 2008; June 18. [Epub ahead of print], doi:10.1007/s10585-008-9176-0.
16. Itano N, Zhuo L, Kimata K. Impact of the hyaluronan-rich tumor microenvironment on cancer initiation and progression. *Cancer Sci* 2008; **99**: 1720–1725.
17. Folkman J. Angiogenesis: an organizing principle for drug discovery? Nat Rev Drug Discov 2007; **6**: 273–286.
18. Angiogenesis Foundation (2008) Understanding Angiogenesis at http://www.angio.org/patients/cancer/understanding_angiogenesis.html
19. Ausprunk DH, Folkman J. Migration and proliferation of endothelial cells in preformed and newly formed blood vessels during tumor angiogenesis. *Microvasc Res* 1977; **15**: 53–65.
20. Sholley MM, Ferguson GP, Seibel HR, Montour JL, Wilson JD. Mechanisms of neovascularization: vascular sprouting can occur without proliferation of endothelial cells. *Lab Invest* 1984; **51**: 624–634.
21. Bouck N, Stellmach V, Hsu SC. How tumors become angiogenic. *Adv Cancer Res* 1996; **69**: 135–174.
22. Kerbel RS, Folkman J. Clinical translation of angiogenesis inhibitors. *Nat Rev Cancer* 2002; **2**: 727–739.
23. Kim ES, Serur A, Huang J, Manley CA, McCrudden KW, Frischer JS, Soffer SZ, Ring L, New T, Zabski S, Rudge JS, Holash J, Yancopoulos GD, Kandel JJ, Yamashiro DJ. Potent VEGF blockade causes regression of coopted vessels in a model of neuroblastoma. *Proc Natl Acad Sci USA* 2002; **99**: 11399–11404.
24. Achilles EG, Fernandez A, Allred EN, Kisker O, Udagawa T, Beecken WD, Flynn E, Folkman J. Heterogeneity of angiogenic activity in a human liposarcoma: A proposed mechanism for 'no take' of human tumors in mice. *J Natl Cancer Inst* 2001; **93**: 1075–1081.
25. Hudlická O. Growth of capillaries in skeletal and cardiac muscle. *Circ Res* 1982; **50**: 451–461.
26. Berges G, Benjamin L. Tumorigenesis and the angiogenic switch. *Nat Rev Cancer* 2002; **3**: 401–410.
27. Hashizume H, Baluk P, Morikawa S, McLean JW, Thurston G, Roberge S, Jain RK, McDonald DM. Openings between defective endothelial cells explain tumor vessel leakiness. *Am J Pathol* 2000; **156**: 1363–1380.
28. Lyden D, Hattori K, Dias S, Costa C, Blaikie P, Butros L, Chadburn A, Heissig B, Marks W, Witte L, Wu Y, Hicklin D, Zhu Z, Hackett NR, Crystal RG, Moore MA, Hajjar KA, Manova K, Benezra R, Rafii S. Impaired recruitment of bone-marrow-derived endothelial and hematopoietic precursor cells blocks tumor angiogenesis and growth. *Nature Med* 2001; 7: 1194–1201.
29. Shi Q, Rafii S, Wu MH, Wijelath ES, Yu C, Ishida A, Fujita Y, Kothari S, Mohle R, Sauvage LR, Moore MA, Storb RF, Hammond WP. Evidence for circulating bone marrow-derived endothelial cells. *Blood* 1998; **92**: 362–367.
30. Hatzopoulos AK, Folkman J, Vasile E, Eiselen GK, Rosenberg RD. Isolation and characterization of endothelial progenitor cells from mouse embryos. *Development* 1998; **125**: 1457–1468.
31. Asahara T, Takahashi T, Masuda H, Kalka C, Chen D, Iwaguro H, Inai Y, Silver M, Isner JM. VEGF contributes to postnatal neovascularization by mobilizing bone marrow-derived endothelial progenitor cells. *Embo J* 1999; **18**: 3964–3972.
32. Murohara T, Ikeda H, Duan J, Shintani S, Sasaki K, Eguchi H, Onitsuka I, Matsui K, Imaizumi T. Transplanted cord blood-derived endothelial precursor cells augment postnatal neovascularization. *J Clin Invest* 2000; **105**: 1527–1536.
33. Rafii S. Circulating endothelial precursors: Mystery, reality, and promise. *J Clin Invest* 2000; **105**: 17–19.
34. Peichev M, Naiyer AJ, Pereira D, Zhu Z, Lane WJ, Williams M, Oz MC, Hicklin DJ, Witte L, Moore MA, Rafii S. Expression of VEGFR-2 and AC133 by circulating human

CD34(+) cells identifies a population of functional endothelial precursors. *Blood* 2000; **95**: 952–958.

35. Gehling UM, Ergün S, Schumacher U, Wagener C, Pantel K, Otte M, Schuch G, Schafhausen P, Mende T, Kilic N, Kluge K, Schäfer B, Hossfeld DK, Fiedler W. In vitro differentiation of endothelial cells from AC133-positive progenitor cells. *Blood* 2000; **95**: 3106–3112.

36. Hattori K, Dias S, Heissig B, Hackett NR, Lyden D, Tateno M, Hicklin DJ, Zhu Z, Witte L, Crystal RG, Moore MA, Rafii S. Vascular endothelial growth factor and angiopoietin-1 stimulate postnatal hematopoiesis by recruitment of vasculogenic and hematopoietic stem cells. *J Exp Med* 2001; **193**: 1005–1014.

37. Hattori K, Heissig B, Tashiro K, Honjo T, Tateno M, Shieh JH, Hackett NR, Quitoriano MS, Crystal RG, Rafii S, Moore MA. Plasma elevation of stromal cell-derived factor-1 induces mobilization of mature and immature hematopoietic progenitor and stem cells. *Blood* 2001; **97**: 3354–3360.

38. Hattori K, Heissig B, Wu Y, Dias S, Tejada R, Ferris B, Hicklin DJ, Zhu Z, Bohlen P, Witte L, Hendrikx J, Hackett NR, Crystal RG, Moore MA, Werb Z, Lyden D, Rafii S. Placental growth factor reconstitutes hematopoiesis by recruiting VEGFR1(+) stem cells from bone marrow microenvironment. *Nature Med* 2002; **8**: 841–849.

39. Heissig B, Hattori K, Dias S, Friedrich M, Ferris B, Hackett NR, Crystal RG, Besmer P, Lyden D, Moore MA, Werb Z, Rafii S. Recruitment of stem and progenitor cells from the bone marrow niche requires MMP-9 mediated release of kit-ligand. *Cell* 2002; **109**: 625–637.

40. Reyes M, Dudek A, Jahagirdar B, Koodie L, Marker PH, Verfaillie CM. Origin of endothelial progenitors in human postnatal bone marrow. *J Clin Invest* 2002; **109**: 337–346.

41. Naik RP, Jin D, Chuang E, Gold EG, Tousimis EA, Moore AL, Christos PJ, de Dalmas T, Donovan D, Rafii S, Vahdat LT. Circulating endothelial progenitor cells correlate to stage in patients with invasive breast cancer. *Breast Cancer Res Treat* 2008; **107**: 133–138.

42. Rafii S, Heissig B, Hattori K. Efficient mobilization and recruitment of marrow-derived endothelial and hematopoietic stem cells by adenoviral vectors expressing angiogenic factors. *Gene Ther* 2002; **9**: 631–641.

43. Kerbel RS, Benezra R, Lyden DC, Hattori K, Heissig B, Nolan DJ, Mittal V, Shaked Y, Dias S, Bertolini F, Rafii S. Endothelial progenitor cells are cellular hubs essential for neoangiogenesis of certain aggressive adenocarcinomas and metastatic transition but not adenomas. *Proc Natl Acad Sci USA* 2008; **105**: E54.

44. Folkman J, Brem H (1992) Angiogenesis and inflammation. In: Gallin JI, Goldstein IM, Snyderman R (eds) Inflammation: Basic principles and clinical correlates, 2nd edn. Raven Press, New York, 1992, pp. 821–839.

45. Polverini P, Leibovich S. Induction of neovascularization in vivo and endothelial proliferation in vitro by tumor-associated macrophages. *Lab Invest* 1984; **51**: 635–642.

46. Bergers G, Brekken R, McMahon G, Vu TH, Itoh T, Tamaki K, Tanzawa K, Thorpe P, Itohara S, Werb Z, Hanahan D. Matrix metalloproteinases-9 triggers the angiogenic switch during carcinogenesis. *Nature Cell Biol* 2000; **2**: 737–744.

47. Coussens LM, Tinkle CL, Hanahan D, Werb Z. MMP-9 supplied by bone marrow-derived cells contributes to skin carcinogenesis. *Cell* 2000; **103**: 481–490. 1998; **10**: 159–164.

48. Fang J, Shing Y, Wiederschain D, Yan L, Butterfield C, Jackson G, Harper J, Tamvakopoulos G, Moses MA. Matrix metalloproteinase-2 (MMP-2) is required for the switch to the angiogenic phenotype in a novel tumor model. *Proc Natl Acad Sci USA* 2000; **97**: 3884–3889.

49. Kadish JL, Butterfield CE, Folkman J. The effect of fibrin on cultured vascular endothelial cells. *Tissue Cell* 1979; **11**: 99–108.

50. Schulze-Osthoff K, Risau W, Vollmer E, Sorg C. In situ detection of basic fibroblast growth factor by highly specific antibodies. *Am J Pathol* 1990; **137**: 85–92.

51. Fukumura D, Xavier R, Sugiura T, Chen Y, Park EC, Lu N, Selig M, Nielsen G, Taksir T, Jain RK, Seed B. Tumor induction of VEGF promotor activity in stromal cells. *Cell* 1998; **94**: 715–725.

52. Holash J, Maisonpierre PC, Compton D, Boland P, Alexander CR, Zagzag D, Yancopoulos GD, Wiegand SJ. Vessel cooption, regression, and growth in tumors mediated by angiopoietins and VEGF. *Science* 1999; **284**: 1994–1998.

53. Möhle R, Green D, Moore MA, Nachman RL, Rafii S. Constitutive production and thrombin-induced release of vascular endothelial growth factor by human megakaryocytes and platelets. *Proc Natl Acad Sci USA* 1997; **94**: 663–668.

54. Verheul HM, Hoekman K, Luykx-de Bakker S, Eekman CA, Folman CC, Broxterman HJ, Pinedo HM. Platelet: transporter of vascular endothelial growth factor. *Clin Cancer Res* 1997; **3**: 2187–2190.

55. Folkman J (1984) Angiogenesis. In: Jaffe EA (ed) *Biology of Endothelial Cells*. Nijhoff, Boston, MA, pp. 412–428.

56. Folkman J, Long DM, Becker FF. Growth and metastasis of tumor in organ culture. *Cancer* 1963; **16**: 453–467.

57. Folkman J, Cole P, Zimmerman S. Tumor behavior in isolated perfused organs: in vitro growth and metastases of biopsy material in rabbit thyroid and canine intestinal segment. *Ann Surg* 1966; **164**: 491–502.

58. Folkman J. Anti-angiogenesis: new concept for therapy of solid tumors. *Ann Surg* 1972; **175**: 409–416.

59. Folkman J. The vascularization of tumors. *Sci Am* 1976; **234**: 58–73.

60. Gimbrone MA Jr, Cotran RS, Folkman J. Human vascular endothelial cells in culture. Growth and DNA synthesis. *J Cell Biol* 1974; **60**: 673–684.

61. Gimbrone MA Jr, Cotran RS, Leapman SB, Folkman J. Tumor growth and neovascularization: An experimental model using the rabbit cornea. *J Natl Cancer Inst* 1974b; **52**: 413–427.

62. Ausprunk DH, Knighton DR, Folkman J. Vascularization of normal and neoplastic tissues grafted to the chick chorioallantois. Role of host and preexisting graft blood vessels. *Am J Pathol* 1975; **79**: 597–628.

63. Langer R, Folkman J. Polymers for the sustained release of proteins and other macromolecules. *Nature* 1976; **263**: 797–800.

64. Auerbach R, Arensman R, Kubai L, Folkman J. Tumor-induced angiogenesis: Lack of inhibition by irradiation. *Int J Cancer* 1975; **15**: 241–245.

65. Brouty-Boyé D, Zetter BR. Inhibition of cell motility by interferon. *Science* 1980; **208**: 516–528.

66. Taylor S, Folkman J. Protamine is an inhibitor of angiogenesis. *Nature* 1982; **297**: 307–312.

67. Crum R, Szabo S, Folkman J. A new class of steroids inhibits angiogenesis in the presence of heparin or a heparin fragment. *Science* 1985; **230**: 1375–1378.

68. Ingber DM, Ingber D, Fujita T, Kishimoto S, Sudo K, Kanamaru T, Brem H, Folkman J. Synthetic analogues of fumagillin that inhibit angiogenesis and suppress tumour growth. *Nature* 1990; **348**: 555–557.

69. O'Reilly MS, Holmgren L, Shing Y, Chen C, Rosenthal RA, Moses M, Lane WS, Cao Y, Sage EH, Folkman J. Angiostatin: A novel angiogenesis inhibitor that mediates the suppression of metastases by a Lewis lung carcinoma. *Cell* 1994; **79**: 315–328.

70. O'Reilly MS, Boehm T, Shing Y, Fukai N, Vasios G, Lane WS, Flynn E, Birkhead JR, Olsen BR, Folkman J. Endostatin: An endogenous inhibitor of angiogenesis and tumor growth. *Cell* 1997; **88**: 277–285.

71. Folkman J. Endogenous angiogenesis inhibitors. *Acta Pathol Microbiol Immunol Scand* 2004; **112**: 496–507.

72. Maeshima Y, Sudhakar A, Lively JC, Ueki K, Kharbanda S, Kahn CR, Sonenberg N, Hynes RO, Kalluri R. Tumstatin. An endothelial cell-specific inhibitor of protein synthesis. *Science* 2002; **295**: 140–143.

73. Fràter-Schröder M, Risau W, Hallmann R, Gautschi, P, Bohlen P. Tumor necrosis factor type α, a potent inhibitor of endothelial cell growth in vitro, is angiogenic in vivo. *Proc Natl Acad Sci USA* 1987; **84**: 5277–5281.

74. Nyberg P, Xie L, Kalluri R. Endogenous inhibitors of angiogenesis. *Cancer Res* 2005; **65**: 3967–3979.

75. Abdollahi A, Hahnfeldt P, Maercker C, Gröne HJ, Debus J, Ansorge W, Folkman J, Hlatky L, Huber PE. Endostatin's antiangiogenic signaling network. *Mol Cell* 2004; **13**: 649–663.

76. Inoue K, Korenaga H, Tanaka NG, Sakamoto N, Kadoya S. The sulfated polysaccharide–peptidoglycan complex potently inhibits embryonic angiogenesis and tumor growth in the presence of cortisone acetate. *Carbohydr Res* 1988; **181**: 135–142.

77. Remembering Judah Folkman (2008) Angiogenesis: Blood Vessel Growth and the Treatment of Disease at http://www.childrenshospital.org/cfapps/research/data_admin/Site2580/mainpageS2580P4.html

78. NIH clinical trials at www.clinicaltrials.gov

79. Boehm T, Folkman J, Browder T, O'Reilly MS. Antiangiogenic therapy of experimental cancer does not induce acquired drug resistance. *Nature* 1997; **390**: 404–407.

80. Kerbel RS. Inhibition of tumour angiogenesis as a strategy to circumvent acquired resistance to anticancer therapeutic agents. *Bioessays* 1991; **13**: 31–36.

81. Kerbel RS, Viloria-Petit A, Okada F, Rak J. Establishing a link between oncogenes and tumor angiogenesis. *Mol Med* 1998; **4**: 286–2895.

82. Rak J, Yu JL, Klement G, Kerbel RS. Oncogenes and angiogenesis: Signaling three-dimensional tumor growth. *J Investig Dermatol Symp Proc* 2000; **5**: 24–33.

83. Rak J, Yu JL, Kerbel RS, Coomber BL. What do oncogenic mutations have to do with angiogenesis/vascular dependence of tumors? *Cancer Res* 2002; **62**: 1931–1934.

84. Arbiser JL, Panigrathy D, Klauber N, Rupnick M, Flynn E, Udagawa T, D'Amato RJ. The antiangiogenic agents TNP-470 and 2-methoxyestradiol inhibit the growth of angiosarcoma in mice. *J Am Acad Dermatol* 1999; **40**: 925–929.

85. Chin L, Tam A, Pomerantz J, Wong M, Holash J, Bardeesy N, Shen Q, O'Hagan R, Pantginis J, Zhou H, Horner JW, 2nd, Cordon-Cardo C, Yancopoulos GD, DePinho RA. Essential role for oncogenic Ras in tumour maintenance. *Nature* 1999; **400**: 468–472.

86. Udagawa T, Fernandez A, Achilles EG, Folkman J, D'Amato RJ. Persistence of microscopic human cancers in mice: alterations in the angiogenic balance accompanies loss of tumor dormancy. *FASEB J* 2002; **16**: 1361–1370.

87. Fernandez A, Udagawa T, Schwesinger C, Beecken W, Achilles-Gerte E, McDonnell T, D'Amato R. Angiogenic potential of prostate carcinoma cells overexpressing bcl-2. *J Natl Cancer Inst* 2001; **93**: 208–213.

88. Petit AM, Rak J, Hung MC, Rockwell P, Goldstein N, Fendly B, Kerbel RS. Neutralizing antibodies against epidermal growth factor and ErB-2/neu receptor tyrosine kinases down-regulate vascular endothelial growth factor production by tumor cells in vitro and in vivo: angiogenic implications for signal transduction therapy of solid tumors. *Am J Pathol* 1997; **151**: 1523–1530.

89. Izumi Y, Xu L, di Tomaso E, Fukumura D, Jain RK. Tumour biology: Herceptin acts as an anti-angiogenic cocktail. *Nature* 2002; **416**: 279–280.

90. Okada F, Rak JW, Croix BS, Lieubeau B, Kaya M, Roncari L, Shirasawa S, Sasazuki T, Kerbel RS. Impact of oncogenes on tumor angiogenesis: mutant K-ras upregulation of VEGF/VPF is necessary but not sufficient for tumorigenicity of human colorectal carcinoma cells. *Proc Natl Acad Sci USA* 1998; **95**: 3609–3614.

91. Ren JG, Jie C, Talbot C. How PEDF prevents angiogenesis: A hypothesized pathway. *Medical Hypotheses* 2005; **64**: 74–78.

92. Gengrinovitch S, Greenberg SM, Cohen T, Gitay-Goren H, Rockwell P, Maione TE, Levi BZ, Neufeld G. Platelet factor-4 inhibits the mitogen activity of VEGF121 and VEGF165 using several concurrent mechanisms. *J Biol Chem* 1995; **270**: 15059–15065.

93. Dvorak HF, Gresser I. Microvascular injury in pathogenesis of interferon-induced necrosis of subcutaneous tumors in mice. *J Natl Cancer Inst* 1989; **81**: 497–502.

94. Sidky YA, Borden EC. Inhibition of angiogenesis by interferons: Effects on tumor- and lymphocyte-induced vascular responses. *Cancer Res* 1987; **47**: 5155–5161.

95. Maione TE, Gray GS, Petro J, Hunt AJ, Donner AL, Bauer SI, Carson HF, Sharpe RJ. Inhibition of angiogenesis by recombinant human platelet factor-4 and related peptides. *Science* 1990; **247**: 77–79.

96. Eder JP Jr, Supko JG, Clark JW, Puchalski TA, Garcia-Carbonero R, Ryan DP, Shulman LN, Proper J, Kirvan M, Rattner B, Connors S, Keogan MT, Janicek MJ, Fogler WE, Schnipper L, Kinchla N, Sidor C, Phillips E, Folkman J, Kufe DW. Phase I clinical trial of recombinant human endostatin administered as a short intravenous infusion repeated daily. *J Clin Oncol* 2002; **20**: 3772–3784.

97. National Cancer Institute (2008) Understanding Cancer Series: Angiogenesis at www.cancer.gov/cancertopics/understandingcancer/angiogenesis/

98. Qian DZ, Kato Y, Shabbeer S, Wei Y, Verheul HM, Salumbides B, Sanni T, Atadja P, Pili R. Targeting tumor angiogenesis with histone deacetylase inhibitors: the hydroxamic acid derivative LBH589. *Clin Cancer Res* 2006; **12**: 634–642.

99. Yeh CH, Peng HC, Yang RS, Huang TF. Rhodostomin, a snake venom disintegrin, inhibits angiogenesis elicited by basic fibroblast growth factor and suppresses tumor growth by a selective alpha (v) beta (3) blockade of endothelial cells. *Mol Pharmacol* 2001; **59**: 1333–1342.

100. Sharma MC, Sharma M. The role of annexin II in angiogenesis and tumor progression: a potential therapeutic target. *Curr Pharm Des* 2007; **13**: 3568–3575.

101. Khan GN, Merajver SD. Modulation of angiogenesis for cancer prevention: strategies based on antioxidants and copper deficiency. *Curr Pharm Des* 2007; **13**: 3584–3590.

102. Senger DR, Galli SJ, Dvorak AM, Perruzzi CA, Harvey VS, Dvorak HF. Tumor cells secrete a vascular permeability factor that promotes accumulation of ascites fluid. *Science* 1983; **219**: 983–985.

103. Dvorak HF. Tumors: Wounds that do not heal. Similarities between tumor stroma generation and wound healing. *N Engl J Med* 1986; **315**: 1650–1659.

104. Ferrara N, Henzel WJ. Pituitary follicular cells secrete a novel heparin-binding growth factor specific for vascular endothelial cells. *Biochem Biophys Res Commun* 1989; **161**: 851–858.

105. Leung DW, Cachianes G, Kuang WJ, Goeddel DV, Ferrara N. Vascular endothelial growth factor is a secreted angiogenic mitogen. *Science* 1989; **246**: 1306–1309.

106. Rosenthal RA, Megyesi JF, Henzel WJ, Ferrara N, Folkman J. Conditioned medium from mouse sarcoma 180 cells contains vascular endothelial growth factor. *Growth Factors* 1990; **4**: 53–59.

107. Connolly DT. Vascular permeability factor: a unique regulator of blood vessel function. *J Cell Biochem* 1991; **47**: 219–223.

108. Dvorak HF, Sioussat TM, Brown LF, Berse B, Nagy JA, Sotrel A, Manseau EJ, Van de Water L, Senger DR. Distribution of vascular permeability factor (vascular endothelial growth factor) in tumors: Concentration in tumor blood vessels. *J Exp Med* 1991; **174**: 1275–1278.

109. Ferrara N, Houck K, Jakeman L, Leung DW. Molecular and biological properties of the vascular endothelial growth factor family of proteins. *Endocr Rev* 1992; **13**: 18–32.

110. Houck KA, Ferrara N, Winer J, Cachianes G, Li B, Leung DW. The vascular endothelial growth factor family: Identification of a fourth molecular species and characterization of alternative splicing of RNA. *Mol Endocrinol* 1991; **5**: 1806–1814.

111. Tischer E, Gospodarowicz D, Mitchell R, Silva M, Schilling J, Lau K, Crisp T, Fiddes JC, Abraham JA. Vascular endothelial growth factor: a new member of the platelet-derived growth factor gene family. *Biochem Biophys Res Commun* 1989; **165**: 1198–1206.

112. Poltorak Z, Cohen T, Sivan R, Kandelis Y, Spira G, Vlodavsky I, Keshet E, Neufeld G. VEGF145, a secreted vascular endothelial growth factor isoform that binds to extracellular matrix. *J Biol Chem* 1997; **272**: 7151–7158.

113. Keyt BA, Berleau LT, Nguyen HV, Chen H, Heinsohn H, Vandlen R, Ferrara N. The carboxyl-terminal domain (111-165) of vascular endothelial growth factor is critical for its mitogenic potency. *J Biol Chem* 1996; **271**: 7788–7795.

114. Soker S, Gollamudi-Payne S, Fidder H, Charmahelli H, Klagsbrun M. Inhibition of vascular endothelial growth factor (VEGF)-induced endothelial cell proliferation by a peptide corresponding to the exon 7-encoded domain of VEGF165. *J Biol Chem* 1997; **272**: 31582–31588.

115. Korpelainen EI, Alitalo K. Signaling angiogenesis and lymphangiogenesis. *Curr Opin Cell Biol* 1998; **10**: 159–164.

116. de Vries C, Escobedo JA, Ueno H, Houck K, Ferrara N, Williams LT. The fms-like tyrosine kinase, a receptor for vascular endothelial growth factor. *Science* 1992; **255**: 989–999.

117. Seetharam L, Gotoh N, Maru Y, Neufeld G, Yamaguchi S, Shibuya M. A unique signal transduction from FLT tyrosine kinase, a receptor for vascular endothelial growth factor VEGF. *Oncogene* 1995; **10**: 135–147.

118. Terman BI, Carrion ME, Kovacs E, Rasmussen BA, Eddy RL, Shows TB. Identification of a new endothelial cell growth factor receptor tyrosine kinase. *Oncogene* 1991; **6**: 1677–1683.

119. Terman BI, Dougher-Vermazen M, Carrion ME, Dimitrov D, Armellino DC, Gospodarowicz D, Bohlen P. Identification of the KDR tyrosine kinase as a receptor for vascular endothelial cell growth factor. *Biochem Biophys Res Commun* 1992; **187**: 1579–1586.

120. Landgren E, Schiller P, Cao Y, Claesson-Welsh L. Placenta growth factor stimulates MAP kinase and mitogenicity but not phospholipase C-gamma and migration of endothelial cells expressing Flt 1. *Oncogene* 1998; **16**: 359–367.

121. Waltenberger J, Claesson-Welsh L, Siegbahn A, Shibuya M, Heldin CH. Different signal transduction properties of KDR and Flt1, two receptors for vascular endothelial growth factor. *J Biol Chem* 1994; **269**: 26988–26995.

122. Bartoli M, Gu X, Tsai NT, Venema RC, Brooks SE, Marrero MB, Caldwell RB. Vascular endothelial growth factor activates STAT proteins in aortic endothelial cells. *J Biol Chem* 2000; **275**: 33189–33192.

123. Millauer B, Shawver LK, Plate KH, Risau W, Ullrich A. Glioblastoma growth inhibited in vivo by a dominant-negative Flk-1 mutant. *Nature* 1994; **367**: 576–579.

124. Millauer B, Longhi MP, Plate KH, Shawver LK, Risau W, Ullrich A, Strawn LM. Dominant-negative inhibition of Flk-1 suppresses the growth of many tumor types in vivo. *Cancer Res* 1996; **56**: 1615–1620.

125. Ferrara N, Carver-Moore K, Chen H, Dowd M, Lu L, O'Shea KS, Powell-Braxton L, Hillan KJ, Moore MW. Heterozygous embryonic lethality induced by targeted inactivation of the VEGF gene. *Nature* 1996; **380**: 439–442.

126. Claffey KP, Brown LF, del Aguila LF, Tognazzi K, Yeo KT, Manseau EJ, Dvorak HF. Expression of vascular permeability factor/vascular endothelial growth factor by melanoma cells increases tumor growth, angiogenesis, and experimental metastasis. *Cancer Res* 1996; **56**: 172–181.

127. Saleh M, Stacker SA, Wilks AF. Inhibition of growth of C6 glioma cells in vivo by expression of antisense vascular endothelial growth factor sequence. *Cancer Res* 1996; **56**: 393–401.

128. Pavco PA, Bouhana KS, Gallegos AM, Agrawal A, Blanchard KS, Grimm SL, Jensen KL, Andrews LE, Wincott FE, Pitot PA, Tressler RJ, Cushman C, Reynolds MA, Parry TJ.

Antitumor and antimetastatic activity of ribozymes targeting the messenger RNA of vascular endothelial growth factor receptors. *Clin Cancer Res* 2000; **6**: 2094–2103.

129. Davidoff AM, Nathwani AC, Spurbeck WW, Ng CY, Zhou J, Vanin EF. rAAV-mediated long-term liver-generated expression of an angiogenesis inhibitor can restrict renal tumor growth in mice. *Cancer Res* 2002; **62**: 3077–3083.

130. Kim KJ, Li B, Winer J, Armanini M, Gillett N, Phillips HS, Ferrara N. Inhibition of vascular endothelial growth factor-induced angiogenesis suppresses tumour growth in vivo. *Nature* 1993; **362**: 841–844.

131. Zhang W, Ran S, Sambade M, Huang X, Thorpe PE. A monoclonal antibody that blocks VEGF binding to VEGFR2 (KDR/Flk-1) inhibits vascular expression of Flk-1 and tumor growth in an orthotopic human breast cancer model. *Angiogenesis* 2002; **5**: 35–44.

132. Prewett M, Huber J, Li Y, Santiago A, O'Connor W, King K, Overholser J, Hooper A, Pytowski B, Witte L, Bohlen P, Hicklin DJ. Antivascular endothelial growth factor receptor (fetal liver kinase 1) monoclonal antibody inhibits tumor angiogenesis and growth of several mouse and human tumors. *Cancer Res* 1999; **59**: 5209–5218.

133. Zhu Z, Rockwell P, Lu D, Kotanides H, Pytowski B, Hicklin DJ, Bohlen P, Witte L. Inhibition of vascular endothelial growth factor-induced receptor activation with anti-kinase insert domain-containing receptor single-chain antibodies from a phage display library. *Cancer Res* 1998; **58**: 3209–3214.

134. Fong TA, Shawver LK, Sun L, Tang C, App H, Powell TJ, Kim YH, Schreck R, Wang X, Risau W, Ullrich A, Hirth KP, McMahon G. SU5416 is a potent and selective inhibitor of the vascular endothelial growth factor receptor (Flk-1/KDR) that inhibits tyrosine kinase catalysis, tumor vascularization, and growth of multiple tumor types. *Cancer Res* 1999; **59**: 99–106.

135. Olofsson B, Jeltsch M, Eriksson U, Alitalo K. Current biology of VEGF-B and VEGF-C. *Curr Opin Biotechnol* 1999; **10**: 528–535.

136. Yancopoulos GD, Davis S, Gale NW, Rudge JS, Wiegand SJ, Holash J. Vascular-specific growth factors and blood vessel formation. *Nature* 2000; **407**: 242–248.

137. Grunstein J, Roberts WG, Mathieu-Costello O, Hanahan D, Johnson RS. Tumor-derived expression of vascular endothelial growth factor is a critical factor in tumor expansion and vascular function. *Cancer Res* 1999; **59**: 1592–1598.

138. Detmar M, Velasco P, Richard L, Claffey KP, Streit M, Riccardi L, Skobe M, Brown LF. Expression of vascular endothelial growth factor induces an invasive phenotype in human squamous cell carcinomas. *Am J Pathol* 2000; **156**: 159–167.

139. Risau W. What, if anything, is an angiogenic factor? *Cancer Metastasis Rev* 1996; **15**: 149–151.

140. Neufeld G, Cohen T, Gengrinovitch S, Poltorak Z. Vascular endothelial growth factor (VEGF) and its receptors. *FASEB J* 1999; **13**: 9–22.

141. Shih SC, Claffey KP. Role of AP-1 and HIF-1 transcription factors in TGF-beta activation of VEGF expression. *Growth Factors* 2001; **19**: 19–34.

142. Hadj-Slimane R, Lepelletier Y, Lopez N, Garbay C, Raynaud F. Short interfering RNA (siRNA), a novel therapeutic tool acting on angiogenesis. *Biochimie* 2007; **89**: 1234–1244.

143. Wang S, Liu H, Ren L, Pan Y, Zhang Y. Inhibiting colorectal carcinoma growth and metastasis by blocking the expression of VEGF using RNA interference. *Neoplasia* 2008; **10**: 399–407.

144. Holash J, Davis S, Papadopoulos N, Croll SD, Ho L, Russell M, Boland P, Leidich R, Hylton D, Burova E, Ioffe E, Huang T, Radziejewski C, Bailey K, Fandl JP, Daly T, Wiegand SJ, Yancopoulos GD, Rudge JS. VEGF-Trap; a VEGF blocker with potent antitumor effects. *Proc Natl Acad Sci USA* 2002; **99**: 11393–11398.

145. Kim LS, Huang S, Lu W, Lev DC, Price JE. Vascular endothelial growth factor expression promotes the growth of breast cancer brain metastases in nude mice. *Clin Exp Metastasis* 2004; **21**: 107–118.

146. Lu Y, Zhang J, Beech DJ, Myers LK, Jennings LK. p16 downregulates VEGF and inhibits angiogenesis in breast cancer cells. *Cancer Ther* 2003; **1**: 143–151.
147. Davidoff AM, Leary MA, Ng CY, Vanin EF. Gene therapy-mediated expression by tumor cells of the angiogenesis inhibitor flk-1 results in inhibition of neuroblastoma growth in vivo. *J Pediatr Surg* 2001; **36**: 30–36.
148. Shing Y, Folkman J, Sullivan R, Butterfield C, Murray J, Klagsbrun M. Heparin affinity: purification of a tumor-derived capillary endothelial cell growth factor. *Science* 1984; **223**: 1296–1298.
149. Hori A, Sasada R, Matsutani E, Naito K, Sakura Y, Fujita T, Kozai Y. Suppression of solid tumor growth by immuno-neutralizing monoclonal antibody against human basic fibroblast growth factor. *Cancer Res* 1991; **51**: 6180–6184.
150. Melder RJ, Koenig GC, Witwer BP, Safabakhsh N, Munn LL, Jain RK. During angiogenesis, vascular endothelial growth factor and basic fibroblast growth factor regulate natural killer cell adhesion to endothelium. *Nature Med* 1996; **2**: 992–997.
151. Griffioen AW, Tromp SC, Hillen HF. Angiogenesis modulates the tumour immune response. *Int J Exp Pathol* 1998; **76**: 363–368.
152. Griffioen AW, Damen CA, Mayo KH, Barendsz-Janson AF, Martinotti S, Blijham GH, Groenewegen G. Angiogenesis inhibitors overcome tumor induced endothelial cell anergy. *Int J Cancer* 1999; **80**: 315–319.
153. Coleman AB, Lugo TG. Normal human melanocytes that express a bFGF transgene still require exogenous bFGF for growth in vitro. *J Invest Dermatol* 1998; **110**: 793–799.
154. Li VW, Folkerth RD, Watanabe H, Yu C, Rupnick M, Barnes P, Scott RM, Black PM, Sallan SE, Folkman J. Microvessel count and cerebrospinal fluid basic fibroblast growth factor in children with brain tumours. *Lancet* 1994; **344**: 82–86.
155. Lin RY, Argenta PA, Sullivan KM, Adzick NS. Diagnostic and prognostic role of basic fibroblast growth factor in Wilm's tumor patients. *Clin Cancer Res* 1995; **1**: 327–331.
156. Nanus DM, Schmitz-Dräger BJ, Motzer RJ, Lee AC, Vlamis V, Cordon-Cardo C, Albino AP, Reuter VE. Expression of basic fibroblast growth factor in primary human renal tumors: correlation with poor survival. *J Natl Cancer Inst* 1993; **85**: 1597–1599.
157. Nguyen M, Watanabe H, Budson AE, Richie JP, Hayes DF, Folkman J. Elevated levels of an angiogenic peptide, basic fibroblast growth factor, in the urine of patients with a wide spectrum of cancers. *J Natl Cancer Inst* 1994; **86**: 356–361.
158. Fennewald SM, Rando RF. Inhibition of high affinity basic fibroblast growth factor binding by oligonucleotides. *J Biol Chem* 1995; **270**: 21718–21721.
159. Hasan J, Clamp A, Whitworth M, Byers R, Bicknell R, Gallagher J, Jayson GC. Inhibition of bFGF activity by size-defined oligosaccharide derivatives of low molecular weight heparin in the sponge angiogenesis assay. *Am Assoc Cancer Res* 2004; **45**: #947.
160. Etscheid M, Beer N, Kress JA, Seitz R, Dodt J. Inhibition of bFGF/EGF-dependent endothelial cell proliferation by the hyaluronan-binding protease from human plasma. *Euro J Cell Biol* 2004; **82**: 597–604.
161. Kaban LB, Mulliken JB, Ezekowitz RA, Ebb D, Smith PS, Folkman J. Antiangiogenic therapy of a recurrent giant cell tumor of the mandible with interferonα-2a. *Pediatrics* 1999; **103**: 1145–1149.
162. Marler JJ, Rubin JB, Trede NS, Connors S, Grier H, Upton J, Mulliken JB, Folkman J. Successful antiangiogenic therapy of giant cell angioblastoma with interferon alfa 2b: report of 2 cases. *Pediatrics* 2002; **109**: 1–5.
163. Hoppeler H, Kayar SR. Capillarity and oxidative capacity of muscles. *News Physiol Sci* 1988; **3**: 113–116.
164. Semenza GL. Targeting HIF-1 for cancer therapy. *Nat Rev Cancer* 2003; **3**: 721–732.
165. Simon JM. Hypoxia and angiogenesis. *Bull Cancer* 2007; **94**: 160–165.
166. Forsythe JA, Jiang BH, Iyer NV, Agani F, Leung SW, Koos RD, Semenza GL. Activation of vascular endothelial growth factor gene transcription by hypoxia-inducible factor 1. *Mol Cell Biol* 1996; **16**: 4604–4613.

167. Warren BA (1979) The vascular morphology of tumors. In:Peterson H-I (ed) *Tumor Blood Circulation: Angiogenesis, Vascular Morphology and Blood Flow of Experimental Human Tumors* CRC Press, Florida, pp. 1–47.
168. Ide AG, Baker NH, Warren SL. Vascularization of the Brown-Pearce rabbit epithelioma transplant as seen in the transparent ear chamber. *AJR Am J Roentgenol* 1939; **42**: 891–899.
169. Iliopoulos O, Levy AP, Jiang C, Kaelin WG Jr, Goldberg MA. Negative regulation of hypoxia-inducible genes by the von Hippel-Lindau protein. *Proc Natl Acad Sci USA* 1996; **93**: 10595–19599.
170. Levy AP, Levy NS, Goldberg MA. Post-transcriptional regulation of vascular endothelial growth factor by hypoxia. *J Biol Chem* 1996; **271**: 2746–2753.
171. Dachs GU, Patterson AV, Firth JD, Ratcliffe PJ, Townsend KM, Stratford IJ, Harris AL. Targeting gene expression to hypoxic tumor cells. *Nat Med* 1997; **3**: 515–520.
172. Folkman J (2002) Angiogenesis in arthritis. In: Smolen J, Lipsky P (eds) *Targeted Therapies in Rheumatology*. Martin Dunitz, London, pp. 111–131.
173. Iervolino A, Trisciuoglio D, Ribatti D, Candiloro A, Biroccio A, Zupi G, Del Bufalo D. Bcl-2 overexpression in human melanoma cells increases angiogenesis through VEGF mRNA stabilization and HIF-1-mediated transcriptional activity. *FASEB J* 2002; **16**: 1453–1455.
174. Blancher C, Moore JW, Talks KL, Houlbrook S, Harris AL. Relationship of hypoxia-inducible factor (HIF)-1alpha and HIF-2alpha expression to vascular endothelial growth factor induction and hypoxia survival in human breast cancer cell lines. *Cancer Res* 2000; **60**: 7106–7113.
175. Chen WT, Huang CJ, Wu MT, Yang SF, Su YC, Chai CY. Hypoxia-inducible factor-1alpha is associated with risk of aggressive behavior and tumor angiogenesis in gastrointestinal stromal tumor. *Jpn J Clin Oncol* 2005; **35**: 207–213.
176. Zhong H, De Marzo AM, Laughner E, Lim M, Hilton DA, Zagzag D, Buechler P, Isaacs WB, Semenza GL, Simons JW. Overexpression of hypoxia-inducible factor 1alpha in common human cancers and their metastases. *Cancer Res* 1999; **59**: 5830–5835.
177. Woelfle U, Cloos J, Sauter G, Riethdorf L, Janicke F, van Diest P, Brakenhoff R, Pantel K. Molecular signature associated with bone marrow micrometastasis in human breast cancer. *Cancer Res* 2003; **63**: 5679–5684.
178. Liao D, Corle C, Seagroves TN, Johnson RS. Hypoxia-inducible factor-1alpha is a key regulator of metastasis in a transgenic model of cancer initiation and progression. *Cancer Res* 2007; **67**: 563–572.
179. Maynard MA, Ohh M. The role of hypoxia-inducible factors in cancer. *Cell Mol Life Sci* 2007; **64**: 2170–2180.
180. Algire GH, Chalkely HW, Legallais FY, Park H. Vascular reactions of normal and malignant tumors in vivo: I. Vascular reactions of mice to wounds and to normal and neoplastic transplants. *J Natl Cancer Inst* 1945; **6**: 73–85.
181. Obermair A, Kucera E, Mayerhofer K, Speiser P, Seifert M, Czerwenka K, Kaider A, Leodolter S, Kainz C, Zeillinger R. Vascular endothelial growth factor (VEGF) in human breast cancer: correlation with disease-free survival. *Int J Cancer* 1997; **74**: 455–458.
182. Gasparini G, Toi M, Gion M, Verderio P, Dittadi R, Hanatani M, Matsubara I, Vinante O, Bonoldi E, Boracchi P, Gatti C, Suzuki, H, Tominaga T. Prognostic significance of vascular endothelial growth factor protein in node-negative breast carcinoma. *J Natl Cancer Inst* 1997; **89**: 139–144.
183. Linderholm B, Tavelin B, Grankvist K, Henriksson R. Vascular endothelial growth factor is of high prognostic value in node-negative breast carcinoma. *J Clin Oncol* 1998; **16**: 3121–3128.

184. Heffelfinger SC, Miller MA, Yassin R, Gear R. Angiogenic growth factors in preinvasive breast disease. *Clin Cancer Res* 1999; **5**: 2867–2876.
185. Ao A, Wang H, Kamarajugadda S, Lu J. Involvement of estrogen-related receptors in transcriptional response to hypoxia and growth of solid tumors. *Proc Natl Acad Sci* 2008; **105**: 7821–7826.
186. Melillo G. Hypoxia-inducible factor 1 inhibitors. *Methods Enzymol* 2007; **435**: 385–402.
187. Welsh S, Williams R, Kirkpatrick L, Paine-Murrieta G, Powis G. Antitumor activity and pharmacodynamic properties of PX-478, an inhibitor of hypoxia-inducible factor-1alpha. *Mol Cancer Ther* 2004; **3**: 233–244.
188. Yeo E-J, Chun Y-S, Park J-W. New anticancer strategies targeting HIF-1. *Biochem Pharmacol* 2004; **68**: 1061–1069.
189. Oh SH, Woo JK, Jin Q, Kang HJ, Jeong JW, Kim KW, Hong WK, Lee HY. Identification of novel antiangiogenic anticancer activities of deguelin targetinghypoxia inducible factor-1 alpha. *Int J Cancer* 2008; **122**: 5–14.
190. Singh RP, Agarwal R. Inducible nitric oxide synthase-vascular endothelial growth factor axis: a potential target to inhibit tumor angiogenesis by dietary agents. *Curr Cancer Drug Targets* 2007; **7**: 475–483.
191. Fang J, Ding M, Yang L, Liu LZ, Jiang BH. PI3K/PTEN/AKT signaling regulates prostate tumor angiogenesis. *Cell Signal* 2007; **19**: 2487–2497.
192. Hampl M, Tanaka T, Albert PS, Lee J, Ferrari N, Fine HA. Therapeutic effects of viral vector-mediated antiangiogenic gene transfer in malignant ascites. *Hum Gene Ther* 2001; **12**: 1713–1729.
193. Colorado PC, Torre A, Kamphaus G, Maeshima Y, Hopfer H, Takahashi K, Volk R, Zamborsky ED, Herman S, Sarkar PK, Ericksen MB, Dhanabal M, Simons M, Post M, Kufe DW, Weichselbaum RR, Sukhatme VP, Kalluri R. Antiangiogenic cues from vascular basement membrane collagen. *Cancer Res* 2000; **60**: 2520–2526.
194. Kamphaus GD, Colorado PC, Panka DJ, Hopfer H, Ramchandran R, Torre A, Maeshima Y, Mier JW, Sukhatme VP, Kalluri R. Canstatin, a novel matrix-derived inhibitor of angiogenesis and tumor growth. *J Biol Chem* 2000; **275**: 1209–1215.
195. Zhang M, Maass N, Magit D, Sager R. Transactivation through Ets and Ap1 transcription sites determines the expression of the tumor-suppressing gene maspin. *Cell Growth Differ* 1997; **8**: 179–186.
196. Watanabe M, Nasu Y, Kashiwakura Y, Kusumi N, Tamayose K, Nagai A, Sasano T, Shimada T, Daida H, Kumon H. Adenoassociated virus 2-mediated intratumoral prostate cancer gene therapy: long-term maspin expression efficiently suppresses tumor growth. *Hum Gene Ther* 2005; **16**: 699–710.
197. Kendall RL, Wang G, Thomas KA. Identification of a natural soluble form of the vascular endothelial growth factorreceptor, FLT-1, and its heterodimerization with KDR. *Biochem Biophys Res Commun* 1996; **226**: 324–328.
198. Griscelli F, Li H, Bennaceur-Griscelli A, Soria J, Opolon P, Soria C, Perricaudet M, Yeh P, Lu H. Angiostatin gene transfer: inhibition of tumor growth in vivo by blockage of endothelial cell proliferation associated with a mitosis arrest. *Proc Natl Acad Sci USA* 1998; **95**: 6367–6372.
199. Indraccolo S, Gola E, Rosato A, Minuzzo S, Habeler W, Tisato V, Roni V, Esposito G, Morini M, Albini A, Noonan DM, Ferrantini M, Amadori A, Chieco-Bianchi L. Differential effects of angiostatin, endostatin and interferon-α (1) gene transfer on in vivo growth of human breast cancer cells. *Gene Ther* 2002; **9**: 867–878.
200. Indraccolo S, Morini M, Gola E, Carrozzino F, Habeler W, Minghelli S, Santi L, Chieco-Bianchi L, Cao Y, Albini A, Noonan DM. Effects of angiostatin gene transfer on functional properties and in vivo growth of Kaposi's sarcoma cells. *Cancer Res* 2001; **61**: 5441–5446.

201. Gyorffy S, Palmer K, Gauldie J. Adenoviral vector expressing murine Angiostatin inhibits a model of breast cancer metastatic growth in the lungs of mice. *Am J Pathol* 2001; **159**: 1137–1147.

202. Sacco MG, Catò EM, Ceruti R, Soldati S, Indraccolo S, Caniatti M, Scanziani E, Vezzoni P. Systemic gene therapy with anti-angiogenic factors inhibits spontaneous breast tumor growth and metastasis in MMTVneu transgenic mice. *Gene Ther* 2001; **8**: 67–70.

203. Ma HI, Lin SZ, Chiang YH, Li J, Chen SL, Tsao YP, Xiao X. Intratumoral gene therapy of malignant brain tumor in a rat model with angiostatin delivered by adeno-associated viral (AAV) vector. *Gene Ther* 2002; **9**: 2–11.

204. Ma HI, Guo P, Li J, Lin SZ, Chiang YH, Xiao X, Cheng SY. Suppression of intracranial human glioma growth after intramuscular administration of an adeno-associated viral vector expressing angiostatin. *Cancer Res* 2002b; **62**: 756–763.

205. Zhang X, Wu J, Fei Z, Gao D, Li X, Liu X, Liang J, Wang X. Angiostatin K (1-3) gene for treatment of human gliomas: an experimental study. *Chin Med J* 2000; **113**: 996–1001.

206. Griscelli F, Li H, Cheong C, Opolon P, Bennaceur-Griscelli A, Vassal G, Soria J, Soria C, Lu H, Perricaudet M, Yeh P. Combined effects of radiotherapy and Angiostatin gene therapy in glioma tumor model. *Proc Natl Acad Sci USA* 2000; **97**: 6698–6703.

207. Rodolfo M, Catò EM, Soldati S, Ceruti R, Asioli M, Scanziani E, Vezzoni P, Parmiani G, Sacco MG. Growth of human melanoma xenografts is suppressed by systemic angiostatin gene therapy. *Cancer Gene Ther* 2001; **8**: 491–496.

208. Matsumoto G, Ohmi Y, Shindo J. Angiostatin gene therapy inhibits the growth of murine squamous cell carcinoma in vivo. *Oral Oncol* 2001; **37**: 369–378.

209. Scappaticci FA, Smith R, Pathak A, Schloss D, Lum B, Cao Y, Johnson F, Engleman EG, Nolan GP. Combination angiostatin and endostatin gene transfer induces synergistic antiangiogenic activity in vitro and antitumor efficacy in leukemia and solid tumors in mice. *Mol Ther* 2001; **3**: 186–196.

210. Scappaticci FA, Contreras A, Smith R, Bonhoure L, Lum B, Cao Y, Engleman EG, Nolan GP. Statin-AE: A novel angiostatin-endostatin fusion protein with enhanced antiangiogenic and antitumor activity. *Angiogenesis* 2001; **4**: 263–268.

211. Shichinohe T, Bochner BH, Mizutani K, Nishida M, Hegerich-Gilliam S, Naldini L, Kasahara N. Development of lentiviral vectors for antiangiogenic gene delivery. *Cancer Gene Ther* 2001; **8**: 879–889.

212. Andrawiss M, Maron A, Beltran W, Opolon P, Connault E, Griscelli F, Yeh P, Perricaudet M, Devauchelle P. Adenovirus-mediated gene transfer in canine eyes: A preclinical study for gene therapy of human uveal melanoma. *J Gene Med* 2001; **3**: 228–239.

213. Harada H, Nakagawa K, Iwata S, Saito M, Kumon Y, Sakaki S, Sato K, Hamada K. Restoration of wild type p16 down-regulates vascular endothelial growth factor expression and inhibits angiogenesis in human gliomas. *Cancer Res* 1999; **59**: 3783–3789.

214. Steiner MS, Zhang Y, Farooq F, Lerner J, Wang Y, Lu Y. Adenoviral vector containing wild type p16 suppresses prostate cancer growth and prolongs survival by inducing cell senescence. *Cancer Gene Ther* 2000; **7**: 360–372.

215. Abe T, Okamura K, Ono M, Kohno K, Mori T, Hori S, Kuwano M. Induction of vascular endothelial tubular morphogenesis by human glioma cells: amodel system for tumor angiogenesis. *J Clin Invest* 1993; **92**: 54–61.

216. Qiu Z, Cui FL, Xu CL, Gu ZQ, Sun YH. Suppression of invasion and angiogenesis in human prostate cancer PC-3 cells by adenovirus-mediated co-transfer of PTEN and P27. *Zhonghua Nan Ke Xue* 2007; **13**: 201–205.

217. Hajitou A, Grignet C, Devy L, Berndt S, Blacher S, Deroanne CF, Bajou K, Fong T, Chiang Y, Foidart JM, Noël A. The antitumoral effect of endostatin and angiostatin is

associated with a down-regulation of vascular endothelial growth factor expression in tumor cell. *FASEB J* 2002; **16**: 1802–1804.

218. te Velde EA, Vogten JM, Gebbink MF, van Gorp JM, Voest EE, Borel Rinkes IH. Enhanced antitumour efficacy by combining conventional chemotherapy with Angiostatin or endostatin in a liver metastasis model. *Br J Surg* 2002; **89**: 1302–1309.

219. Wilczynska U, Kucharska A, Szary J, Szala S. Combined delivery of an antiangiogenic protein (angiostatin) and an immunomodulatory gene (interleukin-12) in the treatment of murine cancer. *Acta Biochim Pol* 2001; **48**: 1077–1084.

220. Matsunaga T, Weihrauch DW, Moniz MC, Tessmer J, Warltier DC, Chilian WM. Angiostatin inhibits coronary angiogenesis during impaired production of nitric oxide. *Circulation* 2002; **105**: 2185–2191.

221. Mauceri HJ, Seetharam S, Beckett MA, Schumm LP, Koons A, Gupta VK, Park JO, Manan A, Lee JY, Montag AG, Kufe DW, Weichselbaum RR. Angiostatin potentiates cyclophosphamide treatment of metastatic disease. *Cancer Chemother Pharmacol* 2002; **50**: 412–418.

222. Tandle A, Blazer DG 3rd, Libutti SK. Antiangiogenic gene therapy of cancer: Recent developments. *J Transl Med* 2004; **2**: 22–42.

223. Abdollahi A, Hlatky L, Huber PE. Endostatin: the logic of antiangiogenic therapy. *Drug Resist Updat* 2005; **8**: 59–74.

224. Camphausen K, Moses MA, Beecken WD, Khan MK, Folkman J, O'Reilly MS. Radiation therapy to a primary tumor accelerates metastatic growth in mice. *Cancer Res* 2001; **61**: 2207–2211.

225. Shibata D. Clonal diversity in tumor progression. *Nat Genet* 2006; **38**: 402–403.

226. Nicolson, G L. Tumor cell instability, diversification, and progression to the metastatic phenotype: from oncogene to oncofetal expression. *Cancer Res* 1987; **47**: 1473–1487.

227. Lazo PA, Klein-Szanto AJP, Tsichlis P N. T-cell lymphoma lines derived from rat thymomas induced by Moloney murine leukemia virus: phenotypic diversity and its implications. *J Virol* 1990; **64**: 3948–3959.

228. Marshall E. Breast cancer research: a special report. Search for a killer: Focus shifts from fat to hormones. *Science* 1993; **259**: 618–621.

229. Steeg PS, Hartsough MT, Clare SE (1998) Nm23, breast differentiation, and cancer metastasis. In: Bowcock AM (ed) *Breast Cancer*. Humana Press, Totowa, New Jersey, 1998, pp. 267–283.

230. Nicolson GL. Cancer metastasis. *Sci Am* 1979; **240**: 66–76.

231. Netland PA, Zetter BR. Organ-specific adhesion of metastatic tumor cells in vitro. *Science* 1984; **224**: 1113–1115.

232. Nicolson GL. Organ specificity of tumor metastasis: role of preferential adhesion, invasion and growth of malignant cells at specific secondary sites. *Cancer Metastasis Rev* 1988; **7**: 143–188.

233. Boxberger HJ, Paweletz N, Spiess E, Kriehuber R. An in vitro model study of BSp73 rat tumour cell invasion into endothelial monolayer. *Anticancer Res* 1989; **9**: 1777–1786.

234. Zetter BR. Angiogenesis and tumor metastasis. *Annu Rev Med* 1998; **49**: 407–424.

235. Weidner N, Semple JP, Welch WR, Folkman J. Tumor angiogenesis correlates with metastasis in invasive breast carcinoma. *N Engl J Med* 1991; **324**: 1–8.

236. Weinstat-Saslow D, Steeg PS. Angiogenesis and colonization in the tumor metastatic process: basic and applied advances. *FASEB J* 1994; **8**: 401–407.

237. Liotta LA, Saidel MG, Kleinerman J. The significance of hematogenous tumor cell clumps in the metastatic process. *Cancer Res* 1976; **36**: 889–894.

238. Dvorak HF, Nagy JA, Dvorak JT, Dvorak AM. Identification and characterization of the blood vessels of solid tumors that are leaky to circulating macromolecules. *Am J Pathol* 1988; **133**: 95–109.

239. Kalebic T, Garbisa S, Glaser B, Liotta LA. Basement membrane collagen: degradation by migrating endothelial cells. *Science* 1983; **221**: 281–283.

240. Nagy JA, Brown LF, Senger DR, Lanir N, Van de Water L, Dvorak AM, Dvorak HF. Pathogenesis of tumor stroma generation: A critical role for leaky blood vessels and fibrin deposition. *Biochem Biophys Acta* 1989; **948**: 305–326.
241. Skinner SA, Tutton PJ, O'Brien PE. Microvascular architecture of experimental colon tumors in the rat. *Cancer Res* 1990; **50**: 2411–2417.
242. Holmgren L, O'Reilly MS, Folkman J. Dormancy of micrometastases: Balanced proliferation and apoptosis in the presence of angiogenesis suppression. *Nat Med* 1995; **1**: 149–153.
243. Folkman J. Angiogenesis in cancer, vascular, rheumatoid and other disease. *Nature Med* 1995; **1**: 27–31.
244. Chambers AF. The metastatic process: basic research and clinical implications. *Oncol Res* 1999; **11**: 161–168.
245. Hanahan D, Christofori G, Naik P, Arbeit J. Transgenic mouse models of tumor angiogenesis: The angiogenic switch, its molecular controls, and prospects for preclinical therapeutic models. *Eur J Cancer* 1996; **32**: 2386–2393.
246. Kandel J, Bossy-Wetzel E, Radvanyi F, Klagsbrun M, Folkman J, Hanahan D. Neovascularization is associated with a switch to the export of bFGF in the multistep development of fibrosarcoma. *Cell* 1991; **66**: 1095–1104.
247. Folkman J, Kalluri R. Tumor Angiogenesis. In: Kufe DW, Pollock RE, Weichselbaum RR, Ralph R, Bast RCJ, Gansler TS, Holland JF, Frei E III. (eds) *Cancer Medicine*, 6th edn. Hamilton, Canada, 2003.
248. Smith-McCune KK, Weidner N. Demonstration and characterization of the angiogenic properties of cervical dysplasia. *Cancer Res* 1994; **54**: 800–804.
249. Hicks RM, Chowaniec J. Experimental induction, histology, and ultrastructure of hyperplasia and neoplasia of the urinary bladder epithelium. *Int Rev Exp Pathol* 1978; **18**: 199–280.
250. Sillman F, Boyce J, Fruchter R. The significance of atypical vessels and neovascularization in cervical neoplasia. *Am J Obstet Gynecol* 1981; **139**: 154–159.
251. Srivastava A, Laidler P, Davies RP, Horfan K. The prognostic significance of tumor vascularity in intermediate-thickness (0.76–4.0 mm thick) skin melanoma. A quantitative histologic study. *Am J Pathol* 1988; **133**: 419–423.
252. Liotta LA, Tryggvason K, Garbisa S, Hart I, Foltz CM, Shafie S. Metastatic potential correlates with enzymatic degradation of basement membrane collagen. *Nature* 1980; **284**: 67–68.
253. Tremblay PL, Huot J, Auger FA. Mechanisms by which E-selectin regulates diapedesis of colon cancer cells under flow conditions. *Cancer Res* 2008; **68**: 5167–5176.
254. Benjamin LE, Bergers G. Angiogenesis: Tumorigenesis and the angiogenic switch. *Nat Rev Cancer* 2003; **3**: 401–410.
255. Brown JM, Giaccia AJ. The Unique Physiology of Solid Tumors: Opportunities (and Problems) for Cancer Therapy. *Cancer Res* 1998; **58**: 1408–1416.
256. Jaffe EA, Nachman RL, Becker CG, Minick CR. Culture of human endothelial cells derived from umbilical veins: identification by morphologic and immunologic criteria. *J Clin Invest* 1972; **52**: 2745–2756.
257. Fukumura D, Jain RK. Tumor microvasculature and microenvironment: targets for anti-angiogenesis and normalization. *Microvasc Res* 2007; **74**: 72–84.
258. Folkman J. Antiangiogenesis. In: DeVita VT Jr, Hellman S, Rosenberg SA (eds) *Biologic Therapy of Cancer*. Lippincott, Philadelphia, 1991, pp. 743–753.
259. Jain RK, Tong RT, Munn LL. Effect of vascular normalization by antiangiogenic therapy on inerstitial hypertension, peritumor edema, and lymphaticmetastasis: insights from a mathematical model. *Cancer Res* 2007; **67**: 2729–2735.
260. Boucher Y, Jain RK. Microvascular pressure is the principal driving force for interstitial hypertension in solid tumors: implications for vascular collapse. *Cancer Res* 1992; **52**: 5110–5114.

261. Winkler F, Kozin SV, Tong RT, Chae SS, Booth MF, Garkavtsev I, Xu L, Hicklin DJ, Fukumura D, di Tomaso E, Munn LL, Jain RK. Kinetics of vascular normalization by VEGFR2 blockade governs brain tumor response to radiation: role of oxygenation, angiopoietin-1, and matrix metalloproteinases. *Cancer Cell* 2004; **6**: 553–563.
262. Ansiaux R, Baudelet C, Jordan BF, Beghein N, Sonveaux P, De Wever J, Martinive P, Grégoire V, Feron O, Gallez B. Thalidomide radiosensitizes tumors through early changes in the tumor microenvironment. *ClinCancer Res* 2005; **11**: 743–750.
263. National Cancer Institute (2008) Executive Summary of the Tumor Microenvironment Think Tank at http://dcb.nci.nih.gov/thinktank/Executive_Summary_of_the_Tumor_Microenvironment_Think_Tank.cfm
264. Ingber DE. Can cancer be reversed by engineering the tumor microenvironment? *Semin Cancer Biol* 2008; **18**: 356–364.
265. Cairns RA, Kalliomaki T, Hill RP. Acute (cyclic) hypoxia enhances spontaneous metastasis of KHT murine tumors. *Cancer Res* 2001; **61**: 8903–8908.
266. Cairns RA, Hill RP. Acute hypoxia enhances spontaneous lymph node metastasis in an orthotopic murine model of humancervical carcinoma. *Cancer Res* 2004; **64**: 2054–2061.
267. Young SD, Marshall RS, Hill RP. Hypoxia induces DNA overreplication and enhances metastatic potential of murine tumor cells. *Proc Natl Acad Sci USA* 1988; **85**: 9533–9537.
268. Stackpole CW, Groszek L, Kalbag SS. Benign-tomalignant B16 melanoma progression induced in two stages in vitro by exposure to hypoxia. *J Natl Cancer Inst* 1994; **86**: 361–367.
269. Rofstad EK, Danielsen T. Hypoxia-induced metastasis of human melanoma cells: involvement of vascular endothelial growth factor-mediated angiogenesis. *Br J Cancer* 1999; **80**: 1697–1707.
270. Semenza GL. Hypoxia-inducible factor 1: Oxygen homeostasis and disease pathophysiology. *Trends Mol Med* 2001; **7**: 345–350.
271. Roth U, Curth K, Unterman TG, Kietzmann T. The transcription factors HIF-1 and HNF-4 and the coactivator p300 are involved in insulin-regulated glucokinase gene expression via the phosphatidylinositol 3-kinase/protein kinase B pathway. *J Biol Chem* 2004; **279**: 2623–2631.
272. Dvorak HF, Nagy JA, Feng D, Brown LF, Dvorak AM. Vascular permeability factor/vascular endothelial growth factor and the significance of microvascular hyperpermeability in angiogenesis. *Curr Top Microbiol Immunol* 1999; **237**: 97–132.
273. Mabjeesh NJ, Amir S. Hypoxia-inducible factor (HIF) in human tumorigenesis. *Histol Histopathol* 2007; **22**: 559–572.
274. Hockel M, Vaupel P. Tumor hypoxia: Definitions and current clinical, biologic, and molecular aspects. *J Natl Cancer Inst* 2001; **93**: 266–276.
275. Dong LW, Wang WY, Yue YT, Li M. Effects of flavones extracted from Portulaca oleracea on ability of hypoxia tolerance in mice and its mechanism. *Zhong Xi Yi Jie He Xue Bao.* 2005 **3**: 450–454.
276. Yeo EJ, Chun YS, Cho YS, Kim J, Lee JC, Kim MS, Park JW. YC-1: a potential anticancer drug targeting hypoxia-inducible factor 1. *J Natl Cancer Inst* 2003; **95**: 516–525.
277. Mabjeesh NJ, Escuin D, LaVallee TM, Pribluda VS, Swartz GM, Johnson MS, Willard MT, Zhong H, Simons JW, Giannakakou P. 2ME2 inhibits tumor growth and angiogenesis by disruptingmicrotubules and dysregulating HIF. *Cancer Cell* 2003; **3**: 363–375.
278. Li X, Lu Y, Liang K, Pan T, Mendelsohn J, Fan Z. Requirement of hypoxia-inducible factor-1alpha down-regulation in mediating the antitumor activity of the anti-epidermal growth factor receptor monoclonal antibody cetuximab. *Mol Cancer Ther* 2008; **7**: 1207–1217.
279. Eyler CE, Rich JN. Survival of the fittest: cancer stem cells in therapeutic resistance and angiogenesis. *J Clin Oncol* 2008; **26**: 2839–2845.

280. Hill RP, Perris R. "Destemming" cancer stem cells. *J Natl Cancer Inst* 2007; **99**: 1435–1440.
281. Craig T, Jordan MLG, Noble M. Cancer stem cells. *N Engl J Med* 2006; **355**: 1253–1261.
282. Clarke MF, Dick JE, Dirks PB, Eaves CJ, Jamieson CH, Jones DL, Visvader J, Weissman IL, Wahl GM. Cancer stem cells – perspectives on current status and future directions: AACRWorkshop on cancer stem cells. *Cancer Res* 2006; **66**: 9339–9344.
283. van Kempen LC, Leenders WP. Tumours can adapt to anti-angiogenic therapy depending on the stromal context: lessons from endothelial cell biology. *Br J Cancer* 2006; **94**: 552–560.
284. Hurwitz H, Fehrenbacher L, Novotny W, Cartwright T, Hainsworth J, Heim W, Berlin J, Baron A, Griffing S, Holmgren E, Ferrara N, Fyfe G, Rogers B, Ross R, Kabbinavar F. Bevacizumab plus irinotecan, fluorouracil, and leucovorin for metastatic colorectal cancer. *N Engl J Med* 2004; **350**: 2335–2342.
285. Casanovas O, Hicklin DJ, Bergers G, Hanahan D. Drug resistance by evasion of antiangiogenic targeting of VEGF signaling in late stage pancreatic islet tumors. *Cancer Cell* 2005; **8**: 299–309.
286. Carmeliet P. Angiogenesis in life, disease and medicine. *Nature* 2005; **438**: 932–936.
287. Shaked Y, Ciarrocchi A, Franco M, Lee CR, Man S, Cheung AM, Hicklin DJ, Chaplin D, Foster FS, Benezra R, Kerbel RS. Therapy-induced acute recruitment of circulating endothelial progenitor cells to tumors. *Science* 2006; **313**: 1785–1787.
288. Willett CG, Boucher Y, Duda DG, di Tomaso E, Munn LL, Tong RT, Kozin SV, Petit L, Jain RK, Chung DC, Sahani DV, Kalva SP, Cohen KS, Scadden DT, Fischman AJ, Clark JW, Ryan DP, Zhu AX, Blaszkowsky LS, Shellito PC, Mino-Kenudson M, Lauwers GY. Surrogate markers for antiangiogenic therapy and dose-limiting toxicities for bevacizumab with radiation and chemotherapy: continued experience of a phase I trial in rectal cancer patients. *J Clin Oncol* 2005; **23**: 8136–8139.
289. O'Reilly MS, Pirie-Shepherd S, Lane WS, Folkman J. Antiangiogenic activity of the cleaved conformation of the Serpin Antithrombin III. *Science* 1999; **285**: 1926–1928.
290. Kerbel RS, Viloria-Petit A, Klement G, Rak J. 'Accidental' anti-angiogenic drugs. Anti-oncogene directed signal transduction inhibitors and conventional chemotherapeutic agents as examples. *Eur J Cancer* 2000; **36**: 1248–1257.
291. Thijssen VL, van Beijnum JR, Mayo KH, Griffioen AW. Identification of Novel Drug Targets for Angiostatic Cancer Therapy; It Takes Two to Tango. *Curr Pharmaceu Design* 2007; **13**: 3576–3583.
292. Lee TY, Lin CT, Kuo SY, Chang DK, Wu HC. Peptide-mediatedtargeting to tumor blood vessels of lung cancer for drug delivery. *Cancer Res* 2007; **67**: 10958–10965.
293. Lo A, Lin CT, Wu HC. Hepatocellular carcinoma cell-specific peptide ligand for targeted drug delivery. *Mol Cancer Ther* 2008; **7**: 579–589.
294. Wu H-C, Huang C-T, Chang D-K. Anti-angiogenic therapeutic drugs for treatment of human cancer. *J Cancer Mol* 2008; **4**: 37–45.
295. Trachtenberg J, Bogaards A, Weersink RA, Haider MA, Evans A, McCluskey SA, Scherz A, Gertner MR, Yue C, Appu S, Aprikian A, Savard J, Wilson BC, Elhilali M. Vascular targeted photodynamic therapy with palladium-bacteriopheophorbide photosensitizer for recurrent prostate cancer following definitive radiation therapy: Assessment of safety and treatment response. *J Urol* 2007; **178**: 1974–1979.
296. Sessa C, Guibal A, Del Conte G, Rüegg C. Biomarkers of angiogenesis for the development of antiangiogenic therapies in oncology: tools or decorations? *Nat Clin Pract Oncol* 2008; **5**: 378–391.
297. Keedy VL, Sandler AB. Inhibition of angiogenesis in the treatment of non-small cell lung cancer. *Cancer Sci* 2007; **98**: 1825–1830.
298. Shimizu K, Asai T, Fuse C, Sadzuka Y, Sonobe T, Ogino K, Taki T, Tanaka T, Oku N. Applicability of anti-neovascular therapy to drug-resistant tumor: suppression of

drug-resistant P388 tumor growth with neovessel-targeted liposomal adriamycin. *Int J Pharm* 2005; **296**: 133–141.

299. Shimizu K, Asai T, Oku N. Antineovascular therapy, a novel antiangiogenic approach. *Expert Opin Ther Targets* 2005; **9**: 63–76.

300. Asai T, Miyazawa S, Maeda N, Hatanaka K, Katanasaka Y, Shimizu K, Shuto S, Oku N. Antineovascular therapy with angiogenic vessel-targeted polyethyleneglycol-shielded liposomal DPP-CNDAC. *Cancer Sci* 2008; **99**: 1029–1033.

301. Maeda N, Miyazawa S, Shimizu K, Asai T, Yonezawa S, Kitazawa S, Namba Y, Tsukada H, Oku N. Enhancement of anticancer activity in antineovascular therapy is based on the intratumoral distribution of the active targeting carrier for anticancer drugs. *Biol Pharm Bull* 2006; **29**: 1936–1940.

302. Shimizu K, Sawazaki Y, Tanaka T, Asai T, Oku N. Chronopharmacologic cancer treatment with an angiogenic vessel-targeted liposomal drug. *Biol Pharm Bull* 2008; **31**: 95–98.

303. Gimmi CD. Current stumbling blocks in oncology drug development. *Ernst Schering Res Found Workshop* 2007; **59**: 135–149.

304. Kwon HJ. Discovery of new small molecules and targets towards angiogenesis via chemical genomics approach. *Curr Drug Targets* 2006; **7**: 397–405.

Anticancer Drug Development

Unique Aspects of Pharmaceutical Development

Ajit S. Narang and Divyakant S. Desai

1 Introduction

Around the world, tremendous resources are being invested in prevention, diagnosis, and treatment of cancer. Cancer is the second leading cause of death in Europe and North America. Discovery and development of anticancer agents are the key focus of several pharmaceutical companies as well as non-profit government and non-government organizations, like the National Cancer Institute (NCI) in the United States, the European Organization for Research and Treatment of Cancer (EORTC), and the British Cancer Research Campaign (CRC).

Identification of cytotoxic compounds led the development of anticancer therapeutics for several decades. Advances in cancer treatment, however, continued to be limited by the identification of unique biochemical aspects of malignancies that could be exploited to selectively target tumor cells. Schwartsmann et al. noted in 1988 that of over 600,000 compounds screened by then, less than 40 agents were routinely used in the clinic [1]. The recent growth in molecular sciences and the advances in genomics and proteomics have generated several potential new drug targets, leading to changes in the paradigms of anticancer drug discovery toward molecularly targeted therapeutics. These shifting paradigms have not only resulted in the greater involvement of biological scientists in the drug discovery process but also required changes in the screening and clinical evaluation of drug candidates. Both small and large molecular compounds continue to be investigated as anticancer agents.

The discovery and development of anticancer drugs, especially cytotoxic agents, differ significantly from the drug development process for any other indication. The unique challenges and opportunities in working with these agents are reflected in each stage of the drug development process. This chapter will highlight the unique aspects of anticancer drug discovery and development.

A.S. Narang (✉)
Bristol-Myers Squibb, Co., New Brunswick, NJ 08901, USA
e-mail: ajit.narang@bms.com

Y. Lu, R.I. Mahato (eds.), *Pharmaceutical Perspectives of Cancer Therapeutics*,
DOI 10.1007/978-1-4419-0131-6_2, © Springer Science+Business Media, LLC 2009

2 Approaches in Anticancer Drug Therapy

Conventional anticancer drug discovery and development have focused on the cytotoxic agents. The drug discovery paradigms selected agents that had significant cytostatic or cytotoxic activity on tumor cell lines and caused tumor regression in murine tumor allografts or xenografts. The anticancer agents were discovered mainly by serendipity or inhibiting metabolic pathways crucial to cell division. Their exact mechanisms of action were often a subject of retrospective investigation. For example, Farber et al. reported the use of folate analogues for the treatment of acute lymphoblastic leukemia (ALL) in 1948 [2], while its mechanism of action, inhibition of the dihydrofolate reductase, was reported by Osborn et al. in 1958 [3, 4]. Similarly, the nitrogen mustard, mustine, was used as a chemotherapeutic agent long before its mechanism of action was understood [5].

Although this strategy has achieved significant success, the recent developments in molecular biology and an understanding of the pharmacology of cancer at a molecular level have challenged researchers to come up with target-based drugs. These are the agents that are pre-designed to inhibit and/or modify a selected molecular marker deemed important in cancer prognosis, growth, and/ or metastasis. Several target-based compounds have emerged in recent years. While most of these compounds are in preclinical testing, several are in clinical trials and a few have been approved in the United States. For example [6],

- Imatinib mesylate (Gleevec®, Novartis) is a small-molecule compound that inhibits a specific tyrosine kinase enzyme, the Bcr–Abl fusion oncoprotein. It is used for gastrointestinal stromal tumor and chronic myeloid leukemia.
- Gefitinib (Iressa®, AstraZeneca & Teva) is a small-molecule inhibitor of the epidermal growth factor receptor's (EGFR, or erbB1) tyrosine kinase domain. It is used for non-small-cell lung cancer.
- Bortezomib (Velcade®, Millenium Pharmaceuticals) is a small-molecule proteasome inhibitor used for the treatment of multiple myeloma refractory to other treatments.
- Rituximab (Rituxan®, Biogen Idec & Genentech) is a monoclonal antibody used in the treatment of B-cell non-Hodgkin's lymphoma and B-cell leukemia. It binds the CD20 antigen on the CD20 + B-cells, causing their apoptosis.
- Trastuzumab (Herceptin®, Genentech) is a monoclonal antibody that binds the cell surface HER2/neu (erbB2) receptor and is used in the therapy of erbB2 + breast cancer.

2.1 Drug Development Paradigms for Molecularly Targeted Agents

Conventional screening models for anticancer agents are geared toward the selection of cytotoxic drugs. The animal screening models predominantly focus on tumor regression and survival advantage, while the early stage human clinical trials are aimed at determining the limiting dose where high drug-related toxicity is observed. Toxicity and tumor-regression effects of cytotoxic agents are based on the same mechanism (Fig. 1A). Thus, these agents are dosed to the allowable maximum levels where serious toxicity is not observed. The molecularly targeted agents, on the other hand, act by mechanisms that may not result in direct and significant toxicity. These agents act on the extra cellular, transmembrane, or nonnuclear intracellular processes and are exemplified by receptor tyrosine kinase inhibitors, farnesyltransferase inhibitors, matrix metalloproteinase (MMP) inhibitors, and angiogenesis inhibitors. For example, compounds such as 5,6-dimethylxanthenone-4-acetic acid (DMXAA) target developing tumor vasculature and have proven useful in cancer treatment when combined with conventional cytotoxic agents [7]. These agents often cause tumor growth inhibition, rather than regression, in animal models. They have better toxicity profiles than cytotoxic drugs and require prolonged administration [8]. The differences between their dose–response and dose–toxicity curves are illustrated in Fig. 1B.

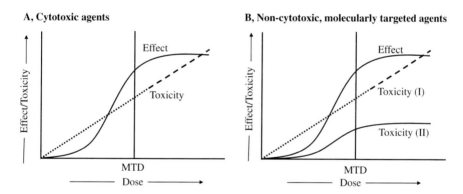

Fig. 1 Hypothetical dose–effect and dose–toxicity curves for cytotoxic (**A**) and non-cytotoxic, molecularly targeted anticancer agents (**B**). The cytotoxic agents are known for their dose-dependent toxicity, which closely follows the dose–effect curve. Non-cytotoxic agents, on the other hand, could have a linear dose–toxicity relationship similar to the cytotoxic agents (I) or a non-linear profile with dose–toxicity curve lower than the dose–effect curve (II). MTD represents the maximum tolerated dose for the cytotoxic agent. Modified from Hoekstra et al. [8]

The discovery and development of molecularly targeted anticancer agents necessitate changes in the anticancer drug preclinical and clinical screening paradigms not only because of the differences in their dose–response and dose–toxicity profiles and mechanisms but also because these agents are discovered with a pre-targeted mechanism of action. Although the development of the molecularly targeted agents is far more complex and demanding, they are being actively pursued with over 1,300 small biotech companies in the United States focusing on molecular targets, of which over half are focusing on cancer treatment. There are estimated at least 395 agents in clinical trials for cancer treatment, more than in any other therapeutic class of medicine [9].

An important element of preclinical and clinical screening of molecularly targeted agents is the investigation of their effects on the specific molecular targets. Even though the drug effects on its molecular target may not be sufficient to demonstrate clinical benefit, it is necessary to validate this model of drug development and to understand the mechanism of drug action. Furthermore, it may be useful as a surrogate marker to guide dose escalation studies in early stage human clinical development. Evaluation of target effects in clinical trials, however, is not trivial. This requires the development and validation of a target specific molecular assay, and the correlation of the molecular target to the tumor type. Furthermore, physiological levels of molecular markers could have high natural variations, leading to difficulty in proving statistically significant drug effects.

Most molecularly targeted agents, however, do not proceed to advanced stages in human clinical trials due to either efficacy or toxicity concerns. The toxicity profile of an agent includes general toxicity and effects explained by its mechanism of action. While the toxicity remains largely unpredictable and difficult to modify, investigations of efficacy of these agents critically depend upon the selection of appropriate molecular targets and clinical trial designs. The latter includes selection of appropriate drug combinations for clinical studies and end points for the demonstration of efficacy.

Combination therapy is particularly important where the actions of target-based drugs are supplemented or potentiated by other agents and where the target-based drugs may act as sensitizers to the cytotoxic agents, e.g., P-glycoprotein (membrane efflux protein responsible for multi-drug resistance in several cases) inhibitors. The clinical end point for demonstration of efficacy has traditionally been the shrinkage of tumor size, as a surrogate for survival. End points for target-based drugs, such as the levels of surrogate molecular markers, changes in tumor markers, growth rate, time to progression, and the improvement in the quality of life (compared to cytotoxic agents), have been difficult to quantify and correlate with therapeutic benefit to the patient. Accordingly, these have been called "soft end points" [10].

Selection of appropriate molecular targets for inhibition or modification, such that the target is tumor specific, non-redundant, and able to influence the outcome of tumor progression, is a significant challenge given the complexity of molecular signaling pathways in cells. Key molecular mechanisms that have been explored for the development of target-based anticancer agents have been discussed in detail by Baguley and Kerr, for example.

2.1.1 Facilitating Apoptosis

Apoptosis is a physiologic intracellular process involving a well-ordered signaling pathway that leads to cell death and clearance of the dead cells by neighboring phagocytes, without inflammation. Cytotoxic drug-induced damage to the cells, especially to the DNA, triggers apoptosis through two signaling mechanisms – the activation and release of mitochondrial pro-apoptotic proteins known as caspases under the control of Bcl-2 family of proteins or upregulated expression of pro-apoptotic receptors on cancer cells, whose subsequent interaction with their ligands activates apoptotic signaling pathways. These receptors include the Fas (also called APO-1 or CD95) and the tumor necrosis factor (TNF)-related apoptosis-inducing ligands (TRAIL) receptors. In addition, anticancer drugs can activate lipid-dependent signaling pathways that result in decreased apoptosis threshold or modulate other cytoprotective pathways such as the nuclear factor-κB (NF-κB), heat shock proteins, and cell cycle regulatory pathways.

2.1.2 Inhibiting Metastasis

Metastasis is the spread of the tumor from one organ or part of the body to another and is attributed to the translocation of cancer cells. This process of tumor cell translocation requires cellular movement as well as the remodeling of the extracellular matrix (ECM) that physically entraps cells and defines the shape of a tissue, at both the initial and the metastasized sites of tumor growth. Extracellular enzymes, matrix metalloproteinases (MMPs), proteases, and plasminogen activators (PAs), have been implicated in this remodeling of the ECM, leading to invasion and dissemination of cancer. Thus, drug candidates targeting proteases and MMP inhibitors have been developed for potential anticancer activity.

2.1.3 Inhibiting Angiogenesis

Angiogenesis, the process of formation of new blood vessels from the existing blood supply, is an essential requirement for the growth of tumor mass as well as its metastasis. Thus, prevention of angiogenesis has the potential to block nutrient and oxygen supply to the tumors, resulting in tumor regression. Three key events involved in tumor angiogenesis include the angiogenesis switch that initiates this process, proliferation and migration of endothelial cells to form the lining of new blood vessels, and remodeling of the ECM. Several cellular signal transduction molecules have been identified to play a role in this process including the angiogenic factors such as the vascular endothelial growth factor (VEGF), the integrins, plasminogen activation system, and the MMPs. Drug targets have been identified to inhibit one or more aspects of these pathways, e.g., VEGF receptor antagonists and VEGF antibodies.

2.1.4 Antibodies Against Tumor-Specific Antigens

Induction of antitumor immune responses by using tumor-specific antigens is a cherished goal in cancer therapeutics since it promises to be free of dose-limiting toxicity. Administration of antibodies against tumor-specific and tumor-associated antigens can be used to target tumors by carrying radioisotopes, toxins, or prodrug converting enzymes. In addition, antibodies per se result in tumor regression by complement fixation or antibody-dependent cellular toxicity (ADCC) through the involvement of natural killer cells, granulocytes, and monocytes. Additional strategies that have been exploited include the expression of target antigens on the antigen-presenting cells (APCs) or dendritic cells to activate body's T-cell immune response.

Thus, preclinical evaluation and clinical development of anticancer agents, especially molecularly targeted therapeutics, present unique challenges – both in the selection of appropriate drug target and in the development of a molecular marker of efficacy. Developing an assay for the surrogate markers and its correlation with antitumor efficacy requires a significant research investment with unpredictable outcome. Also, the molecular understanding of cancer growth and metastasis is still developing and the selection of molecular targets for drug development may not succeed in the clinic. These risks and challenges are inherent in the development of molecularly targeted anticancer agents.

2.2 Pharmacogenetics and Metabolomics

Therapeutic activity and toxicity of cytotoxic drugs are derived from the same molecular mechanisms and usually correlate directly with the dose. To maximize clinical benefits, patients are dosed to the maximum levels that do not result in serious side effects. The resulting narrow therapeutic window of these drugs, along with the serious disease condition of the patients and inter-individual variation in drug response and toxicity, constitutes a significant challenge in their clinical development and use. These considerations, in turn, have generated opportunities for the development of tools for individualization of drug therapy to the patient and monitoring of drug response and toxicity using surrogate markers. Tumor treatment has been individualized for patients based on the tumor type, histology, and the disease state. Pharmacogenetics is an emerging paradigm for individualization of drug therapy using the genetic constitution of the patient.

Pharmacogenetics involves the genotypic and phenotypic imprinting of the individual patient to identify key genes and their proteins that are involved in the pharmacokinetics and/or pharmacodynamics of drug response and/or toxicity. This analysis is expected to reduce the inter-individual variation in drug–response or minimize the side effects by modulating drug doses to adjust for genetic variability in patients. The targets for genotype profiling in patients are usually the drug-metabolizing enzymes or the drug targets. Among the drug-metabolizing enzymes, cytochrome P450 (CYP) superfamily constitutes several isoenzymes that are implicated in the inactivation of anticancer compounds, such as CYP1A2 for flutamide, CYP2A6 for tegafur, CYP2B6 for cyclophosphamide, CYP2C8 for paclitaxel, and CYP2D6 for tamoxifen [11]. Examples of drug targets whose variation impacts anticancer drug treatment include thymidylate synthase with 5-fluorouracil and the epidermal growth factor receptor with the tyrosine kinase inhibitors gefitinib and erlotinib [12]. Screening of patients for markers of specific metabolizing enzymes or drug targets is important not only in the clinical setting to reduce the probability of drug exposure related toxicities but also in the clinical trials of novel anticancer agents with narrow therapeutic index. This approach can help achieve individualization of drug therapy to optimally balance efficacy with toxicity and, thus, contribute to the success of clinical development of novel drug candidates.

Metabolomics, on the other hand, involve the quantitative analyses of metabolites in a cell, tissue, or organism. It could involve two strategies – target analysis and metabolite profiling [13]. While target analysis is restricted to the quantification of a chosen class of compounds (related to a specific pathway, intersecting pathways, or the investigational drug candidate), metabolite profiling involves analyses of a large number of metabolites with the objective of identifying a specific metabolite profile that characterizes a given sample. The analytical techniques used for metabolomic studies include isotopic (e.g., ^{13}C) labeling of chosen metabolites and monitoring their progress through various pathways and assays for low-level quantification in biological samples such as mass spectroscopy (MS), liquid/gas chromatography – tandem MS (LC-MS/MS or GC-MS/MS), and ion cyclotron resonance (ICR).

Metabolic profiling of a system reflects the net effects of genetic and environmental influences, including disease state and drug therapy. Such profiling can help distinguish between the pre-disease, disease, and normal state of cells and tissues. For example, the metabolic phenotype of cancer cells is characterized by high glucose uptake, increased glycolytic activity, low mitochondrial activity, and increased phospholipid turnover [14]. A metabolic profile indicative of any such characteristics can be utilized as a surrogate marker of disease state. Metabolomic profiling can rapidly detect subtle changes in metabolic pathways and shifts in homeostasis much before phenotypic changes can be detected [15]. Although metabolomics is an emerging science that will require significant developments before its successful clinical application, it has potential in drug discovery in the identification and development of biomarkers and classifying patients as responders or nonresponders to a given therapy. For example, Chung et al. identified that the ratio (phosphomonoesters/phosphodiesters), measured using ^{31}P NMR spectroscopy, could be used as a surrogate marker for the antitumor activity of 17-allylamino-17-demethoxygeldanamycin (17 AAG) in cultured tumor cells and xenografts [16].

Narrow therapeutic index combined with the inter-individual variations in drug pharmacokinetics, response, and toxicity adds uncertainty to the clinical trials and use of novel anticancer agents. Pharmacogenetic and metabolomic profiling of the patients promise to at least partly address these concerns, thus helping in the individualization of medication for patients and improved therapeutic outcomes. In addition, these techniques can improve patient selection for clinical trials based on molecular features of the tumor and patient response variables, toward more efficient and cost-effective drug development [17]. For example, it has been suggested that mutations in the epidermal growth factor receptor (EGFR) gene can help predict sensitivity to gefitinib in lung cancer patients [18]. However, the data required for generating such correlations are usually obtained much later in the product development and commercialization cycle. Furthermore, these disciplines are still in their infancy and would need significant further developments before their widespread routine use in drug development and clinical application.

2.3 *Modulators, Sensitizers, and Supportive Cancer-Care Agents*

In addition to the cytotoxic and molecularly targeted anticancer agents, drugs acting through several indirect mechanisms are used in the management of cancer. These include the immunomodulators, chemoprotective agents, multidrug resistance reversing agents, hormonal drugs, photosensitizers, analgesics, anti-emetics, and bone marrow growth factors.

The prospect of developing therapeutic vaccines using immunomodulators for tumor treatment has attracted considerable research interest. Immunomodulators are the drugs that alter the body's immune response to tumor cells. These are based on generating humoral and/or T-cell responses to the specific tumor antigens being targeted. Several strategies have been applied to produce immune-mediated anticancer activity, e.g., enhancing the activity of antigen-presenting cells, the use of cytokines such as interleukin-12 and interferon-α to enhance immune activation, and inhibition of T-cell inhibitory signals [19]. Very few of these agents, however, demonstrated statistically significant improvement in clinical end points in phase III studies [20].

Multi-drug resistance (MDR) is a phenomenon whereby the tumor cells develop resistance to a variety of drug molecules. MDR could be due to the failure of tumor cells to undergo apoptosis in response to chemotherapy or the upregulation of the membrane protein, P-glycoprotein (P-gp). P-gp acts as an efflux pump for a variety of drugs, leading to reduced intracellular concentration and anticancer efficacy. Drugs that inhibit the P-gp efflux pump, therefore, can improve the efficacy of cytotoxic drug treatment. For example, an amlodipine derivative, CJX1, inhibited P-gp and increased the intracellular concentration of doxorubicin, thus reversing doxorubicin resistance of the human myelogenous leukemia cells [21]. Several highly specific P-gp inhibitors, such as tariquidar, zosuquidar, and laniquidar, have entered early stage clinical trials in combination with cytotoxic anticancer agents [22].

Chemoprotective agents are the drugs that can help mitigate the toxic effects of anticancer drugs. For example, the nitrogen mustard ifosfamide causes nephrotoxicity (hemorrhagic cystitis and hematuria), which was attributed to its metabolite, chloroacetaldehyde. Co-administration of the sulfhydryl compound sodium-2-sulfanylethanesulfonate (mesna) neutralizes the active metabolite in renal tubules, thus acting as a chemoprotective agent [23]. Another example of a chemoprotectant is amifostine, which reduces the nephrotoxicity of cisplatin. Amifostine is a thiophosphate prodrug that gets dephosphorylated by alkaline phosphatase in the normal endothelium in vivo to the active sulfhydryl compound [24].

Hormonal drugs and photosensitizers are non-cytotoxic agents that can have anticancer effects in target populations. The use of hormonal drugs as anticancer agents is based on the hormone dependence of certain tumor types, such as endometrial, prostate, ovarian, and breast cancers. Thus, antiestrogens, antiandrogens, and antiprogestins are usually not cytotoxic but may prevent the growth of hormone-dependent tumors by changing the endocrine environment. In many cases, these drugs can be administered by a non-parenteral route, e.g., by oral tablets or transdermal patches.

Photosensitizers are the compounds that are therapeutically inactive until irradiated by light. Laser light irradiation of tumor tissues after photosensitizer administration to the patient leads to the generation of free radicals inside and in the vicinity of the tumor tissue, causing tumor destruction. An example of this class of agents includes the porphyrin precursor 5-aminolaevulinic acid, which has been clinically successful [25]. Longer wavelength laser light is preferred over shorter wavelengths because of less direct tissue damage and deeper penetration. Selectivity of tumor damage is achieved by both the concentration of the photosensitizing agent to the tumor and the localized irradiation.

In addition, supportive cancer-care agents include drugs that help alleviate the serious side effects associated with cytotoxic compounds. This class of drugs includes analgesics, anti-emetics, and growth factors. Examples of these compounds include opiates and fentanyl as analgesics; octreotide for diarrhea; and phenothiazines and butyrophenones as anti-emetics. The bone marrow growth factors such as granulocyte colony stimulating growth factor (Filgastrim®) and granulocyte-macrophage (or monocyte) colony stimulating factor (Sargramostim®) help stimulate white cell production and reduce the risk of serious infection due to myelosuppression [26, 27]. These therapies are aimed at improving the quality of life of cancer patients, increase compliance, and reduce hospitalization due to adverse effects [28]. Many of these agents are available through a wide variety of drug delivery options including immediate and sustained release formulations, transdermal products, and depot formulations.

3 Anticancer Drug Development Process

Conventional anticancer drug development efforts focused on cytostatic or cytotoxic compounds that caused tumor regression. These paradigms have been expanded to include target pre-selection for the discovery of molecularly targeted therapeutic agents. In addition, drug types such as immunomodulators, chemoprotectants, MDR-reversing agents, photosensitizers, and hormonal drugs present an increasing arsenal with unique drug development needs and possibilities of drug combinations to maximize therapeutic outcome. Furthermore, the use of molecular biology technologies such as pharmacogenetics and metabolomics with cytotoxic agents can help control drug toxicity and better predict drug response. Prudent application of these opportunities is significantly influencing the preclinical and clinical development of novel anticancer therapeutics.

The new drug discovery and development process is a systematic approach to identify potential new drug candidates and their evaluation for drug-like properties. Although the discovery and development of anticancer compounds follow the same process as any other new molecular entities (NMEs), they have several unique aspects that impact their development paradigms. The new drug development process typically involves the following stages, not necessarily in a sequential manner:

1. *Acquisition of potential compounds*: This could be achieved by chemical synthesis or by extraction from natural resources. This stage includes the development of analytical methods to confirm identity and purity of the compound, and its stability under real-life and stressed storage conditions. Physicochemical properties of the compound are identified, such as the solid-state form (polymorphism, hydrates, and solvates), melting point, solubility, and stability. Synthesis of the molecule is scaled up as the compound progresses in the development pathway. A formulation suitable for human administration and commercialization is identified and scaled-up.
2. *Drug screening and preclinical pharmacology*: This involves "paper chemistry" whereby the drug structure is compared to those of existing compounds in the databases to identify potential activity, toxicities, degradation pathways, metabolic routes, etc. A preliminary screening in cell culture models is carried out to identify the extent and specificity of its antitumor activity. This is followed by the evaluation of efficacy and toxicity in animal models.
3. *Clinical development*: Clinical development of a drug candidate involves testing in human volunteers to identify the toxicities and the maximum tolerated dose (MTD) in phase I clinical trials. Subsequently, phase II studies are carried out in patients of selected tumor type to quantify efficacy and confirm dosage. Subsequently, larger phase III studies are aimed at head-to-head comparison of the NCE with the then-best-available therapy.

The drug discovery and development process is inherently time and resource consuming with very low success rates, as illustrated in Fig. 2.

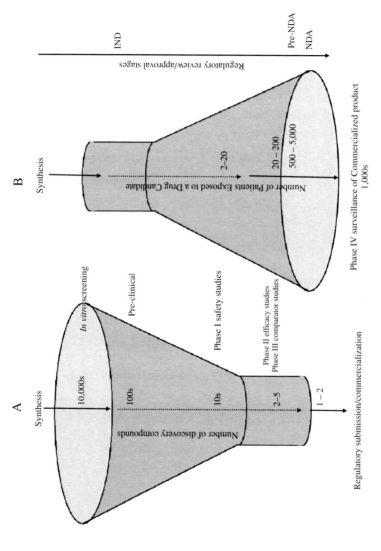

Fig. 2 An example of the funnel of reducing number of compounds progressing through the drug development process (**A**). The progress of a drug candidate through these phases is accompanied by a progressive increase in the number of patients exposed to the drug (**B**). This figure also illustrates the steps where regulatory review and/or approval is required in the United States, such as the Investigational New Drug (IND) application submission before initiating Phase I studies, a pre-NDA meeting with the FDA after the Phase II studies, and New Drug Application (NDA) submission for drug approval for marketing after the completion of Phase III studies

3.1 Historical Background

The history of cancer chemotherapy has been widely described [9, 29, 30]. Most cytotoxic anticancer compounds were discovered by serendipity or as inhibitors of metabolic pathways involved in cell division. For example, nitrogen mustard was discovered in the 1940s upon investigations by Goodman and Gilman of the lymphoid and myeloid suppression observed in soldiers accidentally exposed to the nitrogen mustard gas during the World War II [5]. The utility of hormone therapy in cancer became evident by the works of George Beatson, who documented shrinkage in breast cancers upon removal of the ovaries [31], and Charles Huggins, who showed that the prostate cancer in dogs can be stalled by castration and by estrogen injection [32]. Similarly, the discovery of anticancer properties of platinum coordination compounds, such as cisplatin, is attributed to Barnett Rosenberg, who was investigating the effect of electric field on the growth of bacteria and observed cessation of cell division due to the contamination of the growth medium with the electrolysis product of the platinum electrode [33, 34]. Mitoxantrone was developed from anthracyclines that were originally developed as stable dyes but had the planar ring structure suitable for intercalation in the DNA double strands [35].

Cancer was recognized primarily as a disease of uncontrolled cell division. Hence, all efforts were directed toward the identification of antiproliferative compounds. Accordingly, regression of tumor size has been recognized as the primary, objective end point of effectiveness in preclinical and clinical testing. Murine models of cancer were developed that rapidly grew tumors. Screening of new compounds in the drug discovery programs was focused on testing them in these rapidly growing tumor models. Several clinically important anticancer compounds were identified using this screen. Nevertheless, the selective use of rapidly growing tumor models was implicated as the reason that the successes occurred mainly in the rapidly growing malignancies, e.g., lymphomas, childhood leukemia, and germline tumors. Relatively fewer successes were seen for the slow-growing common solid-tumors of the adults, e.g., lung, breast, and colorectal cancers [36]. These criticisms led investigators to modify the pre-screening and screening protocols to include a variety of cell lines and tumor types. These aspects are discussed further in later sections.

3.2 Discovery of Potential Drug Candidates

The compounds selected for evaluation as potential anticancer agents could be of natural or synthetic origin. Compounds of natural origin have often provided new leads in the novelty of structures with anticancer activity. Mans et al. have enlisted several examples of naturally derived anticancer compounds [35]. For example, vincristine derived from the periwinkle plant *Vinca rosea*, etoposide is derived from the mandrake plant *Podophyllum peltatum*, and taxol, which is derived from the pacific yew, *Taxus brevifolia*. Similarly, doxorubicin and bleomycin are fermentation products of the bacteria *Streptomyces*; L-asparaginase is derived from the broths of *Escherichia coli* or *Erwinia carotovora*; rhizoxin is derived from the fungus *Rhizopus chinensis*; cytarabine was discovered from the marine sponge *Cryptotethya crypta*; and bryostatin from the sea moss *Bugula neritina*.

Analogs of natural compounds have often been synthesized to improve their efficacy or toxicity profiles [35]. For example, carboplatin was developed as an analog of cisplatin with reduced renal toxicity, doxorubicin is an analog of daunomycin that reduces its cardiotoxicity, and topotecan is an analog of camptothecin with better toxicity profile. Analogs of existing drugs have also been synthesized to improve drug targeting and the pharmacokinetic profiles of drug candidates [35]. For example, tauromustine is a nitrosourea anticancer agent coupled to the brain targeting peptide taurine for targeting CNS tumors, and 9-alkyl morpholinyl anthracyclines are analogs of doxorubicin that have been synthesized to reduce drug affinity to the cellular efflux protein, P-glycoprotein. The use of related analogs has also been used to improve drug supply. For example, taxotere was developed to overcome the supply problems with taxol, a natural compound of plant origin with very low yields.

The synthetic compounds could be the analogs of known compounds or novel structures. The process of identifying and selecting these candidates has undergone a sea change in the recent decades with the development of solid-state and combinatorial chemistry and computer modeling of drug–receptor interactions. Discovery of new anticancer agents by laboratory synthesis has evolved from analog evaluation and improvement of new leads to rational design based on drug–receptor or drug–enzyme interactions. Examples of synthetic analogs of natural compounds that demonstrated anticancer activity include the folic acid analog methotrexate and the fluorinated pyrimidine base, 5-fluorouracil. Examples of drugs that have been discovered through the rational design approach by the exploration of molecular mechanisms and interactions with drug targets include EO9, which is a mitomycin C-related indoloquinone and is active against hypoxic tumors; and the ether lipid, ET-10-methoxy-1-octadecyl-2-methyl-rac-glycero-3-phosphocholine, which targets the cell membranes [35].

Invariably, the discovery process leads to far more compounds as potential drug candidates than that can be investigated in the clinic, thus necessitating a screening process for short-listing compounds with the highest potential for clinical success. Computer simulation is used to identify novel and potentially active structures. Selected compounds are tested by cell culture and animal assays to quantify efficacy, identify toxicities, and potentially additional pharmacokinetic and pharmacological properties. These aspects are discussed in the following section.

3.3 Preclinical Evaluation

Screening of drug candidates for anticancer activity is done in several stages, which are designed to create a 'funnel' with reducing number of compounds entering the successive stages of development, as exemplified in Fig. 2A. This screening protocol balances the real-life limitations in the number of drug candidates that can be tested in humans each year with the number of potential new drug candidates that show potential for antitumor activity.

During preclinical development, novel drug candidates are produced in sufficiently large quantities and tested for their physicochemical, biopharmaceutical, and solid-state properties. These include the evaluation of solubility, stability in the solid state and solution, pH solubility and stability studies, identification of degradation pathways, isolation of polymorphic forms and their impact on drug solubility and stability, absorption studies in cell culture models and animals, and the drug-excipient compatibility studies. The anticancer activity is evaluated in vitro in cell culture models by cell growth inhibitory or clonogenic assays, which serves as a pre-screen to identify active compounds. The potential toxicities and early pharmacology of selected compounds are determined in murine allograft or human xenograft mouse models. For example, at the US National Cancer Institute (NCI), new compounds are evaluated for cytostatic or cytotoxic activity against eight cell lines derived from the most common human malignancies. Compounds that show activities in this pre-screen are tested in more detail in a panel of cell lines of the respective tumor type, and subsequently in animal models [37–44].

3.3.1 Preclinical Efficacy Screening

Historically, drug screening in murine models was done in the L1210 mouse leukemia model along with the P388 murine leukemia allograft, and a few other models for special cases such as the sarcoma 180, carcinoma 755, and Lewis lung carcinoma models [45]. The measures of anticancer activity are primarily the (a) reduction of tumor size and (b) increase in the life span of the mice. In addition to the anticancer activity, the in vivo screen provides information on potential toxicities, tolerated doses and dosage regimens, and the spectrum of activity. Drugs that were found effective in this model were evaluated in other rodent models, and, if shown broad activity, were taken up for further development. Several anticancer drugs were identified with activity against lymphomas, leukemias, and some pediatric tumors. However, these models were ineffective to yield drugs against slow-growing adult solid tumors, like the mammary, colon, and lung cancers [37–44, 46].

In 1975, the NCI introduced screening in human tumor xenografts in nude mice, and the P388 model was moved to a pre-screening stage. This approach was further refined in the year 1990 to replace animal testing in the pre-screening stage with a cell culture evaluation in 60 tumor cell lines (called the NCI-60 screen), which are derived from human leukemia, small-cell and non-small-cell lung cancers, and other human carcinomas. These cell lines are continuously being replaced and added and are being characterized for molecular markers and other characteristics relevant to regulation of cell growth, division, and differentiation. This pre-screening stage incorporates a panel of the same cell lines grown as xenograft tumors in nude mice.

The cell culture pre-screen involves inoculation and growth of cells in microtiter plates followed by incubation with different concentrations of the potential anticancer compounds. At the end of incubation, cell growth is measured by a colorimetric assay and the antitumor potential of the compounds is assessed by their cytostatic or cytotoxic activity. Thus, the NCI-60 screen generates a wealth of information with respect to the dose–response curves of potential compounds in several different cell lines, which represent different cancer types and profiles of molecular markers and biochemical pathways. Collectively, this information on the pattern of cell inhibition can be utilized to generate a 'fingerprint' of the compound. Comparing the fingerprint of the novel compound with the library database of compounds with known mechanisms of action can help generate the hypothesis on the mechanism of action of the novel compound.

Kohlhagen et al. provide an example of the application of NCI-60 screen to generate a hypothesis for the mechanism of action of a novel compound, designated NSC-314622 [47]. This process involves generation of dose–response curves for all the NCI-60 cell lines, usually involving four-log dilution range of the drug [48]. A typical dose–response curve is exemplified in Fig. 3. The compound's concentration that inhibits growth by 50% (GI_{50}) for each cell line can be plotted on the x-axis relative to the mean GI_{50} of the panel of 60 cell lines, with bar to the right indicating higher than the mean concentration and the bar to the left indicating lower than the mean [48]. Using these plots to

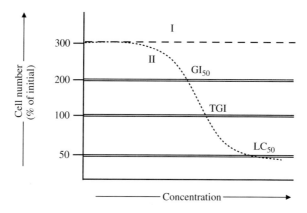

Fig. 3 An illustration of the dose–response curves generated during cell culture pre-screening. This example illustrates the dose-dependent cytotoxic effect of drugs on cells cultured in vitro in cell culture dishes. Cell cultures that are not exposed to the drug (I) grow to a hypothetical three-fold, or 300%, of their initial numbers upon culturing in a growth promoting media for a fixed amount of time. Thus, these cells show 200% growth, or 200% increase in viable cell count. However, the cells exposed to the drug (II) have less number of viable cells upon culture under similar conditions for the same amount of time. The number of viable cells in the drug-exposed culture dish depends upon the drug concentration in a manner illustrated by curve II. The drug concentration at which the viable cell count after culture remains the same as the initial, i.e., at 100%, is defined as the total growth inhibitory (TGI) concentration. Drug concentration that halves the growth of cells in culture, i.e., increase in cell numbers to half of the levels seen without drug (which was 200%), is defined as the GI_{50} (growth inhibition to 50% level). Similarly, the concentration of drug that halves the viable cell count from its initial level (which is 100%) is defined as LC_{50} (lethal concentration to 50% level). Modified from Shoemaker [44]

define a fingerprint of the compound, Kohlhagen et al. observed similarity in the cytotoxicity profiles of NSC-314622 with that of topotecan, camptothecin, and camptothecin derivatives with a Pearson correlation coefficient of 0.74, 0.63, and (0.78–0.84), respectively (Fig. 4). This information helped define the initial hypothesis that NSC-314622 was a topoisomerase I poison, which was then developed further using a battery of tests [47].

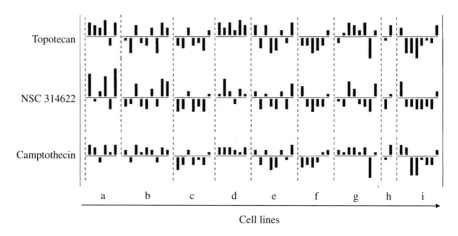

Fig. 4 An example of the use of the NCI-60 screen fingerprint to indicate the mechanism of drug action. This graph displays the drug concentration that inhibits cell growth by 50% (GI_{50}) in the 60 cell lines of the NCI Anticancer Drug Screen, representing different tumor types: (a) leukemia, (b) non-small cell lung cancer, (c) colon cancer, (d) CNS cancer, (e) melanoma, (f) ovarian cancer, (g) renal cancer, (h) prostate cancer, and (i) breast cancer. The y-axis represents the mean GI_{50} in milligram of drug dose as a positive (upwards) or negative (downwards) deviation from the mean. Similarity between different cell lines in their pattern of antitumor efficacy is compared by the Pearson correlation coefficient analyses. In this example, the Pearson correlation coefficient of NSC 314622 with Topotecan was 0.74 and with Camptothecin was 0.63. Modified from Kohlhagen et al [47].

Although the use of cell culture screens has the advantage of cost-effectiveness, high throughput, and minimizing the use of animals; they inherently lack the pharmacological advantages of in vivo assays. These are relevant not only in cases where prodrug activation is required in vivo but also in several cases where cell culture activity may not be a good indicator of in vivo activity. Furthermore, the changing paradigms of anticancer drug development toward molecularly targeted therapeutics sometimes necessitate the utilization of animal models to validate their mechanism of action. For example, drug candidates that act by such specific mechanisms as inhibition of angiogenesis, prevention of metastasis, and induction of differentiation require specialized approaches that are often developed on a case-by-case basis. Thus, several pharmaceutical companies and other research organizations continue to rely on murine allograft and xenograft models for anticancer drug screening.

3.3.2 Preclinical Toxicity Studies

The animal toxicological studies of anticancer agents are aimed at predicting (a) a safe starting dose and dosage regimen for human clinical trials, (b) the toxicities of the compound, and (c) the likely severity and reversibility of drug toxicities. For most cytotoxic anticancer agents, toxicity is expected at standard, therapeutically active, doses. This is because the therapeutic effect and toxicity are attributed to the same mechanism. Therefore, cytotoxic compounds are dosed to the maximum tolerable levels to maximize their anticancer efficacy. Hence, their clinical dosages are determined by their anticipated tolerance.

Toxicological testing is mainly done in small animals under the precept that the common toxicities of cytotoxic agents, such as bone marrow suppression, can be observed in rodent species. The presence and severity of acute toxicities is ascertained in the test organs by histopathology, biochemistry, and hematology investigations shortly after dosing, while the chronic or long-term toxicities are identified by sacrificing and examining the animals several weeks after dosing. Higher animals, such as primates, are avoided in routine animal toxicological studies due to cost and ethical considerations. Drug–dose correlation between different species is usually derived on the basis of body surface area, although other parameters such as age and body weight have also been used.

To determine the phase I entry dose of a cytotoxic anticancer agent, the dose levels that are lethal to 10, 50, and 90% of mice (LD_{10}, LD_{50}, and LD_{90}, respectively) is determined by the same route of administration. Instead of measuring death as an end point, these dose limits could also be defined in terms of doses that cause severe, life-threatening toxicity (severe toxic dose, STD). The projected phase I entry dose is usually $^1/_{10}$th of the LD_{10} or STD_{10}. To minimize the risk associated with human administration of a novel cytotoxic compound, the projected phase I entry dose is first tested in another species, usually rats or dogs, to ascertain lack of significant toxicity. Thus, the preclinical animal toxicology protocol usually involves single- and multiple-dose lethality or severe-toxicity studies in mice, followed by single- and multiple-dose confirmatory toxicity studies in rats or dogs. If serious, irreversible toxicities are exhibited in the non-rodent species at the projected starting dose, then the human starting dose is reduced to the $^1/_6$th of the highest dose tested in the non-rodent species that did not cause any severe, irreversible toxicity.

Evaluation of toxicities of anticancer drugs in animals has several limitations, since anticancer agents are inherently toxic with usually a dose-dependent manifestation of symptoms. The estimation of dose levels in animal toxicology studies that would correspond to the human clinical doses within the therapeutic window is difficult, leading to the possibility of underestimation or overestimation of the drug's toxicological profile. This could be due to species differences in the pharmacokinetics and pharmacodynamic responses of drugs, e.g., due to differences in the metabolic and elimination pathways, protein binding, and the sensitivity of target cells. Furthermore, rare toxicities, e.g., those of cardiovascular or neuromuscular origin, are difficult to detect in animal models. A retrospective study observed 0.5% of toxic deaths in the phase I trials of anticancer agents among ~6,000 participants [49].

An over prediction is highly undesirable for safety reasons. Under prediction, on the other hand, could increase the duration and steps in the dose escalation studies, thus increasing the development costs and time and the unethical administration of ineffective doses to a large number of seriously ill patients [50]. For these reasons, both under and over predictions could result in the dropping out of a molecule from further development. An example of over prediction was seen with the anticancer drug fludarabine. It caused significant bone marrow suppression in phase I studies at the $1/10^{th}$ of mice LD_{10} dose, while dose levels up to 20 times higher than this dose did not cause significant bone marrow suppression in dogs. This difference was explained in terms of species differences in drug pharmacodynamics – higher efficiency of phosphorylation of the drug in human bone marrow cells than those of the dog [51].

Increase in clinical study time due to underestimation of dose is exemplified by brequinar sodium, which needed 19 dose escalation steps over a period of more than 3 years to reach the MTD, since the MTD was 40 times higher than the mouse LD_{10} [52]. Another example is flavone acetic acid, for which the single-dose LD_{10} in mice was similar to that in rats, but dogs and humans tolerated up to four times higher doses. This was attributed to faster drug clearance in the higher species, thus resulting in under prediction of the clinical entry dose [53].

These examples illustrate the need to better estimate drug toxicities in humans to avoid lengthy phase I trials as well as severe drug toxicities. Toward this end, pharmacokinetic analyses are frequently being included in the toxicology protocols. Recently, drug microdosing have been proposed in humans to understand pharmacokinetic properties before projected doses are administered. This aspect is discussed further in Section 3.4.2.

3.4 Clinical Testing

Clinical trials of drug candidates are carried out in three distinct phases: phase I studies to identify safe dose levels and schedules, phase II studies to identify the spectrum of anticancer activity, and phase III studies to compare the NCE with the up-to-then best-available treatment. In addition, post-marketing surveillance phase IV studies continue to monitor drug safety as it is then administered to a significantly greater number of patients. Regulatory involvement is critical at all stages of clinical drug development. As illustrated in Fig. 2, an Investigational New Drug (IND) application is filed with the U.S. Food and Drug Administration (FDA) before the initiation of phase I studies. At the end of phase II studies, usually a pre-NDA meeting is held with the FDA to discuss the results and the plans for the phase III clinical trials. Upon completion of the phase III studies, a New Drug Application (NDA) is filed with the FDA for the grant of marketing authorization.

In the case of anticancer drug development, frequently, drug combinations are evaluated instead of a single compound monotherapy. Phase I studies of anticancer agents are usually conducted in patient, rather than healthy, volunteers. Frequently, this aspect adds to the challenges of developing anticancer compounds since (1) recruitment of tumor-specific patient volunteers becomes difficult and (2) the recruited volunteers are usually in the advanced stages of the disease and refractory to the currently available standard-of-care treatment options. These factors also escalate the clinical costs of drug development.

Phase I clinical trials are carried out at progressively escalating doses to identify the dose-limiting toxicities for cytotoxic compounds and are concluded when the maximum tolerated dose (MTD) is reached. Increments in drug doses in these trials are based on the type, severity, and duration of observed toxicities and their correlation to the expected profile of the given structural class of drugs. Phase I trial concludes when the MTD is reached and the necessary information on the clinical toxicity, pharmacokinetics, and preliminary anti-tumor activity has been gathered.

3.4.1 Dose Escalation Studies

Dose escalation refers to increasing the dose of the drug in phase I clinical trials to identify the maximum tolerated dose. The dose could be increased periodically within the same clinical trial or in each new trial arm. The choice of starting dose and dose escalation steps determine the duration of phase I studies, the number of patients who may be treated with subtherapeutic doses, and the precision of the recommended phase II dose. In the special case of cytotoxic anticancer agents, the likelihood of efficacy is dose dependent. In addition, these agents present a clear dose–toxicity relationship. Therefore, dose-related toxicity is regarded, in general, as a surrogate for efficacy [54]. Thus, the dose escalation process is a careful balance between a conservative approach to ensure safety and a guided approach to ensure early detection of the MTD.

Historically, the most frequently used scheme for phase I dose escalation of cytotoxic agents has been the 'modified Fibonacci search.' This scheme involves dosage increment steps with *increasing decreases* over the previous dose, e.g., (2, 3.3, 5, 7, 9, 12, 16d) as multiples of initial dose (d), or (100, 65, 52, 40, 29, 33, 33%) increases over the previous dose [55]. In contrast to this empirical approach, pharmacologically guided dose escalation (PGDE) scheme proposed by Collins et al. [56] is based on using the preclinical toxicology data to rapidly escalate doses to a target area under the curve (AUC) value obtained from murine pharmacokinetic data.

The PGDE scheme is based on the key assumptions that the drug concentration in the plasma can be used as a predictor for dose-limiting toxicity (DLT) and that the quantitative relationship between toxicity and drug exposure (AUC) is similar across species [56]. Practical limitations of this scheme include the difficulty in obtaining real-time pharmacokinetic data at each dose level, extrapolation of preclinical pharmacokinetic data especially when the dosing schedules were different, and because of the inter-patient variability. In a retrospective evaluation of this dose escalation design, Fuse et al. found that the log AUC for LD_{10} in mice correlated well with the log AUC for MTD in humans for cytotoxic agents whose mechanism of action does not depend upon the cell cycle phase, but not for cell cycle phase-specific agents [57]. Furthermore, accounting for protein binding showed better correlation between the mouse and the human AUC for the unbound drug.

In addition, non-pharmacokinetic statistical modeling approaches have been recommended to guide the dose escalation. These statistical approaches model the dose–toxicity relationship as a sigmoidal curve to predict the MTD. The predicted value of the MTD is adjusted as data on the occurrence or the absence of toxicity accumulate from the clinical trial. Thus, the statistical prediction of the MTD is higher when low toxicity is observed, allowing rapid dose escalation, and the predicted MTD is low when dose-related toxicity is observed, calling for conservative dose escalation steps. This approach of dose escalation has been termed the continual reassessment method (CRM) [54].

3.4.2 Inter-patient Variability and Dose Normalization

Cytotoxic anticancer compounds are inherently toxic and have low therapeutic window. Nevertheless, they are dosed to very high levels, close to but lower than the MTD, to maximize their therapeutic benefit to the patient. Therefore, inter-patient variability in drug exposure has serious implications on drug effectiveness and toxicity to the patients. The variation in drug exposure arises from differences in drug metabolism and elimination. For example, the total body clearance of carboplatin can range from 20 to 200 mL/min due to inter-patient differences in renal function, since most of the drug is eliminated by glomerular filtration through the kidneys [58]. Similarly, topotecan clearance correlates with renal function [59]. On the other hand, clinical drug exposure and toxicity of 6-mercaptopurine are significantly related to the polymorphic phenotype of its metabolizing enzyme, thiopurine methyltransferase [60].

For drugs with clinically established exposure-physiological parameter correlations, dosage adjustment for an individual patient can be done a priori, based on the patient's physiological parameters, such as genotype and/or phenotype of the metabolizing enzymes (pharmacogenetics, see Section 2.2), renal clearance, serum protein, or hepatic function. In addition, for drugs that are dosed repeatedly or continuously, dosage modification can be based on the measurement of drug blood levels and toxicities in the patient. This strategy has been used for continuous intravenous infusions of etoposide and fluorouracil [61]. Another dosage individualization strategy involves administration of a low test dose of the compound to determine the exact pharmacokinetic parameters for an individual patient (microdosing, see Section 3.4.3), followed by modifying the dose to achieve a target drug exposure. Such strategies, however, can only be applied to drugs for which the pharmacokinetic–pharmacodynamic relationships, or relationships between physiological parameters and drug exposure, have been clearly established.

However, many drugs present complex pharmacokinetic relationships, hindering the establishment of such correlations. Furthermore, the clinical experience is usually very limited with new drugs under development. In such situations, clinical oncologists frequently use body surface area (BSA) for drug dose scaling between individuals. Other physiological scaling parameters, such as age, gender, weight, or body mass index, may have also been used in specific circumstances [62].

The use of BSA as a dose-scaling parameter is credited to its early use showing a correlation of BSA with MTD between species [63, 64]. While the use of BSA in preclinical research for scaling between species is well accepted, its use as a scaling parameter has been widely debated and challenged recently [62, 65–69]. For example, BSA correlates well with the total blood volume and the basal metabolic rate, but not with liver function or the glomerular filtration rate [67, 70–71]. Furthermore, BSA varies significantly more among pediatric (0.4–2.0 m^2) than adult (1.6–2.2 m^2) patient populations [62]. The limitations inherent in use of BSA for inter-patient drug scaling are also reflected in the drug–dosage modifications from BSA predicted values. For example, the relative dose per square meter is usually increased in children compared to the adult dose [72], ideal body weight is often used in BSA calculation rather than the actual weight [73], BSA is usually capped at 2 m^2, and dose reduction is undertaken in patients with compromised renal or hepatic function [67]. Nevertheless, the use of BSA as a scaling parameter has shown reduced inter-patient variability in drug exposure in several cases [62, 74] and remains an established clinical practice that usually gives way to or complements the use of more direct correlations as they get established in clinical practice.

Clinical oncologists undertaking new drug development, therefore, need to carefully evaluate the requirement for and the merits and demerits of each modality of inter-patient dose scaling. New drug development programs frequently incorporate measurement of physiological variables, such as the phenotype of key drug-metabolizing enzymes, to establish scaling parameters, where feasible.

3.4.3 Microdosing in Human Clinical Trials

The first-in-human clinical trials of novel cytotoxic compounds constitute a significant safety risk for the patient volunteers. A microdosing strategy has been proposed to mitigate this risk, gather pharmacokinetic data in earlier in clinical development, and to increase the efficiency of drug development. The microdosing concept is based on using extremely low doses of a drug, which are pharmacologically inactive but are able to delineate the pharmacokinetic profile of the drug in humans [75, 76]. This strategy is also expected to reduce the number of participants required for preclinical safety studies and to more accurately predict the first-in-human doses.

The microdose of a small-molecule drug has been defined by the US and European regulatory authorities as "less than $^1/_{100}$th of the dose calculated to yield a pharmacological effect of the test substance to a maximum dose of less than 100 μg." For a protein drug, 30 nmol is considered the maximum dose [77–79]. One key consideration of microdosing studies is the requirement of highly sensitive analytical methods. Such analytical methods include liquid chromatography with tandem mass spectroscopy (LC/MS/MS), positron emission tomography (PET), and accelerated mass spectroscopy (AMS). The use of AMS, however, requires the use of ^{14}C radiolabeled drug, making it less popular.

The American College of Clinical Pharmacology recently issued a position statement on the use of microdosing in the drug development process [80]. In this chapter, Bertino et al. discussed the key considerations for the predictive success and validation of utility of the microdosing protocol. They noted that the success of microdosing strategy depends upon its ability to accurately predict the key pharmacokinetic parameter estimates, e.g., bioavailability, clearance, and the elimination rate, of a drug at much higher therapeutic doses of the drug. The authors noted that only a few studies have reported the comparison of the therapeutic with the microdose data. These studies, however, have used currently marketed drugs and suffer from the limitation of 'prior knowledge', which helps clinical study design in aspects such as the sampling intervals.

A significant limitation of microdosing studies is their inability to predict PK parameters where drugs exhibit nonlinear pharmacokinetics. Nevertheless, this new paradigm of anticancer drug development can complement the existing animal-to-human dose-scaling strategies to improve the safety and the success of early clinical trials.

3.4.4 Drug Combinations and Dosing Strategies

New anticancer agents are categorized in different classes based upon their chemistry, bioactivity profile, and mechanism of action. Furthermore, their clinical use is usually proposed in combination with current therapy, utilizing the established principles and advantages of combination drug therapy to achieve clinical outcomes better than the then-best-available treatment. This section briefly reviews the basis of clinical anticancer drug combinations to understand the drug combinations and dosing strategies utilized during new drug development.

Currently established anticancer drugs include the cytotoxic agents, that damage or kill cells by inhibiting cell division, and hormonal agents, which antagonize hormone action or inhibit its secretion. Hormonal drugs include the glucocorticoids, estrogens, antiestrogens, androgens, and antiandrogens. Cytotoxic agents act as antimetabolites such as pentostatin, 6-mercaptopurine, methotrexate, and 5-fluorouracil; DNA polymerase inhibitors, such as cytarabine; alkylating agents such as cisplatin and mitomycin; RNA synthesis inhibitors, such as doxorubicin, etoposide, and amsacrine; microtubule function inhibitors, such as vinca alkaloids, vincristine and vinblastine; or protein synthesis inhibitors, such as crisantaspase. Based on their action during the cell cycle, these drugs could be classified as being cell cycle active, with or without phase specificity (e.g., G0, G1, M, G2, or S phase of the cell cycle), or non-cell cycle active. Thus, antimetabolites such as 5-fluorouracil and 6-mercaptopurine, and the dihydrofolate reductase inhibitor, methotrexate, are S-phase specific; bleomycin and vinca alkaloids are G2/M-phase specific; alkylating agents (e.g., nitrogen mustard, cyclophosphamide) and doxorubicin are non-phase specific; and corticosteroids such as prednisone and dexamethasone are non-cell cycle active.

Combining drugs in clinical use is a purview of the clinical oncologist and is an ever evolving discipline. Over a hundred clinically used chemotherapy combinations are recognized [81], a detailed discussion of which is beyond the scope of this chapter. Nevertheless, there are a limited set of principles that underlie drug combinations in anticancer treatment [82]. Briefly, the drugs used in combination should possess one or more of the following features:

1. Act by different mechanisms
2. Have some efficacy by themselves
3. Have a different spectrum and/or cell cycle phase specificity of cell kill
4. Have different toxicity profiles
5. Have different mechanisms of resistance development.

Synergistic or additive cell kill, without increasing toxicity, is a frequent goal of drug combinations [83]. The need for higher cell kill is indicated by the first-order nature of this phenomenon, whereby chemotherapy cycles reduce tumor cell number by a given percentage irrespective of the starting cell count. For example, if a drug leads to 99.99% cell kill, it would reduce the tumor cell load of a usually detectable 2 cm solid tumor mass from $\sim10^9$ to $\sim10^5$ cells (the cell kill principle) [84]. The cell kill efficiency of cytotoxic drugs is expressed by the negative log of the fraction of tumor cell population killed by a single course of treatment. Thus, a drug that results in 99.99% cell kill is a 4-log drug, while another drug with 99.9% cell kill would be called a 3-log drug. Additive combination of these drugs, for example, would be expected to result in 7-log cell kill per treatment cycle. Thus, different drugs are given at full doses to increase the percent cell kill toward improved overall clinical outcome and patient survival, while reducing the number of chemotherapy cycles and the emergence of drug resistant cancers.

The principles of chemotherapeutic drug combinations resulting in better clinical outcomes can be exemplified by the use of MOPP combination in Hodgkin's disease and M-BACOP in diffuse lymphoma [85]. The MOPP combination uses nitrogen mustard with vincristine, prednisone, and procarbazine with significantly improved antitumor efficacy and remission rate than any drug alone. It further exemplifies the principles of dose combination, i.e., it uses full dose of drugs with different toxicity profiles (neuropathy with vincristine and typical steroid toxicity with prednisone) and reduced dose of drugs with similar toxicity profiles (bone marrow toxicity of procarbazine and nitrogen mustard). The M-BACOP combination uses methotrexate with bleomycin, adriamycin, cyclophosphamide, vincristine, and prednisone with the same principles of reducing the dose of drugs with overlapping toxicities (bone marrow suppression with adriamycin and cyclophosphamide), but not for different target toxicities (lung toxicity with bleomycin, neuropathy with vincristine, and steroidal toxicity with prednisone).

In addition to drug dosing based on individual and overlapping toxicities of anticancer agents, cytotoxic drugs are dosed in short-duration high-dose cycles rather than a continuous low-dose administration. This is designed to achieve the most cell kill with a high drug dose, while allowing the body to recover from the side effects of chemotherapy between different cycles of treatment. The cell kill efficiency of cytotoxic drugs is the most evident in a solid tumor model (e.g., lung, uterus, and stomach cancer) whereby the tumor consists of actively dividing surface cells overlaying resting cells in the middle, and non-dividing, often non-viable, cells in the core [84].

While short-duration chemotherapy to aggressively kill actively dividing cancer cells is the most common practice, the introduction of novel target-based anticancer agents has allowed changes in the regimens to include continuous, low-dose administration of targeted drugs. For example, Klement et al. report a low-dose anti-angiogenesis regimen utilizing vinblastine combined with an antibody against the VEGF receptor-2 [86]. The authors reported tumor remission without undue toxicity of drug treatment. This approach is particularly applicable to the use of antiangiogenic drugs and has been called low-dose metronomic (LDM) chemotherapy [87].

The clinical development of new anticancer agents builds on the knowledgebase and current practices with existing therapies. Thus, an understanding of drug combinations and dosing relevant to specific disease conditions allows the clinical oncologists to appropriately place new chemical entities in a clinical program to maximize the probability of its beneficial outcome to the patient.

3.4.5 Adverse Effects and Toxicities of Anticancer Drugs

An understanding of toxicities, adverse effects, and special dosing considerations of existing anticancer compounds is important to the design of effective drug combinations and to the interpretation of the toxicological profile of new chemical entities. Most cytotoxic anticancer agents are dosed to maximum tolerated levels to achieve maximum cell kill. The toxicities incumbent with these compounds are often a manifestation of their mechanism of action and killing of the rapidly growing, normal cells such as hair follicle cells, gastrointestinal surface epithelial cells, and stem cells.

The common toxicities of cytotoxic anticancer drugs include the following:

- Bone marrow depression due to damage to the growing stem cells causes reduction in the blood white cell, platelet, and red cell counts. These, in turn, could cause susceptibility to infections, excessive bleeding, and anemia. In addition, certain drugs cause unique and serious bone damage, such as the osteonecrosis of the jaw associated with bisphosphonates [88].

- Damage to growing cells may cause temporary loss of hair (alopecia), skin rashes, changes in the color and texture, or loss of fingernails and toenails. These toxicities are usually reversible.
- Surface epithelial damage to the gastrointestinal tract may result in ulcers, stomatitis, difficulty swallowing (dysphagia), vulnerability to oral infections such as candidiasis, and changes in saliva secretion. In addition, nausea, vomiting, diarrhea, or constipation occur commonly.
- Some drugs may cause kidney damage due to extensive cell destruction, purine catabolism, and deposition of urates in the renal tubules. In addition, liver damage may occur it receives large blood supply. Metabolic conditions of the liver and the kidney are usually monitored for possible correlation to drug blood levels and dosage adjustment, since these are the major drug elimination sites.
- Certain symptoms and side effects associated with cancer could be secondary to disease progression. For example, cancer metastases to the bones could cause chronic pain due to proliferation of cancer cells in the bones and the associated bone remodeling and destruction [89]. Also, tumors that compress veins, the use of central vein catheter [90], and relative immobility of the patient could lead to deep vein thrombosis with potential pulmonary embolism [91].
- Certain drugs, such as paclitaxel and vincristine, could cause peripheral neuropathy [92]. Similarly, anthracyclines are known for rare but serious cardiotoxicity [93, 94].

Thus, adverse drug effects and dose-limiting toxicities of anticancer compounds could be a manifestation of either their mechanisms of action or unrelated toxicities common to a given chemical class of compounds, such as anthracyclines. A close attention to monitor for the emergence of known side effects of anticancer drugs as well as those observed in the preclinical animal toxicology studies ensures patient safety in early oncology drug clinical trials.

3.4.6 Special Patient Populations

Clinical trials in special populations, such as pediatric and geriatrics, nursing and pregnant women, and patients with reduced renal function, are routinely carried out to define the subtleties of clinical application of all drug candidates. These usually involve delineation of a drug's metabolic and elimination pathways, identification of biochemical markers to define the metabolic status of the patient with respect to drug's elimination, genotypic and phenotypic profiling of the patient, defining pharmacokinetic – pharmacodynamic relationships, and dosage adjustment. These principles are practiced with greater vigor for anticancer drugs due to their dose-limiting toxicities, dosing to maximum tolerated levels, and other serious adverse effects.

In addition, pediatric testing of anticancer agents is necessitated by childhood prevalence of fast growing cancers, such as lymphomas, leukemias, and myelomas. Furthermore, regulatory agencies are increasingly encouraging pediatric clinical trials to establish safe and effective doses for pediatric labeling [95, 96]. Phase I clinical trials in children are usually multi-institutional, due to the number of patients available. Ethical considerations further limit the number of levels of dose escalation in children, since treatment with ineffective doses is undesirable. In addition, these trials also enlist patients with intensive prior therapy, which has implications on the maximum tolerated dose determination. Heavily pretreated patients tend to have lower MTDs, especially when DLT involves myelosuppression; which is not the case for patients with minimum prior therapy – thus complicating the determination of MTDs [97].

Pediatric testing of anticancer agents is carried out after the efficacy of these drugs has been established in the adults. A common practice in pediatric oncology is to administer 80% of the MTD determined in adult patients with significant prior therapy and to conduct dose escalation in 30% increments. Further, dose escalation is carried out in successive cohorts of patients since intra-patient dose escalation is usually not permitted and the number of dose escalation steps is sought to be minimized [97]. A retrospective investigation of 69 pediatric oncology trials found that the pediatric MTD strongly correlated with adult MTD and differed by not more than 30% of the dose. They further found that not more than four dose levels were studies in the escalation schemes in over 80% of the trials [98].

3.4.7 Phase II and III Clinical Trials

As a drug candidate progresses through the development stages after the initial proof-of-concept and phase I studies in humans, a reverse funnel of increasing patient exposure to the drug becomes evident (Fig. 2B).

Phase II studies are carried out in a small group of patients with a specific tumor type to determine anticancer efficacy and to define the therapeutic window of the compound. To avoid exposing patients to inactive compounds, these clinical trials use statistical tools to interrupt studies where the in-process data indicate low probability of success. Phase III trials are conducted in a much greater number of patient volunteers of the selected tumor type with prospective and randomized evaluation against the then-available best-possible therapy for the disease, regarded as the standard-of-care in the specific cancer setting. Phase II studies act as a screen of antitumor efficacy to select the most promising agents to enter the pivotal phase III clinical trials. The demonstration of statistically significant improvement in tumor response in large phase III clinical studies against the currently best-available treatment in a tumor type-specific patient population is the ultimate benchmark for regulatory approval and marketing of a novel anticancer agent.

Phase III cancer clinical trials are usually conducted by certain cooperative groups that were founded in the 1960s and later years and include several member institutions participating in a multitude of trials that are actively ongoing at any given time [99]. Examples of these groups include the Children's

Oncology Group, the Eastern Cooperative Oncology Group, and the Cancer and Leukemia Group B [100–102]. Several of these groups are associated with academic institutions. A phase III cancer clinical trial, therefore, is a complex interaction among the cooperative groups involved, their associated academic institutions, the commercial sponsors, and the regulatory agencies.

There are certain key elements of any clinical trial that are incorporated in the study protocol. These include a clear definition of the objectives, end points, inclusion and exclusion criteria for the selection of patient volunteers (study population), treatment plan, clinical assessments, laboratory tests, trial design (including randomization), statistical considerations, data monitoring protocols, and informed consent. Conduct of cancer clinical trials adds unique perspectives and limitations on several of these elements. For example, blinding is often not utilized. This is because of distinct dosing schedules, routes of administration, and toxicity profiles that makes blinding difficult [99]. In addition, often non-inferiority trials are conducted with the goal to prove that the therapeutic benefit of a drug is not lost with a new regimen or treatment approach, such as drug combination or change in the route of administration.

3.4.8 Trial Design

Phase II clinical cancer trials are traditionally designed as single-arm trials utilizing historical controls on the currently best-available treatment, while phase III studies usually use a parallel-arm design. These designs are in contrast to the preference for crossover randomized designs for both phase II and phase III studies in other drug classes. Crossover designs are not preferred for cancer clinical trials to avoid carryover of the treatment effect of the first trial period into the second. The end points used in the cancer clinical trials require that the patients be in the similar overall clinical state at the beginning of both treatment periods. For example, the end point of survival benefit cannot be used in a crossover design. Also, patient tolerance to toxicities may change for the second treatment cycle in the crossover design [99].

Single-arm designs for phase II clinical trials use the proportion of patients who achieve a complete or partial response to the treatment as the primary efficacy measure. This design eliminates truly ineffective therapy and is based on the 'historical control' that only a limited number of tested drugs had any activity [103]. Although this design has served well for cytotoxic drugs, recent high attrition rates in phase III oncology trials has led to its criticism for inability to predict comparative performance vis-à-vis the then-available best-possible, standard-of-care therapeutic option. Furthermore, the molecularly targeted agents, e.g., gefitinib, bevacizumab, and cituximab, may not achieve consistent, high-level tumor regression. These aspects have prompted the consideration of randomized, parallel-arm designs controls and alternative end points [104].

3.4.9 End Points of Cancer Clinical Trials

End point for determining the efficacy in clinical trials of anticancer drugs is an evolving subject. Phase III cancer clinical trials focus on one primary end point to provide evidence of clinical efficacy and one or more secondary end points to delineate biological activity or benefits to the patient, e.g., reduced side effects. Three kinds of end points have been used: (1) objective tumor response, e.g., size regression; (2) time to event end points; and (3) patient-reported outcomes, e.g., palliation of side effects [99].

Tumor regression as an end point is quantified by unidimensional or bidimensional measurement of the size of lesions by clinical examination or imaging-based methods, such as X-ray, computer tomography (CT) and magnetic resonance imaging (MRI) scans, ultrasound, endoscopy, and laparoscopy. The determination of overall tumor response (as complete response, partial response, stable disease, or progressive disease) is based on the observed responses in target and non-target lesions and the appearance of new lesions after treatment [105]. This approach is limited in its inability to account for stable disease and minor response, which could be the only observable direct tumor responses for molecularly targeted agents. In addition, it requires the consideration of inherent variations in biological responses, subjectivity in measurement, and measurement techniques.

Time to event end points measure either of the following [99]:

- Overall survival (OS) is defined as the time from randomization to time of death from any cause. It is often considered an optimal efficacy end point for phase III cancer clinical trials.
- Disease-free survival (DFS) is defined as the time from randomization to disease recurrence or death owing to disease progression. It is frequently used as a primary end point in phase III trials.
- Time to progression (TTP) is defined as the time from randomization to time of progressive disease or death.
- Time to treatment failure (TTF) is defined as the time from randomization to documentation of progressive disease, death, patient discontinuation of study.
- Progression free survival (PFS) is defined as the time from randomization to objective tumor progression or death. It is a preferred regulatory end point since it includes death and may correlate better with overall survival [106].

These studies increasingly also include the quality of life analyses to determine whether the improvements in PFS or survival outweigh the disadvantages of toxicity and inconvenience [107]. The development of newer molecularly targeted anticancer agents is further influencing the paradigms of anticancer efficacy evaluation [8]. Determination of clinical end points for these drugs could be based on the quantifiable pharmacodynamic characteristics such as the target inhibition or the levels of a tumor-specific biochemical marker in the plasma. The use of target markers for determining drug response is exemplified by the measurement of farnesyltransferase activity in buccal scrapings for farnesyltransferase inhibitors [108] and plasma vascular endothelial growth factor (VEGF) concentration for the angiogenesis inhibitor anti-VEGF receptor-2 monoclonal antibody [109]. The use of this strategy, however, requires marker validation and correlation with anticancer response, which is not trivial. For example, while a biologically effective dose of marimastat was defined based on tumor marker levels in plasma in phase I–II clinical studies, the phase III studies did not show substantial benefit [8].

4 Potentials and Practices in Anticancer Drug Delivery

Initial screening of drug candidates in cell culture and animal toxicology studies is usually carried out in the solution form utilizing relatively small quantities. Early stage drug development requires physicochemical characterization of the drug candidate for its solubility and stability characteristics in addition to the chemistry, i.e., proof of structure and control of impurities during synthesis. This stage involves the development of stability indicating analytical methods for the assay of potency and impurity content, and the selection of a solvate or hydrate and the crystal form of the compound. As a compound is funneled down to successively higher stages of drug development, the compound is synthesized in larger quantities with much higher purity and a parallel formulation development effort is undertaken to prepare a dosage form for clinical testing.

Although formulation development of anticancer drugs follows the same precepts as for any drug candidate, special considerations are applicable to the formulation of anticancer compounds for early clinical screening. Formulation choices for anticancer drugs depend upon the physicochemical and biopharmaceutical properties of the drug candidate, its intended dose and route of administration, and the patient and disease factors. An important paradigm for anticancer drug delivery is the preference of the intravenous (IV) route of administration, especially for cytotoxic compounds. The IV route is preferred to avoid any bioavailability issues and problems with oral administration, especially since nausea and vomiting are common side effects of most cytotoxic agents. This also allows accurate dosing, flexibility of dose and dosing schedule, and rapid withdrawal of the drug if undue toxicity is observed. Another important consideration is to minimize the possibility of compromising the therapeutic efficacy of the drug. Thus, preservatives are avoided and excipients are minimized to reduce the possibilities of potential incompatibilities, such as physical adsorption or chemical complexation.

A historical review of formulations most commonly used for anticancer drug delivery indicates that parenteral, especially IV, injection is the first choice, followed by oral tablets or capsules, with only a handful of formulations appearing as gel, implant, or aerosol [110]. Some examples of parenteral formulations and the basis of their selection are included in Table 1 [111].

Table 1 Examples of parenteral formulations of cytotoxic anticancer agents

S. No.	Example of drug	Formulation details	Remarks
Simple aqueous solutions for drugs with high solubility and stability in water			
1	Tetraplatin	Solution in normal saline	Platinum analog
2	CHIP, *cis*-dichloro, *trans*-dihydroxybis-iso-propylamine platinum IV	Solution in normal saline	Platinum analog
3	Topotecan	5 mg/mL base solution in 0.1 M gluconate buffer at pH 3.0	Topoisomerase I inhibitor. Acidic pH of the solution prevents hydrolysis of the lactone ring
Solubility improvement using cosolvent and surfactant			
1	Etoposide (Vepesid®)	Drug formulated with polysorbate 80, PEG 300, and ethanol along with benzyl alcohol as preservative and citric acid for pH adjustment	Large doses of IV ethanol can cause phlebitis. The amount of ethanol that can be administered per hour depends on its rate of metabolism, which is up to 10 g/h
2	Teniposide (Vumon®)	Drug formulation contains N,N-dimethylacetamide, Cremophor EL, and ethanol for solubilization in addition to maleic acid for pH adjustment	High dose teniposide could lead to ethanol intoxication and toxicity due to Cremophor EL
3	Paclitaxel (Taxol®)	Solution in 1:1 mixture of Cremophor EL and ethanol.	IV Cremophor EL can cause hypersensitivity reactions
4	Carzelesin Adozelesin Bizelesin	Uses PEG 400, ethanol, and Tween 80 for solubilization	Must be diluted in the IV infusion fluid before administration
Solubility improvement using cosolvents			
1	Busulfan	Aqueous solutions of 40% PEG 400 in normal saline	
2	2-Amino-5-bromo-6-phenyl-4(3)-pyrimidone (ABPP)	Aqueous solution in sodium carbonate buffer containing N,N-dimethylacetamide (DMA)	

Table 1 (continued)

S. No.	Example of drug	Formulation details	Remarks
3	2-Chloro-2',3'-dideoxyadenosine (2-CIDDA)	Phosphate-buffered solution containing 60% propylene glycol and 10% ethanol	Propylene glycol is hemolytic in vitro and should be administered at less than 40% concentration
4	Melphalan	Aqueous solution containing 60% propylene glycol and 5% ethanol	It is diluted with normal saline before administration
Complexation to improve aqueous solubility and stability			
1	N-nitrosourea-based anticancer agents	Form complex with Tris buffer (Tris(hydroxyethyl)amino ethane)	Rate of degradation of drug in the complex is slower than free drug
2	5-Fluorouracil	Formulated in Tris buffer	Cardiotoxicity observed upon IV administration. Attributed to the presence of adducts of two degradation products of the drug with Tris
3	Erbuzole Benzaldehyde	Complexation with cyclodextrins	
Hydrotropic solubilizing agents			
1	Etoposide	Formulated in sodium salicylate solution. Planar orientation of both the drug and the salicylate salt tend to improve solubility in aqueous solution	
2	Doxorubicin Epirubicin	Use parabens in the lyophilized formulation	Drug has a tendency to form dimeric and polymeric self-aggregates, increasing the time required to dissolve the lyophilized vial. Incorporating parabens facilitates drug-paraben complexation, reduces drug self-aggregation, and facilitates rapid dissolution of the drug

Table 1 (continued)

S. No.	Example of drug	Formulation details	Remarks
Liposomes for improving PK profile, drug activity, and drug targeting			
1	Doxorubicin	Commercially available as a stable, lyophilized liposomal formulation	IV administered liposomes concentrate in fenestrated capillaries such as liver, spleen, and the bone marrow. IV doxorubicin liposomes have been shown to reduce its cardiotoxicity
2	Camptothecin (CPT) 9-Amino CPT (9-ACPT)	Formulated as liposomes of cholesterol, phosphatidyl serine (PS), and phosphatidyl choline (PC)	Freebase of CPT has ~10-fold higher activity than the sodium salt. Therefore, formulation in liposomes provided higher activity
3	Tin protoporphyrin (SnPP)	Formulated as liposomes	IV administration increased drug accumulation in spleen due to its high concentration of reticuloendothelial cells
Microencapsulation for improving toxicity profile, controlled release			
1	Merbarone	Microdispersion of nanoparticles at neutra pH	IV administration of the N-methyl glucamine salt solution at pH 10 caused injection site vasculitis, which was overcome with the nanoparticle formulation
2	Methotrexate	Methotrexate was conjugated with gelatin and incorporated in gelatin microspheres	Reduced renal toxicity compared to the free drug
Parenteral emulsion formulations for improvement in solubility, stability, local irritation or toxicity, and/or compatibility issues			
1	Hexamethyl melamine (HMM)	Ethanol or DMA-solubilized drug to be diluted in Intralipid parenteral emulsion before administration	Overcomes drug solubility problems
2	Perrilla ketone	Drug formulated in propylene glycol, ethanol, and water; to be diluted in a parenteral emulsion before IV administration.	IV administration in 5% dextrose led to loss of 20–60% drug by adsorption to the polyvinylchloride (PVC) of the infusion tubing. This problem was overcome in IV emulsion formulation

Table 1 (continued)

S. No.	Example of drug	Formulation details	Remarks
Lipoproteins for tumor targeting			
1	Prednimustine	Drug microemulsion complexed with the apo **B** receptor of the low-density lipoprotein (LDL) particle.	Its cytotoxic activity against breast cancer cells was higher than the free drug. This was attributed to the upregulation of LDL receptors on tumor cells
2	Vincristine	LDL-associated vincristine compared with free drug.	Reduced neurotoxicity with the LDL formulation
Prodrug approaches to increase drug activity and aqueous solubility			
1	1-β-D-arabinofuranosylcytosine (ara-C)	Lipophilic prodrug prepared by conjugation with phosphatidic acid	Significant increase in the life span of mice with L1210 and P388 leukemia
2	Chlorambucil	Drug conjugation to α, β-poly(N-hydroxyethyl-DL-aspartamide) by ester linkage.	Increased water solubility
Lyophilization to improve drug stability			
1	Bryostatin I	Bryostatin lyophilized from butanolic solution with povidone; to be dissolved in PEG 400, ethanol, and Tween 80 mixture (PET diluent) followed by dilution in normal saline immediately before administration	Improved drug solubility with reduced requirement of cosolvents for administration and improved shelf-life of the lyophilized formulation
2	Tumor necrosis factor-α (TNF-α)	Lyophilized solution with mannitol and the sugar based amorphous protectant dextran, sucrose, or cyclodextrin in citrate buffer	Stabilization of solution from tendency for dimeric and polymeric self-aggregation, leading to the formation of particulates in solution

One of the blessings of having anticancer drugs in the pipeline is the fact that these drugs allow the exploration of sophisticated and unconventional formulation approaches due to their urgent need in the clinic and the special circumstances of the care of cancer patients. For example, the water-insoluble and unstable nitrogen mustard, carmustine, is supplied in lyophilized vials with sterile drug. Separately, vials with sterile, dried ethanol and sterile water for injection are provided. At the time of use, the drug is dissolved in ethanol and further diluted with water before injection. Another example of a water-insoluble and water-unstable drug administered unconventionally is spiromustine. It is supplied as a lyophilized drug in vials, which is first dissolved in sterile ethanol and then dispersed in a sterile emulsion for intravenous administration. Commercially available IV nutrition emulsions, such as those of soybean oil, e.g., Intralipid®, or safflower oil, e.g., Liposyn®, are used for this purpose.

The investigational drug carzelesin offers another example of the unique drug delivery possibilities with anticancer therapeutics. Carzelesin is highly insoluble and is available as a solution in polyethylene glycol 400, ethanol, and polysorbate 80 for dilution in the IV infusion fluid immediately before administration. However, due to its tendency for rapid crystallization, it is administered to patients with a two-pump infusion system such that the drug solution and the infusion solution come in contact with each other for a very brief period before entering the bloodstream.

The use of unconventional drug delivery systems often presents unique drug development challenges. For example, paclitaxel is formulated in a 1:1 mixture with the surfactant cremophor and ethanol (Taxol®). Intravenous administration of this agent resulted in local toxicity and systemic hypersensitivity reactions when the drug was infused over a 3 hour period [112]. This resulted in prolongation of the infusion rate of taxol to 6 hours or longer [113]. Further clinical studies to define the appropriate rate and amount of drug administration to minimize systemic toxicity resulted in a clinical protocol that identified a low-dose, low-duration (135–175 mg/m^2 infused in less than 6 hours) administration regimen with superior hematologic toxicity and neurotoxicity profile than a similar or higher dose, longer duration (170 mg/m^2 or more infused over 24 hours) administration [114]. Thus, sophisticated formulations can potentially lead to toxicity to the patients, resulting in increased clinical testing, delays, and possibly the drug development program.

A significant requirement of anticancer drug development is the extraordinarily high amount of safety precautions necessary in the handling of these drug substances from the first discovery stages through commercial production. These safety precautions often slow down the pace of drug development and necessitate infrastructural investments to explore technologies that minimize potential exposure and hazard to the employees. Pharmaceutical companies actively engaged in anticancer drug development commonly have special containment areas and ventilation hoods for the handling of these substances. An example of investment in technologies for employee safety reasons is the adoption of single-pot processors for wet granulation, which enables granulation followed by drying in the same mixer [115]. Several of these equipments are now commercially available [116].

Increasingly, oral drug formulations of anticancer agents are being developed. The incentives for oral drug formulation of anticancer agents include improved safety, efficacy, quality of life, reduced cost, and the ability to deliver chemotherapy at home and to apply drug schedules that maximize an agent's efficacy [117]. The development of oral drug formulations is constrained by restrictions in dose size, bioavailability concerns, and patient compliance – especially for drugs that cause nausea and vomiting. The preference for oral route of administration is reflected in the increasing number of drugs being formulated as tablets or capsules. Examples of anticancer compounds that have been marketed as oral solid dosage forms include anastrozole, dasatinib, gefitinib, tamoxifen, mercaptopurine, 6-mercaptopurine, estramustine, cyclophosphamide, levamisole, toremifene, letrozole, capecitabine, and exemestane [110].

5 Regulatory Considerations

Anticancer drug development brings forth unique perspectives and their regulation has evolved to accommodate and address those unique aspects. One key driving force for anticancer drugs is the urgent patient need for the development of new agents and the need to rapidly move the promising agents into clinical trials. Another is the recognition that these agents are dosed to toxic levels, close to the maximum tolerated dose, MTD, with the precept that the side effects of drug therapy would be less threatening to the patient than their disease. Control of clinical toxicity is sought by careful dosing, monitoring, and prompt treatment of toxicity, or drug withdrawal.

The regulatory requirements for anticancer compounds focus on drug safety evaluation in preclinical toxicology studies, based on the intended use and mechanism of action of the drug, and the target patient population. As DeGeorge et al. point out, in situations where the potential benefits of therapy are the greatest, e.g., advanced, life-threatening disease, the greater risks of treatment toxicity can be accepted and the requirements for preclinical testing can be minimal [118]. Nevertheless, in cases where the patient population is free of known disease, e.g., adjuvant therapy, chemoprevention, or healthy volunteers, the acceptable risks are much less and preclinical evaluation is more extensive.

As discussed before, two acute preclinical toxicity studies are required. The first is in a rodent species to identify doses that result in lethality or life-threatening toxicities to derive the clinical phase I entry dose. The second study is conducted in a non-rodent species to confirm that the selected dose is not lethal and does not cause serious or irreversible toxicity. It is highly desirable that these preclinical toxicology studies be conducted with the same schedule, duration, formulation, and route of administration of the drug as proposed in the clinical trials. The requirements for preclinical studies depend upon the nature of the drug being developed.

Cytotoxic anticancer agents are administered in short-term phases and thus need acute preclinical toxicity studies (generally, less than 28 days). On the other hand, non-cytotoxic agents, such as immunomodulators or hormonal drugs, are intended for long-term use with continuous daily administration. Thus, the preclinical toxicology study requirements for non-cytotoxic drugs are equivalent to the duration of intended therapeutic use in patients, up to 6 months in rodent and 12 months in a non-rodent species. In addition, genotoxicity, carcinogenicity, and reproductive toxicity studies are required for the new drug application (NDA) submission. Special toxicity studies may be needed in cases where compound or drug-class-specific toxicities are known. For example, anthracyclines are known for their cardiotoxic potential and platinum-based drugs are likely to exhibit ototoxicity [119]. The dosing of non-cytotoxic agents, such as immunomodulators, is aimed to a pharmacodynamically active range, usually much lower than the MTD.

In addition, pharmacokinetic and pharmacodynamic studies are recommended to support the safety profile of the drug, which may help in deciding the starting dose, route, schedule, the dose escalation steps, and optimum plasma concentrations for the phase I clinical trials. Combinations of cytotoxic agents generally do not need preclinical toxicology testing if the agents have individually been used in humans and have an established safety profile, unless there is a reason to believe there could be synergistic interactions that might lead to increased toxicity [118].

Preclinical toxicological evaluation of non-cytotoxic agents depends on the kind of agents and therapeutic options being investigated. For example, photosensitizers require special testing protocols because of their unique modes of action and toxicity. Photosensitizers form free radicals upon absorption of light energy, which are then responsible for site-specific tumor destruction. Exposure of the patients to sunlight could cause retinal damage or phototoxicity similar to sunburn [120]. Therefore, toxicological evaluation of photosensitizers involves photosensitivity assessment as a function of the dose of light (total energy of irradiant light) in relation to that of the drug, and the correlation of photosensitivity to the plasma levels of the photosensitizer. Also, knowledge of the elimination half-life of the compound may be used to determine the duration of time a patient needs to take precautions against exposure to intense light.

Regulatory preclinical testing requirements for specialized drug delivery systems such as antibody-drug conjugates, liposomes, and depot formulations include the proof-of-concept studies that the claimed advantage of these systems is indeed being derived without additional toxicity burden. For example, safety concerns for antibody-drug conjugates include the potential for toxicity from abrupt release of the drug and the potential for unexpected specific toxicity in normal human tissues [118]. Thus, in addition to the standard toxicity testing, investigations of the stability of the conjugate as a function of the release mechanism and the reactivity of the conjugate with a complete panel of human tissues (with and without the target antigen expression) are recommended. In addition, pharmacokinetic studies that distinguish between the conjugate, free antibody, and the free drug are desirable [118].

Toxicology studies for hormonal drugs, e.g., antiestrogens, antiprogestins, antiandrogens, aromatase inhibitors, and gonadotropin releasing hormone agonists, are recommended using the same route, formulation, schedule, and duration of treatment. In addition, preclinical evaluation of both sexes is recommended, even though these drugs are usually prescribed for sex-specific indications, to delineate the toxicities unrelated to the primary hormonal action of the drug. In addition, genotoxicity, reproductive toxicity, and carcinogenicity studies are indicated [118].

Agents that target the multi-drug resistance (MDR) of the tumors to anti cancer drugs may lead to increased toxicity of the combination. Thus, preclinical toxicity evaluation of new MDR-reversing agents is recommended in combination with the cytotoxic drug at both minimally and significantly toxic doses, in addition to the toxicological evaluation of the agent alone. Similar approach is applied for chemotherapy sensitizers [118]. In brief, the preclinical toxicology evaluations of novel agents are based on the mechanism of action and the potential additional toxicities that may emanate from the modalities of drug administration.

6 Conclusions

The clinical application of anticancer drugs brings forth unique perspectives that are evident in their discovery and development. Historical development of cytotoxic compounds, with significant contributions from serendipity, and the currently shifting focus on target-based drug discovery is evident in the evolving paradigms of preclinical and clinical evaluation of new drug candidates. Current challenges of anticancer drug development include the significant time and cost involvement, and the low success rates. These have led to increasing efforts of the pharmaceutical industry toward increasing the effectiveness of the drug discovery and development process and to minimize failure of drug candidates at later stages of development. These efforts include development of high throughput preclinical screening methods and biological assays with greater specificity and predictability. Increasing emphasis is being placed on developing a mechanistic understanding of the physicochemical and biological phenomena involved in drug development such as chemical and polymorph stability, and pharmacokinetics. The use of mathematical models to explain the mechanisms of drug degradation and predict the outcomes of formulation and process changes and scale-up is increasingly being adopted. The paradigm of continuous improvement is now incorporating a risk-based approach, where the risk to the patient is continuously evaluated through the course of drug development. The level of risk is mitigated or minimized by appropriate measures. The critical product quality attributes (CQAs) are defined and a design space is created around all the formulation and process variables with demonstrated, reproducible achievement of the product CQAs.

This chapter has attempted to highlight the unique aspects of anticancer drugs from a pharmaceutical development viewpoint, some of which are highlighted in Table 2. The evolving paradigms of anticancer drug development demonstrate the increasing influence of scientific advancements in diverse fields and increased understanding of the disease process. These trends are expected to continue with the hope for more effective and less toxic therapeutic options.

Table 2 Blessings and liabilities of anticancer drugs in the pipeline from a pharmaceutical development viewpoint

Development aspect	Blessings	Liabilities
Drug discovery	Well-established objective screens for cytotoxic drug evaluation in both cell cultures and animal models are available	Animal and cell culture models for drug discovery screening are not representative of all tumor types and are constantly evolving
Material handling during the lifecycle of the product		Extraordinarily high safety precautions for the protection of the employees, patients, and the general population
		Cost of the active pharmaceutical ingredient (API) is usually high
		Availability of the API for development use is usually very limited
Pharmaceutical development	Sophisticated and unusual formulation choices can be made depending on the potential of the drug candidate and the disease condition	Most cytotoxic agents have low solubility, dissolution rate, stability, and bioavailability
	Most cytotoxic compounds are formulated as IV parenterals, thus obviating bioavailability issues	Usually the amount of material available for development use is very limited and the development timelines accelerated for promising candidates
		Safety considerations require specialized manufacturing processes and facilities to be used
Clinical trials	Patient willingness to participate in the clinical trials may be higher depending upon the severity of the disease condition and availability of alternative therapies	For cytotoxic compounds, clinical trials usually need to be done in patients rather than healthy volunteers
		This increases the cost and time involved in clinical testing

Table 2 (continued)

Development aspect	Blessings	Liabilities
	Potential for making the greatest contribution to the most needy patients. These drugs help 'extend and enhance human life' (Bristol-Myers Squibb, Co.'s mission statement, http://www.bms.com).	Safety of the clinical trial participants is a significant concern for cytotoxic compounds since toxicity and efficacy are usually closely dose related
Regulatory considerations	Relatively rapid regulatory review times because of the urgent need of these therapies for the patients Regulatory tolerance of the side effects of cytotoxic agents depending upon indication and the current patient need for the drug	Higher regulatory proof-of-concept and preclinical toxicology requirements, especially for target-based anticancer agents and specialized drug delivery systems
Patient and marketing considerations		The drug development programs are expensive and the drugs have high costs to the patient, often with marginal benefit over pre-existing drugs in terms of extending human life and/or improving the quality of life

References

1. Schwartsmann G, Winograd B, Pinedo HM. The main steps in the development of anticancer agents. *Radiother Oncol* 1988; **12**: 301–313.
2. Farber S et al. Temporary remissions in acute leukemia in children produced by folic acid antagonist, 4-aminopteroylglutamic acid (aminopterin). *N Engl J Med* 1948; **238**: 787–793.
3. Osborn MJ, Freeman M, Huennekens FM. Inhibition of dihydrofolic reductase by aminopterin and amethopterin. *Proc Soc Exp Biol Med* 1958; **97**: 429–431.
4. Osborn MJ, Huennekens FM. Enzymatic reduction of dihydrofolic acid. *J Biol Chem* 1958; **233**: 969–974.
5. Goodman LS et al. Landmark article Sept. 21, 1946: Nitrogen mustard therapy. Use of methyl-bis(beta-chloroethyl)amine hydrochloride and tris(beta-chloroethyl)amine hydrochloride for Hodgkin's disease, lymphosarcoma, leukemia and certain allied and miscellaneous disorders. By Louis S. Goodman, Maxwell M. Wintrobe, William Dameshek, Morton J. Goodman, Alfred Gilman and Margaret T. McLennan. *JAMA* 1984; **251**: 2255–2261.
6. Institute, National Cancer. Targeted Cancer Therapies, 2008. http://www.cancer.gov/cancertopics/factsheet/Therapy/targeted.
7. McKeage MJ. The potential of DMXAA (ASA404) in combination with docetaxel in advanced prostate cancer. *Expert Opin Investig Drugs* 2008; **17**: 23–29.
8. Hoekstra R, Verweij J, Eskens FA. Clinical trial design for target specific anticancer agents. *Invest New Drugs* 2003; **21**: 243–250.
9. Chabner BA, Roberts TG Jr. Timeline: Chemotherapy and the war on cancer. *Nat Rev Cancer* 2005; **5**: 65–72.

10. Saijo N, Tamura T, Nishio K. Strategy for the development of novel anticancer drugs. *Cancer Chemother Pharmacol* 2003; **52 Suppl 1**: S97–S101.
11. Van Schaik RH. Cancer treatment and pharmacogenetics of cytochrome P450 enzymes. *Invest New Drugs* 2005; **23**: 513–522.
12. Yong WP, Innocenti F, Ratain MJ. The role of pharmacogenetics in cancer therapeutics. *Br J Clin Pharmacol* 2006; **62**: 35–46.
13. Claudino WM et al. Metabolomics: available results, current research projects in breast cancer, and future applications. *J Clin Oncol* 2007; **25**: 2840–2846.
14. Serkova NJ, Spratlin JL, Eckhardt SG. NMR-based metabolomics: translational application and treatment of cancer. *Curr Opin Mol Ther* 2007; **9**: 572–585.
15. Kim YS, Maruvada P. Frontiers in metabolomics for cancer research: Proceedings of a National Cancer Institute workshop. *Metabolomics* 2008; **4**: 105–113.
16. Chung YL et al. Magnetic resonance spectroscopic pharmacodynamic markers of the heat shock protein 90 inhibitor 17-allylamino,17-demethoxygeldanamycin (17AAG) in human colon cancer models. *J Natl Cancer Inst* 2003; **95**: 1624–1633.
17. Roberts TG Jr, Chabner BA. Beyond fast track for drug approvals. *N Engl J Med* 2004; **351**: 501–505.
18. Paez JG et al. EGFR mutations in lung cancer: Correlation with clinical response to gefitinib therapy. *Science* 2004; **304**: 1497–1500.
19. Berinstein NL. Enhancing cancer vaccines with immunomodulators. *Vaccine* 2007; **25 Suppl 2**: B72–B88.
20. Finke LH et al. Lessons from randomized phase III studies with active cancer immunotherapies – outcomes from the 2006 meeting of the Cancer Vaccine Consortium (CVC). *Vaccine* 2007; **25 Suppl 2**: B97–B109.
21. Ji BS, He L, Liu GQ. Reversal of p-glycoprotein-mediated multidrug resistance by CJX1, an amlodipine derivative, in doxorubicin-resistant human myelogenous leukemia (K562/DOX) cells. *Life Sci* 2005; **77**: 2221–2232.
22. Ross DD. Modulation of drug resistance transporters as a strategy for treating myelodysplastic syndrome. *Best Pract Res Clin Haematol* 2004; **17**: 641–651.
23. Skinner R, Sharkey IM, Pearson AD, Craft AW. Ifosfamide, mesna, and nephrotoxicity in children. *J Clin Oncol* 1993; **11**: 173–190.
24. Kouvaris JR, Kouloulias VE, Vlahos LJ. Amifostine: the first selective-target and broad-spectrum radioprotector. *Oncologist* 2007; **12**: 738–747.
25. Wainwright M. Photodynamic therapy: the development of new photosensitisers. *Anti-Cancer Agents Med Chem* 2008; **8**: 280–291.
26. Lieschke GJ, Burgess AW. Granulocyte colony-stimulating factor and granulocyte-macrophage colony-stimulating factor. *New Engl J Med* 1992; **327**: 28–35.
27. Lieschke GJ, Burgess AW. Granulocyte colony-stimulating factor and granulocyte-macrophage colony-stimulating factor (2). *New Engl J Med* 1992; **327**: 99–106.
28. Houston D. Supportive therapies for cancer chemotherapy patients and the role of the oncology nurse. *Cancer Nurs* 1997; **20**: 409–413.
29. Wikipedia. History of Cancer Chemotherapy, 2008. http://en.wikipedia.org/wiki/History_of_cancer_chemotherapy.
30. Foundation, The Chemical Heritage. Magic Bullets: Chemistry Vs. Cancer, 2008. http://www.chemheritage.org/EducationalServices/pharm/chemo/readings/ages.htm.
31. Beaston G. On the treatment of inoperable cases of carcinoma of the mamma: Suggestions for a new method of treatment, with illustrative cases. *Lancet* 1896; **2**: 104–107.
32. Huggins C, Clark PJ. Quantitative studies of prostatic secretions. II. The effect of castration and of estrogen injection on the normal and on the hyperplastic prostate glands of dogs. *J Exp Med* 1940; **72**: 747–762.
33. Rosenberg B, Vancamp L, Krigas T. Inhibition of cell division in Escherichia Coli by electrolysis products from a platinum electrode. *Nature* 1965; **205**: 698–699.

34. Rosenberg B. Biological effects of platinum compounds. New agents for the control of tumors. *Platinum Metals Rev* 1971; **15**: 42–51.

35. Mans DRA, Jung FA, Schwartsmann G. Anticancer drug discovery and development. *J Brazilian Assoc Advancement Sci* 1994; **46**: 70–81.

36. Suggitt M, Bibby MC. 50 years of preclinical anticancer drug screening: Empirical to target-driven approaches. *Clin Cancer Res* 2005; **11**: 971–981.

37. Amundson SA et al. Integrating global gene expression and radiation survival parameters across the 60 cell lines of the National Cancer Institute Anticancer Drug Screen. *Cancer Res* 2008; **68**: 415–424.

38. Covell DG, Huang R, Wallqvist A. Anticancer medicines in development: assessment of bioactivity profiles within the National Cancer Institute anticancer screening data. *Mol Cancer Ther* 2007; **6**: 2261–2270.

39. Takimoto CH. Anticancer drug development at the US National Cancer Institute. *Cancer Chemother Pharmacol* 2003; **52 Suppl 1**: S29–S33.

40. Frei E 3rd. The National Cancer Chemotherapy Program. *Science* 1982; **217**: 600–606.

41. Venditti JM. The National Cancer Institute antitumor drug discovery program, current and future perspectives: A commentary. *Cancer Treat Rep* 1983; **67**: 767–772.

42. Venditti JM. Preclinical drug development: Rationale and methods. *Semin Oncol* 1981; **8**: 349–361.

43. Zubrod CG. Origins and development of chemotherapy research at the National Cancer Institute. *Cancer Treat Rep* 1984; **68**: 9–19.

44. Shoemaker RH et al. Development of human tumor cell line panels for use in disease-oriented drug screening. *Prog Clin Biol Res* 1988; **276**: 265–286.

45. National Cancer Institute NIoH. Developmental Therapeutics Program, 2008.

46. Talmadge JE, Singh RK, Fidler IJ, Raz A. Murine models to evaluate novel and conventional therapeutic strategies for cancer. *Am J Pathol* 2007; **170**: 793 804.

47. Kohlhagen G et al. Protein-linked DNA strand breaks induced by NSC 314622, a novel noncamptothecin topoisomerase I poison. *Mol Pharmacol* 1998; **54**: 50–58.

48. Shoemaker RH. The NCI60 human tumour cell line anticancer drug screen. *Nat Rev Cancer* 2006; **6**: 813–823.

49. Decoster G, Stein G, Holdener EE. Responses and toxic deaths in phase I clinical trials. *Ann Oncol* 1990; **1**: 175–181.

50. Grunwald HW. Ethical and design issues of phase I clinical trials in cancer patients. *Cancer Invest* 2007; **25**: 124–126.

51. Grieshaber CK, Marsoni S. Relation of preclinical toxicology to findings in early clinical trials. *Cancer Treat Rep* 1986; **70**: 65–72.

52. Newell DR. Phase I clinical studies with cytotoxic drugs: Pharmacokinetic and pharmacodynamic considerations. *Br J Cancer* 1990; **61**: 189–191.

53. Zaharko DS, Grieshaber CK, Plowman J, Cradock JC. Therapeutic and pharmacokinetic relationships of flavone acetic acid: an agent with activity against solid tumors. *Cancer Treat Rep* 1986; **70**: 1415–1421.

54. Eisenhauer EA, O'Dwyer PJ, Christian M, Humphrey JS. Phase I clinical trial design in cancer drug development. *J Clin Oncol* 2000; **18**: 684–692.

55. Omura GA. Modified Fibonacci search. *J Clin Oncol* 2003; **21**: 3177.

56. Collins JM, Grieshaber CK, Chabner BA. Pharmacologically guided phase I clinical trials based upon preclinical drug development. *J Natl Cancer Inst* 1990; **82**: 1321–1326.

57. Fuse E et al. Application of pharmacokinetically guided dose escalation with respect to cell cycle phase specificity. *J Natl Cancer Inst* 1994; **86**: 989–996.

58. Chatelut E et al. Prediction of carboplatin clearance from standard morphological and biological patient characteristics. *J Natl Cancer Inst* 1995; **87**: 573–580.

59. O'Reilly S et al. Phase I and pharmacologic studies of topotecan in patients with impaired hepatic function. *J Natl Cancer Inst* 1996; **88**: 817–824.

60. Lennard L. The clinical pharmacology of 6-mercaptopurine. *Eur J Clin Pharmacol* 1992; **43**: 329–339.
61. Canal P, Chatelut E, Guichard S. Practical treatment guide for dose individualisation in cancer chemotherapy. *Drugs* 1998; **56**: 1019–1038.
62. Hempel G, Boos J. Flat-fixed dosing versus body surface area based dosing of anticancer drugs: there is a difference. *Oncologist* 2007; **12**: 924–926.
63. Pinkel D. The use of body surface area as a criterion of drug dosage in cancer chemotherapy. *Cancer Res* 1958; **18**: 853–856.
64. Freireich EJ et al. Quantitative comparison of toxicity of anticancer agents in mouse, rat, hamster, dog, monkey, and man. *Cancer Chemother Rep* 1966; **50**: 219–244.
65. Baker SD et al. Role of body surface area in dosing of investigational anticancer agents in adults, 1991–2001. *J Natl Cancer Inst* 2002; **94**: 1883–1888.
66. Grochow LB, Baraldi C, Noe D. Is dose normalization to weight or body surface area useful in adults? *J Natl Cancer Inst* 1990; **82**: 323–325.
67. Gurney H. Dose calculation of anticancer drugs: A review of the current practice and introduction of an alternative. *J Clin Oncol* 1996; **14**: 2590–2611.
68. Gurney HP, Ackland S, Gebski V, Farrell G. Factors affecting epirubicin pharmacokinetics and toxicity: evidence against using body-surface area for dose calculation. *J Clin Oncol* 1998; **16**: 2299–2304.
69. Reilly JJ, Workman P. Normalisation of anti-cancer drug dosage using body weight and surface area: is it worthwhile? A review of theoretical and practical considerations. *Cancer Chemother Pharmacol* 1993; **32**: 411–418.
70. Dooley MJ, Poole SG. Poor correlation between body surface area and glomerular filtration rate. *Cancer Chemother Pharmacol* 2000; **46**: 523–526.
71. Miller AA. Body surface area in dosing anticancer agents: Scratch the surface! *J Natl Cancer Inst* 2002; **94**: 1822–1823.
72. Marsoni S et al. Tolerance to antineoplastic agents in children and adults. *Cancer Treat Rep* 1985; **69**: 1263–1269.
73. Gelman RS et al. Actual versus ideal weight in the calculation of surface area: Effects on dose of 11 chemotherapy agents. *Cancer Treat Rep* 1987; **71**: 907–911.
74. Smorenburg CH et al. Randomized cross-over evaluation of body-surface area-based dosing versus flat-fixed dosing of paclitaxel. *J Clin Oncol* 2003; **21**: 197–202.
75. McLean MA et al. Accelerating drug development: Methodology to support first-in-man pharmacokinetic studies by the use of drug candidate microdosing. *Drug Dev Res* 2007; **68**: 14–22.
76. Garner RC. Less is more: the human microdosing concept. *Drug Discov Today* 2005; **10**: 449–451.
77. Administration, US Food and Drug. Radioactive Drugs for Certain Research, 2007. http://www.accessdata.fda.gov/scripts/cdrh/cfdocs/cfcfr/CFRSearch.cfm?fr = 361.1.
78. Administration, US Food and Drug. Guidance for Industry, Investigators, and Reviewers. Exploratory IND Studies including Human Microdose Studies, 2006. http://www.fda.gov/CDER/guidance/7086fnl.htm.
79. Agency EM. Position Paper on Non-clinical Safety Studies to Support Clinical Trials with a Single Microdose, 2004.
80. Bertino JS Jr, Greenberg HE, Reed MD. American College of Clinical Pharmacology position statement on the use of microdosing in the drug development process. *J Clin Pharmacol* 2007; **47**: 418–422.
81. Leather H, George TJ. Hematology/Oncology Handbook. The University of Florida Shands Cancer Center, 2007.
82. Goldin A. Combined chemotherapy. *Oncology* 1980; **37 Suppl 1**: 3–8.
83. Mori T et al. Prediction of cell kill kinetics of anticancer agents using the collagen gel droplet embedded-culture drug sensitivity test. *Oncol Reports* 2002; **9**: 301–305.
84. Rang HP, Dale MM, Ritter JM. Cancer Chemotherapy. In: Rang HP, Dale MM, Ritter JM (eds) *Pharmacology*. Churchill Livingstone: New York, 1995, pp. 696–700.

85. Canellos GP, Lister TA, Skarin AT. Chemotherapy of the non-Hodgkin's lymphomas. *Cancer* 1978; **42**: 932–940.
86. Klement G et al. Continuous low-dose therapy with vinblastine and VEGF receptor-2 antibody induces sustained tumor regression without overt toxicity. *J Clin Invest* 2000; **105**: R15–R24.
87. Stempak D, Seely D, Baruchel S. Metronomic dosing of chemotherapy: Applications in pediatric oncology. *Cancer Invest* 2006; **24**: 432–443.
88. Sarin J, DeRossi SS, Akintoye SO. Updates on bisphosphonates and potential pathobiology of bisphosphonate-induced jaw osteonecrosis. *Oral Dis* 2008; **14**: 277–285.
89. Sabino MAC et al. Simultaneous reduction in cancer pain, bone destruction, and tumor growth by selective inhibition of cyclooxygenase-2. *Cancer Res* 2002; **62**: 7343–7349.
90. Verso M et al. Risk factors for upper limb deep vein thrombosis associated with the use of central vein catheter in cancer patients. *Intern Emerg Med* 2008; **3**: 117–122.
91. Falanga A, Zacharski L. Deep vein thrombosis in cancer: the scale of the problem and approaches to management. *Ann Oncol* 2005; **16**: 696–701.
92. Siau C, Xiao W, Bennett GJ. Paclitaxel- and vincristine-evoked painful peripheral neuropathies: loss of epidermal innervation and activation of Langerhans cells. *Exp Neurol* 2006; **201**: 507–514.
93. Sereno M et al. Cardiac toxicity: Old and new issues in anti-cancer drugs. *Clin Transl Oncol* 2008; **10**: 35–46.
94. Schimmel KJ, Richel DJ, van den Brink RB, Guchelaar HJ. Cardiotoxicity of cytotoxic drugs. *Cancer Treat Rev* 2004; **30**: 181–191.
95. Schachter AD, Ramoni MF. Paediatric drug development. *Nat Rev Drug Discov* 2007; **6**: 429–430.
96. Schreiner MS. Pediatric clinical trials: Redressing the imbalance. *Nat Rev Drug Discov* 2003; **2**: 949–961.
97. Smith M et al. Conduct of phase I trials in children with cancer. *J Clin Oncol* 1998; **16**: 966–978.
98. Lee DP, Skolnik JM, Adamson PC. Pediatric phase I trials in oncology: An analysis of study conduct efficiency. *J Clin Oncol* 2005; **23**: 8431–8441.
99. Dagher RN, Pazdur R. The Phase III Clinical Cancer Trial. In: Teicher BA, Andrews PA (eds) *Cancer Drug Discovery and Development: Anticancer Drug Development Guide: Preclinical Screening, Clinical Trials, and Approval.* Humana Press, Inc., Totowa, NJ, 2004.
100. Cancer and Leukemia Group B. 2008. http://www.calgb.org/.
101. Children's Oncology Group. 2008. http://www.childrensoncologygroup.org/.
102. Eastern Cooperative Oncology Group. 2008. http://ecog.dfci.harvard.edu/.
103. Karrison TG, Maitland ML, Stadler WM, Ratain MJ. Design of phase II cancer trials using a continuous endpoint of change in tumor size: application to a study of sorafenib and erlotinib in non small-cell lung cancer. *J Natl Cancer Inst* 2007; **99**: 1455–1461.
104. Ratain MJ, Eckhardt SG. Phase II studies of modern drugs directed against new targets: If you are fazed, too, then resist RECIST. *J Clin Oncol* 2004; **22**: 4442–4445.
105. Therasse P et al. New guidelines to evaluate the response to treatment in solid tumors. European Organization for Research and Treatment of Cancer, National Cancer Institute of the United States, National Cancer Institute of Canada. *J Natl Cancer Inst* 2000; **92**: 205–216.
106. Pazdur R. Endpoints for assessing drug activity in clinical trials. *The oncologist* 2008; **13 Suppl 2**: 19–21.
107. Ferrans CE. Differences in what quality-of-life instruments measure. *J Natl Cancer Inst Monogr* 2007: 22–26.
108. Adjei AA et al. A Phase I trial of the farnesyl transferase inhibitor SCH66336: Evidence for biological and clinical activity. *Cancer Res* 2000; **60**: 1871–1877.

109. Bocci G et al. Increased plasma vascular endothelial growth factor (VEGF) as a surrogate marker for optimal therapeutic dosing of VEGF receptor-2 monoclonal antibodies. *Cancer Res* 2004; **64**: 6616–6625.
110. Administration, U. S. Food and Drug. Approval Statistics of Oncology Drugs, 2008. http://www.accessdata.fda.gov/scripts/cder/onctools/statistics.cfm.
111. Vries JDJ, Flora KP, Bult A, Beijnen JH. Pharmaceutical Development of (Investigational) Anticancer Agents for Parenteral Use – A Review. *Drug Dev Ind Pharm* 1996; **22**: 475–494.
112. Kris MG et al. Phase I trial of taxol given as a 3-hour infusion every 21 days. *Cancer Treatment Reports* 1986; **70**: 605–607.
113. Brown T et al. A phase I trial of taxol given by a 6-hour intravenous infusion. *J clin Oncol* 1991; **9**: 1261–1267.
114. Canetta RM, Eisenhauer E, Rozencsweig M. Methods for administration of taxol for cancer treatment with reduced toxicity. (Bristol-Myers Squibb Co., USA). Application: AU, 1994, 38 pp.
115. Cuschler G, Carius W, Bauer KH. Single-step Granulation: Development of a Vacuum-based IR Drying Method (pilot scale results). *Drug Dev Ind Pharm* 1997; **23**: 119–126.
116. Giry K et al. Multiphase versus Single Pot Granulation Process: Influence of Process and Granulation Parameters on Granule Properties. *Drug Dev Ind Pharm* 2006; **32**: 509–530.
117. Bleyer WA, Danielson MG. Oral cancer chemotherapy in paediatric patients: Obstacles and potential for development and utilisation. *Drugs* 1999; **58 Suppl 3**: 133–140.
118. DeGeorge JJ et al. Regulatory considerations for preclinical development of anticancer drugs. *Cancer Chemother Pharmacol* 1998; **41**: 173–185.
119. Peck CC et al. Opportunities for integration of pharmacokinetics, pharmacodynamics, and toxico kinetics in rational drug development. *Clin Pharmacol Ther* 1992; **51**: 465–473.
120. Dougherty TJ. Photodynamic therapy. *Photochem Photobiol* 1993; **58**: 895–900.

Tumor-Targeted Macromolecular Drug Delivery Based on the Enhanced Permeability and Retention Effect in Solid Tumor

Takahiro Seki, Jun Fang, and Hiroshi Maeda

1 Introduction

1.1 Status Quo

Cancer remains the first or second main cause of death in developed countries. In the world, 7.6 million people died of cancer in 2005 [1]. However, the cure for advanced cancer in major cancers has not improved in the past 50 years, although chemotherapy is supposed to be a last resort, if not all [2, 3]. One of the recent successful stories in cancer chemotherapy is imatinib (Gleevec®), a drug for chronic myeloid leukemia (CML) which is an inhibitor of BCR/ABL tyrosine kinase, a product of oncogene. Imatinib shows a remarkable therapeutic effect against CML while a natural course of life span of CML patients is about 5 years. However, upon blastic period when the leukemic cell growth becomes exponential, majority of patients developed drug resistance within 6 months. Therefore, one can conclude that imatinib contributes only 10% prolongation of the life span. In addition, some more fashionable molecular target drugs, such as trastuzumab (Herceptin®) which is a humanized monoclonal antibody for treatment of HER2-positive breast cancer [4] and sorafenib (Torisel™); sunitinib (Sutent®) and temsirolimus (Nexavar®) for treatment of advanced renal cell carcinoma; and bevacizumab (Avastin®) as an inhibitor of vascular endothelial cell growth factor [5], have received great attention in recent years.

H. Maeda (✉)
Laboratory of Microbiology and Oncology, Faculty of Pharmaceutical Sciences, Sojo University, Kumamoto 860-0082, Japan; BioDynamics Research Laboratory, Kumamoto University, Innovative Collaborative Organization, Cooperative Research Laboratory, Kumamoto 861-2202, Japan
e-mail: hirmaeda@ph.sojo-u.ac.jp

Y. Lu, R.I. Mahato (eds.), *Pharmaceutical Perspectives of Cancer Therapeutics*, DOI 10.1007/978-1-4419-0131-6_3, © Springer Science+Business Media, LLC 2009

1.2 Problems

However, experimental data based on cancer genomics showed that above-mentioned strategies may have only limited efficacy. Regardless of the monoclonality or polyclonality of human cancer origin, the tumor of a cancer patient has a large number of mutations in their cancer cells. In fact, it was reported that 13,023 genes of an individual tumor in 11 breast and 11 colorectal cancer patients revealed an average of about 90 mutant genes, and contained a wide range of uncommon mutant genes [6, 7]. It thus indicated potential difficulty in limiting a single epitopic target in cancer treatment. In addition, emergence of drug-resistant cancer cells during the treatment greatly hampers the efficacy of the treatment.

In consistent with the above account, clinical evaluation of these molecular target drugs or antibody drugs was found to be effective only for 4–5% of the patients, and now they were considered meaningful only as an adjuvant therapy, as many reported in the American Society of Clinical Oncology Meeting in recent years. To make it worse, the cost of manufacturing is so high, although polyethylene glycol (PEG)-conjugated interferon α (IFN-α) of MW 50 kDa can make better cost/performance benefit compared with native IFN-α. A recent report from the UK said Avastin® was rejected for reimbursement from national insurance system [8]. The only incentive of such expensive drugs is that they are financially lucrative for megasize pharmaceutical companies. In Japan large pharmaceutical companies have now shifted the gear toward anti-tumor molecular target drug development, although the social insurance system may become at risk financially, while the cost of clinical development is soaring which will be transferred to the price of the drugs. In any case the improvement of survival span with these drugs may be only a limited percent, meantime various burdens such as severe side effects, cost, and quality of life (QOL) to patients impose another problem [9].

In the Editorial of recent issue of *The Lancet*, criticism was raised by NICE (National Institute for Health and Clinical Excellence of UK) chairman, Michael Rawlins, on the pricing strategy and profit motives of pharmaceutical industry, and he suggested another parameter "QALY (quality adjusted life year) for drug appraisal" [10]. Similarly, Office of Fair Trading of UK released a report expressing a concern of pricing mechanism involving Pharmaceutical Price Regulation System [11].

As to the efficacy of current chemotherapy, critical evaluation of traditional chemotherapy was undertaken in the breast cancer patients who underwent surgery, with or without chemotherapy. The benefit of survival gain by adjuvant chemotherapy is marginal, 5% in 60 months despite the severe side effects, cost, and moribund QOL [12]. Speaking of response rate in chemotherapy, even Herceptin® is not a miracle agent for the breast cancer. Its primary target is the estrogen receptor-positive breast cancer patients which comprises about 20% of total breast cancer patients, and 20% of them show good response. The overall efficacy of Herceptin in breast cancer is only 4–5%.

In the normal business transaction of any commodity, the case which meets the requirement of customer less than 20% or less may be considered undesirable if not fraudulent [13]. It is thus necessary to develop anticancer drugs with more universal, more tumor selective, or pinpoint targeting potential, which may not be as specific as antibody, but cover universal characteristics of solid tumor, and are thus capable of eradicating total cancer cells without damaging systemic immune and other vital functions. We believe a clue for this tumor-selective delivery is seen in the EPR effect-based drug development, and its further augmentation is technically possible.

1.3 Population Dynamics of Cancer Cells and Recurrence of Cancer

When cancer is detected as palpable or by X-ray imaging, most cancer mass consists of as many as 10^9-10^{12} cells. Conventional chemotherapy for cancer treatment using low molecular weight cytotoxic agents cannot reduce the number of cells to less than 0.01–0.001%, but most likely 60–90% per one cycle in clinical setting. This means common treatment leaves at least 10^7-10^{10} cancer cells escaping from the treatment and survive. When we inoculate $10^5-5 \times 10^6$ cancer cells to healthy mice, tumor will grow within a few weeks, and it is formidable to treat when the size is more than 2 cm in diameter. Further conventional chemotherapy often causes serious side effects that lead to dysfunction of vital organs, such as the heart, kidney, and bone marrow, as well as nausea, vomiting, neurotoxicity, diarrhea, and loss of hair or appetite [9, 12]. To overcome these problems, we need to develop more tumor-selective anticancer drugs, because this method would improve the therapeutic efficacy and reduce the side effectsto normal organs. Conventional low molecular weight anticancer agents can indiscriminately diffuse into normal and cancer tissues throughout the whole body, thereby causing severe systemic side effects.

Although traditional approach yielded a few successes it is not a real remedy. Under these circumstances, we see a light in *the enhanced permeability and retention* (EPR) effect based on pinpoint targeting of the drug to tumor which utilizes a unique characteristic of blood vessels of solid tumors [14–16]. We have studied abnormalities in vascular pathophysiology of solid tumor, in particular, vascular permeability in tumors: abnormal extravasation of macromolecules or lipidic particles, which are then retained in the interstitium of tumor tissues for extended periods, and the EPR effect was thus discovered. The tumor-selective targeting drugs are gaining more attention as one of the most important therapeutic modalities, and thus it becomes one of the hallmark concepts which is applied for cancer drug development. Under these circumstances we witnessed an increase in the number of citations of EPR effect progressively in the past few years (Fig. 1).

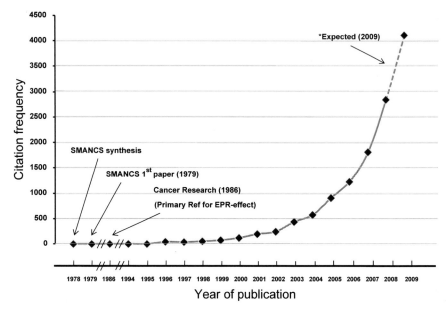

Fig. 1 Numbers of citations of the enhanced permeability and retention (EPR) effect. The number has increased progressively in the last few years (provided form Elsevier Science Publisher and THOMSON/ISI)

1.4 Proof of Evidence and Forward

The best and most efficient utilization of the EPR effect, as an example under clinical setting, is administration of polymeric drug (e.g., SMANCS) into the tumor-feeding artery, e.g., the hepatic artery for hepatoma or the renal artery for renal tumor as oily (Lipiodol®) formulation [16]. The location of Lipiodol®, which is iodinated poppy seed oil, can be visualized by CT scan clearly because of its high electron density [16–22]. SMANCS is dissolved in Lipiodol, being a lipophilic drug, and is infused into the blood vessels. SMANCS/Lipiodol®, being a macromolecular lipid particle, is retained exclusively in tumor very well for prolonged period (Fig. 2A), while very little washout will occur within a few days [19]. As a consequence, the drug concentration of SMANCS/Lipiodol® in the tumor is more than 2000-fold of that in the plasma and it remains in tumor for several weeks (Fig. 2A, B) [19]. This approach of SMANCS/Lipiodol® injection via the arterial route was demonstrated at first in hepatocellular carcinoma, and SMANCS/Lipodol® therapy was approved in 1993 and used for thousands of patients in Japan. The approval of SMANCS for solid tumor heralded the birth of tumor targeting with macromolecular anticancer agents, and led us to discover the EPR effect. Another clinical example is lately obtained using ^{111}In-diethylenetriaminepentaacetic (DTPA)-labeled PEG liposome which clearly showed tumor accumulation [23].

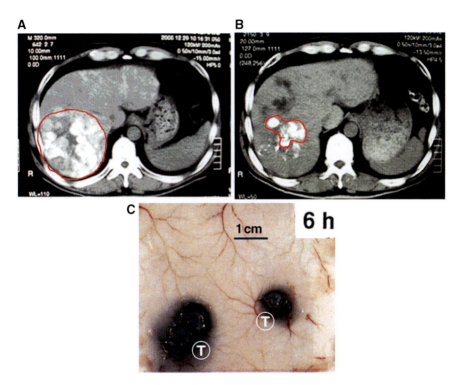

Fig. 2 EPR effect and drug accumulation in solid tumor. (**A**) and (**B**) CT scan of human liver with hepatocellular carcinoma. When SMANCS/Lipiodol® was infused arterially it was selectively taken up in the tumor. CT scan of (**A**) was obtained 2 days after the initial arterial infusion via a catheter, in which SMANCS/Lipiodol® was selectively accumulated in the massive carcinoma seen as *white area* in the liver (due to high electron density of Lipiodol®). After 6 months with intermitted infusions of SMANCS two more times, tumor size (containing SMANCS) has remarkably regressed (**B**). (**C**) EPR effect in mouse sarcoma S-180 in mouse skin. Two *dark blue circular areas* are tumors marked by Ⓣ, where putative macromolecular drug, Evans blue/albumin (MW 70 kDa), accumulated selectively. Note that the background of the normal skin shows no uptake of blue albumin. Mouse was killed at 6 h after the injection of Evans blue and it was quantified after extraction

Another clinical example of the EPR effect is the gallium scintigraphy. In this case radioactive ^{67}gallium citrate is injected intravenously. Then, $^{67}Ga^{2+}$ will bind to plasma protein transferrin (MW 90 kDa) in the blood, thus radioactive (^{67}Ga) transferrin will accumulate in the tumor during next few days by EPR effect. Subsequently, radio-scintigram is obtained 2–3 days after injection of $^{67}Ga^{2+}$ so as to improve signal/noise ratio. The clearance of ^{67}Ga-transferrin from the normal tissue will take place for a few days via the lymphatic system in contrast to tumor tissue.

In this chapter we focus on the pathophysiology and factors involved in the EPR effect in tumor tissues, lymphotropic nature of macromolecular drugs, and control of lymphatic metastasis. Furthermore, suggestions and future perspectives to utilize this technology for enhanced EPR effect are also discussed. Some examples of potentially promising polymeric anticancer agents under development are also discussed.

2 Mechanisms of the EPR Effect

2.1 Pathophysiology and Architecture of Neovasculature of Cancer

Angiogenesis is induced when cluster of tumor cells reach a diameter of 1–2 mm: new blood vessel (neovasculature) thus formed is to supply ever increasing demand of cancer cells for nutrients and oxygen [24, 25]. These newly formed blood vessels in tumors are uniquely different from normal blood vessels, i.e., irregular in shape, dilated, fenestra, sinusoids, lack of smooth muscle layer, large gaps in endothelial cell–cell junctions, and lack of or fewer receptors for angiotensin (AT)-II [26–28]. These architectural differences at physioanatomical level can be demonstrated by scanning electron microscopy (SEM) shown in Fig. 3A–D vs. E, F. Namely, when water-soluble acrylic monomer that forms polymeric resin was injected into blood vessel, one can

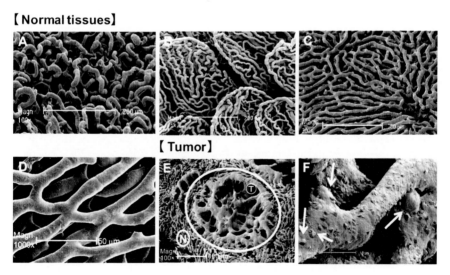

Fig. 3 Scanning electron microscope images of blood vessels in normal tissues and blood vessels of tumor. Normal capillary of the pancreas (**A**), colon (intestinal villi) (**B**), and liver (sinusoid) (**C**), and enlarged image of blood capillary of normal liver (**D**) are shown. (**E**) Metastatic tumor nodule (area Ⓣ) in the normal liver is shown. (**F**) Tumor vessels at capillary level (larger magnification) and showing rough surface, and early phase of extravasating vessels (shown by *arrows*). No leakage of polymer is seen in normal tissues (**A–D**), whereas tumor-selective extravasation of polymer (by EPR effect) is seen clearly in the tumor nodule (**E**)

obtain the plastic cast of the blood vessels. As shown in Fig. 3A–D, capillaries of normal tissues are regularly aligned, and the leakage of plastic polymeric resin is not observed in the normal blood vessels. On the contrary, the polymer is exclusively extravasated outside of blood vessels of tumor nodule (Fig. 3E); tumor nodules are almost filled with polymeric resin (Fig. 3 circled Ⓣ area), or it is about to leak out (Fig. 3F). These electron micrograms clearly show completely different vascular features in tumor compared with normal tissues. Furthermore, this is consistent with the observation of tumor-selective extravasation of macromolecules (blue albumin) shown in Fig. 2C, and lipidic particle (SMANCS/Lipiodol$^{\text{®}}$) as seen by CT scan in Fig. 2A and B. Thus, the neovasculature having excessive permeability in tumor tissues makes nutrients and oxygen readily available for tumor cells and sustains their rapid growth, while this phenomenon greatly facilitates the accumulation of macromolecular drugs in tumor.

Carcinogenesis or tumor metastasis occurs in the normal tissue at first, and the periphery of growing tumor nodule is also the normal tissue. Thus tumor cells need to obtain those nutrients and oxygen from the normal milieu. Under such circumstances many vascular factors, as listed in Table 1, affect the permeability of normal vessels of surrounding tumors and thus sustain tumor growth; these factors in the normal tissue result in the same effect to the EPR effect.

Table 1 Factors affecting enhanced permeability and retention effect that influence the accumulation of macromolecular drugs in solid tumors

Anatomical or biochemical	Unique characteristics and factors

Architectural differences and functions	☐ Active angiogenesis and high vascular density
	 ☐ Extensive production of vascular mediators that facilitate extravasation
	 ☐ Defective vascular architecture:
	     Lack of smooth muscle layer
	     Lack of or fewer receptors for angiotensin II
	     Large gap in endothelial cell–cell junctions and fenestration
	     Anomalous conformation of tumor vasculature (e.g., branching or stretching)
	 ☐ Defective lymphatic clearance of macromolecules and lipids from interstitial tissue (prolonged retention of these substances)
	 ☐ Whimsical blood flow and bidirectional blood flow

Factors affecting endothelial cell gaps and permeability	☐ Bradykinin (BK) and/or 3-hydroxypropyl BK ☐ Nitric oxide (NO) ☐ Vascular endothelial growth factor (VPF/VEGF) ☐ Prostaglandins (PGE$_2$, PGI$_2$) ☐ Collagenases (matrix metalloproteinases or MMPs) ☐ Peroxynitrite per se, and this activates MMPs ☐ Other proteinases (involving kallikrein system) ☐ Other inflammatory cytokines (TNF-α, IL-1, IL-6, IL-8, etc.)

In addition to the extravasating situation, the lymphatic system of tumor tissue is mostly dysfunctional. As a consequence, once these macromolecules or nanoparticles permeate into tumor tissues, they will be retained there over a long period of time (weeks) [14–22, 29–31]. Under these circumstances the concept of the EPR effect for cancer drug development becomes one of the most important principles for passive targeting to the tumor. However, it is not just a passive targeting. The sustained presence of the drugs in tumor tissue is of critical importance. One can demonstrate passive tumor targeting with a water-soluble contrast agent by angiography infusing via the tumor-feeding artery. During the bolus intraarterial infusion of the contrast agent, series of X-ray pictures are continuously taken, e.g., 10 pictures per second for 10–20 s. Then one can visualize the flow of contract dye from the upstream arteriole to the capillary, then to the venous side. When tumor mass or nodule exists, more densely stained spot or area will appear. This demonstrates passive delivery to tumor; however, this tumor stain will last no more than 10 s. It is a great contrast to the angiographic procedure using Lipodol®-containing SMANCS. Lipiodol® will remain more selectively in the tumor for more than several weeks (Fig. 2A, B) [17–20, 31]. This means passive drug targeting alone is not enough which lacks retention as seen in EPR effect.

The EPR effect can be observed with macromolecules having apparent molecular size larger than 40–800 kDa [14–22, 29–31], or more to the size of bacteria [32]. Namely, biocompatible polymeric drugs having size larger than the renal clearance threshold (more than 40 kDa) exhibit the EPR effect [14–22].

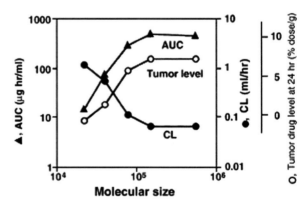

Fig. 4 Relationship between macromolecular drugs of various molecular sizes and tumor accumulation, plasma concentration (AUC), renal clearance (CL) in mice. Putative polymer drugs are ^{125}I-Tyr-HPMA-copolymers of various molecular sizes given intravenously in S-180 tumor model (taken from [29] after modification)

As stated above, low molecular weight drugs can permeate to tumor tissue, but then they will rapidly diffuse into the circulating blood within a short time, and reaching equilibrium throughout the body. Therefore, it is essentially difficult for these low molecular weight drugs to remain in the tumor tissue unless they have a specific receptor with very high association constant.

2.2 Factors That Mediate EPR Effect

We have extensively studied these vascular mediators and generation of such mediator triggered by cancer cells directly or indirectly. It is interesting to note that they are common to inflammatory mediators; consequently, one can observe that cancer is like inflammation that never ceases but grows.

2.2.1 Bradykinin (kinin)

We had initially identified that bradykinin (BK) was generated in all bacterial infections [33–35]. An intrinsic proteolytic cascade system yields BK and this system is triggered by microbial proteases. BK is an important mediator of hyperalgesia, inflammatory reaction, asthma, pain, increased vascular permeability, and vasodilatation. Hageman factor (or factor XII) of coagulation cascade is the uppermost protease of the kallikrein–kinin system. Activation of factor XII is followed by activation of prekallikrein to kallikrein. Kallikrein generates BK directly from kininogen. BK is the most potent pain-inducing peptide in plasma with half-life of a few second which is constantly generated at the site of infection and will facilitate vascular permeability in the tissue. It is interesting to note that many tumors, if not all, induce pain, and it is another physiological effect of BK associated with inflammation, infection, and cancer (Fig. 5). In other words, BK is a common mediator between cancer and inflammation.

We demonstrated that BK is an important mediator of EPR effect in cancer [36]. Figure 5 shows network of BK and other mediators involving in EPR effect. BK interacts with various proinflammatory factors involving vascular permeability. For instance, it is also known to activate endothelial cell-type nitric oxide synthase (eNOS), which is one of the primary enzymes to produce NO from L-arginine. We have reported that the BK-generating cascade is activated in tumor tissues [36]. More importantly, malignant ascetic and pleural fluids would be caused by activation of kallikrein–kinin system in carcinomatosis [37].

BK is degraded by many peptidases, especially angiotensin-converting enzyme (ACE). ACE inhibitor can thus block kinin degeneration as well as AT-II formation (hence resulting in blood lowering effect). BK in most cancer patients, if not all cases, contains hydroxyproline at the third position in place of proline, and both BK and 3-hydroxyprolyl-BK are liberated from kininogen by kallikrein [38]. Both Bhoola's and our groups reported the presence of excessive levels of BK receptor (B2) in various human and rodent solid tumors [39, 40], which would affect the EPR effect (Fig. 5).

2.2.2 Nitric Oxide

Nitric oxide (NO) is generated by three isoforms of NOS, and the most potent isoform is inducible-type NOS (iNOS) which is produced in macrophages and

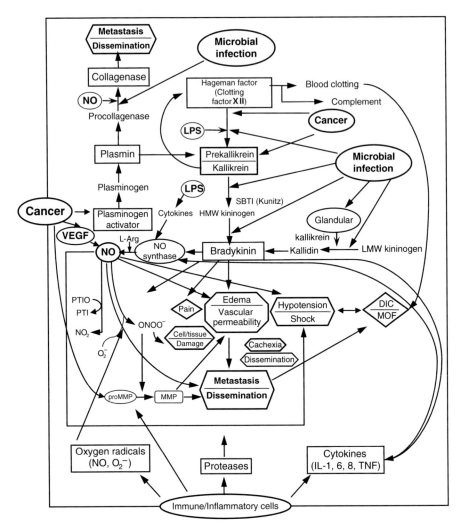

Fig. 5 A comprehensive network of vascular mediators: bradykinin, NO, and others are involving EPR effect in infection, inflammation, and cancer (taken from [117] after modification)

neutrophiles. These leukocytes are known to infiltrate into tumor tissues extensively. One of the most important physiological functions of NO, mediated by NO-cGMP signaling, is vasorelaxation of vascular smooth muscle cells and hence lowering of the blood pressure. NO also influences tumor vascular permeability and plays a crucial role as a mediator of the EPR effect in solid tumor [41, 42]. As an evidence, NOS inhibitors, N^ω-monomethyl-L-arginine (L-NMMA) and N^ω-nitro-L-arginine methylester (L-NAME), as well as NO scavenger, 2-phenyl-4,4,5,5-tetramethylimidazoline-1-oxyl-3-oxide (PTIO), suppressed the vascular permeability in solid tumors [41–43]. When the contribution of NO in EPR effect was quantified by scavenging NO using PTIO and analyzed according to tumor size, the extent of EPR effect, based on uptake of Evans blue albumin, was found proportionally dependent on the tumor size up to 0.25 g. Further increase in tumor size leads to the decreased contribution of NO in EPR effect. This means NO may play more important role at early phase of tumor growth (Fig. 6).

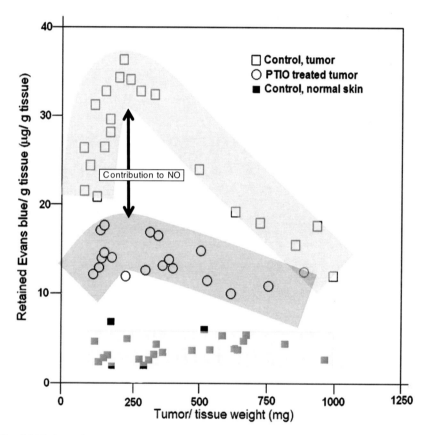

Fig. 6 NO-dependent vascular permeability of solid tumors (S-180) as quantified by uptake of Evans blue albumin complex in tumor of various sizes in mice. Mice were administered with NO scavenger 2-phenyl-4,4,5,5-tetramethylimidazoline-1-oxyl 3-oxide (PTIO) orally (dose: PTIO, 125 mg/kg Í 4 in 8 h). Note that EPR effect is greatly suppressed by PTIO, which is a fraction of NO contributing to EPR effect. Further note that when the tumor size is larger than 0.25 g, the contribution of NO in EPR effect is less pronounced. This implicates the importance of NO at the early stages of tumor growth (see text) (from [42] after modification)

Meyer et al. also found that NOS inhibitor irreversibly attenuated blood flow in R3230Ac rat mammary adenocarcinoma [44]. Similarly, Tozer et al. demonstrated a selective reduction in tumor blood flow with another NOS inhibitor, N^{ω}-nitro-L-arginine in P22 tumor-bearing rats [45]. In different context we further identified its involvement of NO in collagenase activation for EPR effect. Namely, NO reacts rapidly with superoxide anion, which is predominantly produced by leukocytes, to generate peroxynitrite ($ONOO^-$). $ONOO^-$ can activate precursors of matrix metalloproteinase (proMMP) to become MMP by oxidizing zinc-cystein switch of proMMP [46]. Proteases in tumor are known to contribute to tumor growth and metastasis, and MMPs play an important role in tumor metastasis [47, 48]. On the other hand, $ONOO^-$ per se and the subsequently activated MMP also appear to contribute to EPR effect [49, 50].

2.2.3 VEGF

Vascular endothelial cell-derived growth factor (VEGF) was previously identified as the vascular permeability factor (VPF) by Dvorak et al. [51, 52]. Table 2 shows quantification of VEGF in various tumors and normal tissues in mice [50]. The amount of VEGF in tumor was 2- to 30- fold higher than that of normal tissues with the exception of the lung.

Table 2 Amount of kinin in ascetic (A) and VEGF in normal and tumor tissues of mice (B)

A. Amount of VEGF in various tissues and tumors

Tissues	pg/mg[a]		Species/strain
<Normal tissue>			
Kidney	15.42±2.14		Mouse/AKR
Liver	2.68±0.39	8.81±2.66	Mouse/AKR
Heart	12.08±1.39		Mouse/AKR
Testis	5.04±1.09		Mouse/AKR
Lung	67.3±38.30	20.50±11.92	Mouse/AKR
<Tumor tissue>			
Sarcoma 180[b]	34.68±14.46		Mouse/ddY
Lewis lung carcinoma[b]	45.00±2.08	53.54±14.02	Mouse/C57BL6/J
Colon carcinoma 38[b]	80.95±22.15		Mouse/C57BL6/J

B. Amount of kinin in cancer

Ascites	Bioassay (ng/ml)[c]	ELISA(ng/ml)[c]
S-180 (mouse)[d]	1–4	0.625–2.5
AH-130 (rat)[d]	1–8	0.625–2.0
Pancreas cancer (human)[e]	1	0.625
Stomach cancer (human)[e]	30–40	8–10
Lung cancer (human)[e]	40	20
Hepatoma with liver cirrhosis[e](human)	2.5	Not done
Ovarian cancer (human)[e]	2.5	Not done

[a] $n = 3\sim6$ for all experimental data: values are mean ± S.E.
[b] All tumors were implanted at the dorsal skin. From Ref. [50].
[c] Synthetic bradykinin was used as standard.
[d] Values are from several rodent ascites. Different ascite samples were used for bioassay and ELISA.
[e] Individual cases. From Ref. [36]

Regarding the involvement of VEGF in EPR effect, we examined the extravasation of Evans blue in guinea pig skin by intradermally injecting VEGF as well as BK. VEGF like BK significantly enhanced the extravasation of Evans blue (albumin) in a dose-dependent manner, as shown in Fig. 7. Therefore, VEGF may also play an important role in the EPR effect [50].

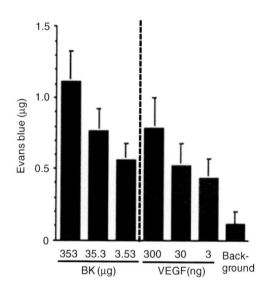

Fig. 7 Enhanced vascular permeability induced by exogenous BK and VEGF in normal guinea pig dorsal skin. Various amounts of BK and VEGF were injected intradermally into the dorsal skin of guinea pigs at doses given in the figure. The amount of Evans blue extravasated into the skin was extracted and quantified. Data are mean ± S.E., n = 6 (from [50])

2.2.4 Others

Inducible form of cyclooxygenase 2 (COX-2), which is also induced by inflammatory cytokines (TNF-α, IL-1β, IL-8, etc.), can increase the generation of prostaglandins (PGs) (PGE$_2$, PGI$_2$, etc.), thus enhancing the EPR effect [41, 43, 53].

3 Development of EPR Effect: Past and Future

3.1 Background

Based on the EPR effect it is now possible to achieve very high local drug concentrations in tumor using macromolecular size drugs, i.e., polymer conjugates, micellar or liposomal drugs, or nanomedicine [14–16, 30, 31, 54–58]. Plasma proteins with molecular weight larger than 40 kDa such as non-antibody IgG can also exhibit high tumor targeting efficiency [14, 15, 59].

Initially, Maeda et al. conjugated an antitumor protein neocarzinostatin (NCS, MW 12 kDa) with copolymer of styrene–maleic acid–half-*n*-butylate (SMA) [59–61]. The conjugation of protein (NCS) with SMA called SMANCS did confer number of advantages: hydrophobicity, enlarging molecular size, capacity with albumin binding, oily formulation, higher stability, and stealth character against phagocytosis. Accordingly, SMANCS exhibited much improved physicochemical, biochemical, and pharmacological properties than parental NCS, and most importantly, it also behaved in a tumor-selective manner in vivo [30, 59].

3.2 Augmentation of EPR Effect: Development for Future

3.2.1 Under Angiotensin (AT)-II-Induced Hypertension

The anatomical architecture of blood vessels of tumor is quite different from that of normal tissue as described above. Normal blood vessels maintain vascular blood flow volume constant regardless of the blood pressure applied by a homeostatic mechanism. Namely, when hypertension is induced by vascular mediators, i.e., vasoconstrictor AT-II, the blood vessels will constrict resulting in higher blood pressure, accompanying faster velocity of blood flow per area of cross section in normal vasculature. The cross section being now smaller, the blood flow volume thus remains constant [62, 63]. Contrary to normal vasculature, there is no homeostatic blood flow regulation in the tumor vasculature. In 1981, Suzuki et al. found that raising the systolic blood pressure by infusing AT-II into tumor-bearing rats caused a selective increase of blood flow volume in tumor about 2- to 6-fold; the degree of increase depends on the induced blood pressure [62].

We thus anticipated that the EPR effect could be augmented by AT-II-induced hypertensive state, thereby increasing macromolecular drug delivery. ^{51}Cr-labeled SMANCS or other putative macromolecular drug (bovine serum albumin, ^{14}C-BSA) was infused i.v. into the rats bearing tumor, followed by immediate infusion of AT-II via i.v. route, thus elevating the systolic blood pressure from 100 to 150 mmHg, which was maintained for 15 min. We found the accumulation of both radioactive BSA and SMANCS increased in tumor tissues to 1.3- to 3-fold [64]. In contrast to tumor, the amount of these drugs delivered to normal organs such as kidney, intestine, and bone marrow was reduced because of the vasoconstriction (tightening of endothelial cell gap junction). Namely, the extravasation of nanoparticle size larger than 40 kDa in normal tissues was more suppressed due to tighter endothelial intercellular junction. Consequently, less damage was found in the bone marrow and the intestine as judged by the bone marrow cellularity and the degree of diarrhea [64]. It should also be noted that conventional low molecular weight anticancer agents are not applicable to this strategy due to the rapid washout. In normotensive state, it is difficult to achieve more than 2- to 3-fold higher tumor delivery by increasing the dose due to dose-limiting toxicity. However, it now becomes possible by AT-II-induced hypertensive state. Therefore, the AT-II-induced hypertensive state makes it possible to achieve a significantly higher tumor-selective accumulation without increase in the drug dosage. Consequently, a better therapeutic effect was observed clinically by using this method for SMANCS/Lipiodol[®] (e.g., SMANCS dynamic therapy), which is administered intraarterially against cholangiocarcinoma, metastatic liver cancer, renal cell carcinoma, pancreatic cancer, as well as hepatocellular carcinoma [21, 22, 30]. As expected, the present procedure showed much fewer side effects.

3.2.2 Local Increase of Bradykinin Level by ACE Inhibitor

Maeda's group demonstrated that inhibition of ACE by systemic administration of ACE inhibitors caused local increase of BK levels at the tumor site, because BK generation was occurring exclusively in tumor tissue unless inflammation existed elsewhere. ACE inhibitors are benign and commonly used as antihypertensive agents, and they do not affect normotensive patients. Most of them are orally administered and show very long plasma half-life (>4 h). On the basis of these data, we used the ACE inhibitors enalapril and temocapril to inhibit BK degradation and showed that the elevated BK level resulted in further enhancement of vascular permeability or the EPR effect [36, 41]. ACE inhibitors thus increased the delivery of macromolecular drugs to tumors, even in normotensive patients. Experimental and clinical effects to enhance both drug delivery and the antitumor effects by use of ACE inhibitor need to be validated along this line using macromolecular drugs.

3.2.3 By Using Prostacyclin Agonists

Prostaglandins (PGs) are formed by cyclooxygenases (COX-1 and COX-2), and PGEs production is markedly elevated in human and experimental tumors [66, 67]. We showed that COX inhibitor, indomethacin, significantly suppressed vascular permeability in S-180 and other solid tumor models [41]. In addition, we found that injection of beraprost sodium, a stable prostaglandin I_2 (PGI_2) agonist, which has much longer in vivo $t_{1/2}$ than PGI_2(60 min vs. a few seconds), resulted in about 2-fold enhancement of the EPR effect, similar to the situation for ACE inhibitors [53, 65]. As an incidental finding, beraprost reduced downstream blood flow to an almost negligible degree (about 10%) while enhancing vascular leakage of tumor [53]. As a consequence, macromolecular tumor-imaging agents may be further concentrated in tumor tissues by combination with beraprost, although this possibility must be demonstrated in clinical settings.

3.2.4 Increasing NO Concentration in Tumor by Use of NO-Releasing Agents

We found that the NO-releasing agent isosorbide dinitrate (ISDN, Nitrol[®]) enhanced antitumor activity of SMANCS/Lipiodol[®] when they were infused into the tumor-feeding bronchial artery of lung cancer using a catheter preceding to the infusion of SMANCS arterially. This ISDN infusion enhanced opening of the feeding artery, followed by increase of blood flow; thus, more drugs were delivered in the tumor as revealed by CT scan image [22]. This enhanced vascular flow may also ameliorate the state of hypoxia, followed by suppressing hypoxia-inducible factor (HIF-1α), which will otherwise induce angiogenesis and tumor growth. Further, it may also suppress the production of VEGF since HIF-1α is known to induce VEGF.

Recently, we found that EPR effect is further enhanced by applying nitroglycerin ointment onto the skin of superficial tumors including breast cancer induced by chemical carcinogen, 7,12-dimethylbenz[a]anthracene (DMBA) in rats, and also transplanted mice tumors (Seki and Maeda, in preparation). The increase of Evans blue/albumin delivered into the solid tumors was 2- to 3-fold of that without nitroglycerin [68].

4 Important Issues on Nanomedicine: Intracellular Uptake of Macromolecular Drugs, Drug Release Rate from the Complex, and Drug Resistance

4.1 Access to Tumor and Intracellular Uptake, and to the Molecular Target

Two major steps in drug delivery are commonly considered: first step is the tissue vascular level (organ), accomplished by EPR effect for polymer therapeutics (nanomedicine) which can traverse the vascular wall to the tumor interstitium, where EPR effect plays the single most important role [69].

Second step is to reach to the molecular target after binding to cell membrane, followed by internalization across the cell membrane. This can be better accomplished more frequently by a specific receptor/ligand binding followed by internalization, which is possible with specific antigenic site using antibody, or the ligands (agonists) and receptor, or the unique probe molecules, respectively. Even without a unique or specific epitope receptor, the endocytotic mechanism for macromolecules would take place more generally. Subsequently, free diffusion of low molecular weight drugs would proceed after release from micelles or liposomes at the vicinity of molecular target in the tumor cells or tumor tissues.

4.1.1 Free Drug Diffusion

A significant distance will be covered by free diffusion, for both low and high molecular weight drugs to access tumor cells after extravasating from blood vessels. This non-static/dynamic state in biological in vivo system should not be overlooked. For instance, distance of diffusion of IgG (MW 160 kDa) can be easily detected several millimeters during overnight incubation at room temperature in the classic agar immuno-diffusion experiment. Also in antibiotic drug assays using agar plate, we routinely observed the mobility of about 10 mm or more in the agar diffusion of antibiotics overnight. Therefore whatever the mechanism, biologically active molecules can reach about 10–100 μm distance easily to tumor cells outside the capillary in the interstitial matrix of tumor tissue and get access to tumor cells within the distance of free diffusion.

4.1.2 Cellular Uptake

Macromolecular drugs are less likely to traverse into cells by simple diffusion across cell membranes because of their size; therefore, endocytosis (fluid-phase endocytosis or pinocytosis, receptor-mediated endocytosis, phagocytosis, transcytosis) appears to be the usual means of internalization [70–72]. Efficient endocytotic internalization occurs after specific binding to receptors (upregulation of receptor). It is well known that many receptors such as transferrin, low-density lipoprotein (LDL), and folate are highly upregulated on tumor cells and corresponding ligand-linked drugs will be effectively internalized to the tumor [73, 74]. In this connection it is known that dividing tumor cells have more active intracellular uptake (endocytosis) than non-dividing cells [75], indicating a higher uptake efficiency of macromolecular drugs by dividing cancer cells.

4.1.3 Access to Submolecular Target

This offers another step of selectivity. After internalization of the drugs into the cytoplasm via phagosomes, the phagosomes fuse with lysosomes, which are rich in proteolytic and hydrolytic enzymes (e.g., rich in cathepsin B in tumor [76]), of which low pH optimum fits to that of tumor tissue (pH 5.5–6.5) rather than normal tissues. Then active principle is hydrolysed and released in this milieu. This confers the third step of advantage. Therefore, for many pendant-type linked drugs, the types of chemical bonds become important: the peptidyl linkers must be selected to facilitate easy cleavage in cancer cells to fit the substrate requirement of a specific cathepsin or other specific enzymes [77–79]. For example, linker cleaved by cathepsin B is ideal, which is probably the case of OPAXIO^{TM} (Xylotax, CT-2103). In this case, polyglutamyl carboxyl group is linked to 2'-hydroxyl of paclitaxel by ester linkage.

In the case of SMANCS, it is essentially taken up into the cell by endocytosis, and acidic pH (<6) of phago-lysosome liberates the active component (NCS) by spontaneous hydrolysis of the maleylamide bond. Then chromophore of NCS diffuses into the cytoplasm or to the nucleus, where the drug action to DNA would occur [70, 71]. Another acid-labile bond is azide bond which is discussed by other researchers [80].

In our SMA micelles of pirarubicin or doxorubicin constant release of the anthracycline from micelles was observed, the rate was much slower than the endocytotic process, which showed a release rate of 4–5%/day. In these cases, once the micelles are taken up into the tumor cells, active principle of free drugs will be continuously released. However, pirarubicin, which exhibits higher intracellular uptake than doxorubicin [81], resulted in better therapeutic effect than doxorubicin [81, 82]. Some micellar drugs exhibiting too fast (e.g., NK911 [83]) or too slow (e.g., Doxil® [84]) release rates will potentially affect their side effect or anticancer effect.

4.2 Against Multidrug Resistance

In a different context, after intracellular uptake of macromolecular drugs, P-glycoprotein (Pgp)-dependent efflux system of multidrug-resistant (MDR) cells is not operative for macromolecular drugs [85–89]. This result suggests that EPR-mediated targeting of polymeric anticancer drugs cannot be nullified by Pgp-dependent system until it becomes free drug such as doxorubicin, thus ensuring higher intracellular activity against MDR-positive cancer cells.

As another advantage of nanomedicine for managing MDR problem, Minko et al. reported that HPMA-block copolymer-doxorubicin conjugated circumvent MDR issue by modulating intracellular signaling leading to apoptosis in MDR cells [88, 89].

5 Recent Developments of Macromolecular Anticancer Agents for Tumor-Targeted Delivery Utilizing EPR Effect: Potential Drugs for Future

5.1 OPAXIO^{TM}, Poly(L-Glutamic Acid)-Paclitaxel Conjugates

Paclitaxel (PTX) is a conventional anticancer agent for various cancers such as tumors of the ovary, the breast, and the lung. The drug was first isolated in 1967, and approved by FDA for ovarian cancer in 1992. However, the major difficulty in the clinical application of PTX was poor water solubility and usual toxicity of neutropenia and peripheral sensory neuropathy. To overcome these problems, Li et al. developed a conjugate of poly(L-glutamic acid) and PTX via ester bonds (OPAXIO^{TM}, formerly known as XYOTAX, CT-2103) [90]. The conjugate has a molecular weight of approximately 49 kDa, containing 35% of PTX (w/w), and exhibits prolonged plasma and tumor half-life. It is taken up by endocytosis and free PTX is liberated by cathepsin B cleavage. Further, OPAXIO^{TM} exhibited greater antitumor activity against both murine tumors and human tumor xenografts compared to PTX [90, 91]. Phase III trials were performed in patients with non-small cell lung cancer (NSCLC). OPAXIO^{TM} showed significant decrease of many side effects, such as alopecia, infection, and cardiac symptoms, compared to PTX (control), and exhibited 40% improvement of overall survival compared to vinorelbine which is used for comparison group in the treatment of NSCLC, and it was recently approved by EU Medicines Agency.

5.2 NK012, SN-38-Encapsulated Micelles

7-Ethyl-10-hydroxy-camptothecin (SN-38) is an active principle of irinotecan hydrochloride (CPT-11) generated by hydrolysis of carboxy esterase. SN-38 exhibits up to 1000-fold more potent cytotoxic activity against various cancer cells in vitro than CPT-11 [92]. Although camptothecin exhibited antitumor activity both in vitro and in vivo in experimental studies, it is used only in limited extent clinically because of its low therapeutic efficacy and severe side effect including severe diarrhea and liver toxicity [93, 94]. Although SN-38 per se showed a potent antitumor activity, it is not soluble in water, the same problem as PTX. To overcome this problem, SN-38-loaded polymeric micelle (NK012) was developed by the self-assembly of an amphiphilic block copolymer which consists of PEG and partially modified polyglutamate [95]. NK012 has molecular weight of 19 kDa and a mean particle size of 20 nm in diameter, and contained about 20% (w/w) of SN-38 in the micelle. The releasing rates of SN-38 in 5% glucose solution at 37°C were 1 and 3% at 24 and 48 h, respectively. Therefore, NK012 is stable in micelle under physiological condition, and is expected to show the EPR effect. Further, it showed potent cytotoxicity 43- to 340-fold higher than that of CPT-11 in various tumor cells and 2.3- to 5.8-fold higher than that of free SN-38 in various cells in vitro. NK012 showed more potent antitumor activity than CPT-11 in vivo against two human small cell lung cancer cell lines, SBC/Neo and SBC/VEGF in human xenograft mice models [96]. Phase I study of the NK012 is now undergoing in Japan.

5.3 NK105, Paclitaxel-Encapsulated Micelle

NK105 was developed by Kataoka et al. in early 1990s, designed to utilize the EPR effect [97, 98]. NK105 is a block copolymer micelle composed of PEG and polyaspartate. The polymer has a molecular weight of approximately 20 kDa, and contains 23% of PTX (w/w). NK105 dramatically improved aforementioned toxicity problems. Further, NK105 exhibited slower clearance from the plasma than PTX, and remained in plasma up to 72 h, whereas free PTX was not detected 24 h after injection. The antitumor effect of NK105 is more potent than that of PTX, while body weight loss was not observed in the mice by administration of NK105 at 100 mg/kg (PTX equivalent). These encouraging experimental results in vivo led to clinical trials currently under Phase II study in Japan [99, 100].

5.4 NC6004, Cisplatin-Encapsulated Micelle and MBP-426, Oxaliplatin Containing Transferrin-Coated Stealth Liposomes

cis-Dichlorodiammineplatinum (II) (cisplatin, CDDP) is an important agent in cancer chemotherapy. Polymeric micelle containing CDDP utilizing EPR effect was also developed by Kataoka et al. in early 1990s [101, 102]. Similar to the development of NK105, NC6004 is a micellar drug which consists of PEG-poly(glutamic acid) block copolymer encapsulating CDDP. The micelle has a molecular weight of 18 kDa, and a mean distribution size of 30 nm [101]. The micelles are stable and the release rates of CDDP from NC6004 were 19.6 and 47.8% at 24 and 96 h, respectively. NC6004 showed significant tumor growth suppression in the human gastric cancer xenograft mice, while it did not induce decrease of body weight in contrast to CDDP at 5 mg/kg. Phase I clinical trial of NC6004 is now undergoing in the UK and will be started soon in the National Cancer Center Hospital, Japan [101].

Maruyama et al. developed transferrin-targeted PEG-stealth liposome [103] containing *trans*-L-diaminocyclohexane oxalatoplatinum (oxaliplatin), MBP-426, and designed to utilize EPR effect as well as transferrin receptor which is highly expressed on tumor cells, for active targeting. The size of transferrin-PEG-liposome is about 180 nm in diameter, and it contains oxaliplatin of 14.8 μg/mg liposomal lipid [104]. The transferrin-liposome showed about 16-fold more tumor accumulation than parent-free oxaliplatin in colon 26 tumor at 30 h after injection [104]. Further, it remained about 2-fold higher in concentration in tumor at 72 h after i.v. than that of liposome without transferrin. The transferrin-PEG-liposome at 5 mg/kg oxaliplatin equivalent suppressed colon 26 tumor growth significantly compared to free oxaliplatin (about 80% suppression) and the liposome without transferrin [104]. Phase I clinical study is currently undergoing in the USA.

5.5 Camptothecin Conjugates

Camptothecin is a potent cytotoxic agent first isolated from plant *Camptotheca accuminata*. Besides low specificity to tumor cells as many other low-MW anticancer drugs, camptothecin possesses two major drawbacks: weak solubility in water and a high affinity for human serum albumin via a reaction that renders the drug inactive. $20(S)$-camptothecin contains a lactone ring that is essential for cytotoxic effect and binding to topoisomerase I. The camptothecin usually exists in equilibrium with lactone ring and open-ended carboxylate form, which reacts with human albumin at physiological pH, then the drug is converted into the inactive form. Similar to the modification of free PTX for OPAXIO^{TM}, camptothecin was conjugated with poly-L-glutamatic acid, which made it soluble in water as well as stabilization of the labile lactone ring, so that the conjugate could benefit from EPR effect. Indeed, this conjugate showed improved pharmacokinetics and higher intratumor accumulation as a result of the EPR effect [101]. A Phase I/II study is now underway in the USA and Europe. This conjugate offers a marked advantage compared with free camptothecin as are other polymeric drugs.

5.6 PEG- and SMA-Conjugated Zinc Protoporphyrin IX

Zinc protoporphyrin IX (ZnPP) shows specific inhibition of heme oxygenase-1 (HO-1), which is also known as heat shock protein 32 (Hsp32). HO-1 plays a key role in regulating the intracellular heme level by catalyzing initial oxidation of heme to generate billiverdin, carbon oxide (CO), and free iron, which is the rate-limiting step of heme degradation. Billiverdin will further be converted to bilirubin by billiverdin reductase. Bilirubin is one of the most potent antioxidants which cancer cells utilize, and CO is now known as an important anti-oxidative and anti-apoptotic molecule. Consequently, induction of HO-1 (or Hsp32) parallels to the anti-apoptotic and proliferative activity of cancer cells. HO-1 (Hsp32) is thus referred as a survival factor of cancer cells. All neoplastic cells we tested found high expression of HO-1 mRNA and HO-1 protein, including experimental solid tumors as well as leukemic cells [105–109]. Therefore, HO-1 may be a good anticancer target, and its inhibitor, such as ZnPP, would be a good candidate of a new anticancer strategy. Indeed, we demonstrated ZnPP has potent antitumor activity in vivo. [107, 110] However, the problem is that ZnPP is not readily water soluble. Therefore, we developed a water-soluble PEG-conjugated ZnPP (PZP). In another series of experiments we prepared SMA micelles containing ZnPP (SZP). Both PZP and SZP showed high tumor targeting and antitumor effect [107, 110, 111]. Obviously, these polymeric drugs achieved tumor-targeted delivery based on EPR effect. Thus, inhibition of the enzyme HO-1 with PZP in tumor would result in marked increase in reactive oxygen species (ROS), or the oxystress in tumor cells that would lead to apoptosis and marked antitumor effects [107, 109].

In combination with ROS, PZP pretreatment suppressed tumor growth in mice more significantly [111]. Further combination with other anticancer agents such as [111] showed additive or synergistic antitumor effect with PZP pretreatment compared with either treatment alone.

In addition to oxystress/apoptosis hypothesis induced by PZP, Peter Valent et al. [105, 112, 113] showed remarkable downregulation of oncogene *BCR/ABL* in CML which led to apoptosis. PZP or SZP exhibits also growth suppressing effect on imanitib-resistant CML as well as acute lymphoblastic leukemia (ALL) [105, 112–114]. These findings suggest that HO-1 (Hsp-32) is an attractive target for chemotherapeutic intervention for combination therapy.

We recently found that SZP and PZP generated singlet oxygen, another ROS, upon xenon light (>400 nm) irradiation [115, 116] and consequently exhibited cytotoxic effect in Jurkat cells and KYSE (human esophageal carcinoma cells) in vitro [115], and S-180 tumor growth and DMBA-induced breast cancer in rodents upon irradiation of conventional endoscopic light [116]. Because of its unique tumoritropic nature by EPR and singlet oxygen generation by endoscopic xenon light, the anticancer effect of PZP and SZP will become 2- to 3-fold interesting, and will be applicable for all GI cancers

including esophageal, and superficial cancers, such as breast, skin, broncho-
genic, urinary, and cervical cancers.

6 Conclusions

Discovery of EPR effect represents a major milestone in the history of cancer
targeting chemotherapy. EPR effect is commonly observed for macromolecular
drugs in most of solid tumors, and thus this spontaneous tumor targeting
character of macromolecular drugs makes great breakthrough. Various promising macromolecular drugs have been developed based on the EPR effect
[54– 58, 100, 107], and they showed greatly improved characteristics, such as
prolonged half-life in plasma and tumor, lesser systemic toxicity, and increased
distribution to tumor, accompanied by prolonged retention in the tumor tissues. We expect that EPR effect-based targeting of anticancer drugs ensure a
better QOL, improved compliance of patients as well as low manufacturing
cost, which is more critically discussed recently [10].

EPR effect can be augmented by modulating blood pressure and increase of
local blood flow using AT-II-induced hypertension in most solid tumors and
NO-releasing agent (ISDN or GTN) in the lung and ductal cancer and superficial cancer and others. Thus, the delivery of macromolecular drugs will be
increased further 1.5- to 3-fold. Accordingly improved efficacy will be warranted. Therefore, augmentation of the EPR effect-dependent macromolecular
drugs delivery to tumor will be an important strategy for cancer therapy in
future.

Taken together, we believe the EPR effect-based drugs design and its artificial augmentation will open up new door for future cancer chemotherapy.

Acknowledgments Authors thank Ms Daruwalla J and Prof. Christophi C, Department of
Surgery, Austin Health Hospital, University of Melbourne, Australia, for supplying the SEM
pictures of blood capillaries used in Fig. 2A–F. Authors are indebted to all collaborators (to
H. Maeda) for their painstaking assistance or support.

References

1. "World Health Organization" report. 2008. Available from: http://www.who.int/cancer/en/
2. Leaf CF. Why we are losing the war on cancer and how to win it. *Fortune* 2005; **149**: 76–97.
3. Miklos, GLG. The human cancer genome project-one more misstep in the war on cancer.
   Nat Biotechnol 2005; **23**: 535–537.
4. Hind D, Pilgrim H, Ward S. Questions about adjuvant trastuzumab still remain. *The Lancet*
   2007; **369**: 3–5.
5. Allen TM. Ligand-targeted therapeutics in anticancer therapy. *Nat Rev Cancer* 2002; **2**:
   750–765.
6. Sjöblom T, Jones S, Wood LD, Parsons W, Lin J, Barber TD, Mandelker D, Leary RJ,
   Ptak J, Silliman N, Szabo S, Buckhaults P, Farrell C, Meeh P, Markowitz SD, Willis J,
   Dawson D, Willson JKV, Gazdar AF, Hartigan J, Wu L, Liu C, Parmigiani G, Park BH,

Bachman KE, Papadopoulos N, Vogelstein B, Kinzler KW, Velculescu VE. The consensus coding sequences of human breast and colorectal cancers. *Science* 2006; **314**: 268–274.

7. Wood LD, Parsons DW, Jones S, Lin J, Sjöblom T, Leary RJ, Shen D, Boca SM, Barber T, Ptak J, Silliman N, Szabo S, Dezso Z, Ustyanksky V, Nikolskaya T, Nikolsky Y, Karchin R, Wilson PA, Kaminker JS, Zhang Z, Croshaw R, Willis J, Dawson D, Shipitsin M, Willson JKV, Sukumar S, Polyak K, Park BH, Pethiyagoda CL, Pant PVK, Ballinger DG, Sparks AB, Hartigan J, Smith DR, Suh E, Papadopoulos N, Buckhaults P, Markowitz SD, Parmigiani G, Kinzler KW, Velculescu VE, Vogelstein B. *Science* 2007; **318**: 1108–1113.

8. Jack A, Simonian H. Roche to switch to primary care force. *Financial Times, European Ed.* 2008; July 2: 18.

9. Rabinovitch D. Take Off Your Dress. London, Simon & Schuster; 2007.

10. Editorial. Welcome clinical leadership at NICE. *The Lancet* 2008; **372**: 601.

11. Office of Fair Trading report. 2007. [Available from: http://www.oft.gov.uk/shared_oft/reports/comp_policy/oft885.pdf]

12. Hassett MJ, O'Malley J, Pakes JR, Newhouse JP, Earle CC. *J Natl Cancer Inst* 2006; **98**: 1108–1117.

13. Angell M. *The Truth About the Drug Companies.* New York, Random House, 2004.

14. Matsumura Y, Maeda H. A new concept for macromolecular therapeutics in cancer chemotherapy: mechanism of tumoritropic accumulation of proteins and the antitumor agent smancs. *Cancer Res* 1986; **46**: 6387–6392.

15. Maeda H, Matsumura Y. Tumoritropic and lymphotropic principles of macromolecular drugs. *Crit Rev Ther Drug Carrier Syst* 1989; **6**: 193–210.

16. Maeda H, Sawa T, Konno T. Mechanism of tumor-targeted delivery of macromolecular drugs, including the EPR effect in solid tumor and clinical overview of the prototype polymeric drug SMANCS. *J Control Release* 2001; **74**: 47–61.

17. K. Iwai, Maeda H, Konno T. Use of oily contrast medium for selective drug targeting to tumor: enhanced therapeutic effect and X-ray image. *Cancer Res* 1984; **44**: 2115–2121.

18. Iwai K, Maeda H, Konno T, Matsumura Y, Yamashita R, Yamasaki K, Hirayama S, Miyauchi Y. Tumor targeting by arterial administration of lipids: rabbit model with VX2 carcinoma in the liver. *Anticancer Res* 1987; **7**: 321–327.

19. Konno T, Maeda H, Iwai K, Maki S, Tashiro S, Uchida M, Miyauchi Y. *Cancer* 1984; **54**: 2367–2374.

20. Maki S, Konno T, Maeda H. Image enhancement in computerized tomography for selective diagnosis of liver cancer and semiquantitation of tumor selective drug targeting with oily contrast medium. *Cancer* 1985; **56**: 751–757.

21. Greish K, Fang J, Inutsuka T, Nagamitsu A, Maeda H. Macromolecular Therapeutics: Advantages and prospects with special emphasis on solid tumour targeting. *Clin Pharmacokinet* 2003; **42**: 1089–1105.

22. Nagamitsu A, Inuzuka T, Greish K, Maeda H. SMANCS dynamic therapy for various advanced solid tumors and promising clinical effects: Enhanced drug delivery by hydrodynamic modulation with vascular mediators, particularly angiotensin II, during arterial infusion. *Drug Deliv Sys* 2007; **22-5**: 510–521. In Japanese.

23. Harrington KJ, Mohammadtaghi S, Uster PS, Glass D, Peters AM, Vile RG, Stewart JSW. Effective targeting of solid tumors in patients with locally advanced cancers by radiolabeled pegylated liposomes. *Clin Cancer Res* 2001; **7**: 243–254.

24. Folkman J. What is the evidence that tumors are angiogenesis dependent? *J Natl Cancer Inst* 1990; **82**: 4–6.

25. Folkman J. Angiogenesis in cancer, vascular, rheumatoid and other disease. *Nat Med* 1995; **1**: 27–30.

26. Skinner SA, Tutton PJM, O'Brien PE. Microvascular architecture of experimental colon tumors in the rat. *Cancer Res* 1990; **50**: 2411–2417.

27. Brock TA, Dvorak HF, Sengar DR. Tumor-secreted vascular permeability factor increases cytosolic Ca^{2+} and von Willebrand factor release in human endothelial cells. *Am J Pathol* 1991; **138**: 213–221.

28. Hashizume H, Baluk P, Morikawa S, McLean JW, Thurston G, Roberge S, Jain RK, McDonald DM. Openings between defective endothelial cells explain tumor vessel leakiness. *Am J Pathol* 2000; **156**: 1363–1380.

29. Noguchi Y, Wu J, Duncan R, Strohalm J, Ulbrich K, Akaike T, Maeda H. Early phase tumor accumulation of macromolecules: A great difference in clearance rate between tumor and normal tissues. *Jpn J Cancer Res* 1998; **89**: 307–314.

30. Maeda H. SMANCS and polymer-conjugated macromolecular drugs: advantages in cancer chemotherapy. *Adv Drug Deliv Rev* 2001; **46**: 169–185.

31. Maeda H, Wu J, Sawa T, Matsumura Y, Hori K. Tumor vascular permeability and the EPR effects in macromolecular therapeutics: a review. *J Control Release* 2000; **65**: 271–284.

32. Kimura NT, Taniguchi S, Aoki K, Baba T. Selective localization and growth of *Bifidobacterium bifidum* in mouse tumors following intravenous administration. *Cancer Res* 1980; **40**: 2061–2068.

33. Matsumoto K, Yamamoto T, Kamata R, Maeda H. Pathogenesis of serratial infection: activation of the Hageman factor-prekallikrein cascade by serratial protease. *J Biochem* 1984; **96**: 739–749.

34. Molla A, Yamamoto T, Akaike T, Miyoshi S, Maeda H. Activation of Hageman factor and prekallikrein and generation of kinin by various microbial proteinases. *J Biol Chem* 1989; **264**: 10589–10594.

35. Maruo K, Akaike T, Inada Y, Ohkubo I, Ono T, Maeda H. Effect of microbial and mite proteases on low and high molecular weight kininogens. *J Biol Chem* 1993; **268**: 17711–17715.

36. Matsumura Y, Kimura M, Yamamoto T, Maeda H. Involvement of the kinin-generating cascade in enhanced vascular permeability in tumor tissue. *Jpn J Cancer Res* 1988; **79**: 1327–1334.

37. Matsumura Y, Maruo K, Kimura M, Yamamoto T, Konno T, Maeda H. Kinin-generating cascade in advanced cancer patients and in vitro study. *Jpn J Cancer Res* 1991; **82**: 732–741.

38. Maeda H, Matsumura Y, Kato H. Purification and identification of [hydroxyprolyl³]-bradykinin in ascetic fluid from a patient with gastric cancer. *J Biol Chem* 1988; **263**: 16051–16054.

39. Plendl J, Snyman C, Naidoo S, Sawant S, Mahabeer R, Bhoola KD. Expression of tissue kallikrein and kinin receptors in angiogenic microvascular endothelial cells. *Biol Chem* 2000; **381**: 1103–1115.

40. Wu J Akaike T, Hayashida K, Miyamoto Y, Nakagawa T, Miyakawa K, Müller-Esterl W and Maeda H. Identification of bradykinin receptors in clinical cancer specimens and murine tumor tissues. *Int J Cancer* 2002; **98**: 29–35.

41. Wu J, Akaike T, Maeda H. Modulation of enhanced vascular permeability in tumors by a bradykinin antagonist, a cyclooxygenase inhibitor, and nitric oxide scavenger. *Cancer Res* 1998; **58**: 159–165.

42. Maeda H, Noguchi Y, Sato K, Akaike T. Enhanced vascular permeability in solid tumor is mediated by nitric oxide and inhibited by both new nitric oxide scavenger and nitric oxide synthase inhibitor. *Jpn J Cancer Res* 1994; **85**: 331–334.

43. Maeda H, Wu J, Okamoto T, Maruo K, Akaike T. Kallikrein-kinin in infection and cancer. *Immunopharmacology* 1999; **43**: 115–128.

44. Meyer RE, Shan S, DeAngelo J, Dodge RK, Bonaventura J, Ong ET, Dewhirst MW. Nitric oxide synthase inhibition irreversibly decreases perfusion in the R3230Ac rat mammary adenocarcinoma. *Br J Cancer* 1995; **71**: 1169–1174.

45. Tozer GM, Prise VE, Chaplin DJ. Inhibition of nitric oxide synthase induces a selective reduction in tumor blood flow that is reversible with L-arginine. *Cancer Res* 1997; **57**: 948–955.

46. Okamoto T, Akaike T, Sawa T, Miyamoto Y, van der Vliet A, Maeda H. Activation of matrix metalloproteinases by peroxynitrite-induced protein S-glutathiolation via disulfide S-oxide formation. *J Biol Chem* 2001; **276**: 29596–29602.
47. Liotta LA, Kohn EC. Invasion and metastases. In: RC Bast Jr, JF HollanD, E Frei, et al. (eds) *Cancer Medicine*, ed. 5. Hamilton: B.C. Decker Inc, pp. 121–131, 2000.
48. Chambers AF, Matrisian LM. Changing views of the role of matrix metalloproteinases in metastasis. *J Natl Cancer Inst* 1997; **89**: 1260–1270.
49. Wu J, Akaike T, Hayashida K, Okamoto T, Okuyama A and Maeda H. Enhanced vascular permeability in solid tumor involving peroxynitrite and matrix metalloproteinases. *Jpn J Cancer Res* 2001; **92**: 439–451.
50. H. Maeda, Fang J, Inutsuka T, Kitamoto Y. Vascular permeability enhancement in solid tumor: various factors, mechanisms involved and its implications. *Int Immunopharmacol* 2003; **3**: 319–328.
51. Senger DR, Galli SJ, Dvorak AM, Perruzzi CA, Harvey VS, Dvorak HF. Tumor cells secrete a vascular permeability factor that promotes accumulation of ascites fluid. *Science* 1983; **219**: 983–985.
52. Dvorak HF, Nagy JA, Feng D, Brown LF, Dvorak AM. Vascular permeability factor/vascular endothelial growth factor and the significance of microvascular hyperpermeability in angiogenesis. *Curr Top Microbiol Immunol* 1999; **237**: 97–132.
53. Tanaka S, Akaike T, Wu J, Fang J, Sawa T, Ogawa M, Beppu T, Maeda H. Modulation of tumor-selective vascular blood flow and extravasation by the stable prostaglandin I_2 analogue beraprost sodium. *J Drug Target* 2003; **1**: 45–52.
54. Duncan R. Polymer conjugates as anticancer nanomedicines. *Nat Rev Cancer* 2006; **6**: 688–701.
55. Peer D, Karp JM, Hong S, Farokhzad OC, Margalit R, Langer R. Nanocarriers as an emerging platform for cancer therapy. *Nat Nanotech* 2007; **2**: 751–760.
56. Kakizawa Y, Kataoka K. Block copolymer micelles for delivery of gene and related compounds. *Adv Drug Deliv Rev* 2002; **54**: 203–222.
57. Davis ME, Chen Z, Shin DM. Nanoparticle therapeutics: an emerging treatment modality for cancer. *Nat Rev Drug Discov* 2008; **7**: 771–782.
58. Vicent MJ, Duncan R. Polymer conjugates: Nanosized medicines for treating cancer. *Trend Biotechnol* 2006; **24**: 39–47.
59. Maeda H, Matsumoto T, Konno T, Iwai K, Ueda M. Tailor-making of protein drugs by polymer conjugation for tumor targeting: A brief review on smancs. *J Protein Chem* 1984; **3**: 181–193.
60. Maeda H, Takeshita J, Kanamaru R. A lipophilic derivative of neocarzinostatin. A polymer conjugation of an antitumor protein antibiotic. *Int J Pept Protein Res* 1979; **14**: 81–87.
61. Maeda H, Ueda M, Morinaga T, Matsumoto T. Conjugation of poly(styrene-co-maleic acid) derivatives to the antitumor protein neocarzinostatin: Pronounced improvements in pharmacological properties. *J Med Chem* 1985; **28**: 455–461.
62. Suzuki M, Hori K, Abe I, Saito S, Sato H. A new approach to cancer chemotherapy: A selective enhancement of tumor blood flow with angiotensin II. *J Natl Cancer Inst* 1981; **67**: 663–669.
63. Hori K, Suzuki M, Tanda S, Saito D, Shinozaki M, Zhang QH. Fluctuations in tumor blood flow under normotension and the effect of angiotensin II-induced hypertension. *Jpn J Cancer Res* 1991; **82**: 1309–1316.
64. Li CJ, Miyamoto Y, Kojima Y, Maeda H. Augmentation of tumour delivery of macromolecular drugs with reduced bone marrow delivery by elevating blood pressure. *Br J Cancer* 1993; **67**: 975–980.
65. Hori K, Saito S, Takahashi H, Sato H, Maeda H, Sato Y. Tumor-selective blood flow decrease induced by an angiotensin converting enzyme inhibitor, temocapril hydrochloride. *Jpn J Cancer Res* 2000; **91**: 261–269.

66. Strausser HR, Humes JL. Prostaglandin synthesis inhibition: Effect on bone changes and sarcoma tumor induction in balb/c mice. *Int J Cancer* 1975; **15**: 724–730.
67. Trevisani A, Ferretti E, Capuzzo A, Tomasi V. Elevated levels of prostaglandin E2 in Yoshida hepatoma and the inhibition of tumour growth by non-steroidal anti-inflammatory drugs. *Br J Cancer* 1980; **41**: 341–347.
68. Seki T, Fang J, and Maeda H. Enhanced antitumor drug-delivery by topical applications of nitroglycerine on superficial tumors. *Nitric Oxide* 2008; **19**: S68.
69. Torchilin VP. Drug targeting. *Eur J Pharmaceut Sci* 2000; **11**: S81–S91.
70. Maeda H, Aikawa S, Yamashita A. Subcellular fate of protein antibiotic neocarzinostatin in culture of a lymphoid cell line from Burkitt's lymphoma. *Cancer Res* 1975; **35**: 554–559.
71. Oda T, Maeda H. Binding to and internalization by cultured cells of neocarzinostatin and enhancement of its actions by conjugation with lipophilic styrene-maleic acid copolymer. *Cancer Res* 1987; **47**: 3206–3211.
72. Miyamoto Y, Oda T, Maeda H. Comparison of the cytotoxic effects of the high- and low-molecular-weight anticancer agents on multidrug-resistant Chinese hamster ovary cells *in vitro*. *Cancer Res* 1990; **50**: 1571–1575.
73. Leamon CP, Reddy JA, Vlahov IR, Kleindl PJ, Vetzel M, Westrick E. Synthesis and biological evaluation of EC140: A novel folate-targeted vinca alkaloid conjugate. *Bioconjug Chem* 2006; **17**: 1226–1232.
74. Miyajima Y, Nakamura H, Kuwata Y, Lee JD, Masunaga S, Ono K, Maruyama K. Transferrin-loaded *nido*-carborane liposomes: Tumor-targeting boron delivery system for neutron capture therapy. *Bioconjug Chem* 2006; **17**: 1314–1320.
75. Pellegrin P, Fernandez A, Lamb NJC, Bennes R. Macromolecular uptake is a spontaneous event during mitosis in cultured fibroblasts: Implications for vector-dependent plasmid transfection. *Mol Biol Cell* 2002; **13**: 570–578.
76. Shaffer SA, Baker-Lee C, Kennedy J, Lai MS, de Vries P, Buhler K, Singer JW. In vitro and in vivo metabolism of paclitaxel poliglumex: identification of metabolites and active proteases. *Cancer Chemother Pharmacol* 2007; **59**: 537–548.
77. Duncan R. Polymer conjugates for tumour targeting and intracytoplasmic delivery. The EPR effect as a common gateway? *Pharm Sci Technol Today* 1999; **2**: 441–449.
78. Duncan R. The dawning era of polymer therapeutics. *Nat Rev Drug Discov* 2003; **2**: 347–360.
79. Duncan R, Gac-Breton S, Keane R, Musila R, Sat YN, Satchi R, Searle F. Polymer-drug conjugates, PDEPT and PELT: Basic principles for design and transfer from the laboratory to clinic. *J Control Release* 2001; **74**: 135–146.
80. Ferruti P, Marchisio MA, Duncan R. Poly(amido-amine)s: Biomedical applications. *Macromol Rapid Commun* 2002; **23**: 332–355.
81. Greish K, Nagamitsu A, Fang J, Maeda H. Copoly(styrene-maleic acid)-pirarubicin micelles: High tumor-targeting efficiency with little toxicity. *Bioconjug Chem* 2005; **16**: 230–236.
82. Greish K, Sawa T, Fang J, Akaike T, Maeda H. SMA-doxorubicin, a new polymeric micellar drug for effective targeting to solid tumours. *J Control Release* 2004; **97**: 219–230.
83. Matsumura Y, Hamaguchi T, Ura T, Muro K, Yamada Y, Shimada Y, Shirao K, Okusaka T, Ueno H, Ikeda M, Watanabe N. Phase I clinical trial and pharmacokinetic evaluation of NK911 amicelle-encapsulated doxorubicin. *Br J Cancer* 2004; **91**: 1775–1781.
84. Gabizon A, Shmeeda H, Barenholz Y. Pharmacokinetics of pegylated liposomal doxorubicin. *Clin Pharmacokinet* 2003; **42**: 419–436.
85. Miyamoto Y, Maeda H. Enhancement by verapamil of neocarzinostatin action on multidrug-resistant Chinese ovary cells: Possible release of nonprotein chromophore in cells. *Jpn J Cancer Res* 1991; **82**: 351–356.
86. Šťastný M, Strohalm J, Plocová D, Ulbrich K, Říhová B. A possibility to overcome P-glycoprotein (PGP)-mediated multidrug resistance by antibody-targeted drugs conjugated to N-(2-hydroxypropyl)methacrylamide (HPMA) copolymer carrier. *Eur J Cancer* 1999; **35**: 459–466.

87. Minko T, Kopečková P, Pozharov V, Kopeček J. HPMA copolymer bound adriamycin overcomes *MDR1* gene encoded resistance in a human ovarian carcinoma cell line. *J Control Release* 1998; **54**: 223–233.
88. Minko T, Batrakova EV, Li S, Li Y, Pakunlu RI, Alakhov VY, Kabanov AV. Pluronic block copolymers alter apoptotic signal transduction of doxorubicin in drug-resistant cancer cells. *J Control Release* 2005; **105**: 269–278.
89. Zalipsky S, Saad M, Kiwan R, Ber E, Yu N, Minko T. Antitumor activity of new liposomal prodrug of mitomycin C in multidrug resistant solid tumor: Insights of the mechanism of action. *J Drug Target* 2007; **15**: 518–530.
90. Li C, Yu DF, Newman RA, Cabral F, Stephens LC, Hunter N, Milas L, Wallace S. Complete regression of well-established tumors using a novel water-soluble poly(L-glutamic acid)-paclitaxel conjugate. *Cancer Res* 1998; **58**: 2404–2409.
91. Li C, Ke S, Wu QP, Tansey W, Hunter N, Buchmiller LM, Milas L, Charnsangavej C, Wallace S. Tumor irradiation enhances the tumor-specific distribution of poly(L-glutamic acid)-conjugated paclitaxel and its antitumor efficacy. *Clin Cancer Res* 2000; **6**: 2829–2834.
92. Matsumura Y. Preclinical and clinical studies of anticancer drug-incorporated polymeric micelles. *J Drug Target* 2007; **15**: 507–517.
93. Li LH, Fraser TJ, Olin EJ, Bhuyan BK. Action of camptothecin on mammalian cells in culture. *Cancer Res* 1972; **32**: 2643–2650.
94. Gallo RC, Whang-Peng J, Adamson RH. Studies on the antitumor activity, mechanism of action, and cell cycle effects of camptothecin. *J Natl Cancer Inst* 1971; **46**: 789–795.
95. Yokoyama M, Okano T, Sakurai Y, Ekimoto H, Shibazaki C, Kataoka K. Toxicity and antitumor activity against solid tumors of micelle-forming polymeric anticancer drug and its extremely long circulation in blood. *Cancer Res* 1991; **51**: 3229–3236.
96. Koizumi F, Kitagawa M, Negishi T, Onda T, Matsumoto S, Hamaguchi T, Matsumura Y. Novel SN-38-incorporating polymeric micelles, NK012, eradicate vascular endothelial growth factor-secreting bulky tumors. *Cancer Res* 2006; **66**: 10048–10056.
97. Yokoyama M, Miyauchi M, Yamada N, Okano T, Sakurai Y, Kataoka K, Inoue S. Polymer micelles as novel drug carrier: Adriamycin-conjugated poly(ethylene glycol)-poly(aspartic acid) block copolymer. *J Control Release* 1990; **11**: 269–278.
98. Kataoka K, Kwon GS, Yokoyama M, Okano T, Sakurai Y. Block copolymer micelles as vehicles for drug delivery. *J Control Release* 1993; **24**: 119–132.
99. Hamaguchi T, Kato K, Yasui H, Morizane C, Ikeda M, Ueno H, Muro K, Yamada Y, Okusaka T, Shirao K, Shimada Y, Nakahama H, Matsumura Y. A phase I and pharmacokinetic study of NK105, a paclitaxel-incorporating micellar nanoparticle formulation. *Br J Cancer* 2007; **97**: 170–176.
100. Mastumura Y. Poly(amino acid) micelle nanocarriers in preclinical and clinical studies. *Adv Drug Del Rev* 2008; **60**: 899–914.
101. Nishiyama N, Okazaki S, Cabral H, Miyamoto M, Kato Y, Sugiyama Y, Nishio K, Matsumura Y, Kataoka K. Novel cisplatin-incorporated polymeric micelles can eradicate solid tumors in mice. *Cancer Res* 2003; **63**: 8977–8983.
102. Uchino H, Matsumura Y, Negishi T, Koizumi F, Hayashi T, Honda T, Nishiyama N, Kataoka K, Naito S, Kakizoe T. Cisplatin-incorporating polymeric micelles (NC-6004) can reduce nephrotoxicity and neurotoxicity of cisplatin in rats. *Br J Cancer* 2005; **93**: 678–687.
103. Ishida O, Maruyama K, Tanahashi H, Iwatsuru M, Sasaki K, Eriguchi M, Yanagie H. Liposomes bearing polyethyleneglycol-coupled transferrin with intracellular targeting property to the solid tumors in vivo. *Pharmaceutical Res* 2001; **18**: 1042–1048.
104. Suzuki R, Takizawa T, Kuwata Y, Mutoh M, Ishiguro N, Utoguchi N, Shinohara A, Eriguchi M, Yanagie H, Maruyama K. Effective anti-tumor activity of oxaliplatin encapsulated in transferrin-PEG-liposome. *Int J Pharm* 2008; **346**: 143–150.

105. Kondo R, Gleixner KV, Mayerhofer M, Vales A, Gruze A, Samorapoompichit P, Greish K, Krauth MT, Aichberger KJ, Pickl WF, Esterbauer H, Sillaber C, Maeda H, Valent P. Identification of heat shock protein 32 (Hsp32) as a novel survival factor and therapeutic target in neoplastic mast cells. *Blood* 2007; **110**: 661–669.
106. Doi K, Akaike T, Fujii S, Tanaka S, Ikebe N, Beppu T, Shibahara S, Ogawa M, Maeda H. Induction of haem oxygenase-1 by nitric oxide and ischaemia in experimental solid tumours and implications for tumour growth. *Br J Cancer* 1999; **80**: 1945–1954.
107. Fang J, Sawa T, Akaike T, Akuta T, Sahoo SK, Khaled G, Hamada A, Maeda H. In vivo antitumor activity of pegylated zinc protoporphyrin: Targeted inhibition of heme oxygenase in solid tumor. *Cancer Res* 2003; **63**: 3567–3574.
108. Tanaka S, Akaike T, Fang J, Beppu T, Ogawa M, Tamura F, Miyamoto Y, Maeda H. Antiapoptotic effect of haem oxygenase-1 induced by nitric oxide in experimental solid tumour. *Br J Cancer* 2003; **88**: 902–909.
109. Fang J, Akaike T, Maeda H. Antiapoptotic role of heme oxygenase (HO) and the potential of HO as a target in anticancer treatment. *Apoptosis* 2004; **9**: 27–35.
110. Sahoo SK, Sawa T, Fang J, Tanaka S, Miyamoto Y, Akaike T, Maeda H. Pegylated zinc protoporphyrin: A water-soluble heme oxygenase inhibitor with tumor-targeting capacity. *Bioconjug Chem* 2002; **13**: 1031–1038.
111. Fang J, Sawa T, Akaike T, Greish K, Maeda H. Enhancement of chemotherapeutic response of tumor cells by a heme oxygenase inhibitor, pegylated zinc protoporphyrin. *Int J Cancer* 2004; **109**: 1–8.
112. Mayerhofer M, Gleixner KV, Mayerhofer J, Hoermann G, Jaeger E, Aichberger KJ, Ott RG, Greish K, Nakamura H, Derdak S, Samorapoompichit P, Pickl WF, Sexl V, Esterbauer H, Schwarzinger I, Sillaber C, Maeda H, Valent P. Targeting of heat shock protein 32 (Hsp32)/heme oxygenase-1 (HO-1) in leukemic cells in chronic myeloid leukemia: a novel approach to overcome resistance against imatinib. *Blood* 2008; **111**: 2200–2210.
113. Hadzijusufovic E, Rebuzzi L, Gleixner KV, Ferenc V, Peter B, Kondo R, Gruze A, Kneidinger M, Krauth MT, Mayerhofer M, Samorapoompichit P, Greish K, Iyer AK, Pickl WF, Maeda H, Willmann M, Valent P. Targeting of heat-shock protein 32/heme oxygenase-1 in canine mastocytoma cells is associated with reduced growth and induction of apoptosis. *Exp Hematol* 2008; **36**: 1461–1470.
114. Gleixner KV, Mayerhofer M, Vales A, Gruze A, Pickl WF, Lackner E, Sillaber C, Zielinski CC, Maeda H, Valent P. The Hsp32/HO-1-targeted drug SMA-ZnPP counteracts the proliferation and viability of neoplastic cells in solid tumors and hematologic neoplasms. *J Clin Oncol* 2007; **25**: 14122.
115. Regehly M, Greish K, Rancan F, Maeda H, Böhm F, Röder B. Water-soluble polymer conjugates of ZnPP for photodynamic therapy. *Bioconjug Chem* 2007; **18**: 494–499.
116. Iyer AK, Greish K, Seki T, Okazaki S, Fang J, Takeshita K, Maeda H. Polymeric micelles of zinc protoporphyrin for tumor targeted delivery based on EPR effect and singlet oxygen generation. *J Drug Target* 2007; **15**: 496–506.
117. Maeda H. Role of microbial proteases in pathogenesis. *Microbiol Immunol* 1996; **40**: 685–699.

Multidrug Resistance in Solid Tumor and Its Reversal

Ho Lun Wong, Xiao Yu Wu, and Reina Bendayan

1 Introduction

Chemotherapy was first used for the treatment of advanced lymphomas in the 1940s [1]. Since then several classes of chemotherapeutic compounds such as alkylating agents, antimetabolites, anthracyclines, plant alkaloids, and later topoisomerase inhibitors and taxanes have been identified or synthesized to treat various forms of cancer [2, 3]. Although numerous in vitro and animal studies have demonstrated their effectiveness in inducing cancer cell death (cytotoxic) or cell growth arrest (cytostatic), these promising anticancer activities seen in the controlled environment of the laboratory frequently do not translate well into the expected clinical outcomes [4–8].

Some cancer types such as hepatocellular cancer and thyroid cancer basically do not respond to chemotherapy [9]. These cancers are intrinsically drug-resistant. For most of the other cancer types, chemotherapy is occasionally curative when the cancers are still in the early stage and remain localized, but once the diseases progress into the advanced stage and metastasize, the cure rates will significantly decline [9, 10]. This is particularly true for solid tumors including prostate cancer, breast cancer, ovarian cancer, colorectal cancer, bladder cancer, osteosarcoma, and head and neck cancers. For example, the 10-year survival rate for localized prostate cancer (stage A1) was estimated as 95%, whereas fewer than 1% of patients with stage D2 (metastasized) will be cured [10]. A similar trend is seen in the node-negative breast cancer patients, in which chemotherapy produced an absolute survival benefit of 5.7%, which drops to 2.3% when the cancer spreads to the lymph nodes, and when the cancer becomes metastatic, it is essentially incurable [11]. These cancers can acquire drug resistance during the course of treatment. In order to develop effective strategies to overcome the drug resistance, its underlying mechanisms must be identified and understood.

H.L. Wong (✉)
School of Pharmacy, Temple University, 3307 North Broad Street, Philadelphia,
PA 19140, USA
e-mail: ho-lun.wong@temple.edu

Y. Lu, R.I. Mahato (eds.), *Pharmaceutical Perspectives of Cancer Therapeutics*,
DOI 10.1007/978-1-4419-0131-6_4, © Springer Science+Business Media, LLC 2009

"Multidrug resistance" (MDR) phenotype is one of the first studied elements that underlie the observed clinical drug resistance. MDR in cancer is defined as the cross-resistance or insensitivity of cancer cells to the cytotoxic or cytostatic activity of a broad spectrum of anticancer compounds which are structurally or functionally distinct and have different molecular targets [12]. The first correlation between this phenomenon and membrane drug transporters was established in mid-1970s [13], and later these membrane-bound transporters were purified and shown to be the members of the ATP-binding cassette (ABC) transporter superfamily [14, 15]. P-glycoprotein (P-gp) is the first and probably most characterized ABC transporter that is related to the MDR phenotype. By causing efflux of drug molecules from cancer cells, P-gp can effectively lower the intracellular drug concentration and protect the cells from the drug actions [16, 17]. The discovery of this P-gp-mediated "classical" MDR phenotype quickly triggered extensive research in this field, and it was soon found that other ABC transporters such as multidrug resistance-associated proteins (MRP) [18] and breast cancer resistance protein (BCRP) [19] also contribute to drug resistance in a similar manner.

Meanwhile, more alternative drug resistance mechanisms in cancer were revealed. The majority of these mechanisms involve dysfunctional or altered molecular pathways which lead to diminished anticancer drug effects [20–22]. Table 1 provides an update of some of these mechanisms and the therapeutic agents for overcoming these forms of resistance. In this chapter, our focus will be on the ABC transporter mechanism. In order to overcome MDR, chemical entities that reverse the MDR mechanisms mainly by inhibition of the ABC transporter functions, sometimes known as "chemosensitizers" or "MDR reversal agents" [23], have been discovered or designed with the purpose to restore the sensitivity of cancer to chemotherapy. Although promising findings were obtained with some of these compounds, in general this class of drugs is less effective than expected. However, with better understanding of cancer biology such as the role of cancer progenitor/stem cells, and the tremendous advances made in the development of novel therapeutics such as nanomedicine and molecular targeting strategies in the past few years [22, 23], there are strong signs indicating the revival of the interest in MDR reversal treatment.

2 Multidrug Resistance Mediated by ATP-Binding Cassette (ABC) Transporters

2.1 ABC Transporters – Classification, Structure, and Drug Efflux Mechanism

The ABC transporter superfamily consists of a variety of transmembrane proteins, many of them responsible for the transport of diverse classes of substrates that include not only anticancer drug molecules but also lipids, sterols, polypeptides, ions, and metabolic products across extracellular and

Table 1 Cellular drug resistance mechanisms

Type of drug resistance	Mechanism	Therapeutic agents to overcome drug resistance
Increased cellular drug efflux	Overexpression of ABC transporters, e.g., P-gp, MRP1, BCRP	MDR reversal agents (e.g., PSC833, XR9576, GG918)
Apoptosis evasion	Reduced sphingolipid ceramide generation or enhanced ceramide metabolism	Ceramide generation activator (e.g., gefitinib); ceramide metabolism inhibitors (e.g., LCL204, N-oleoylethanolamine)
	Increased level of surviving	Antisense oligonucleotide
	Overexpression of antiapoptotic Bcl-2 protein	Bcl-2 inhibitor (e.g., ABT-737), antisense therapy (e.g., Genasense G3139)
Increased survival signaling	Overexpressed and aberrantly activated EGFR	EGFR antibody (e.g., mAb-C225), antisense oligonucleotide
	Sustained or altered Wnt signaling	Anti-Wnt antibody
	Activated hedgehog signaling pathway	SMO inhibitor cyclopamine
	BCR-ABL expression	Tyrosine kinase inhibitors (e.g., Imatinib, dasatinib)
Drug detoxification	Overexpression of glutathione S-transferase	γ-Glutamylcysteine synthetase
Altered drug target	Mutation of tubulin	Not known
Enhanced DNA repair	Increased level of O^6-alkylguanine-DNA alkyltransferase	Not known

ABC, ATP-binding cassette; BCRP, breast cancer resistance protein; MRP1, multidrug resistance-associated proteins 1; P-gp, P-glycoprotein; Wnt, Wingless signaling pathway.

intracellular membranes [24]. They have been shown to play several physiological and pathological roles. In addition to cancer MDR, these transporters are also implicated in bacterial drug resistance, cystic fibrosis, and a number of inherited diseases [14]. So far 50 human ABC transporter members have been identified [25, 26]. Human Genome Organization classified these transporters into seven families based on the organization and sequence of their ATP-binding domain(s), also known as nucleotide-binding folds. Table 2 shows a list of human ABC transporters involved in MDR and their chemotherapeutic drug substrates.

Overall, all ABC transporters contain one or two ATP-binding domains located at the cytosolic side of the membranes and one or two transmembrane domains, each consists of 6–11 α-helices spanning across the phospholipids bilayer of the membrane several times [27, 28]. Ligand-binding site is found between the transmembrane domains. Recent studies have revealed the presence of several single nucleotide polymorphisms in the ABC transporter genes [29, 30]. However, the significance of these findings is not precisely known. ABC transporters are also sometimes classified into full transporters or half

Table 2 ABC transporter superfamily members associated with drug resistance

Gene	Transporter	Chemotherapeutic drug substrates
ABCA2	ABCA2	Estramustine
ABCA3	ABCA3	Doxorubicin, methotrexate, vinblastine
ABCB1/	P-gp /	Actinomycin-D, colchicine, daunorubicin, docetaxel,
mdr1	MDR1	doxorubicin, epirubicin, etoposide, methotrexate, mitomycin-C, mitoxantrone, paclitaxel, teniposide, vinblastine, vincristine
ABCC1	MRP1	Camptothecins, colchicine, daunorubicin, doxorubicin, etoposide, methotrexate, paclitaxel, vincristine, vinblastine
ABCC2	MRP2	Cisplatin, doxorubicin, etoposide, irinotecan, methotrexate, SN-38 (metabolite of irinotecan), vincristine, vinblastine
ABCC3	MRP3	Etoposide, methotrexate
ABCC4	MRP4	6-mercaptopurine, 6-thioguanine, methotrexate,
ABCC5	MRP5	6-mercaptopurine, 6-thioguanine
ABCC6	MRP6	Etoposide
ABCC11	MRP8	5-Fluorouracil
ABCG2	BCRP / MXR	Bisantrene, daunorubicin, doxorubicin, epirubicin, etoposide, flavopiridol, imatinib, irinotecan, methotrexate, mitoxantrone, SN-38, topotecan

ABC, ATP-binding cassette; BCRP, breast cancer resistance protein; MDR1, multidrug resistance 1; MRP1–MRP8, multidrug resistance-associated proteins 1–8; MXR, mitoxantrone resistance protein; P-gp, P-glycoprotein.

transporters. A full ABC transporter consists of two transmembrane domains and two ATP-binding domains, whereas a half transporter consists of only one of each [26]. Because two transmembrane domains and two ATP-binding domains are required for a transporter to be functional, half transporters need to form dimers to gain functionality.

The mechanism of drug transport by the ABC transporters has not been fully elucidated. It is known that when an ATP molecule binds to the ATP-binding domains, ATP hydrolysis occurs and a conformational change in these domains is induced. This change is eventually communicated to the transmembrane domains to alter the translocation pathway, so substrate transport is achieved [31–36]. However, how this series of events exactly happen is not completely known. Some groups hypothesized that an ABC transporter allows drug molecules to be transported through a central pore, but recent lines of evidence suggested that these transporters may more likely act like a hydrophobic "vacuum cleaner" or "flippase" [34, 35]. In this proposed scheme, substrate molecules crossing the membrane are intercepted by the transporters inside the phospholipid bilayers and "flipped" back to outside. It should be noted that this is an active process driven by the energy derived from ATP hydrolysis. ABC transporters are therefore able to create and maintain a thermodynamically unfavorable concentration gradient of their drug substrates across the cell membrane, and allow cancer cells overexpressing them to maintain a relatively drug-free intracellular environment during chemotherapy (see Fig. 1 for the scheme illustrating these events).

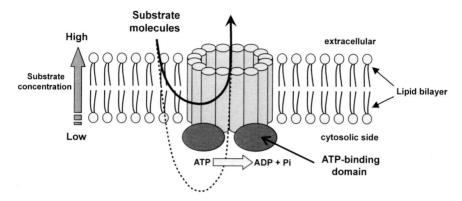

Fig. 1 Schematic representation of drug efflux by an ABC transporter. There are two possible ways substrates can be pumped out: substrates that enter the cytosolic compartment may be pumped out through the pore of the transporter (*dashed line*) or they may be intercepted by the pump in the lipid bilayer and flipped out (*solid line*). Hydrolysis of ATP provides the energy required for the drug efflux against the substrate concentration gradient across the membrane. Only the transmembrane domains and ATP-binding domains are shown in this scheme

2.2 P-glycoprotein (P-gp)

Among all ABC transporters, P-gp, also known as MDR1 protein, ABCB1 or CD243, is probably the most studied and characterized member. It was first found as a 170-kDa ATP-dependent membrane glycoprotein that acts as a drug efflux pump [15]. P-gp is a broad-spectrum transporter, capable of transporting several structurally and functionally unrelated substrate molecules. Its substrates are typically hydrophobic, amphipathic products, including many chemotherapeutic compounds used for cancer treatment, e.g., vinca alkaloids (vincristine, vinblastine), taxanes (paclitaxel, docetaxel), epipodophyllotoxins (etoposide, teniposide), anthracyclines (doxorubicin, daunorubicin, epirubicin), topotecan, dactinomycin, and mitomycin-C [37].

Although P-gp is best known for its contribution to MDR in cancer, this transporter is also recognized for its involvement in a variety of physiological functions, including removal of toxic metabolites and xenobiotics from healthy tissues into bile, intestinal lumen, and urine, maintenance of the barrier function of a number of sanctuary site tissues such as blood–brain barrier (BBB), placenta, and blood–testis barrier, and protection of hematopoietic stem cells from harmful substances [38–42]. In addition, P-gp was also found on the nuclear envelope and the membranes of several cytoplasmic organelles (e.g., endoplasmic reticulum, Golgi apparatus) in both normal and cancer cells [43, 44]. It is possible that these P-gp transporters may regulate the intracellular distribution of drug molecules, e.g., sequestration of anticancer drug molecules from important cell organelles to give the cancer cells additional drug resistance.

Experimental and clinical evidence points to the significance of P-gp in MDR. Mouse fibroblasts lacking functional P-gp were several times (3- to 16-fold) more sensitive to paclitaxel, anthracyclines, and vinca alkaloids than the P-gp-expressing parental cells [45]. Meanwhile, overexpression of P-gp is generally associated with increased cancer drug resistance. In humans, P-gp is the product of *MDR1* gene. Transfection of drug-sensitive, wild-type cancer cells with *MDR1* gene can lead to the subline manifesting MDR phenotype (e.g., drug-sensitive MDA435 human breast cancer cells into drug-resistant MDA435/LCC6/ MDR1 subline) [46]. It was shown that the MDR phenotype conferred by P-gp may be intrinsic or acquired. In epithelial cells of liver, colon, adrenal, pancreas, and kidneys, P-gp is normally expressed without previous exposure to chemotherapeutic agents. This ultimately results in the high basal levels of multidrug resistance in the cancers which affect these organs [9, 37, 47]. Genetic changes resulting in amplification of the *MDR1* gene may also be rapidly induced by exposure to high doses of chemotherapeutic drugs [48]. Alternatively, P-gp upregulation can be induced by prolonged exposure to suboptimal drug levels, or according to the "clonal selection" theory, it may also favor the proliferation of P-gp-overexpressing cells under the stress of cytotoxic drug exposure [49–51].

2.3 Other ABC Transporters Related to MDR

In addition to P-gp, there are other ABC transporters that may confer MDR phenotype to cancer cells. Like P-gp, multidrug resistance-associated proteins (MRPs), belonging to the ABCC subfamily, are ABC transporters normally expressed in the canalicular part of the hepatocyte where they play an important role in biliary transport [52]. Unlike P-gp, studies have shown that multiple members of MRP (MRP-1–MRP-8) are involved in cancer drug resistance (Table 2). Each member is responsible for the resistance to a number of anticancer compounds, including 5-fluorouracil, anthracyclines, vincristine, methotrexate, camptothecins, and etoposide. MRP also transport neutral or mildly anionic drug conjugates [53]. Many substrates of MRP are drug conjugates of lipophilic anions (e.g., glucuronate or glutathione conjugates).

BCRP (also known as ABCG2) is a half ABC transporter. It is sometimes known as mitoxantrone resistance protein (MXR) because of its elevated expression in many cancer cell lines selected with mitoxantrone [54]. BCRP was first identified in breast cancer, but it is also found in several normal tissues, including placenta, liver canaliculi, small intestine, colon, the bronchial epithelial layer in the lung, and endothelial cells [55]. Its level is also elevated in other cancer types. For instance, an analysis of 150 untreated tumors with immunohistochemical technique demonstrated a high incidence of BCRP overexpression particularly in tumors of gastrointestinal origin [56]. Elevated BCRP level is consistently associated with the phenotype that includes strong resistance to mitoxantrone, moderate resistance to anthracyclines, and sensitivity to paclitaxel, cisplatin, and vinca alkaloids, and is also implicated in drug resistance to newer anticancer compounds such as SN-38, topotecan, and etoposide [54, 57, 58–61].

Other less known ABC transporters such as ABCA2 and ABCA3 are also implicated in MDR. These two membrane transporters are members of the ABC1 subfamily. A high level of ABCA2 transporter is associated with the resistance to mitoxantrone and estramustine in small-cell lung cancer and ovarian cancer cell lines [62, 63], respectively. In these studies, ABCA2 transporter was found localized in the endolysosomal compartment. It was therefore suggested that ABCA2 transporter contributed to the MDR phenomenon by lysosomal detoxification instead of the most commonly seen drug efflux mechanism. In addition, increased levels of ABCA2 and ABCA3 transporters were also detected in pediatric T-cell acute lymphoblastic leukemia and acute myeloid leukemia using microarray and real-time polymerase chain reaction analyses [64, 65]. These cancer cells were shown more resistant to vinblastine, doxorubicin, and methotrexate.

3 Therapeutic Strategies Reversing Multidrug Resistance

3.1 MDR Reversal Agents Targeting ABC Transporters

Since 1980s a number of "MDR reversal agents" (Table 3) have been identified or synthesized to target different steps of the transporter-mediated MDR mechanism. The "first-generation" MDR reversal agents including verapamil, quinidine, cyclosporin A, tamoxifen, and a number of calmodulin antagonists are drugs commonly used for other therapeutic indications but found to possess P-gp modulatory activities [37]. In comparison, the MDR reversal agents of the newer generations were specifically designed for overcoming MDR. They are more potent and P-gp selective than the first-generation compounds. The second-generation agents including dex-verapamil, Valspodar (PSC833), and Biricodar (VX710) are novel analogs of the first-generation agents [67], whereas the third-generation agents including Tariquidar (XR9576) [68], Zosuquidar (LY335979) [69], Laniquidar (R101933) [70], ONT093 [71], and Elacridar (GF120918/GG918) [72] are synthetic molecules developed using structure–activity relationship and combinatorial chemistry. Some of these newer generation agents are effective in blocking the cellular drug efflux at micro- and even nano-molar ranges for extended time [68, 73]. In an in vitro study, the P-gp transporters remained blocked for more than 22 h after Tariquidar treatment had been withdrawn [74]. The in vivo activity of the second and third generation compounds has also been confirmed. Significantly increased tumor accumulation of P-gp substrates such as ^{99}m-Tc-Sestamibi was detected in patients treated with dex-verapamil, PSC833, or XR9576 [75–77].

The clinical efficacy of MDR reversal agents is less proven. A number of clinical trials have led to unsatisfactory outcomes [37] with several causes of failure identified. Because the first-generation agents often require high doses to

Table 3 MDR reversal agents for inhibition of ABC transporters

Primary target	MDR reversal agents	Notes
P-gp	First generation	
	Verapamil	Clinical benefit seen in breast cancer and NSCLC patients, but as a calcium channel blocker to lower blood pressure, frequent hypotension, and other intolerable cardiovascular side effects observed
	Cyclosporin A	As an immunomodulatory agent, may lead to nephrotoxicity. Moderately significant improvement seen in AML patients
	Quinidine	Frequent GI disturbances
	Tamoxifen	Also inhibit BCRP
	Second generation	
	Dex-verapamil	P-gp specific analog of verapamil
	PSC833 (Valspodar)	Non-immunosuppressive analog of cyclosporin A. Likely the most studied new-generation P-gp inhibitor. Some limited success in treating refractory cancers
	VX710 (Biricodar)	Also inhibit MRP1
	Third generation	
	GG918 (GF120918, Elacridar)	Also inhibit BCRP
	XR9576 (Tariquidar)	Also inhibit BCRP
	R101933 (Laniquidar)	
	LY335979 (Zosuquidar)	
	ONT093 (OC144093)	
	CBT1	
	Miscellaneous	
	Flavonoids	May inhibit other ABC transporters
	UIC2 monoclonal antibody	
MRP1	Tolmetin	
	NSAIDs	
BCRP	Gefitinib	
	Prazosin	
	C11033	

ABC, ATP-binding cassette; AML, acute mylogenous leukemia; NSCLC, non-small-cell lung cancer; NSAIDs, non-steroidal anti-inflammatory drugs; BCRP, breast cancer resistance protein; MDR1, multidrug resistance 1; MRP, multidrug resistance-associated proteins; P-gp, P-glycoprotein.

achieve the desired chemosensitization effect, they all carry high risks of toxicity (see Table 3). These agents and their second-generation analogs are also substrates for other important metabolic enzymes (e.g., cytochrome-P450) and transporter systems (e.g., organic cationic transporter), so undesirable pharmacokinetic interactions occasionally happened when they were combined with other anticancer agents [78]. For instance, increased serum concentrations of paclitaxel and vinblastine were observed when PSC833 was co-administered [79]. These interactions are usually too unpredictable to cope with by dose adjustment. The biggest challenge against the use of MDR reversal agents for cancer treatment relates to the clinical significance of MDR reversal. Some clinicians argued that P-gp overexpression is merely a prognostic indicator reflecting the aggressiveness of the cancer cells [80, 81]. Following this argument, inhibition of P-gp can only relieve a symptom, but cannot cure the cancer disease itself.

On the other hand, moderate but significant clinical benefits of MDR reversal agents were indeed observed in a few trials. For instance, the addition of cyclosporin A to the regimen of cytarabine and daunorubicin in acute myelogenous leukemia patients significantly improved the relapse-free survival (34% vs. 9%) and overall survival rates (22% vs. 12%) [82], with the best outcomes obtained in the subgroup showing the highest P-gp levels. A similar study with PSC833, the potent analog of cyclosporine-A, also resulted in significant improvement in the P-gp-overexpressing subgroup [83]. In a phase II trial conducted to study VX710 in patients with locally advanced or metastatic breast cancer resistant to paclitaxel, an 11% response rate was observed, although this was accompanied by a 40% incidence of grade 4 neutropenia [84].

Up to date, the clinical results of the third-generation compounds are pending. The data obtained so far have been inconclusive but showing signs of promise. At a minimum, most phase I trials indicate that they are safe and rarely lead to significant pharmacokinetic interactions [85]. Some adverse effects including mild cases of neutropenia and cardiac toxicity were detected in the trial of GG918, but they were generally moderate and reversible [86]. There are suggestions that treatment failures may be derived from the fact that these MDR reversal agents are unable to inhibit all of the ABC transporters responsible for the clinical drug resistance. This prompts some researchers to combine different MDR reversal agents at low doses, and improvement of efficacy was observed [87]. Finally, there were also researchers arguing that MDR reversal agents should be used together with other molecular targeting agents and in the context of cancer stem cell theory to be truly effective [22, 66]. It is obvious that further studies are required to determine how exactly MDR reversal agents should be used to achieve the optimal chemosensitizing effects in the clinical settings.

3.2 Reversal of MDR with Drug Carrier of Nano- or Micro-meter Size

Studies have shown that drug delivery systems such as microspheres, nanoparticles, and liposomes are able to improve the therapeutic index of cancer chemotherapy. These systems offer several advantages over the conventionally used free drug solution. (1) Drug carrier of submicron size can take advantage of the "enhanced permeability and retention (EPR)" effect [88] (also refer to Chapter 6 for details). These small carriers tend to extravasate into the tumor site and stay longer at this site, resulting in prolonged elevation of local tumor drug level. (2) The physicochemical parameters of a drug carrier, e.g., particle size, surface charge, and surface hydrophobicity/hydrophilicity, can be conveniently modified to achieve the optimal EPR effect and minimal binding to the body tissues and serum proteins. (3) A drug carrier can be further optimized by surface engineering for cancer targeting. For example, the carrier surface can be grafted with polyethylene glycol chains to achieve immunosurveillance evasion [89] or labeled with molecular targeting agents for enhanced specificity for the tumor cells expressing the corresponding surface targets [90]. For further information about the use of nanomedicine for cancer therapy refer to Chapter 21. Here we will focus on their use for overcoming MDR.

In general, particulate drug carriers can be used to reverse MDR by three ways: (1) intrinsic MDR reversal activities of drug carriers; (2) encapsulation and delivery of MDR reversal agents; (3) delivery of combinational therapy or unconventional anticancer agents; and (4) bypassing the membrane transporter resistance mechanisms. Some researchers also combined more than one of these approaches to obtain additional MDR reversal activity.

3.2.1 Intrinsic MDR Reversal Activities of Drug Carriers

It has long been recognized that nanoparticles are able to circumvent the effect of P-gp and deliver compounds across the P-gp-rich BBB without damaging its structural integrity [91, 92]. There are also reports of improved drug accumulation in the drug-resistant cancer cells in the absence of additional MDR reversal agents as long as the drugs are delivered by nanoparticle or liposomal systems [93, 94]. In addition, studies performed on both non-cancerous and cancerous tissues have demonstrated that some particulate formulations, even without any loaded drug, can inhibit the functions of membrane transporters [95, 96]. This suggests that some drug carriers possess their own intrinsic chemosensitizing properties.

Many drug carriers are made of hydrophobic materials such as lipids and poly(butyl cyanoacrylate). It will be thermodynamically unstable for submicron particles made of these materials to remain dispersed in an aqueous environment such as blood circulation. Surfactants or block co-polymers are therefore routinely included in these formulations to prevent particle aggregation. Studies showed that a number of these agents, most noticeably the nonionic surfactants such as polysorbates (also known as Tweens) and Tritons and block co-polymers such as poloxamers (also known as Pluronics), may inhibit the ABC transporters [97–99]. As previously discussed, ABC transporters interact with their substrates in the lipid bilayers of the plasma membrane. Surfactants can disrupt the arrangement of the lipid bilayer expressing the transporters and subsequently inhibit their drug efflux activities [97, 100]. It was shown that Triton-X-100-immobilized dextran microspheres can enhance vinblastine accumulation by Chinese hamster ovary cells by twofold [101].

Extensive studies have been conducted on the use of poloxamers for the delivery of anticancer drugs to MDR cells [99]. Poloxamers are non-ionic, amphiphilic polymers with surfactant properties. They can be used for nano-particle coating or directly as a chemosensitizer or form micelles for drug delivery [102, 103]. Studies conducted using the drug-resistant SKVLB ovarian cancer cell line showed that concurrent treatment with Pluronic P85 could lead to 80- to 1090-fold increases in the cellular accumulation of a range of che-motherapeutic compounds including daunorubicin, cisplatin, mitomycin-C, methotrexate, and vinblastine [104], and up to 2–3 orders of magnitude increase in the cytotoxicity. It was suggested that in addition to causing inhibition of the ABC transporters, poloxamer-based carriers also compromise a number of alternative drug resistance mechanisms, including prevention of drug seques-tration by acidic vesicles, inhibition of glutathione/glutathione S-transferase detoxification system, and reduction in the intracellular ATP levels in the MDR cells [105, 106]. The last mechanism is noteworthy as drug resistance is a multi-factorial phenomenon, and many of the mechanisms involved, e.g., ABC trans-porters, are ATP-dependent. By depleting their common energy source, the drug resistance problem could be more effectively controlled.

3.2.2 Encapsulation and Delivery of MDR Reversal Agents

The use of MDR reversal agents is frequently limited by their side effects, risk of inducing drug interactions, and unfavorable physicochemical properties. It was reasoned that these limitations can be at least in part overcome by encapsulat-ing and delivering these agents with drug carriers. Using the previously men-tioned Triton-linked microsphere system as an example, significant reduction in the toxicity was achieved by immobilization of Triton-X-100 molecules on dextran particles [101]. In addition, some MDR reversal agents are poorly soluble in water, and are therefore more efficiently administered using lipid-based or hydrophobic polymer carrier systems. For example, cyclosporin A could be easily delivered using solid lipid nanoparticles [107]. The analog of cyclosporin A, PSC833, was delivered by liposomes made of intralipids for in vivo inhibition of P-gp at the BBB in primates [108]. In this study the AUC_{brain}/AUC_{blood} ratio of ^{11}C-verapmail(as a P-gp substrate) radioactivity was increased 2.3-fold with the addition of PSC833-liposomes.

Recently, the concept of simultaneous delivery of cytotoxic anticancer com-pounds and MDR reversal agents has been studied. Polymer–lipid hybrid nanoparticle (PLN) systems co-loaded with doxorubicin (cytotoxic compound) and verapamil (as MDR reversal agent) or GG918 were prepared [109]. It was found that the dual-loaded system resulted in the highest accumulation of doxorubicin in the drug-resistant MDA435/MDR1 breast cancer. The doxor-ubicin-mediated cell kill was also improved by nearly an order of magnitude when compared to the combination of free doxorubicin and GG918 solution.

These studies also showed that when the cytotoxic drug/MDR reversal agent combination was delivered in a single drug carrier instead of two separate carrier systems, the anticancer effect as measured by clonogenic assays was several times stronger. It was suggested that the use of cytotoxic drug/chemosensitizer co-loaded carrier system may provide enhanced MDR reversal effect due to elevated local levels of both agents near the membrane transporters (Fig. 2). Additional chemosensitization may also be achieved by particle endocytosis.

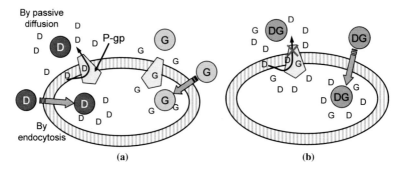

Fig. 2 Schematic illustration of the proposed mechanism of importance of the precise spatial distribution of encapsulated cytotoxic drug and chemosensitizer in the combinational treatment. (**a**) Single agent-loaded PLNs, (**b**) dual agent-loaded PLN. D – cytotoxic drug doxorubicin, G – chemosensitizer GG918, DG – doxorubicin and GG918 co-loaded (adapted from Wong et al. [110])

3.2.3 Delivery of Combinational Therapy or Unconventional Anticancer Agents

Synergistic anticancer effects can sometimes be achieved by combining multiple chemotherapeutic compounds in the chemotherapy (i.e., polytherapy), especially when these compounds use different cytotoxic mechanisms, e.g., doxorubicin and mitomycin-C [111]. Cancer cells are less likely to develop several different drug resistance mechanisms to counteract the therapy. The main drawback of this strategy is the increased risk of side effects [3]. This risk may be reduced by delivering the polytherapy with drug carrier. In recent studies, it was shown that PLN delivering both doxorubicin and mitomycin-C could reduce the colony-forming ability of the P-gp overexpressing MDA435/MDR1 breast cancer cells to nearly 1%. This effect was particularly strong when the two agents were dual loaded and delivered using the same PLN. As shown in Fig. 3, significantly higher DNA double-strand breaks were obtained with the dual-loaded PLN.

Instead of treating drug-resistant cancers with multiple chemotherapeutic compounds to achieve better cytotoxic effect, some researchers turn to novel therapeutic agents which remain effective against MDR cells. Many of these unconventional therapeutic agents such as oligonucleotides and small-interfering RNA (i.e., siRNA) are often fairly unstable in vivo [113, 114]. This problem can be overcome by encapsulating them in drug carriers. Recently our group has been

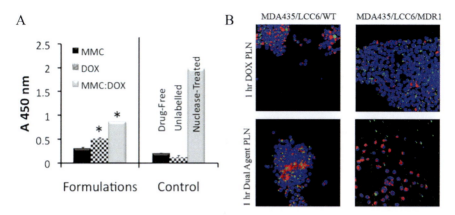

Fig. 3 Induction of DNA double-strand breaks by single and dual agent PLN formulations. (**A**) MDA435/LCC6/WT cells were treated with drug–PLN formulation containing 1.2 μM DOX and 0.6 μM MMC for 1 h prior to processing by the TUNEL assay for DNA double-strand break induction. Data are the mean ± standard deviations of three independent trials. *Significant increase in DNA double-strand breaks relative to drug-free control ($p<0.05$). (**B**) Qualitative determination of the source of DNA double-strand breaks as drug- or apoptosis-induced by immunocytochemistry. DNA double-strand breaks are indicated by activated Phospho γH2AX staining (*red*), apoptosis was detected through staining against active Caspase 3 (*green*) and nuclei were stained *blue*. Cells were treated with drug–PLN formulation containing 1.2 μM DOX and 0.6 μM MMC for 1 h prior to processing. Images were acquired with 20× objective lens (adapted from Shuhendler et al. [111])

studying the use of microspheres encapsulated with glucose oxidase (GOX) for MDR cancer treatment [115]. We found that cancer cells can be extensively killed by the reactive oxidative species generated by the encapsulated GOX enzyme. The most appealing feature of this therapy is that the GOX-mediated cytotoxic effect is essentially unaffected by the MDR phenotype (Fig. 4). Further studies will be conducted to optimize this strategy.

3.2.4 Bypassing Membrane Transporter Resistance Mechanism by Endocytosis

Drug delivery to cancer cells commonly involves release of drug molecules from the drug carrier located at the proximity of the cells, and diffusion of these released free drug molecules across the cell membrane to reach the cytosol. However, when a drug carrier is of submicron size, it can alternatively take the endocytotic routes to deliver its full load of drugs to the cytoplasmic compartment [116]. In this manner, the drug molecules may bypass the interception by the membrane transporters and avoid efflux.

Several mechanisms of endocytotic pathways exist. These include clathrin-mediated endocytosis, caveolae-mediated endocytosis, macropinocytosis, and non-clathrin receptor-mediated endocytosis (Table 4). All of these pathways can be exploited for drug trafficking into resistant cancer cells. For example, the

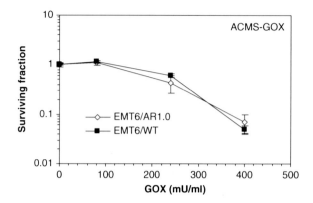

Fig. 4 Comparison of survival fractions of EMT6/WT and EMT6/AR1.0 cells treated for 1 h with different doses of ACMS-GOX. 5×10^5 cells were seeded in 10 cm Petri dishes containing 10 ml of growth medium 24 h before the treatment. The data points and error bars represent mean ± SD of at least three independent experiments, where not shown, the SDs lie within the symbols (ACMS-GOX: glucose oxidase-encapsulated alginate–chitosan microspheres) (adapted from Liu [115])

Table 4 Endocytotic pathways and their use for drug trafficking into drug-resistant cancer cells

Endocytotic pathways	Features	Examples of endocytotic transport	Applications for drug trafficking
Clathrin-mediated endocytosis	• Major and best characterized pathway • May involve receptors, trigger formation of clathrin-coated pits • Vesicles 100–150 nm, fuse with lysosomes (acidic/enzymatic process) • Highly regulated, energy-dependent	• Most of the receptor-mediated transport	• Targeting of LDL receptors at BBB with apolipoprotein-coated carriers for brain tumor treatment
Caveolae-mediated endocytosis	• Form flask-shaped invaginations of membrane (caveolae). Associate with cholesterol-binding proteins called caveolins • Common in endothelial cells • Smaller (50–60 nm) vesicles	• Cholesterol and glycosphingolipid transport • Transcytosis/endocytosis of some viruses	• Viral delivery of genes

Table 4 (continued)

Endocytotic pathways	Features	Examples of endocytotic transport	Applications for drug trafficking
	• Direct transport to ER and Golgi bodies. Non-acidic process		
Macropinocytosis	• Actin-driven evagination (ruffling) of plasma membrane • Form large (up to 5 μm) and leaky vesicles of irregular size and shape • No coat formed, no concentration of receptors. Vesicles do not fuse with lysosomes. Less acidic	• Fluid-phase endocytosis • Non-selective endocytosis of macromolecules	• TAT peptide-mediated delivery • Gene delivery with increased efficiency and stability • Potential use for carriers of larger size (e.g., SLN, PLN)
(Non-clathrin) receptor-mediated endocytosis	• Specific receptors • Clathrin independent	• Interleukin uptake into lymphocytes • Folate receptor-mediated uptake	• Delivery of imaging or therapeutic agents with folate-coated carriers (e.g., quantum dots, SLN)

BBB, blood–brain barrier; LDL, low-density lipoprotein; PLN, polymer–lipid hybrid nano-particles; SLN, solid lipid nanoparticles.

clathrin-mediated endocytotic pathway has been targeted to enhance the penetration of drug carrier into the BBB. In the studies by Kreuter et al., poly(butyl cyanoacrylate) nanoparticles coated with polysorbate-80 were formulated to treat brain diseases that are highly resistant to drug therapy [117]. The polysorbate-80 molecules on the carrier surface not only directly inhibited the P-gp at the BBB but also promoted apolipoproteins B and E adsorption on the nanoparticle surface [118]. These adsorbed apolipoproteins then in turn bound to the low-density-lipoprotein receptors on the endothelial cells forming the BBB and triggered clathrin-mediated endocytosis of the nanoparticles. As a result, these polysorbate-coated nanoparticles were able to efficiently deliver doxorubicin across the BBB, resulting in a significantly elevated AUC of doxorubicin in the brain and stronger anticancer effect against the intracranial glioblastoma in rat models [118].

Caveolae-mediated endocytosis is involved in viral transfection. This route can therefore be used for the delivery of oncolytic genetic materials by a viral vector [120]. Macropinocytosis is a relatively non-specific process which allows uptake of large particles up to the micron size range [121]. It is likely useful for the delivery of systems like solid lipid nanoparticles and PLN, which are frequently 200–300 nm in diameter. Macropinocytosis is also related to the uptake of TAT peptides [122]. One recent trend is the delivery of TAT-fusion products containing anticancer moieties to cancer cells. Significant anticancer activities were observed both in vitro and in vivo. In addition, macropinocytotic pathway leads to the formation of relatively leaky and non-acidic vesicles [123], and this feature has drawn scientists' interest to develop new forms of gene therapy which can escape into the cytoplasm with relative ease. Receptor-mediated endocytosis such as folate receptor-mediated uptake has also been studied for drug-resistant cancer targeting. Several drug-resistant cancers express elevated levels of folate receptors [124]. By linking to folate molecules, increased cellular uptake of quantum dots and solid lipid nanoparticles carrying cancer imaging agents and anticancer compounds have been demonstrated [125, 126].

It is now recognized that there are several therapeutic advantages of targeting the endocytotic routes for drug-resistant cancer therapy besides evasion of membrane transporters. It was suggested that when an anticancer compound is delivered by a particulate carrier, drug molecules can stay longer in the cytoplasmic compartment as it is unlikely for the membrane transporters to eliminate the particulate components. Figure 5 illustrates this strategy. P-gp-overexpressing breast cancer cells were treated with doxorubicin in free solution or nanoparticles. Two hours following the end of the treatment a high level of doxorubicin, a P-gp substrate, was shown mostly retained in the cancer cells when the drug was administered by nanoparticles, whereas most doxorubicin administered as free

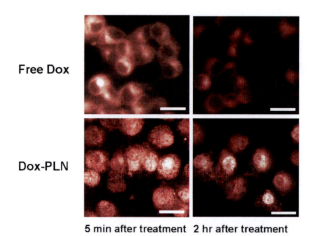

5 min after treatment 2 hr after treatment

Fig. 5 Fluorescence microscope images demonstrating the effect of drug carrier on the retention and intracellular distribution of doxorubicin (Dox) in MDA435/LCC6/MDR1 human breast cancer cells overexpressing P-gp. Cells were all incubated with Dox solution or nanoparticles containing Dox (Dox-PLN) for 2 h. Images were taken either within 5 min after the end of treatment or 2 h after the end of treatment and re-incubation in drug-free EBSS medium at 37°C. Enhanced retention of drugs and particles were observed when delivered in PLN form. Magnification of objective = 100×. Bars represent 20 μm (adapted from Wong et al. [127])

solution has been removed from the cytoplasm by P-gp [127]. By prolonging the retention time of the chemotherapeutic compounds in the cytoplasm, additional anticancer effects may be achieved.

In another study, doxorubicin was conjugated with the copolymer of *N*-(2-hydroxypropyl)methacrylamide (pHPMA). This conjugate was not equally efficaciousagainst both MDR and non-MDR cancers; long-term treatment of cancer cells with it also did not lead to the acquired MDR phenotype [128]. A recent study further indicated that pHPMA–doxorubicin could induce additional caspase-dependent apoptosis signaling pathways to trigger a stronger apoptotic response in cancer when compared to the free drug [129]. Overall, with better understanding of the endocytotic mechanisms, it is expected that more reasonable and efficient designs of drug carrier will be developed for effective therapy of chemoresistant cancers.

4 New Perspectives on Overcoming Multidrug Resistance in Solid Tumors

With better understanding of cancer biology, the role of ABC transporters has been recently redefined. It is now becoming clear that the drug resistance conferred by these membrane transporters needs to be considered within the context of the function of cancer progenitor cells and other forms of drug resistance such as non-cellular resistance in solid malignancies. Along this trend, it is also important to re-examine the field of MDR reversal and improve its therapeutic value.

4.1 Cancer Progenitor/Stem Cells and Multidrug Resistance

Cancer progenitor cells and their early progeny (e.g., cancer stem cells) are critical in generating a heterogeneous population of differentiated cancer cells to form a complete tumor [130–133]. Cancer stem cells are also capable of self-renewal when the size of their cell pool is reduced (refer to Chapter 16). From the therapeutic viewpoint, it is the response of the progenitor/stem cells, not their more differentiated descendants, to the treatment that determines whether a cancer is curable or not. If these groups of cells persist after treatment, they will eventually regenerate the differentiated cell subpopulations to reinitiate the malignant disease. Meanwhile, cancer progenitor/stem cells have been shown to be more susceptible to genetic mutations and can easily acquire the drug-resistant and aggressive phenotypes. This explains a number of phenomena including the acquired MDR phenotypes and the suboptimal clinical efficacy of many anticancer compounds that perform well in in vitro experiments. These cancer progenitor/stem cells are highly adaptive and can "get tough" during the course of chemotherapy. If they are not killed early, the risk of encountering drug resistance in the advanced stage will be far higher [66].

New paradigms for the treatment of drug-resistant cancer therefore need to incorporate the concepts of cancer progenitor/stem cells. Instead of reversing drug resistance of cancer cells in general, the inhibitors of drug resistance mechanisms such as the ABC transporters should be designed to specifically target the cancer progenitor/stem cells. There are many possibilities: (1) It was shown that cancer stem cells express high levels of different ABC transporter members, as indicated by the high efflux rates of a broad range of ABC transporter substrates including Hoechst dye, doxorubicin, 5-fluorouracil, gemcitabine, and mitoxantrone [134]. Among these transporters, BCRP are especially abundant [135]. MDR reversal agents that inhibit multiple transporters including BCRP (e.g., GG-918 and tariquidar) are therefore potentially more effective than the inhibitors that are too specific for one transporter. (2) It is also possible to directly link these MDR reversal agents to a progenitor/stem cell targeting agent such as antibody against the stem cell surface markers to enhance the treatment specificity and reduce the systemic toxicity. (3) Along this line of thoughts, the MDR reversal agents can be encapsulated and delivered using nanosized drug carrier surface engineered for cancer progenitor/stem cell targeting [66].

4.2 Other Molecular Pathways and Multidrug Resistance

A growing body of evidence shows that ABC transporters likely work in an integrated and interactive manner with other drug resistance pathways. By targeting these molecular pathways, it is sometimes possible to indirectly modulate the ABC transporters to achieve additional drug resistance reversal effects. For example, the activity of glucosylceramide synthase (GCS) was found elevated in some resistant forms of cancer [136]. GCS is an enzyme converting the pro-apoptotic ceramide into glucosylceramide, and a higher activity of GCS will decrease the cellular ceramide level and hence prevent the apoptotic death of cancer cells. It was found that inhibition of GCS by novel agents such as siRNA and D,L-threo-1-phenyl-2-palmitoylamino-3-morpholino-1-propanol also downregulated the overexpressed P-gp and enhanced the cellular uptake and activity of chemotherapeutic compounds [137, 138]. Another example is the epidermal growth factor receptor (EGFR) signaling pathway, which triggers the progression of several aggressive and resistant forms of cancer when activated. It was found that the use of gefitinib to modulate the dysfunctional EGFR signaling pathway may also inhibit the membrane transporter-mediated drug efflux. Sensitivity to several chemotherapeutic compounds such as mitoxantrone, topotecan, and SN-38 was restored in cancer cell lines selected to overexpress P-gp and/or BCRP [139, 140]. Cox-2 activity has also been recently linked to P-gp expression. Inhibition of Cox-2 with its inhibitor celecoxib was able to inhibit P-gp [141]. In the first of the above three examples, it was additionally shown that the inhibition of P-gp by PSC833 also stimulated the ceramide synthesis pathway, so the cancer cells became more vulnerable to apoptosis-inducing agents. It is apparent that this effect can spread between different drug resistance pathways in a two-way manner. When an ABC transporter is being targeted, attention must also be paid to whether additional chemosensitization effect is achieved via other pathways.

4.3 Solid Tumors and Multidrug Resistance

It was argued that this tumor microenvironment cannot be overlooked in the discussion of drug resistance and the related therapy. Solid tumors are not simple aggregates of tumor cells, but possess heterogeneous and structurally complex organ-like structures [142]. They are generally less sensitive to chemotherapy than malignancies consisting of circulating single cells, e.g., leukemia. This phenomenon is likely related to the unique microenvironment of solid tumors, including the formation of inaccessible spots in the tumor as a result of its poorly organized vasculature, impediment of drug diffusion by the high cell density in solid tumors, prevention of efficient convective flow from the blood vessel to the tumor by the elevated interstitial fluid pressure inside the tumor, deactivation of anticancer compounds by the acidic environment in the tumor core, the presence of extracellular matrix that may prevent drug penetration and increase the resistance of cancer cells to apoptosis, and the development of various resistance mechanisms in the hypoxic cancer cells located inside the tumor (e.g., entering quiescent state) [142]. In brief, the microenvironment in a solid tumor can both reduce the amount of drugs getting inside (pharmacokinetic barrier) and render the drugs that reach the target less active (pharmacodynamic barrier).

In the context of drug resistance and cancer stem cell theory, it is not hard to see that the task of killing cancer progenitor/stem cells can only get more difficult when these cells are packed densely together with their differentiated descendants in the solid tumor microenvironment. A significant portion of a solid tumor will inevitably receive drug therapy at sub-therapeutic concentrations. This is compounded by the fact that cancer progenitor/stem cells are intrinsically more drug resistant. Although recent studies showed that these cells might prefer to locate near the blood vessels [143], it was also found that some of the cells distal to blood vessels can repopulate tumors after chemotherapy, revealing the presence of some cancer stem cells situated deep inside the tumor mass [144]. A number of drug resistance reversal strategies are therefore developed to improve drug penetration, so these cells can become accessible to the therapy. Some of these strategies are listed in Table 5. Some exciting findings have been obtained. For example, a single dose of lipid nanoparticles for sustained release of doxorubicin injected intratumorally into a highly invasive EMT6 breast cancer was able to cause extensive cell death within the tumor core, and the subsequent growth of tumor was delayed by nearly 100% [145]. Nonetheless, in general, the use of these strategies is still largely in experimental stage. Whether these promising findings will translate into clinical use remains to be seen.

Table 5 Strategies to overcome the resistance to drug therapy by solid tumor

Strategy	Method used	References
Intratumoral therapy	Administration of nanoparticles intratumorally for sustained release of anticancer compounds	145
Tumor-priming	Pre-treatment of solid tumor with apoptosis-inducing agents (e.g., paclitaxel) to reduce cell density and trigger cell shrinkage, so subsequent nanoparticle/macromolecule treatment can penetrate better	146
Normalization of tumor vasculature	Targeting vascular endothelial growth factor (VEGF) receptors to prune the immature, abnormal blood vessels, so more efficient drug penetration is achieved	147
Degradation of extracellular matrix (ECM)	Collagenase or relaxin causes enzymatic degradation of ECM	148

5 Conclusion and Future Directions

Although the discovery of ABC transporters and their inhibitors represents an exciting approach to drug resistance reversal in cancer, this task is far from completion. It must be emphasized that clinical drug resistance is the result of multiple inter-related mechanisms interplaying in an integrated manner. However, with proper adjustment of the current paradigm for MDR reversal, this form of treatment will still prove to be extremely valuable. Further studies should provide us a better understanding of the interaction between the ABC transporter-mediated resistance mechanism and other drug resistance pathways. The MDR reversal therapy can be properly integrated with the agents targeting these pathways to achieve synergistic effects. More detailed characterization of cancer stem/progenitor cells and better understanding of the role of membrane transporter mechanisms in these cells is also needed. MDR reversal therapy should be designed to target these cancer cell subpopulations. To reach this goal the current MDR reversal therapy should be more effective. In addition to further improvement of the MDR reversal agents, the advances made in the development of novel experimental therapeutics such as nanomedicines and various solid tumor permeabilization techniques should also be considered. Further works will lead to the development of a more holistic and effective form of drug resistance reversal therapy.

References

1. Goodman LS, Wintrobe MM, Dameshek W, Goodman MJ, Gilman A, McLennan MT. Nitrogen mustard therapy. *JAMA* 1946; **132**: 126–132.
2. Hirsch J. An anniversary for cancer chemotherapy. *JAMA* 2006; **296**: 1518–1520.
3. Ewesuedo RB, Ratain MJ. Principles of cancer chemotherapy. In: Vokes EE, Golomb HM (ed). *Oncologic Therapies*. Springer, New York. 2003; pp. 19–67.

4. Baird RD, Kaye SB. Drug resistance reversal – are we getting closer. *Eur J Cancer* 2003; **39**: 2450–2461.
5. Mimeault M, Brand RE, Sasson AA, Batra SK. Recent advances on the molecular mechanisms involved in pancreatic cancer progression and therapies. *Pancreas* 2005; **31**: 301–316.
6. Mimeault M, Batra SK. Recent advances on multiple tumorigenic cascades involved in prostatic cancer progress and targeting therapies. *Carcinogenesis* 2006; **24**: 1–22.
7. Carrick S, Parker S, Wilcken N, Ghersi D, Marzo M, Simes J. Single agent versus combination chemotherapy for metastatic breast cancer. In: The Cochrane library (ed). *The Cochrane Database of Systematic Reviews.* John Wiley and Sons, Chichester, 2005.
8. Gieseler F, Rudolph P, Kloeppel G, Foelsch UR. Resistance mechanisms of gastrointestinal cancers: why does conventional chemotherapy fail? *Int J Colorectal Disease* 2003; **18**: 470–480.
9. Balmer CM, Valley AW, Iannucci A. Cancer treatment and chemotherapy. In: DiPiro JT, Talbert RL, Yee GC et al. (ed). *Pharmacotherapy: A Pathophysiologic Approach.* McGraw-Hill, New York, 2005; pp. 2279–2328.
10. Scardinao PT, Weaver R, Hudson MA. Early detection of prostate cancer. *Hum Pathol* 1992; **23**: 211–222.
11. NIH Consensus Development Conference Statement. Adjuvant therapy for breast cancer 2000, NIH. http://www.nih.gov. Accessed Sept. 25, 2008.
12. Biedler JL, Riehm H. Cellular resistance to actinomycin D in Chinese hamster cells in vitro: cross-resistance, radioautographic, and cytogenic studies. *Cancer Res* 1970; **30**: 1174–1184.
13. Juliano RL, Ling V. A surface glycoprotein modulating drug permeability in Chinese hamster ovary cell mutants. *Biochim Acta*1976; **455**: 152–162.
14. Glavinas H, Krajcsi P, Cserepes J, Sarkadi B. The role of ABC transporters in drug resistance, metabolism and toxicity. *Curr Drug Deliv* 2004; **1**: 27–42.
15. Riordan JR, Ling V. Purification of P-glycoprotein from plasma membrane vesicles of Chinese hamster ovary cell mutants with reduced colchicine permeability. *J Biol Chem* 1979; **254**: 12701–12705.
16. Riordan JR, Deuchars KK, Norbert AN, Noa A, Jeffrey T, Ling V. Amplification of P-glycoprotein genes in multidrug-resistant mammalian cell lines. *Nature* 1985; **316**: 817–819.
17. Debenham PG, Kartner N, Siminovitch L, Riordan JR, Ling V. DNA-mediated transfer of multiple drug resistance and plasma membrane glycoprotein expression. *Mol Cell Biol* 1982; **2**: 881–889.
18. Cole SP, Bhardwaj G, Gerlach JH, Mackie JE, Grant CE, Almquist KC, Stewart AJ, Kurz EU, Duncan AMV, Deeley RG. Overexpression of a transporter gene in a multi-drug-resistant human lung-cancer cell-line. *Science*1992; **258**: 1650–1654.
19. Doyle LA, Ross DD. Multidrug resistance mediated by the breast cancer resistance protein BCRP (ABCG2). *Oncogene* 2003; **22**: 7340–7358.
20. Mellor HR, Callaghan R. Resistance to chemotherapy in cancer: A complex and integrated cellular response. *Pharmacology* 2008; **81**: 275–300.
21. Chien AJ, Moasser MM. Cellular mechanisms of resistance to anthracyclines and taxanes in cancer: Intrinsic and acquired. *Semin Oncol* 2008; **35**: S1–S14.
22. Mimeault M, Hauke R, Batra SK. Recent advances on the molecular mechanisms involved in the drug resistance of cancer cells and novel targeting therapies. *Clin Pharmacol Therapeutics* 2008; **83**: 673–691.
23. Thomas H, Coley HM. Overcoming multidrug resistance in cancer: an update on the clinical strategy of inhibiting P-glycoprotein. *Cancer Control* 2003; **10**: 159–165.
24. Gottesman MM, Fojo T, Bates SE. Multidrug resistance in cancer: role of ATP-dependent transporters. *Natl Rev Cancer* 2003; **2**: 48–58.
25. Dean M, Rzhetsky A, Allikmets R. The human ATP-binding cassette (ABC) transporter superfamily. *Genome Res* 2001; **11**: 1156–1166.

26. Dean M. The human ATP-binding cassette (ABC) transporter superfamily. National Library of Medicine (US), NCBI. http://www.ncbi.nlm.nih.gov/bookshelf/br.fcgi?book=mono_001&part=A137. 2002, Accessed 4 October 2008.

27. Hollenstein K, Frei DC, Locher KP. Structure of an ABC transporter in complex with its binding protein. *Nature* 2007; **446**: 213–216.

28. Davidson AL, Maloney PC. ABC transporters: how small machines do a big job. *Trends Microbiol* 2007; **15**: 448–455.

29. Tamura A, Watanabe M, Saito H, Nakagawa H, Kamachi T, Okura I, Ishikawa T. Functional validation of the genetic polymorphisms of human ATP-binding cassette (ABC) transporter ABCG2: identification of alleles that are defective in porphyrin transport. *Mol Pharmacol* 2006; **70**: 287–296.

30. Fromm MF. The influence of MDR1 polymorphisms on P-glycoprotein expression and function in humans. *Adv Drug Deliv Rev* 2003; **54**: 1295–1310.

31. Gottesman MM. Mechanisms of cancer drug resistance. *Ann Rev Med* 2002; **53**: 615–627.

32. Ambudkar SV, Kimchi-Sarfaty C, Sauna ZE, Gottesman MM. P-glycoprotein: from genomics to mechanism. *Oncogene* 2003; **22**: 7468–7485.

33. Varadi A, Szakacs G, Bakos E, Sarkadi B. P-glycoprotein and the mechanism of multidrug resistance. *Novartis Foundation Symposium* 2002; **243**: 54–65.

34. Eckford PD, Sharom FJ. The reconstituted P-glycoprotein multidrug transporter is a flippase for glucosylceramide and other simple glycosphingolipids. *Biochem J* 2005; **389**: 517–526.

35. Al-Shawi MK, Omote H. The remarkable transport mechanism of P-glycoprotein: a multidrug transporter. *J Bioenerg Biomembr* 2006; **37**: 489–496.

36. Orlowski S, Martin S, Escargueil A. P-glycoprotein and 'lipid rafts': some ambiguous mutual relationships (floating on them, building them or meeting them by chance?) *Cell Mol Life Sci* 2006; **63**: 1038–1059.

37. Krishna R, Mayer LD. Multidrug resistance (MDR) in cancer. mechanisms, reversal using modulators of MDR and the role of MDR modulators in influencing the pharmacokinetics of anticancer drugs. *Eur J Pharm Sci* 2000; **11**: 265–283.

38. Jeffrey P, Summerfield SG. Challenges for blood–brain barrier (BBB) screening. *Xenobiotica* 2007; **37**: 1135–1151.

39. Gedeon C, Behravan J, Koren G, Piquette-Miller M. Transport of glyburide by placental ABC transporters: implications in fetal drug exposure. *Placenta* 2006; **27**: 1096–1010.

40. Melaine N, Liénard M, Dorval I, Le Goascogne C, Lejeune H, Jégou B. Multidrug resistance genes and P-glycoprotein in the testis of the rat, mouse, guinea pig, and human. *Biol Reprod* 2002; **67**: 1699–1707.

41. Bunting KD, Zhou S, Lu T, Brian P. Enforced P-glycoprotein pump function in murine bone marrow cells results in expansion of side population stem cells in vitro and repopulating cells in vivo. *Blood* 2000; **96**: 902–909.

42. Johnstone RW, Ruefli AA, Smyth MJ. Multiple physiological functions for multidrug transporter P-glycoprotein. *Tr Biochem Sci* 2000; **25**: 1–6.

43. Ronaldson PT, Bendayan M, Gingras D, Piquette-Miller M, Bendayan R. Cellular localization and functional expression of P-glycoprotein in rat astrocyte cultures. *J Neurochem* 2004; **89**: 788–800.

44. Babakhanian K, Bendayan M, Bendayan R. Localization of P-glycoprotein at the nuclear envelope of rat brain cells. *Biochem Biophys Res Commun* 2007; **361**: 301–306.

45. Allen JD, Brinkhuis RF, van Deemter L, Wijnholds J, Schinkel AH. Extensive contribution of the multidrug transporters P-glycoprotein and Mrp1 to basal drug resistance. *Cancer Res* 2000; **60**: 5761–5766.

46. Leonessa F, Green D, Licht T, Wijinholds J, Schinkel AH. MDA435/LCC6/WT and MDA435/LCC6/mdr1: ascites models of human breast cancer. *Br J Cancer* 1996; **73**: 154–161.

47. Arceci RJ. Can multidrug resistance mechanisms be modified? *Brit J Haematol* 2000; **110**: 285–291.

48. Endicott JA, Ling V. The biochemistry of P-glycoprotein-mediated multidrug resistance. *Ann Rev Biochem* 1989; **58**: 137–171.
49. Johnson WW. P-glycoprotein-mediated efflux as a major factor in the variance of absorption and distribution of drugs: modulation of chemotherapy resistance. *Methods Find Exp Clin Pharmacol* 2002; **24**: 501–514.
50. Campone M, Vavasseur F, Le Cabellec MT, Meflah K, Vallette FM, Oliver L. Induction of chemoresistance in HL-60 cells concomitantly causes a resistance to apoptosis and the synthesis of P-glycoprotein. *Leukemia* 2001; **15**: 1377–1387.
51. Hahn SM, Russo A, Cook JA, Mitchell JB. A multidrug-resistant breast cancer line induced by weekly exposure to doxorubicin. *Int J Oncol* 1999; **14**: 273–279.
52. Mayer R, Kartenbeck J, Buchler M, Jedlitschky G, Leier I, Keppler D. Expression of the MRP gene-encoded conjugate export pump in liver and its selective absence from the canalicular membrane in transport- deficient mutant hepatocytes. *J Cell Biol* 1995; **131**: 137–150.
53. Evers R, Kool M, van Deemter L, Janssen H, Calafat J, Oomen LC, Paulusma CC, Oude Elferink RP, Baas F, Schinkel AH, Borst P. Drug export activity of the human canalicular multispecific organic anion transporter in polarized kidney MDCK cells expressing cMOAT (MRP2) cDNA. *J Clin Invest* 1998; **101**: 1310–1319.
54. Doyle LA, Yang W, Abruzzo LV. A multidrug resistance transporter from human MCF-7 breast cancer cells. *Proc Natl Acad Sci USA* 1998; **95**: 15665–15670.
55. Maliepaard M, Scheffer GL, Faneyte IF, van Gastelen MA, Pijnenborg AC, Schinkel AH, van De Vijver MJ, Scheper RJ, Schellens JH. Subcellular localization and distribution of the breast cancer resistance protein transporter in normal human tissues. *Cancer Res* 2001; **61**: 3458–3464.
56. Diestra JE, Scheffer GL, Catala II, Maliepaard M, Schellens JH, Scheper RJ, Germà-Lluch JR, Izquierdo MA. Frequent expression of the multi-drug resistance-associated protein BCRP/MXR/ABCP/ABCG2 in human tumours detected by the BXP-21 monoclonal antibody in paraffin-embedded material. *J Pathol* 2002; **198**: 213–219.
57. Brangi M, Litman T, Ciotti M, Nishiyama K, Kohlhagen G, Takimoto C, Robey R, Pommier Y, Fojo T, Bates SE. Camptothecin resistance: role of the ATP-binding cassette (ABC), mitoxantrone-resistance half-transporter (MXR), and potential for glucuronidation in MXR-expressing cells. *Cancer Res* 1999; **59**: 5938–5946.
58. Maliepaard M, van Gastelen MA, de Jong LA, Pluim D, van Waardenburg RC, Ruevekamp-Helmers MC, Floot BG, Schellens JH. Overexpression of the BCRP/MXR/ABCP gene in a topotecan-selected ovarian tumor cell line. *Cancer Res* 1999; **59**: 4559–4563.
59. Ross DD, Yang W, Abruzzo LV, Dalton WS, Schneider E, Lage H, Dietel M, Greenberger L, Cole SP, Doyle LA. Atypical multidrug resistance: breast cancer resistance protein messenger RNA expression in mitoxantrone-selected cell lines. *J Natl Cancer Inst* 1999; **91**: 429–433.
60. Krishnamurthy P, Schuetz JD. Role of ABCG2/BCRP in biology and medicine. *Annu Rev Pharmcol Toxicol* 2006; **46**: 381–410.
61. Sugimoto Y, Tsukahara S, Ishikawa E, Mitsuhashi J. Breast cancer resistance protein: molecular target for anticancer drug resistance and pharmacokinetics/pharmacodynamics. *Cancer Sci* 2005; **96**: 457–465.
62. Boonstra R, Timmer-Bosscha H, van Echten-Arends J, van der Kolk DM, van den Berg A, de Jong B, Tew KD, Poppema S, de Vries EGE. Mitoxantrone resistance in a small cell lung cancer cell line is associated with ABCA2 upregulation. *Brit J Cancer* 2004; **90**: 2411–2417.
63. Mack JT, Beljanski V, Tew KD, Townsend DM. The ATP-binding cassette transporter ABCA2 as a mediator of intracellular trafficking. *Biomed Pharmacother* 2006; **60**: 587–592.
64. Efferth T, Gillet JP, Sauerbrey A, Bertholet V, de Longueville FO, Remacle J, Steinbach D. Expression profiling of ATP-binding cassette transporters in childhood T-cell acute lymphoblastic leukemia. *Mol Cancer Ther* 2006; **5**: 1986–1994.

65. Steinbach D, Gillet JP, Sauerbrey A, Bernd Gruhn, Dawczynski K, Bertholet V, de Longueville F, Zintl F, Remacle J, Efferth T. ABCA3 as a possible cause of drug resistance in childhood acute myeloid leukemia. *Clin Cancer Res* 2006; **12**: 4357–4363.
66. Dean M, Fojo T, Bates S. Tumour stem cells and drug resistance. *Nat Rev Cancer* 2005; **5**: 275–284.
67. Klopman G, Shi LM, Ramu A. Quantitative structure–activity relationship of multidrug resistance reversal agents. *Mol Pharmacol* 1997; **52**: 323–334.
68. Roe M, Folkes A, Ashworth P Brumwell J, Chima L, Hunjan S, Pretswell I, Dangerfield W, Ryder H, Charlton P. Reversal of P-glycoprotein mediated multidrug resistance by novel anthranilamide derivatives. *Bioorg Med Chem Lett* 1999; **9**: 595–600.
69. Starling JJ, Shepard RL, Cao J, Law KL, Norman BH, Kroin JS, Ehlhardt WJ, Baughman TM, Winter MA, Bell MG, Shih C, Gruber J, Elmquist WF, Dantzig AH. Pharmacological characterization of LY335979: A potent cyclopropyldibenzosuberane modulator of P-glycoprotein. *Adv Enzyme Regul* 1997; **37**: 335–347.
70. van Zuylen L, Nooter K, Sparreboom A, Verweij J. Development of multidrug-resistance convertors: sense or nonsense? *Invest New Drugs* 2000; **18**: 205–220.
71. Newman MJ, Rodarte JC, Benbatoul KD, Romano SJ, Zhang C, Krane S, Moran EJ, Uyeda RT, Dixon R, Guns ES, Mayer LD. Discovery and characterization of OC144-093, a novel inhibitor of P-glycoprotein-mediated multidrug resistance. *Cancer Res* 2000; **60**: 2964–2972.
72. Wallstab A, Koester M, Bohme M, Keppler D. Selective inhibition of MDR1 P-glycoprotein-mediated transport by the acridone carboxamide derivative GG918. *Br J Cancer* 1999; **79**: 1053–1060.
73. Coley HM, Verrill MW, Gregson SE. Incidence of P-glycoprotein over expression and multidrug resistance (MDR) reversal in adult soft tissue sarcoma. *Eur J Cancer* 2000; **36**: 881–888.
74. Mistry P, Stewart AJ, Dangerfield W, Okiji S, Liddle C, Bootle D, Plumb JA, Templeton D, Charlton P. In vitro and in vivo reversal of P-glycoprotein-mediated multidrug resistance by a novel potent modulator, XR9576. *Cancer Res* 2001; **61**: 749–758.
75. Agrawal M, Abraham J, Balis FM, Edgerly M, Stein WD, Bates S, Fojo T, Chen CC. Increased 99m-Tc-sestamibi accumulation in normal liver and drug-resistant tumors after the administration of the glycoprotein inhibitor, XR9576 *Clin Cancer Res* 2003; **9**: 650–656.
76. Bakker M, van der Graaf WT, Piers DA, Franssen EJ, Groen HJ, Smit EF, Kool W, Hollema H, Muller EA, deVries EG. 99mTc-Sestamibi scanning with SDZ PSC 833 as a functional detection method for resistance modulation in patients with solid tumours. *Anticancer Res* 1999; **19**: 2349–2353.
77. Peck RA, Hewett J, Harding MW, Wang YM, Chaturvedi PR, Bhatnagar A, Ziessman H, Atkins F, Hawkins MJ. Phase I and pharmacokinetic study of the novel MDR1 and MRP1 inhibitor biricodar administered alone and in combination with doxorubicin. *J Clin Oncol* 2001; **19**: 3130–3141.
78. Fischer V, Rodriguez-Gascon A, Heitz F, Tynes R, Hauck C, Cohen D, Vickers AEM. The multidrug resistance modulator valspodar (PSC 833) is metabolized by human cytochrome P450 3A: Implications for drug-drug interactions and pharmacological activity of the main metabolite. *Drug Metab Dispos* 1998; **26**: 802–811.
79. Wandel C, Kim RB, Kajiji S, Guengerich FP, Wilkinson GR, Wood AJJ. P-glycoprotein and cytochrome P450 3A inhibition: dissociation of inhibitory potencies. *Cancer Res* 1999; **59**: 3944–3948.
80. Nobili S, Landini I, Giglioni B, Mini E. Pharmacological strategies for overcoming multidrug resistance. *Current Drug Targets* 2006; **7**: 861–879.
81. Duhem C, Ries F, Dicato M. What does Multidrug Resistance (MDR) Expression Mean in the Clinic? *The Oncologist* 1996; **1**: 151–158.
82. Sonneveld P, Suciu S, Weijermans P, Beksac M, Neuwirtova R, Solbu G, Lokhorst H, Van der lelie J, Dohner H, Gerhartz H, Segeren CM, Willemze R, Lowenberg B.

Cyclosporin A combined with vincristine, doxorubicin and dexamethasone (VAD) compared with VAD alone in patients with advanced refractory multiple myeloma: an EORTC-HOVON randomized phase III study (06914). *Br J Haematol* 2001; **115**: 895–902.

83. Baer MR, George SL, Dodge RK, O'Loughlin KL, Minderman H, Caligiuri MA, Anastasi J, Powell BL, Kolitz JE, Schiffer CA, Bloomfield CD, Larson RA. Phase 3 study of the multidrug resistance modulator PSC-833 in previously untreated patients 60 years of age and older with acute myeloid leukemia: Cancer and Leukemia Group B Study 9720. *Blood* 2002; **100**: 1224–1232.

84. Toppmeyer D, Seidman AD, Pollak M, Russell C, Tkaczuk K, Verma S, Overmoyer B, Garg V, Ette E, Harding MW, Demetri GD. Safety and efficacy of the multidrug resistance inhibitor Incel (biricodar; VX-710) in combination with paclitaxel for advanced breast cancer refractory to paclitaxel. *Clin Cancer Res* 2002; **8**: 670–678.

85. Stavrovskaya AA. Cellular mechanisms of multidrug resistance of tumor cells. *Biochemistry* 2000; **65**: 95–106.

86. Sparreboom A, Planting AS, Jewell RC, van der Burg ME, van der Gaast A, de Bruijin P, Loos WJ, Nooter K, Chndler LH, Paul EM, Wissel PS, Verweij J. Clinical pharmacokinetics of doxorubicin in combination with GF120918, a potent inhibitor of MDR1 P-glycoprotein. *Anticancer Drugs* 1999; **10**: 719–728.

87. Aszalos A, Ladanyi A, Bocsi J, Szende B. Induction of apoptosis in MDR1 expressing cells by daunorubicin with combinations of suboptimal concentrations of P-glycoprotein modulators. *Cancer Let* 2001; **167**: 157–162.

88. Matsumura Y, Maeda H. A new concept for macromolecular therapeutics in cancer chemotherapy: Mechanism of tumoritropic accumulation of proteins and the antitumor agent SMANCS. *Cancer Res* 1986; **6**: 193–210.

89. Northfelt DW, Dezube BJ, Thommes JA, Miller BJ, Fischl MA, Friedman-Kien A, Kaplan LD, Du Mond C, Mamelok RD, Henry DH. Efficacy of pegylated-liposomal doxorubicin in the treatment of AIDS-related Kaposi's sarcoma after failure of standard chemotherapy. *J Clin Oncol* 1997; **15**: 653–659.

90. Park JW. Liposome-based drug delivery in breast cancer treatment. *Breast Cancer Res* 2002; **4**: 95–99.

91. Popovic N, Brundin P. Therapeutic potential of controlled drug delivery systems in neurodegenerative diseases. *Int J Pharmaceut* 2006; **314**: 120–126.

92. Koziara JM, Lockman PR, Allen DD, Mumper RJ. Paclitaxel nanoparticles for the potential treatment of brain tumors. *J Control Release* 2004; **99**: 259–269.

93. Wong HL, Rauth AM, Bendayan R, Manias JL, Ramaswamy M, Liu Z, Erhan SZ, Wu XY. A new polymer-lipid hybrid nanoparticle system increases cytotoxicity of doxorubicin against multidrug resistant human breast cancer cells. *Pharm Res* 2006; **23**: 1574–1585.

94. Mamot C, Drummond DC, Hong K, Kirpotin DB, Park JW. Liposome-based approaches to overcome anticancer drug resistance. *Drug Res Update* 2003; **6**: 271–279.

95. Hagiwara A, Sakakura C, Shirasu M, Togawa T, Sonoyama Y, Fujiyama J, Ebihara Y, Itoh T, Yamagishi H. Intraperitoneal injection of dextran sulfate as an anti-adherent drug for the prevention of peritoneal metastasis of cancer shows low toxicity in animals. *Anti-Cancer Drugs* 2000; **11**: 393–399.

96. Hu YP, Jarillon S, Dubernet C, Couvreur P, Robert J. On the mechanism of action of doxorubicin encapsulation in nanospheres for the reversal of multidrug resistance. *Cancer Chemother Pharmacol* 1996; **37**: 556–560.

97. Drori S, Eytan GD, Assaraf YG. Potentiation of anticancer-drug cytotoxicity by multidrug-resistance chemosensitizers involves alterations in membrane fluidity leading to increased membrane permeability. *Eur J Biochem* 1995; **228**: 1020–1029.

98. Riehm H, Biedler JL. Potentiation of drug effect by Tween 80 in Chinese Hamster cells resistant to actinomycin D and daunomycin. *Cancer Res* 1972; **32**: 1195–1200.

99. Kabanov AV, Batrakova EV, Alakhov VY. Pluronic block copolymers for overcoming drug resistance in cancer. *Adv Drug Del Rev* 2002; **54**: 759–779.
100. Doige CA, Yu X, Sharom FJ. The effects of lipids and detergents on ATPase activity of P-glycoprotein. *Biochim Biophys Acta* 1993; **1146**: 65–72.
101. Liu Z, Bendayan R, Wu XY. Triton-X-100-modified polymer and microspheres for reversal of multidrug resistance. *J Pharm Pharmacol* 2001; **53**: 1–12.
102. Batrakova EV, Han HY, Miller DW, Kabanov AV. Effects of pluronic P85 unimers and micelles on drug permeability in polarized BBMEC and Caco-2 cells. *Pharm Res* 1998; **15**: 1525–1532.
103. Alakhov VY, Kabanov AV. Block copolymeric biotransport carriers as versatile vehicles for drug delivery. *Exp Opin Invest Drugs* 1998; **7**: 1453–1473.
104. Alakhov VY, Moskaleva EY, Batrakova EV. Hypersensitization of multidrug resistant human ovarian carcinoma cells by pluronic P85 block copolymer. *Bioconjug Chem* 1996; **7**: 209–216.
105. Kabonov AV, Batrakova EV, Alakhov VY. An essential relationship between ATP depletion and chemosensitizing activity of pluronic block copolymers. *J Control Release* 2003; **91**: 75–83.
106. Batrakova EV, Li S, Vinogradov SV, Alakhov VY, Miller DW, Kabanov AV. Mechanism of pluronic effect on p-glycoprotein efflux system in blood brain barrier: contributions of energy depletion and membrane fluidization. *J Pharmacol Exp Ther* 2001; **299**: 483–493.
107. Ugazio E, Cavali R, Gasco MR. Incorporation of cyclosporin A in solid lipid nanoparticles (SLN). *Int J Pharm* 2002; **241**: 341–344.
108. Lo YL, Liu FI, Cheung JY. Effect of PSC 833 liposomes and intralipid on the transport of epirubicin in Caco-2 cells and rat intestines. *J Control Release* 2001; **76**: 1–10.
109. Wong HL, Bendayan R, Rauth AM, Wu XY. Development of solid lipid nanoparticles containing ionically-complexed chemotherapeutic drugs and chemosensitizers. *J Pharm Sci* 2004; **93**: 1993–2004.
110. Wong HL, Rauth AM, Bendayan R, Wu XY. Combinational treatment with doxorubicin and GG918 (Elacridar) using polymer-lipid hybrid nanoparticles (PLN) and evaluation of strategies for multidrug-resistance reversal in human breast cancer cells. *J Control Release* 2006; **116**: 275–284.
111. Shuhendler AJ, O'Brien P, Rauth AM, Wu XY. On the synergistic effect of doxorubicin and mitomycin C against breast cancer cells. *Drug Metabol Drug Interactions* 2008; **22**: 201–233.
112. Shuhendler AJ, Chung R, Manias J, Connor A, Rauth AM, Wu XY. A novel doxorubicin-mitomycin C co-encapsulated nanoparticle formulation exhibits anti-cancer synergy in multidrug resistant human breast cancer cells. *Breast Cancer Res Treatment*, submitted in 2008.
113. Dass CR, Choong PFM. Selective gene delivery for cancer therapy using cationic liposomes: In vivo proof of applicability. *J Control Release* 2006; **113**: 155–163.
114. Behlke M. Progress towards in vivo use of siRNAs. *Mol Therapy* 2006; **13**: 645–670.
115. Qun (Tony) Liu. *Enzyme Microencapsulation and Its Application for Overcoming Multidrug Resistance in Breast Cancer Treatment*, Ph.D.Thesis, University of Toronto, Toronto, Canada, 2008.
116. Khalil IA, Kogure K, Akita H. Uptake pathways and subsequent intracellular trafficking in nonviral gene delivery. *Pharmacol Rev* 2006; **58**: 32–45.
117. Kreuter J, Ramge P, Petrov V, Hamm S, Gelperina SE, Engelhardt B, Alyautdin R, von Briesen H, Begley DJ. Direct evidence that polysorbate-80-coated poly (butylcyanoacrylate) nanoparticles deliver drugs to the CNS via specific mechanisms requiring prior binding of drug to the nanoparticles. *Pharm Res* 2003; **20**: 409–416.
118. Kreuter J, Shamenkov D, Petrov V, Ramge P, Cychutek K, Koch-Brandt C, Alyautdin R. Apolipoprotein-mediated transport of nanoparticle-bound drugs across the blood–brain barrier. *J Drug Target* 2002; **10**: 317–325.

119. Steiniger SC, Kreuter J, Khalansky AS, Skidan IN, Bobruskin AI, Smirnova ZS, Severin SE, Uhl R, Kock M, Geiger KD, Gelperina SE. Chemotherapy of glioblastoma in rats using doxorubicin-loaded nanoparticles. *Int J Cancer* 2004; **109**: 59–767.

120. Pelkmans L, Kartenbeck J, Helenius A. Caveolar endocytosis of simian virus 40 reveals a new two-step vesicular-transport pathway to the ER. *Nat Cell Biol* 2001; **3**: 473–483.

121. Amyere M, Mettlen M, van der Smissen P, Platek A, Payrastre B, Veithen A, Courtoy PJ. Origin, originality, functions, subversions and molecular signaling of macropinocytosis. *Int J Med Microbiol* 2002; **291**: 487–494.

122. Kaplan IM, Wadia JS, Dowdy SF. Cationic TAT peptide transduction domain enters cells by macropinocytosis. *J Control Release* 2005; **102**: 247–253.

123. Khalil IA, Kogure K, Futaki S, Harashima H. High density of octaarginine stimulates macropinocytosis leading to efficient intracellular trafficking for gene expression. *J Biol Chem* 2006; **6**: 3544–3551.

124. Cho KC, Kim SH, Jeong JH, Park TG. Folate receptor-mediated gene delivery using folate-poly(ethylene glycol)-poly(L-lysine) conjugate. *Macromol Biosci* 2005; **5**: 512–519.

125. Zhang H, Yee D, Wang C. Quantum Dots for Cancer Diagnosis and Therapy. *Biol Clin Perspectives* 2008; **3**: 83–91.

126. Stevens PJ, Sekido M, Lee RJ. A folate-receptor-targeted lipid nanoparticle formulation for a lipophilic paclitaxel prodrug. *Pharm Res* 2004; **21**: 2153–2157.

127. Wong HL, Bendayan R, Rauth AM, Xue HY, Babakhanian K, Wu XY. A mechanistic study of enhanced doxorubicin uptake and retention in multidrug resistant breast cancer cells using a polymer-lipid hybrid nanoparticle (PLN) system. *J Pharmacol Exp Ther* 2006; **317**: 1372–1381.

128. Kopecek J, Kopeckova P, Minko T, Lu ZR. HPMA copolymer–anticancer drug conjugates: design, activity, and mechanism of action. *Eur J Pharm Biopharm* 2000; **50**: 61–81.

129. Kopecek J, Kopeckova P, Minko T, Lu ZR, Peterson CM. Water soluble polymers in tumor targeted delivery. *J Control Release* 2001; **74**: 147–158.

130. Bonnet D, Dick JE. Human acute myeloid leukemia is organized as a hierarchy that originates from a primitive hematopoietic cell. *Nat Med* 1997; **3**: 730–737.

131. Li C, Heidt DG, Dalerba P, Burant CF, Zhang L, Adsay V, Wicha M, Clarke MF, Simeone DM. Identification of pancreatic cancer stem cells. *Cancer Res* 2007; **67**: 1030–1037.

132. Singh SK, Clarke ID, Terasaki M, Bonn VE, Hawkins C, Squire J, Dirks PB. Identification of a cancer stem cell in human brain tumors. *Cancer Res* 2003; **63**: 5821–5828.

133. O'Brien CA, Pollett A, Gallinger S, Dick JE. A human colon cancer cell capable of initiating tumour growth in immunodeficient mice. *Nature* 2007; **445**: 106–110.

134. Donnenberg VS, Donnenberg AD. Multiple drug resistance in cancer revisited: the cancer stem cell hypothesis. *J Clin Pharmacol* 2005; **45**: 872–877.

135. Hirschmann-Jax C, Foster AE, Wulf GG. A distinct "side population" of cells with high drug efflux capacity in human tumor cells. *Proc Natl Acad Sci USA* 2004; **101**: 14228–14233.

136. Gouaze V, Yu JY, Bleicher RJ, Han TY, Liu YY, Wang H, Michael M, Gottesman MM, Bitterman A, Giuliano AE, Cabot MC. Overexpression of glucosylceramide synthase and P-glycoprotein in cancer cells selected for resistance to natural product chemotherapy. *Mol Cancer Ther* 2004; **3**: 633–639.

137. Gouaze V, Liu YY, Prickett CS, Yu JY, Giuliano AE, Cabot MC. Glucosylceramide synthase blockade down-regulates P-glycoprotein and resensitizes multidrug-resistant breast cancer cells to anticancer drugs. *Cancer Res* 2005; **65**: 3861–3867.

138. Sun YL, Zhou GY, Li KN, Gao P, Zhang QH, Zhen JH, Bai YH, Zhang XF. Suppression of glucosylceramide synthase by RNA interference reverses multidrug resistance in human breast cancer cells. *Neoplasma* 2006; **53**: 1–8.

139. Nakamura Y, Oka M, Soda H, Shiozawa K, Yoshikawa M, Itoh A, Ikegami Y, Tsurutani J, Nakatomi K, Kitazaki T, Doi S, Yoshida H, Kohno Sn. Gefitinib ("Iressa" ZD1839), an epidermal growth factor receptor tyrosine kinase inhibitor, reverses breast cancer resistance protein/ABCG2-mediated drug resistance. *Cancer Res* 2005; **65**: 1541–1546.

140. Yanase K, Tsukahara S, Asada S, Ishikawa E, Imai Y, Sugimoto Y. Gefitinib reverses breast cancer resistance protein-mediated drug resistance. *Mol Cancer Ther* 2004; **3**: 1119–1125.

141. Fantappiè O, Solazzo M, Lasagna N, Platini F, Tessitore L, Mazzant R. P-glycoprotein mediates celecoxib-induced apoptosis in multiple drug-resistant cell lines. *Cancer Res* 2007; **67**: 4915–4923.

142. Tredan O, Galmarini CM, Patel K, Tannock IF. Drug resistance and the solid tumor microenvironment. *J Natl Cancer Inst* 2007; **99**: 1441–1454.

143. Calabrese C, Poppleton H, Kocak M, Hogg TL, Fuller C, Haner B Oh EY, Gaber MW, Finklestein D, Allen M, Frank A, Bayazitov IT, Zakharenko SS, Gajjar A, Davidoff A, Gilbertson RJ. A perivascular niche for brain tumor stem cells. *Cancer Cell* 2007; **11**: 69–82.

144. Kim JJ, Tannock IF. Repopulation of cancer cells during therapy: An important cause of treatment failure. *Nat Rev Cancer* 2005; **5**: 516–525.

145. Wong HL, Rauth AM, Bendayan R, Wu XY. Evaluation of the in vivo efficacy, toxicity and lymphatic drainage of loco-regional administered polymer-lipid hybrid nanoparticles (PLN) loaded with doxorubicin in a murine solid tumor model. *Eur J Pharm Biopharm* 2007; **65**: 300–308.

146. Jang SH, Wientjes MG, Au JL. Enhancement of paclitaxel delivery to solid tumors by apoptosis-inducing pretreatment: effect of treatment schedule. *J Pharmacol Exp Ther* 2001; **296**: 1035–1042.

147. Winkler F, Kozin SV, Tong RT, Chae S, Booth M, Garkavtsev I, Xu L, Hicklin D, Fukumura D, Tomaso ED. Kinetics of vascular normalization by VEGFR2 blockade governs brain tumor response to radiation: role of oxygenation, angiopoietin-1, and matrix metalloproteinases. *Cancer Cell* 2004; **6**: 553–563.

148. Brown E, Mckee T, diTomaso, Pluen A, Seed B, Boucher Y, Rakesh K. Jain RK. Dynamic imaging of collagen and its modulation in tumors in vivo using second-harmonic generation. *Nat Med* 2003; **9**: 796–800.

Targeting of Apoptosis Signaling Pathways and Their Mediators for Cancer Therapy

Arun K. Rishi, Xinbo Zhang, and Anil Wali

1 Introduction

Apoptosis, also known as programmed cell death, is essential for the regulation of development, the generation of the immune system, and is a central mechanism for maintenance of cellular homeostasis in eukaryotes. This phenomenon of cellular death was described for almost a century, and was named apoptosis only recently to differentiate naturally occurring cell death during development from the acute injury associated necrotic cell death [1]. The apoptosis processes function to maintain equilibrium between cell proliferation and death, while dysregulated apoptosis is involved in development and etiology of many pathological disorders. The acute pathological conditions such as stroke, heart attack, or liver failure as well as chronic neurodegenerative disorders are associated with increased apoptosis resulting in sudden or progressive death of the target tissues. The pathologies of auto-immune disorders and carcinogenesis, on the other hand, arise due in part to the loss or reduced rate of apoptosis. Approximately half of the known clinical pathologies are estimated to arise due to either too little or too much apoptosis. Apoptosis is considered a major mechanism of chemotherapy-induced cell death, and many currently utilized cytotoxic anti-cancer agents are known to function by promoting apoptosis in the target cells. Although the precise mechanisms of actions of many anti-cancer agents are yet to be elucidated, the apoptosis by most agents is often initiated by either damage to the cellular DNA or key signaling mediators that regulate cell survival [2]. The defects in apoptosis signaling pathways in the cancer cells therefore contribute to reduction or abrogation of the initial stress response signals and apoptosis, resulting in development of drug-resistant phenotypes. Since, adequate therapies for many disorders are lacking, the apoptosis signaling pathways therefore can be exploited in the preclinical

A.K. Rishi (✉)
Karmanos Cancer Institute, Department of Internal Medicine, Wayne State
University, Room B4334, John D. Dingell VA Medical Center, 4646 Detroit,
MI 48201, USA
e-mail: rishia@karmanos.org

Y. Lu, R.I. Mahato (eds.), *Pharmaceutical Perspectives of Cancer Therapeutics*,
DOI 10.1007/978-1-4419-0131-6_5, © Springer Science+Business Media, LLC 2009

drug discovery investigations to develop effective and perhaps novel agents for treatment of diverse pathologies including cancer.

Apoptosis signaling is transduced by two distinct molecular pathways that consist of the *intrinsic*, or mitochondria-mediated pathway, and the *extrinsic*, or extracellular receptor-activated pathway [3–5]. The morphologic characteristics of the cells undergoing apoptosis include cell membrane blebbing, cell shrinkage, chromatin condensation, and nucleosomal fragmentation. The neighboring healthy cells of the tissue or the macrophages eventually devour the fractionated remains of the apoptotic cells. The intracellular stress signals including DNA damage and high levels of reactive oxygen species (ROS), as well as viral infection and activation of oncogenes induce intrinsic apoptosis pathway. The extrinsic pathway on the other hand is activated by the binding of an extracellular ligand to a receptor on the plasma membrane. The eventual breakdown of the cellular proteins, organelles, and cell architecture is accomplished by proteolytic enzymes called caspases that are activated by both the extrinsic and intrinsic pathways (Fig. 1). The caspases are

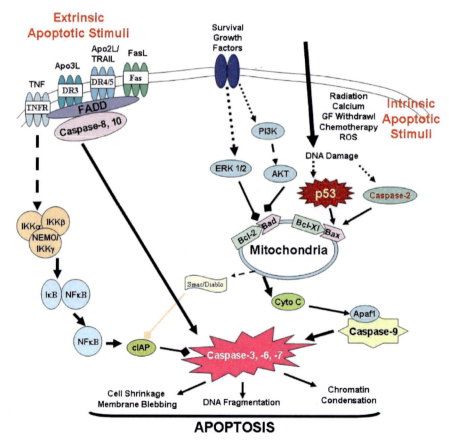

Fig. 1 Schematic of apoptosis signaling pathways. Lines with *arrowheads* indicate activation and lines with *diamondheads* indicate inhibition of a target gene. Cyto C, cytochrome *c*; ROS, reactive oxygen species; GF, growth factors

normally expressed as inactive precursors and the apoptosis signals target them for post-translational modifications and cleavage to form active oligomers [6, 7]. Two broad groups of caspases consist of the initiator/apical caspases (caspase-8, caspase-9, and caspase-10) and the effector/executioner caspases (caspase-3, caspase-6, and caspase-7). The autocatalytic mechanisms often activate the initiator caspases, while the effector caspases are generally dependent on the initiator caspases for their cleavage and activation.

2 Apoptosis Pathways

2.1 The Extrinsic Pathway

The activation of extrinsic apoptosis is normally accomplished by binding of the tumor necrosis factor (TNF) family of ligands to their cognate cell surface TNFR and/or death receptors. The TNF family consists of 18 ligands that are thought to target 29 cell surface receptors [8]. The receptors that have been well characterized for their roles in apoptosis signaling include TNFR1 (aka DR1, CD120a, p55, and p60), Fas (aka CD95, DR2, Apo-1), DR3 (aka APO-3, LARD, TRAMP, and WSL1), TNF-related apoptosis-inducing ligand (TRAIL) receptor 1 (aka DR4, APO-2), TRAILR2 (aka DR5, KILLER and TRICK2), DR6, ectodysplasin A receptor (EDAR), and nerve growth factor receptor (NGFR). These receptors harbor a distinct cytoplasmic domain termed death domain (DD). A subclass of receptors known as decoy receptors (DcRs) that do not have DD include TRAILR3 (aka DcR1), TRAILR4 (aka DcR2), DcR3, and osteoprotegrin (OPG). The DcRs also bind to various ligands but do not form intracellular signaling complexes [9]. Binding of the TNF to TNFRs generally activates cell survival and pro-inflammatory signaling. Many ligands of this family are also known to induce apoptosis signaling. In this context, the stimulation of apoptosis signaling by the ligands such as TRAIL/Apo2L and the FasL/CD95L is well documented [10, 11]. The extrinsic apoptosis signaling is central to maintaining immune homeostasis, development of autoimmunity, and orderly regulation of lymphogenesis [12]. This pathway is extensively utilized to derive cells from the progenitor cells (CD8$^+$ T cells, natural killer cells [NK], dendritic cells) during processes of hematopoiesis. Further, induction of FasL, TNF, and TRAIL following antigen stimulation of T cells is critical in promoting contact-dependent destruction of T-cell target cells [13–17]. The caspase-like proteases known as granzymes that are often released by cytotoxic immune cells enter the target cells and activate apoptosis through both caspase-dependent and caspase-independent mechanisms [18].

The signaling induced following ligation of TRAIL and FasL to the cell surface receptors is similar and leads to apoptosis; the TNF-dependent signaling, however, is more complex and often results in either cell survival or apoptosis outcomes [19]. The apoptosis signaling by these ligands promotes recruitment of initiating caspases and various adaptor proteins at the cytoplasmic death domains of the receptors. For example, the binding of FasL or TRAIL to the death receptors (DR4 and DR5) results in recruitment of the adapter protein Fas-associated death domain-containing protein (FADD) followed by the initiator caspase-8 and caspase-10 [20]. This assembly of proteins (death receptors, FADD, and caspases) is known as the death-inducing signaling complex (DISC). The assembly of DISC induces autoproteolytic cleavage of the caspase-8/10 [21–23]. This autoproteolytic cleavage of caspase-8/10 is often blocked by binding of a FADD-like interleukin-1β-converting enzyme inhibitory protein (FLIP) with caspase-8/10. Thus, FLIP functions as a dominant-negative inhibitor of autocatalytic activation of these caspases. The activated caspase-8/10 either directly target the effector caspases-3/6/7 [24] or activate the BH3-only protein Bid to target mitochondria. The activated caspase-8 cleaves Bid, and the truncated Bid (tBid) then targets mitochondria [25, 26], thereby connecting the extrinsic pathway to mitochondria-dependent intrinsic apoptosis pathway (see below). The activated caspase-6 is also known to feedback-activate extrinsic pathway by cleaving caspase-8 [27].

2.2 The Intrinsic Pathway

The mitochondria are the key intracellular targets of the intrinsic apoptosis signaling pathways. Bcl-2 family of proteins (discussed in detail below) function to transduce the intrinsic apoptosis signals by regulating mitochondrial outer membrane potential (MOMP) and release of the apoptogenic factors from mitochondria. Bcl-2 proteins contain from one to four Bcl-2 homology (BH) domains which mediate protein interactions [28]. The proteins with four BH domains are usually associated with cell survival and have anti-apoptotic properties. The pro-apoptotic members of this family either have BH1-3 domains or have only the BH3 domain. The pro-survival members of the Bcl-2 family function by binding to and antagonizing pro-apoptotic members, while the BH3-only members promote apoptosis by binding and antagonizing the pro-survival proteins [29]. On the basis of the death-promoting and antagonistic interactions of various Bcl-2 family of proteins, a rheostat model was proposed in which the ratio of the pro- and the anti-apoptotic proteins was suggested to control the cell fate [30]. The tumor suppressor p53 or post-translational mechanisms such as phosphorylation also control the activity of several members of this family of proteins. For example, the cell survival and/or growth factor signals phosphorylate the BH-only protein Bad to promote its sequestration by 14-3-3 proteins, resulting in prevention of its mitochondrial targeting [31]. On the other hand, cellular stresses, such as ionizing radiation (IR) or chemotherapy, activate a DNA damage response that enhances p53 stability. The increased p53, in turn, transcriptionally activates cyclin-dependent kinase (CDKI) p21 to promote cell cycle arrest to allow cells time to repair the damage. In an event the damage cannot be repaired, the elevated p53 mediates apoptotic cell death by either activating transcription of a number of pro-apoptotic Bcl-2 family members or by binding with anti-apoptotic Bcl-2 family members to facilitate activation of MOMP [32–34].

The intrinsic apoptosis signals promote oligomerization of pro-apoptotic Bcl-2 family members in the mitochondrial outer membrane to activate MOMP. For example, the pro-apoptotic, BH1-3 domain Bax and Bak proteins normally exist as inactive monomers. Bax resides in the cytosol or loosely attached to intracellular membranes [35], and Bak is bound by Mcl-1, Bcl-xL, or voltage-dependent anion channel protein 2 (VDAC-2) in the mitochondrial outer membrane [36–38]. The oligomerization of Bax and Bak causes release of the mitochondrial apoptogenic factors. These factors include cytochrome c, second mitochondria-derived activator of caspase/direct inhibitor of apoptosis (IAP) binding protein with low pI (Smac/DIA-BLO), and Omi stress-regulated endoprotease/high-temperature requirement protein A2 (Omi/HtrA2). These mitochondrial factors then bind with apoptotic protease-activating factor 1 (Apaf-1), which recruits pro-caspase-9, promoting its self-activation. Activated caspase-9 then targets the downstream effectors caspase-3, caspase-7, to promote their cleavage and activation to transduce apoptosis signaling. Several inhibitors of apoptosis (IAP) proteins (discussed in detail in a separate section later) antagonize activation of the effector caspases by inhibiting the active sites of caspase-3, caspase-7, and caspase-9. A dynamic interplay of protein–protein interactions of the mitochondrial factors and the IAPs in turn regulate activation of effector caspases and apoptosis. When released from mitochondria, Smac/DIA-BLO and Omi/HtrA2 can bind these IAPs and prevent their inhibition of the activated caspases [38–40].

3 Targeting of the Extrinsic Pathway

The extrinsic pathway often serves as an attractive target for intervention in chemo-resistant cancers that have defects in their mitochondrial/intrinsic apoptosis signaling. Most of the strategies are directed to inducing apoptosis signals by activating TNF family of receptors. Although some TNF family receptors function in transducing cell survival and inflammation-associated signaling and blocking these receptors has been useful in lymphoid malignancies, the interactions of a number of TNF family of ligands with their receptors are known to stimulate apoptosis. Here, the cancer therapeutics applications causing activation of extrinsic pathway have predominantly focused on TNFR1, Fas, and the death receptors 4 and 5. Two broad strategies have thus far been pursued to activate extrinsic apoptosis and include expression of recombinant ligands with only extracellular domains of type 2 receptors, and agonistic small molecules as well as monoclonal antibodies. Additional strategies have focused on targeting various intracellular effectors/mediators of this pathway.

Apoptosis signaling following ligation of TNF or FasL is a well-documented mechanism of attenuating cancer cell growth in vitro; the utility of these ligands as systemic anti-cancer therapies, however, has been limited due mainly to their toxic side effects that include septic shock and lethal liver injuries [41–43]. Although not widely used in clinics, TNF in combination with certain chemotherapeutic agents such as melphalan have been useful for localized treatments of sarcomas and melanomas where it is thought to promote destruction of tumor vasculature [44, 45]. In contrast to TNF or Fasl, TRAIL was not found to be cytotoxic for a variety of normal human cells including fibroblasts, epithelial, endothelial, smooth muscle cells as well as astrocytes [46–48], while some toxic effects were noted in hepatocytes and brain tissues [49, 50]. Interestingly, systemic administration of recombinant human TRAIL in rodents and primates was found to be safe with minimal toxicities [46]. However, recombinant soluble TRAIL stimulated apoptosis in a variety of cancer cells in vitro as well as attenuated growth of different human cancer cell-derived tumor xenografts in vivo [10].

Monoclonal antibodies that targeted TRAILR1 (DR4) or TRAILR2 (DR5) elicited potent antitumor activities against variety of cancer cells in vitro and in preclinical cancer models [51, 52]. TRAILR2 antibody (TRA-8) has been proven to be cytotoxic to the hepatocellular carcinoma cells while sparing the normal hepatocytes. The reduced sensitivity of this antibody to the normal cells was attributed to generally low to absent levels of the DR4 in the normal cells. Another TRAILR1/DR4 antibody (HGS-ETR1) has been utilized in the phase 2 clinical trials for treatment of colon cancer, nonsmall cell lung cancer, and non-Hodgkins lymphomas. A number of studies further demonstrated utility of TRAIL in combination with chemotherapy (IFN-γ, cyclooxygenase-2 inhibitors, genotoxic agents such as doxorubicin, cisplatin, etoposide) or radiotherapy [53–57]. The TRAIL in combination with chemotherapy or radiotherapy was found to attenuate tumor growth as well as progression in part by simultaneously inducing intrinsic as well as extrinsic apoptosis pathways. The underlying mechanisms vary from the tumor cell type, the TRAIL sensitization to chemotherapies nevertheless includes elevated expression/transcription of DR4 and DR5 receptors, enhanced assembly of the cell surface death receptors, downregulation of intracellular anti-apoptosis effectors such as Bcl-2, Bcl-X_L, or FLIP, and/or upregulation/activation of pro-apoptosis effectors such as caspases or FADD [58–65]. In this context, agents that diminish/reduce FLIP expression have been found to sensitize tumor cells for TRAIL treatment. Reduced expression of FLIP by actinomycin D caused enhanced sensitivity of various tumor cells to receptor-induced apoptosis. In addition, other molecules such as PPARα ligands and proteasome inhibitors have been found to sensitize cancer cells to TRAIL-dependent apoptosis in part by selectively inhibiting FLIP expression [66–68].

4 Caspases and Strategies for Targeting Their Activation

Genetic and cell lineage studies in the nematode *Caenorhabditis elegans* revealed involvement of both positive and negative regulators of apoptosis in the nematode's developmental program [69]. Four genes, egl-1, *ced*-3, *ced*-4, and *ced*-9, encode proteins required for the general apoptosis program. The initiation of apoptosis is regulated by transcriptional upregulation of egl-1 [70]. Binding of egl-1 to anti-apoptotic *ced*-9 relieves the inhibition that ced-9 exerts on the adaptor *ced*-4, allowing *ced*-4 to bind and activate the cysteine (Cys) protease *ced*-3, which in turn cleaves multiple-specific cellular substrates to execute cell death. Multiple mammalian homologs of each class of the *C. elegans* ced proteins, known as caspases, regulate a complex apoptosis program. The caspase family includes 13 members that are classified into three groups [71]: initiators (caspase-2, caspase-8, caspase-9, caspase-10, and caspase-12), which initiate the caspase cascade in apoptosis; executioners (caspase-3, caspase-6, and caspase-7), which act in the downstream execution steps of the process; and inflammatory caspases (caspase-1, caspase-5 and caspase-11), which mediate cell death and inflammatory responses. Caspases are a family of Cys proteases that cleave their substrates after Asp residues. Caspases contain three main domains: a prodomain and large (p20) and small (p10) catalytic subunits. The large domain contains the active site Cys residue. Activation of caspases involves the proteolytic cleavage of zymogens, the removal of the prodomain and separation of the p20 and p10 subunits, or allosteric conformational changes. The prodomains of activator and inflammatory caspases contain protein–protein interaction domains (such as the caspase-recruitment domain (CARD) and the death-effector domain (DED)) that link them to apoptosis signaling molecules [7]. The termination of the caspase activity, on the other hand, generally involves their removal from the cell by the ubiquitin-targeted proteasome degradation machinery or direct inhibition of their enzymatic activities. Intriguingly, there is evidence that members of the inhibitor of apoptosis protein (IAP) family are capable of both functions [72–74].

In light of the fact that caspase family of proteases plays important roles in both the signaling and execution phases of apoptosis, it is conceivable that low expression or dysregulation of caspase function might influence the apoptosis process and result in inappropriate cell proliferation [75]. Expression of execution caspases in tumor cells has been investigated in detail, but the results are conflicting. For example, spontaneous regression and differentiation of neuroblastoma are associated with the translocation of both ICE and CPP32 from the cytoplasm into the nuclei [76]. In contrast, the expression of ICE and CPP32 was significantly downregulated in the tissues of human hepatocellular carcinomas compared to non-tumor parts, indicating that reduced expression of CPP32 may contribute to resistance against apoptosis in human hepatocellular carcinomas [77]. In addition, the nuclear expression of caspase-3 was significantly higher in noninvasive than in invasive tumors of intraductal papillary-mucinous tumor of the pancreas (IPMT) [78]. Since IPMT is a unique tumor that grows intraductally with rare stromal invasion, high expression of caspase-3 may reflect the benign biological behavior of IPMT. Two reports describe that high level of caspase-3, measured by immunohistochemistry and/or western blot analysis, might be an indicator of a good prognosis for non-small cell lung carcinomas [79, 80]. However, in vitro detection of enzymatic caspase-3 activity in colorectal carcinomas revealed that high activity of caspase-3 correlated with poor prognosis [81]. The caspase-3 expression index in human gastric carcinoma correlated significantly with lymph node metastasis and the lower caspase-3 expression index group had a better prognosis than the higher group [82]. A deficiency of caspase-8 has recently been described in small cell lung cancer (SCLC) and in neuroblastomas [83, 84]. The reported observations of caspase-8 changes in cancer cells, including gene deletion, methylation, and point mutation, identify mechanisms by which some tumors, including lung carcinoma, Ewing tumors, neuroblastoma and melanomas, may escape caspase-8-mediated cell death. The gene of caspase-8 is silenced through DNA methylation as well as through gene deletion. Treatment with the demethylation agent 5-aza-2'-deoxycytidine (5-dAzaC) reversed hypermethylation of caspase-8, resulting in restoration of caspase-8 expression and recruitment and activation of caspase-8 at the CD95 DISC upon receptor cross-linking thereby sensitizing for death receptor, and importantly, also for drug-induced apoptosis [85]. In addition to the DNA methylation, three mutation sites in caspase-8 have recently been reported. A mutation modifies the stop codon and adds an Alu repeat to the coding region, thereby lengthening the protein by 88 amino acids in head and neck cancer cell lines [86]. Another missense mutation (alanine to valine) at the caspase-8 codon 96 was found in a neuroblastoma cell line lacking caspase-8 expression [87]. Deletion of the leucine 62 in caspase-8, which was observed in human vulval squamous carcinoma cells, dramatically altered the pro-apoptosis function of caspase-8 [88]. This mutation prevents interaction of pro-caspase-8 with FADD and, hence, the activation of the caspase cascade.

Strategies to target caspase activation or inhibition have been subjects of intense scientific investigation for drug development. A spectrum of caspase inhibitors have been identified and developed for potential applications in diseases and pathologic conditions such as alcoholic liver disease, ischemic kidney and brain injury, myocardial injury, and inflammatory diseases where prevention of tissue/cellular loss is desired [89]. Selective activation of caspases, on the other hand, is considered a valuable strategy for development of anticancer therapies (Table 1). A number of gene delivery approaches have been described. These include activation of inducible caspases by adenoviral gene transfer [90, 91] or their tissue/tumor-specific activation [92–94]. Additionally, tumor-selective activation of caspase-3 or caspase-6 by delivering their anti-Her2/erbB2 antibody fusions in a variety of Her-2-positive tumors in vitro and in xenograft mouse models have also been reported [95, 96]. Tse and Rabbitts

Table 1 Select anti-cancer experimental strategies targeting caspases

Agent	Mechanism of action	Experimental effects	Clinical status	References
Immunocasp-3 Immunocasp-6	Cell-permeable caspase-3 or -6 fusion with anti-HER2 monoclonal antibody	Inhibits growth of HER2-positive mouse xenografts	Preclinical	95, 96
Ad-G/iCasp 3	Chemically inducible caspase-3 adenoviruses	Attenuates tumor growth in a prostate cancer mouse model	Preclinical	91
PEF-F8.CP3	Construct encoding Sc-antibody fused caspase-3	Induces apoptosis in antigendependent fashion	Preclinical	97
FKBP 12/cesp-9 fusion protein	Chemically inducible caspase-9	Caspase-9 dimerization cause anti-angiogenic effects in mouse models	Preclinical	93
RGD peptides	Tripeptide sequencer close to caspase-3 active site	Disrupts intramolecular interaction resulting in caspase-3 activation	Clinical use as antithorobic agent Potenteial use as anti-angiogenic agent	98
Dichlorobenyl carbamates Indolones	Small molecule mimetics targeting caspase-3	Induce apoptosis by activating caspase-3	In vitro testing	100
Gambogic acid derivatives	Activators of caspase-3	Induce apoptosis by activating caspase-3 in syngeneic prostate animal model	Preclinical	101

Part of this table adapted from Fisher and Schulze-Osthoff (2005)

[97] developed a single-chain antibody-caspase-3 fusion gene that conferred toxicity in an antigen-specific manner since binding of the fusion protein to a multivalent antigen led to autoactivation of caspase-3. The effective tumor targeting could potentially involve this reagent in combination with the antibodies against tumor-specific antigens. Unfortunately, the success of the gene delivery approaches has thus far been limited, thus provoking interest in development of cell-permeable, small molecule pharmacological activators of caspases for potential anti-cancer utility. In this context, Buckley et al. [98] reported identification of soluble RGD peptides that promote apoptosis by direct intracellular activation of caspase-3. The naturally occurring RGD tripeptide sequence near the active site of caspase-3 is thought to regulate the quiescent state of this caspase, and the presence of the RGD peptide disrupts the intramolecular interaction and leads to the activation of the protease. These peptides are currently in clinical use as anti-thrombic agents, and are being further explored as candidate drugs to inhibit formation of new tumor blood vessels. High-throughput screening (HTS) approaches are also currently being pursued to identify inducers of caspase activity in living cells or in vitro models. A small molecule activator of caspase-3 was identified by HTS of chemical libraries [99]. This molecule, α-(trichloro-methyl)-4-pyridineethanol (PETCM), although activated caspase-3 in cell extracts, has a requirement of high concentrations (200 μM) for in vitro activation of caspase-3 that unfortunately precludes its therapeutic utility. A similar HTS approach by Nguyen and Wells [100] reported identification of dichlorobenzyl carbamates and indolones as strong caspase activators. An indolone compound potently activated caspase-3 and cell death with an IC_{50} of 4–50 μM in various tumor cell lines in vitro. Further, Zhang et al. [101] reported caspase-activating gambogic acid derivatives that were shown to promote apoptosis in a variety of cancer cells and also in a syngeneic prostate animal cancer model that are currently being evaluated for their anti-cancer potential.

5 Inhibitors of Apoptosis as Potential Targets for Therapeutic Intervention

Viruses are unable to grow or reproduce outside a host cell, but infection of viruses causes disruption of healthy homeostasis, resulting in cell death. Thus, viruses have to keep the host cell alive long enough for viral replication to occur. What is the mechanism by which viruses prevent premature cell death during infection? Normally, replication of baculovirus in host insect cell results in the formation of polyhedra at around 24-h post-infection. However, infection of p35 mutant virus causes cell death beginning at around 9–12 h post-infection, and no polyhedra are formed [102]. This discovery opened a new avenue to identify a family of proteins called inhibitors of apoptosis (IAPs).

The IAP family has at least eight members, including XIAP, cIAP-1, cIAP-2, Ts-IAP, NAIP, survivin, Livin/ML-IAP, and Apollon/Bruce [73, 103–105]. In contrast to Bcl-2 family proteins, all IAPs constitute a family of anti-apoptotic proteins that possess between one and three zinc-binding baculo-viral IAP repeat (BIR) domains that are required for the suppression of apoptosis. Some family members also have a RING finger domain for the ubiquitination and degradation of caspases or caspase-associated recruitment domain (CARD) at the C-terminus [74, 103, 106]. The IAP proteins have been divided into three classes based on the presence or absence of a RING finger and the homology of their BIR domains [107]. Class 1 IAPs (e.g., XIAP, cIAP-1, cIAP-2, Livin/ML-IAP) contain homologous BIR domains and a RING finger motif. The Class 2 IAP family member NAIP has three BIR domains but no RING finger motif [108]. Class 3 IAP members, such as survivin, contain only a single BIR domain and no RING finger [109]. BIRs are regions of ∼70 amino acids that contain the signature sequence CX2CX16HX6C (C, cysteine; H, histidine; and X, any amino acid) and fold as three-stranded β sheets surrounded by four α helices [110–112]. BIRs function mainly by regulating protein–protein interaction. In XIAP, BIR3 (the third BIR domain) potently inhibits the activity of the active caspase-9, whereas the linker region between BIR1 and BIR2, as well as the BIR2 domain itself, selectively targets active caspase-3 or caspase-7 [133, 114]. Thus, IAP suppresses apoptosis by binding to and inhibiting upstream (e.g., caspase-9) and downstream caspases (e.g., caspase-3 and caspase-7) through BIR domains [73, 103, 115]. IAPs inhibit both the intrinsic and the extrinsic pathways for initiation of caspase activation, as well as influence a third minor pathway in which granzyme B directly activates caspase-3 [18, 116]. In apoptotic cells, caspase inhibition by IAP is negatively regulated by a mitochondrial protein, second mitochondria-derived activator of caspase (Smac). Smac physically interacts with multiple IAPs through a conserved N-terminal IAP-binding motif (IBM) and relieves their inhibitory effect on caspase-3, caspase-7, and caspase-9. Smac binds to the BIR3 domain of XIAP through four N-terminal residues (AVPI) that recognize a surface groove on BIR3. These four amino acids are conserved in three *Drosophila* proteins (Reaper, Grim, and Hid) that induce apoptosis by eliminating the binding of *Drosophila* IAP to caspases [117, 118]. Studies by Eckelman et al. [119] revealed that XIAP BIR2 and a short preceding peptide strand bind the substrate-binding cleft of caspase-3 and caspase-7, with the peptide strand in reverse orientation to that of substrate ("back and front"). In contrast, BIR3 inhibits caspase-9 by a novel allosteric mechanism in which its distal helix forces caspase-9 into an inactive monomeric conformation by interposition between the caspase dimerization interfaces [120]. Unlike BIR2 and BIR3, the BIR1 domain of XIAP, c-IAP1, and c-IAP2 functions in several signaling pathways via oligomerization of binding partner instead of binding caspase or IBM proteins such as Smac. For example, when overexpressed, XIAP BIR1 interacts with TGF-β activating

Kinase 1 associating subunit 1 to induce NF-κB activation [121]. These findings provide an example of functional diversity within BIRs.

Many studies have revealed that IAPs are preferentially expressed in malignant cells and are prognostically important. For example, survivin a 16.5 kDa protein is overexpressed in almost all malignancies but rarely detected in normal differentiated adult tissues [109, 122], and its expression correlates with poor prognosis leading to the hypothesis that IAP overexpression might be an oncogenic event [122, 123]. XIAP is also overexpressed in many cancer cell lines and cancer tissues. High XIAP expression has been correlated with resistance to chemotherapy and radiotherapy and to poor clinical outcomes [124]. However, knocking out XIAP with siRNA or antisense oligonucleotides restores chemosensitivity in a variety of cancer cells [125–128]. Given possible importance of IAPs in tumorigenesis, strategies summarized in Table 2 have been developed to target IAPs by downregulating their expression with different techniques including gene knockdown (antisense oligonucleotides and RNA interference), gene therapy, small molecule antagonist, and immunotherapy (DNA vaccine). Mesri et al. [129] reported generation of adenoviruses expressing nonphosphorylatable mutant of survivin that induced apoptosis in cancer cells by interfering with survivin function and suppressed breast cancer xenograft growth in animal models. The antisense molecules targeting depletion of IAPs used in research studies and clinical trial include DNA oligonucleotides or RNA oligonucleotides or mixture of DNA and RNA oligonucleotides. The antisense molecule inhibits its target by forming a duplex with the native mRNA. In this double-stranded conformation, intracellular RNAase H cleaves the native mRNA while leaving the antisense intact. The antisense is released back into the cytoplasm where it is capable of binding additional target mRNA. Thus, antisense oligonucleotides knock down their targets by promoting the degradation of native mRNA rather than by directly inhibiting translation. In preclinical studies, antisense oligonucleotides against either XIAP [128, 130, 131] or survivin [132] directly induced apoptosis and sensitized malignant cells to chemotherapy and γ-irradiation. Antisense oligonucleotide compounds against XIAP (AEG35156) and survivin (YM-155 and LY-2181308) are already in Phase I/II trials for treatment of a variety of cancers (http://clinicaltrials.gov). The discovery that synthetic 21–23 nucleotide RNA duplexes can trigger an RNA interference (RNAi) response in mammalian cells and induce strong inhibition of specific gene expression has opened the door to the therapeutic use of small interfering RNAs (siRNAs) [133]. Several studies using chemically synthesized siRNAs or plasmid/viral vectors encoding short hairpin RNAs showed that RNAi-mediated survivin knockdown was able to reduce tumor cell proliferative potential and induce caspase-dependent apoptosis in a variety of human tumor cell models, as well as to decrease the formation of new tumors and the growth of already established lesions in nude mice [134].

An alternate approach to inhibiting IAPs involves small molecules that block active sites on the IAP protein. Structural and functional studies have

Table 2 Select anti-cancer agents targeting inhibitor of apoptosis proteins

Agent	Mechanisma of action	Experimental effects	Clinical status	Reference/company
BIR3 antagonists	Small molecule antagonists of IAPs	Cause apoptosis in cancer cell lines	Preclinical	Idun Pharmaceuticals, Inc.
Capped tripeptide XIAP antagonists	XIAP ligands that target BIR3 domain	Inhibit growth of cancer cells and breast cancer xenografts	Preclinical	Abbott Laboratories [135]
TWX024	Nonpeptidic small molecule that inhibits BIR2/caspase-3 interaction	Induces apoptosis in cancer cells, synergizes with anti-CD95 and TRAIL	Preclinical	138
Polyphenylurea derivatives	Specific BIR2 inhibitors	Activate caspases, suppress growth of xenografted tumors	Preclinical	140
SMAC mimetics	XIAP-binding Smac mimetics	Enhance cisplatin-induced apoptosis in prostate cancer cells	Preclinical	136
XIAP RNAi plasmids and antisense oligos	Blocl XIAP expression	Induce apoptosis in cancer cells, synergize with chemotheraopy in mouse models	Preclinical	128, 130, 131
AEG35156/GEM640	XIAP antisense oligonucleotide	Inhibits growth of xenografted cancers alone or in combination with chemotherapeutics	Phase 1	Aegera Therapeutics Inc. and Hybridon
Small molecule Smac mimetics	Cell-permeable inhibitors of XIAP, cIAP-1, cIAP-2	Potentiate apoptosis in combination with TRIAL and TNF	Preclinical	137
LY2181308	Construct expressing survivin antisense	Anti-tumor activity in a broad range of cancers	Phase 1	ISIS Pharmaceuticals, Inc. and Eli Lilly & Company
Ad-survivin T34A	Adenovirus expressing nonphosphroylatable mutant of survivin	Induces apoptosis in cancer cells, and suppresses breast cancer xenograft growth	Preclinical	129

demonstrated BIR 3 domain of XIAP binds and inhibits caspase-9, two surfaces on the BIR 2 domain bind and inhibit active caspase-3 and caspase-7, and Smac binds the BIRs of IAPs and neutralizes their anti-apoptotic activity. Different groups of small molecules have been identified using methods such as high-throughput fluorescent polarization competitive binding assay [135, 136], computer-based rational drug design [137], high-throughput enzymatic de-repression assay [138], and computational structure-based herbal library screening [139]. Schimmer et al. [140] utilized an enzyme de-repression assay to screen for polyphenylurea-based XIAP antagonists. These polyphenylurea derivatives induced apoptosis in leukemia cells as well as suppressed growth of xenografted colon cancer cells in animal models. These molecules bind the active sites of IAPs and inhibit the interaction between IAPs and caspases and thereby repress IAP-mediated inhibition of caspases. Results indicate that all these small molecule compounds specifically bind to their targets and induce apoptosis and sensitize cells to anti-cancer treatment. Based on the crystallization of XIAP BIR3 in a complex with Smac, small compounds or peptide that mimic Smac function have also been reported [141]. These Smac peptides not only neutralize IAP inhibition of caspase activity in vitro but they also sensitize primary cancer cells to death receptor or chemotherapy-induced apoptosis [142, 143].

Two main gene therapy approaches targeting survivin have been successfully developed. One is based on the use of plasmids or viral vectors to deliver dominant-negative survivin mutants to tumor cells [144, 145]. The second gene therapy approach involves the use of the survivin gene promoter to drive the expression of cytotoxic genes in tumor cells [146, 147]. Survivin is a tumor-associated antigen [148]. Autoantibody against survivin has been detected in cancer patients [149]. Survivin-specific cytotoxic T lymphocytes induced by HLA-A2-binding peptide and dendritic cells from healthy donors efficiently lysed target cells, indicating that survivin epitopes are presented on a broad variety of malignancies and can be applied in vaccination therapies [150, 151]. These approaches are now in clinical testing [152].

6 The Anti-apoptotic BCL-2 Family of Proteins as Targets for Anti-cancer Strategies

In the multi-cellular organisms cells are normally protected from early death in part by the Bcl-2 family of anti- and pro-apoptotic regulators that mediate intrinsic pathway of apoptosis. BCL-2 (for B-cell lymphoma-2) was first identified at the chromosomal breakpoint of t(14;18) bearing human follicular B-cell lymphoma [153–155]. Bcl-2-transfected B cells were shown to be resistant toward a default death process normally induced in B cells by IL-3 withdrawal [156]. Further experiments have demonstrated that overexpression of the human bcl-2 gene in the nematode *C. elegans* reduced the number of programmed cell deaths [157], and that ced-9 and bcl-2 are homologs, indicating the molecular mechanisms of apoptosis are highly conserved within the animal kingdom [158]. These pioneer research work revealed that cell growth and survival were under independent genetic control and that Bcl-2-mediated pathway toward tumorigenesis depends not only on the ability to escape growth control but also depends on the ability to prevent apoptosis.

At least 15 Bcl-2 family members have been identified in mammalian cells and several others in viruses [5]. As indicated before, all members possess at least one of four conserved motifs known as Bcl-2 homology domains (BH1–BH4). Based on the content of BH, the family numbers are classified into three groups [3]. Anti-apoptotic members (e.g., BCL-2, BCL-X_L, BCL-w, MCL-1, and A1) contain all four BH domains defined by their similarity among the members of the family and promote cell survival by inhibiting the function of the pro-apoptotic Bcl-2 family members. In addition, all anti-apoptotic members of the Bcl-2 family have an N-terminal BH4 domain [159, 160]. The "multidomain" pro-apoptotic proteins (BAX, BAK, and Bok) contain BH domains 1–3. BH3-only proteins of pro-apoptotic members (e.g., BID, BAD, BIM, BIK, PUMA, and NOXA) contain only BH domain 3 (BH3) and are structurally diverse [161]. The 3D structure of Bcl-X_L [162, 163] has revealed that several Bcl-2 family members share striking structural similarity to the pore-forming domains of bacterial toxins thus sparking a series of subsequent studies that demonstrated an ability of Bcl-X_L, Bcl-2, and Bax to form ion channels in synthetic membranes [164–166]. Although it is still unclear if these channels are functionally involved in apoptosis, pore formation by Bcl-2 proteins has been hypothesized to be important for regulating the release of cytochrome c and perturbing mitochondrial physiology [167]. Point mutations and domain deletion experiments indicate that the BH4 domain is essential for pro-survival protein such as Bcl-2, Bcl-xL, and Bcl-w and that this domain functions by binding, sequestering, and inactivating apoptotic peptidase-activating factor 1 (Apaf-1) [160]. The BH3 domain in all pro-apoptotic Bcl-2 proteins is critical for their interaction with death suppressors. The BH1, BH2, and BH3 domains are single amphipathic alpha helices and form a hydrophobic pocket. This pocket is thought to act as a binding site for BH3-only death-promoting proteins [168].

An exact mechanism by which Bcl-2 regulates intrinsic pathway is still unclear, but there are at least three different models to explain how different stimuli trigger apoptosis [169]. In the first model, the pro-apoptotic Bax and Bak are in an inactive conformation through direct interactions with one or two different anti-apoptotic Bcl-2 proteins. In response to an apoptosis stimulus, BH3-only proteins bind to and neutralize the anti-apoptotic Bcl-2 proteins, thereby releasing Bax and Bak [37, 170]. Alternatively, it has been shown that certain BH3-only proteins can interact with the pro-apoptotic proteins and trigger apoptosis by binding directly to Bax and Bak [171]. Finally, recent data suggest that anti-apoptotic Bcl-2 family members sequester BH3-only proteins, preventing the activation of pro-apoptotic Bax and Bak. Eventually, the activated BH3-only protein will overcome the anti-apoptotic Bcl-2 protein, thereby triggering the death process by direct activation of Bax/Bak or, possibly, activation of some other unknown factor in the cytosol or mitochondria required for Bax/Bak activation [172]. Interestingly, in some circumstances, Bcl-2 and Bcl-X_L are targets of caspases, and cleavage of these proteins converts them from pro-survival to pro-apoptotic molecules that are able to induce cytochrome c release from the mitochondria, which could be the fourth model of Bcl2-regulated apoptosis [173–175]. Once pro-apoptotic proteins (Bax or Bak) translocate to the mitochondria cytochrome c release and caspase activation occur [176]. Cytochrome c release was highly associated with induction of the mitochondrial permeability transition and disruption of the mitochondrial inner transmembrane potential ($\Delta\Psi_m$) [177]. Cytochrome c released from mitochondria forms a complex with Apaf-1 in the cytosol and inactive caspase-9 [178–180]. In the presence of dATP or ATP, this complex processes and activates the caspase-9, which in turn triggers a cascade by processing and activating other caspases (in particular, caspase-3, caspase-6, and caspase-7) [180, 181]. These activated caspases then cleave key substrates and coordinate the process of apoptotic cell death.

Bcl-2 overexpression is a common phenomenon in many malignant tumors such as non-Hodgkin's follicular B-cell lymphoma, prostate cancer, colon cancer, lung cancer, breast cancer, gastric cancer, renal cancer, neuroblastoma, acute and chronic leukemia, and skin cancer [182]. Bcl-2 inhibition of cytochrome c release and stabilization of mitochondrial function are associated with the resistance to chemotherapy- and radiation-induced apoptosis [3]. Therefore, strategies targeting the intrinsic apoptosis pathway have focused on Bcl-2 family proteins [183]. To date, several approaches have been used to target the proteins of Bcl-2 family [184], and a select group of strategies that have shown promise in preclinical as well as clinical studies are indicated in Table 3. In general, various strategies thus far have been focused in either downregulating expression of anti-apoptotic Bcl-2 family of protein by means of antisense-dependent methods, peptide or small molecule mimetics of BH3 domain, or small molecule agents to interfere with Bcl-2 functions. Since Bcl-2 does not protect against GSH-dependent loss of $\Delta\Psi_m$ and cell death induced by the thiol-crosslinking agent diazenedicarboxylic acid bis $5N,N$-dimethylamide or the GSH-depleting agent diethylmaleate [185, 186] a potential way to overcome the anti-apoptotic action of Bcl-2 may be to develop drugs designed to deplete mitochondrial GSH levels and induce mitochondrial protein oxidation and cell death [184]. It has been reported that PK11195, prototypic ligand of the mitochondrial benzodiazepine receptor, has been able to reverse the resistance to apoptosis in cells that overexpress Bcl-2 by activating the mitochondrial permeability transition [187], suggesting a novel strategy for enhancing the susceptibility of cells to apoptosis induction and, concomitantly, for reversing Bcl-2-mediated cytoprotection. Bcl-2-targeted antisense therapy represents a promising new apoptosis-modulating strategy [188, 189]. For example, Zangemeister-Wittke et al. [190] identified a bispecific antisense oligonucleotide

Table 3 Select anti-cancer strategies targeting Bcl-2 proteins

Agent	Mechanisma of action	Experimental effects	Clinical status	Reference/company
Bcl-2 blocker	Small molecule antagonists of Bcl-2/Bcl-X$_L$	Cause apoptosis in cancer cells	Preclinical	Idun Pharmaceuticals, Inc. Abbott Laboratories
GX01 compounds	Small molecule inhibitors binding Bcl-2 proteins	Cause apoptosis in cancer cells	Preclinical	Gemin X Biotechnologies
Bcl-2 antagonists	Structure-based small molecule Bcl-2 antagonists		Preclinical	Structural Bioinformatics Inc.
Tetrocarcin-A derivatives	Natural fungal compound inhibitor of Bcl-2	Induces apoptosis by inhibiting mitochondrial functions of Bcl-2	Preclinical	199
Chelerythrime	Plant alkaloid inhibitor of Bcl-2/Bax interaction	Induces death in Bcl-2 and Bcl-X$_L$-overexpressing cancer cells	Preclinical	203
Antimycin A derivatives	Natural and synthetic inhibitors of Bcl-2/Bcl-X$_L$	Induce apoptosis by binding to the BH3 pocket of Bcl-2 and Bcl-X$_L$	Preclinical	201
Synthetic compound	Chemical compound binding the BH3 pocket of Bcl-2	Induces deatj in Bcl-2 overexpressing cancer cells	Preclinical	
Genasemse/ oblimersen	18-mer Bcl-2 antisense oligonucleotide	Kills drug-resistant chroniclumphocytic leukemia (CLL) cells, delays development of fetal lymphoma in mice, enhances dacarbasine efficacy in melanoma models	Phase 3 for melanoma, multiple myeloma, CLL NSCLC Phase 2 for hormone refractory prostate cancer	Aventis, Genta Inc.

Table 3 (continued)

Agent	Mechanisma of action	Experimental effects	Clinical status	Reference/company
SAHBs	Bax/Bak oilgomerization-inducing BH-3 peptidomimetics	Induce apoptosis in cancer cells and suppress leukemic xenograft growth	Preclinical	196
BH3Is	Compounds interfering with Bzk-BH3/Bcl-X$_L$ interaction	Induce apoptosis	Preclinical	202

Adapted from Fisher and Schulze-Osthoff (2005)

corresponding to a sequence that is highly homologous in Bcl-2 and Bcl-X$_L$ mRNAs but missing in Bcl-X$_S$ mRNA. This antisense oligonucleotide effectively killed a diverse type of cancer cells. Another approach by Taylor et al. [191] exploited the fact that Bcl-X gene is differentially spliced to give rise to Bcl-X$_L$ and Bcl-X$_S$ mRNAs encoding the anti- and pro-apoptotic proteins, respectively. The antisense targeting the region proximal to the splice donor site essential for the generation of mature Bcl-X$_L$ mRNA triggered the splicing complex to produce mainly the mRNA for short (Bcl-X$_S$) variant. This agent caused reduced Bcl-X$_L$/Bcl-X$_S$ ratio, and sensitized cancer cells to UV- and chemotherapy-induced apoptosis. The most clinically advanced anti-Bcl-2 therapy, the antisense agent oblimersen, has reached phase III development. Results have been encouraging in patients with chronic lymphocytic leukemia, with improved response and remission rates and prolonged progression-free survival [189]. Other promising results have been observed among patients with advanced, relapsed melanoma, with the evidence of prolonged overall survival [192].

An alternative to inhibiting Bcl-2 to activate apoptosis has been to target pro-apoptotic Bcl-2 proteins and peptides to mitochondria. For example, gene therapy employing adenoviral Bax-delivering vectors has been successful in activating mitochondrial apoptosis [193–195]. Because protein interaction between BCL-2 members is a prominent mechanism of control and is mediated through the amphipathic alpha-helical BH3 segment, an essential death domain the stapled peptides, called "stabilized alpha-helix of BCL-2 domains" are designed to specifically bind to multidomain BCL-2 member pockets to block the action of Bcl-2 and activate Bax and Bak [196]. Multiple studies have focused on developing peptide mimetics of the BH3 domains and their delivery by cationic lipids as well as their conjugation with protein transduction domains [197], fatty acids. Direct delivery of Bad peptide together with decanoic acid to enhance cell permeability was found to induce apoptosis in tumor cells without harming normal human peripheral lymphocytes [198].

High-throughput screening (HTS) of chemical libraries has yielded several small molecules to target functions of the Bcl-2 family proteins. For instance, tetrocarcin-A (TC-A), an antibiotic from *Actinomyces* was isolated and found to sensitize Bcl-2-overexpressing HeLa cells to death receptor- and staurosporine-mediated apoptosis [199]. Wang et al. [200] identified a compound (HA14-1) that competed with Bak for binding with Bcl-2 and in turn induced apoptosis in HL60 cells. Similar approaches resulted in identification of antimycin A3, an inhibitor of mitochondrial electron transport chain, that targeted the BH3 pocket and induced apoptosis in Bcl-2- and Bcl-X$_L$-overexpressing cancer cells [201]. HTS of a library of pre-selected compounds yielded BH3 inhibitors that disrupt Bcl-X$_L$ complex and cause decreased mitochondrial membrane potential to promote apoptosis [202], while Chan et al. [203] similarly identified a natural alkaloid chelerythrine that inhibited Bcl-X$_L$/Bak-BH3 interaction and suppressed growth of Bcl-2- and Bcl-X$_L$-overexpressing cells. In addition, several promising small molecule antagonists of Bcl-2 are in early development. The R-(-)-gossypol derivative AT-101, a BH3 mimetic, is in phase I testing, as is ABT-263, a small molecule that binds with subnanomolar affinity to Bcl-2, Bcl-X_L, and Bcl-W. Both molecules have demonstrated single-agent activity and an additive effect in combination with cytotoxic agents in preclinical studies [204, 205]. GX-15-070 (obatoclax), which is reported to inhibit all five members of the Bcl-2 family, is in phase II clinical trials [206].

7 P53 and Strategies Targeting Its Functional Activation

P53, commonly referred to as the gatekeeper of the genome, was discovered in 1979 and subsequently classified as a tumor suppressor protein. This classification was based on a large body of experimental evidence derived from a wealth of in vitro and in vivo studies demonstrating loss of p53 or presence of its mutations in a variety of tumors, along with the observations showing suppression of cell growth and transformation following ectopic overexpression of p53 [207]. Thus, loss of p53 function, and the fact that different stress and DNA damaging signals often activate p53 to induce cell cycle arrest and/or apoptosis, led to emergence of approaches to restore wild-type p53 functions in tumors harboring mutant p53. These include targeting of p53 mutants by small molecules to induce conformational changes that favor its growth inhibitory functions [208], synthetic peptides derived from its C-terminus that interact with the core domain of the mutant p53 and restore growth-inhibitory transcriptional functions of p53 [209, 210]. Additional strategies have been reported to deliver functional p53 by using the protein transduction domains (PTD) or the anti-DNA monoclonal antibodies in order to restore tumor suppressor function of p53 in vitro as well as in preclinical mouse model of colon cancer metastasis [211–214].

Strategies to stabilize p53 and to restore its tumor suppressor function have also included targeting its binding with the negative regulator Mdm2. The E3 ligase activity of Mdm2 protein is responsible for proteasomal degradation of Mdm2-bound p53 that results in loss of p53 expression and consequent function. In addition, E6 protein of human papillomaviruses (HPV) induces p53 degradation with the help of cellular E3 ligase. Hence, targeting of Mdm2 binding with p53 and/or E3 ligase function of Mdm2 to prevent p53 degradation are therefore attractive approaches to restoring p53 function. Synthetic peptide aptamers that compete for HPV E6 binding with p53 have been found to promote apoptosis-inducing function of p53 in HPV-positive cervical cancers [215] while small molecule antagonists of Mdm2 E3 ligase function have been identified and evaluated as potential anti-cancer agents [216]. Several peptide-based mimetics that specifically interfere with p53–Mdm2 interactions have also been reported and tested for their anti-cancer properties in vitro as well as animal xenograft models [217]. Virtual database screening strategies identified a number of non-peptide small molecule inhibitors of p53–Mdm2 interaction. The prominent examples include the imidazoline compounds called nutlins [218, 219], a benzodiazepine-based inhibitor [220], and spiro-oxindole-based inhibitor [221]. NCI compound library search further yielded a furan derivative termed RITA that was found to interfere with p53–Mdm2 binding in vitro and in vivo, and attenuated growth of colon cancer xenografts in mice [222]. Considering the facts that almost 50% of all cancers have p53 function modified by mutations or deletions [223] and the mutant p53 proteins generally do not bind Mdm2, the approaches directed to restore the function of wild-type p53 nonetheless are expected to have significant impact in designing future anti-cancer therapeutic strategies in 50% of cancers with wild-type p53.

The apoptotic functions of p53 are complex and involve transcriptional regulation of pro-apoptotic genes, direct targeting of the anti- and pro-apoptotic Bcl2 family of proteins as well as the mitochondria [224]. Although p53 lacks classical mitochondrial targeting epitopes and the precise signal on p53 for its mitochondrial translocation is unknown, a variety of stress signals nevertheless are known to induce p53 translocation to mitochondria and promote outer mitochondrial membrane (OMM) permeabilization, an event necessary for mitochondria-dependent apoptosis signaling. In light of the fact that the mutant p53 is known to accumulate in tumors and functions in part by antagonizing other members of its family to promote tumor growth, pharmacological targeting of heat shock protein-90 to promote proteasomal degradation of p53 mutants unfortunately had limited success due primarily to toxic side effects of HSP inhibitors [225]. Moreover, a number of studies over the last decade have suggested an intriguing, two-faced nature of the p53 protein [226]. It appears that mutations in p53 not only promote loss of its tumor suppression property but the mutant forms of p53 protein also tend to be oncogenic and a combination of loss of tumor suppression and gain of oncogenic functions contribute to development of tumors. These emergent apoptotic as well as oncogenic functions of p53 thus present novel avenues/challenges to rationally target p53 to not only restore its wild-type functions but also, perhaps concomitantly, to effectively block oncogenic functions of its mutants.

8 Novel and Emerging Apoptosis Transducers as Targets for Anti-cancer Strategies

8.1 Nur77/TR3

Nur77 (aka TR3, NGFI-B, TIS1, and NAK-1) belongs to a subfamily within the nuclear receptor superfamily. The members of this subfamily are often classified as orphan receptors because they have no known physiological ligands [227, 228]. The other closely related members of this subfamily are Nur1 (aka RNR-1, TINUR, and HZF-3) and NOR-1 (aka MINOR, CHN, and TEC). Structural analyses of these orphan receptors revealed absence of classical ligand pockets in their ligand-binding domains indicating that their biological functions are likely independent of the ligand binding [229, 230]. The various members of this subfamily are known to transduce diverse signals including survival, differentiation, and apoptosis. Their function/activities are regulated by their subcellular distribution, expression, post-translational modifications as well as their ability to heterodimerize with the retinoid X receptors [224]. A number of reports have revealed cell survival and oncogenic functions of these receptors. Nur77 is a target of growth factor and mitogenic signaling since it is overexpressed in diverse cancer cell lines as well as in prostate cancers [231], its ectopic overexpression conferred resistance to retinoids in lung cancer cells [232], while its suppression inhibited transformed phenotype of several cancer cells in part by promoting apoptosis [233].

Apoptosis signals are also known to target the Nur77 family of receptors as indicated by studies showing their crucial involvement in the T-cell receptor-dependent apoptosis [234, 235]. The Nur77 family members are induced by antigen-receptor engagement, ischemic stress, and function in part by promoting apoptosis of the affected cells [236]. A large number of investigations subsequently revealed induction of Nur77 by a variety of apoptosis-promoting agents in cancer cells [175, 237–240]. The potential clinical relevance of Nur77 functions was further highlighted by the studies showing expression of its family member Nor-1 was one of the outcome predictors and was found to correlate with cured as opposed to fatal/refractory diffuse large B-cell lymphomas [241]. Although transcriptional function of Nur77 is thought to be critical for T-cell apoptosis, several studies indicated apoptosis signaling by Nur77 by mechanisms independent of its transcriptional functions. In this context, activation of apoptosis signaling has been shown to cause increased phosphorylation as well as translocation of Nur77 from nucleus to cytosolic compartment where it interacts with a number of Bcl-2 family members that include Bcl-2, Bcl-B, Bfl-1, and the complex targets the mitochondria for Nur77-dependent apoptosis [175, 242, 243]. Several variations in cytoplasmic Nur77-dependent apoptosis signaling have also been reported. For example, in colon cancer cells, the cytoplasmic relocation of Nur77 is thought to indirectly activate mitochondrial pathway by promoting Bax localization to mitochondria [244]. The mitochondrial targeting by Nur77 has also been implicated in the neuronal cell death pathways [245].

Diverse signaling pathways regulate Nur77 function and its nuclear-cytoplasmic shuttling by either targeting phosphorylation of its N-terminal A/B region or its heterodimerization with RXRs [175, 242]. Although the precise mechanisms of Nur77 shuttling and mitochondrial targeting are yet to be elucidated, its interactions with RXRs are thought to facilitate its nuclear export in part via the nuclear export sequences (NES) of the RXRα [175]. In this context, the growth inhibitory effects of 9-*cis*-retinoic acid (an RXR ligand), its metabolites, and insulin-like growth factor-binding protein (IGFBP)-3 are thought to regulate Nur77-RXRα interactions, cytoplasmic translocation, and mitochondrial targeting by this receptor [175, 246, 247]. Since both Nur77 and Bcl-2 family of proteins are often overexpressed in many cancers, the mechanisms regulating their interactions, translocation, and mitochondrial targeting are therefore excellent opportunities for development of anti-cancer agents that will mimic aspect(s) of apoptosis-promoting functions of Nur77. To this end, binding of Nur77 with Bcl-2 was exploited to design a Nur77-mimicking peptide that inhibited growth of myeloma cells in vitro, and the binding of this peptide with Bcl-B was recently utilized for high-throughput screening to identify novel small molecule Bcl-B inhibitors [243, 248].

8.2 CARP-1/CCAR1

Cell cycle and apoptosis regulatory protein (CARP)-1, also known as CCAR1, is a novel regulator of apoptosis signaling. The GenBank database indicates CARP-1 proteins deduced from the nucleotide sequences of diverse species including mouse, rat, dog, chimpanzee, gallus (fowl), xenopus, honey bee, and *C. elegans*. Human CARP-1 gene is located at the long arm of chromosome 10 (10q21–10q22). CARP-1 transduces diverse growth inhibitory signaling, and functions in a manner independent of tumor suppressor p53 [249, 250]. CARP-1 expression correlated inversely with the breast cancer tumor grades (Table 4), and its loss in breast cancers was due in part to methylation-dependent gene silencing mechanisms [251]. Loss of CARP-1 interferes with cell growth inhibition induced by adriamycin, etoposide but not by cisplatin, suggesting that CARP-1 is an important mediator of signaling by adriamycin [249]. Genetic studies in *C. elegans* revealed CARP-1 ortholog Lst3 is a transducer of Notch signaling that functions as a counteractor of the EGFR–MAPK pathway [252]. This function of CARP-1 as EGFR signaling antagonist was also supported in studies by Rishi et al. [250] where CARP-1 was found to regulate growth of diverse cancer cells following inhibition of EGFRs. The apoptosis signaling by EGFRs stimulated tyrosine phosphorylation of CARP-1 and targeted CARP-1 tyrosine 192, while CARP-1-dependent apoptosis in turn involved activation of stress-activated MAPK (SAPK) p38 and caspase-9 [250]. Breast cancer cells overexpressing CARP-1, that were generated following transfection of plasmid encoding wild-type CARP-1, formed reduced-sized tumors in the severely compromised immunodeficient (SCID) mice when compared with the tumors formed by their vector-expressing or wild-type counterparts (Fig. 2). Whether

Table 4 CARP-1 expression inversely correlates with the breast cancer histologic grade (Fisher's exact P = 0.00000378)

Tumor histologic grade (N = 100)	CARP-1 expression	
	Low (%)	High (%)
Low	16	27
High	47	10

Adapted from Zhang et al., (2007)

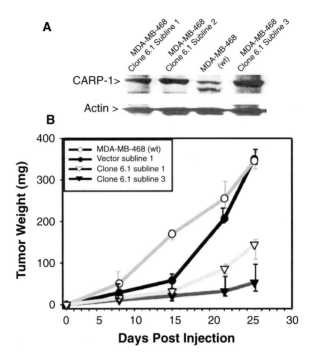

Fig. 2 CARP-1 expression in breast cancer cells results in their reduced growth as xenografted tumors in SCID mice. (A) Western immunoblot of wild-type human breast cancer cells and their sublines that were transfected with plasmid clone 6.1 for expression of CARP-1-myc-His fusion protein. The cells were lysed and the total proteins were analyzed by SDS-PAGE followed by their transfer to nitrocellulose membrane and probing the membrane with anti-CARP-1 (α1) antibodies or anti-actin antibodies. **(B)**Histogram of growth of tumor xenografts derived from the wild-type, the vector-expressing, or CARP-1-myc-His fusion protein-expressing breast cancer cells. Points, average of tumor weights from two independent experiments; bars, SE (adapted from Zhang et al. [251])

CARP-1 expression inhibited breast cancer cell growth was further studied by utilizing various cell-permeable, TAT-tagged CARP-1 peptides including the peptide having CARP-1 amino-terminal 1–198 amino acids that contained the epitope targeted by EGFR signaling. Consistent with the perinuclear presence of CARP-1, incubation of breast cancer cells with these affinity-purified, denatured TAT-tagged CARP-1 peptides resulted in the predominant localization of these peptides to the cytoplasmic/perinuclear region. The TAT-tagged CARP-1 (1–198) peptide, but not its tyrosine 192 to phenylalanine variant or TAT-tagged eGFP protein, inhibited growth of the breast cancer cells in part by inducing apoptosis in a time-dependent manner [251]. The affinity-purified, TAT-tagged CARP-1 (1–198) peptide, but not its tyrosine 192 to phenylalanine variant, also suppressed growth of breast cancer cell-derived xenografted tumors in SCID mice (Fig. 3), in part, by promoting apoptosis as evidenced by elevated TUNEL staining as well as presence of activated (phosphorylated)

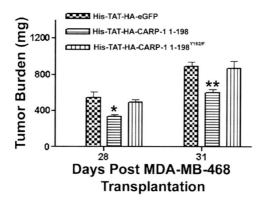

Fig. 3 His-TAT-HA-CARP-1 (1-198) protein inhibits growth of human breast cancer cell-derived tumor xenografts in SCID mice. The wild-type breast cancer cells were xenografted subcutaneously in each flank. After the palpable tumors developed, the proteins were injected intratumorally at a dose of 25 μg/tumor/day for 5 consecutive days and tumor growth monitored for additional 20 days. Histogram columns represent mean tumor weight and the standard deviation is indicated by bars. *P = 0.0015; **P = 0.003 compared with the corresponding His-TAT-HA-eGFP-treated tumors (adapted from Zhang et al. [251])

p38 stress-activated protein kinase (SAPK) in the xenograft biopsies (Fig. 4). The facts that EGFR signaling targeted CARP-1 tyrosine 192 and suppression of cell growth following attenuation of EGFRs involved elevated tyrosine phosphorylation of CARP-1 [250] strongly support a breast cancer cell growth inhibitory function of CARP-1. Phosphopeptide mapping studies further revealed that CARP-1 is a serine phospho-protein, and although the epidermal growth factor (EGF) as well as the ATM kinase signaling phosphorylates specific serine residues of CARP-1 [253–255], the extent this CARP-1 serine phosphorylation modulates its function in regulating cell growth is yet to be clarified. In light of the fact that serine/threonine phosphorylation of pro-apoptotic Bcl-2 family of proteins often promotes their binding with and sequestration by the 14-3-3 proteins to allow cell growth and survival and the facts that CARP-1 binds with 14-3-3 [249] and is also a part of the NFκB proteome [256], it remains to be elucidated whether its serine phosphorylation is crucial for its interactions with 14-3-3 and the extent this interaction regulates NFκB signaling. Mutagenesis studies nonetheless revealed the presence of multiple, non-redundant apoptosis-promoting epitopes within CARP-1, suggesting that diverse apoptosis signals likely target this protein [250].

Consistent with the perinuclear presence of CARP-1, a broader role of CARP-1 in transcriptional regulation has also been recently described [257]. These studies not only elaborated CARP-1 as a key regulator of mediator complex recruitment to the estrogen receptor (ER)-α and glucocorticoid receptor for nuclear receptor target gene activation but was also found to be a co-activator of tumor suppressor p53 in regulating DNA damage-induced

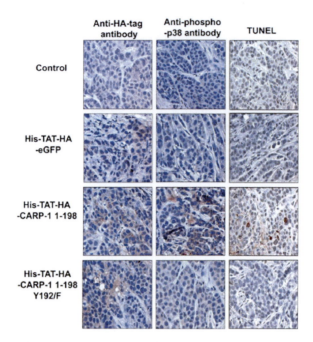

Fig. 4 Inhibition of human breast cancer cell-derived xenograft growth by His-TAT-HA-CARP-1 (1-198) protein involves elevated apoptosis. The formalin-fixed tumor xenograft biopsies from the experiment in Fig. 3 were paraffin embedded, processed, and subsequently subjected to immunohistochemical staining for determination of apoptosis. The representative photomicrographs showing intratumoral presence (*brown color*) of respective peptides are indicated by staining with anti-HA-tag antibodies (*left*). Representative photomicrographs are also presented showing apoptosis in xenografted tumors following their staining with anti-phospho-p38 antibodies (*middle*) using terminal deoxynucleotidyl transferase-mediated nick-end labeling (TUNEL) assay (*right*) (adapted from Zhang et al. [251])

transcriptional upregulation of cyclin-dependent kinase inhibitor p21$^{\text{WAF1/CIP1}}$. Thus, like Nur77, the studies by Kim et al. [257] reveal a dual role for CARP-1 in supporting hormone-dependent transcriptional activation for cell proliferation as well as in apoptosis induction following DNA damage. The fact that peptides derived from CARP-1 inhibit growth of breast cancer cells in vitro and xeno-grafted tumors in part by inducing apoptosis [251] suggests that the apoptosis signaling mechanisms by CARP-1 could potentially be exploited to identify/ develop strategies for effective targeting of a range of cancers. Given that ∼50% of all cancers harbor mutant p53, the mutant forms of p53 are often oncogenic with altered transcriptional activation of target genes and contribute to malignant phenotype [226], and in cancers where nuclear receptor signaling is compromised such as the triple negative (i.e., lacking ER, HER-2, and progester-one receptor) as well as hormone-resistant breast cancers, the elucidation of the molecular basis of diverse cell growth and apoptosis signaling by CARP-1 could potentially help in designing improved perhaps novel strategies for effective targeting of these cancers.

9 Concluding Remarks

A wealth of scientific investigations that have focused on elucidating the mechanisms regulating cell growth and proliferation suggest that cancer cells have activated and/or dysregulated signaling for growth and proliferation. Although cancer cell homeostasis involves different modes of cell death that include necrosis, autophagy, mitotic catastrophe, and apoptosis, increasing body of evidence indicates that inhibitory pathways such as apoptosis are often compromised in a variety of cancers. These conclusions are based, in part, on the fact that a preponderance of the current chemotherapeutics eliminates cancer cells by activating intrinsic and/or extrinsic apoptosis programs. It is therefore, not entirely surprising to find that a significant number of drug-resistant cancer phenotypes often arise due to defects in the intrinsic or extrinsic apoptosis programs. Accordingly, elucidating/understanding of the mechanisms activating chemotherapy-dependent apoptosis signaling networks in cancer cells, tumors, and animal models can be exploited to develop novel apoptosis-based anti-cancer strategies. Identification of cancer cell apoptosis defects by comparative DNA as well as proteomic analyses together with novel mediators/effectors of apoptosis signaling will permit development of agents for use alone or in combination with current therapeutics to effectively eliminate cancer cells and, in turn, restore sensitivity of the resistant forms of cancers.

Acknowledgments The authors gratefully acknowledge the grants support from the Department of Veterans Affairs Merit Review (AKR, AW) and the Susan G Komen Breast Cancer Foundation (AKR).

References

1. Kerr JF, Wyllie AH, Currie AR. Apoptosis: a basic biological phenomenon with wide-ranging implications in tissue kinetics. Br J Cancer 1972; 26: 239–257.
2. Johnstone RW, Rufeli AA, Lowe SW. Apoptosis: a link between cancer genetics and chemotherapy. Cell 2002; 108: 153–164.
3. Danial NN, Korsmeyer SJ. Cell death: critical control points. Cell 2004; 116: 205–219.
4. Nagata S. Apoptosis by death factor. Cell 1997; 88: 355–365.
5. Cory S, Adams JM. The Bcl2 family: regulators of the cellular life-or-death switch. Nat Rev Cancer 2002; 2: 647–656.
6. Thornberry NA, Lazebnik Y. Caspases: enemies within. Science 1998; 281: 1312–1316.
7. Degterev A, Yuan J. Expansion and evolution of cell death programmes. Nat Rev Mol Cell Biol 2008; 9: 378–390.
8. Locksley RM, Killeen N, Lenardo MJ. The TNF and TNF receptor superfamilies: integrating mammalian biology. Cell 2001; 104: 487–501.

9. Laverik I, Golks A, Krammer PH. Death receptor signaling. J Cell Sci 2005; 118: 265–267.

10. LeBlanc HN, Ashkenazi A. Apo2L/TRAIL and its death and decoy receptors. Cell Death Differ 2003; 10: 66–75.

11. Peter ME, Krammer PH. The CD95(APO-1/Fas) DISC and beyond. Cell Death Differ 2003; 10: 26–35.

12. Bidere N, Su HC, Lenardo MJ. Genetic disorders of programmed cell death in the immune system. Annu Rev Immunol 2006; 24: 321–352.

13. Brunner T, Mogil RJ, LaFace D et al. Cell-autonomous Fas (CD95)/Fas-ligand interaction mediates activation-induced apoptosis in T-cell hybridomas. Nature 1995; 373: 441–444.

14. Dhein J, Walczak H, Baumler C et al. Autocrine T-cell suicide mediated by APO-1/(Fas/CD95). Nature 1995; 373: 438–441.

15. Ju ST, Panka DJ, Cui H et al. Fas(CD95)/FasL interactions required for programmed cell death after T-cell activation. Nature 1995; 373: 444–448.

16. Zheng L, Fisher G, Miller RE et al. Induction of apoptosis in mature T cells by tumour necrosis factor. Nature 1995; 377: 348–351.

17. Janssen EM, Droin NM, Lemmens EE et al. CD4[+] T-cell help controls CD8[+] T-cell memory via TRAIL-mediated activation-induced cell death. Nature 2005; 434: 88–93.

18. Barry M, Bleackley RC. Cytotoxic T lymphocytes: all roads lead to death. Nat Rev Immunol 2002; 2: 401–409.

19. Wajant H, Pfizenmaier K, Scheurich P. Tumor necrosis factor signaling. Cell Death Differ 2003; 10: 45–65.

20. Chinnaiyan AM, O'Rourke K, Tewari M et al. FADD, a novel death domain-containing protein, interacts with the death domain of Fas and initiates apoptosis. Cell 1995; 81: 505–512.

21. Kischkel FC, Hellbardt S, Behrmann I et al. Cytotoxicity-dependent APO-1 (Fas/CD95)-associated proteins form a death-inducing signaling complex (DISC) with the receptor. EMBO J 1995; 14: 5579–5588.

22. Donepudi M, Mac Sweeney A, Briand C et al. Insights into the regulatory mechanism for caspase-8 activation. Mol Cell 2003; 11: 543–549.

23. Boatright KM, Renatus M, Scott FL et al. A unified model for apical caspase activation. Mol Cell 2003; 11: 529–541.

24. Scaffidi C, Fulda S, Srinivasan A et al. Two CD95 (APO-1/Fas) signaling pathways. EMBO J 1998; 17: 1675–1687.

25. Li H, Zhu H, Xu CJ et al. Cleavage of BID by caspase 8 mediates the mitochondrial damage in the Fas pathway of apoptosis. Cell 1998; 94: 491–501.

26. Luo X, Budihardjo I, Zou H et al. Bid, a Bcl2 interacting protein, mediates cytochrome c release from mitochondria in response to activation of cell surface death receptors. Cell 1998; 94: 481–490.

27. Cowling V, Downward J. Caspase-6 is the direct activator of caspase-8 in the cytochrome c-induced apoptosis pathway: absolute requirement for removal of caspase-6 prodomain. Cell Death and Differentiation 2002; 9: 1046–1056.

28. Cory S, Huang DC, Adams JM. The Bcl-2 family: roles in cell survival and oncogenesis. Oncogene 2003; 22(53): 8590–8607.

29. Bouillet P, Strasser A. BH3-only proteins – evolutionarily conserved proapoptotic Bcl-2 family members essential for initiating programmed cell death. J Cell Sci 2002; 115: 1567–1574.

30. Korsmeyer SJ, Shutter JR, Veis DJ, Merry DE, Oltvai ZN. Bcl-2/Bax: a rheostat that regulates an anti-oxidant pathway and cell death. Semin. Cancer Biol. 1993; 4: 327–332.

31. Yang E, Zha J, Jockel J, Boise LH, Thompson CB, Korsmeyer SJ. Bad, a heterodimeric partner for Bcl-XL and Bcl-2, displaces Bax and promotes cell death. Cell 1995; 80: 285–291.

32. El-Deiry WS. The role of p53 in chemosensitivity and radiosensitivity. Oncogene 2003; 22: 7486–7495.
33. Leu JI, Dumont P, Hafey M et al. Mitochondrial p53 activates Bak and causes disruption of a Bak-Mcl1 complex. Nat Cell Biol 2004; 6: 443–450.
34. Mihara M, Erster S, Zaika A et al. p53 has a direct apoptogenic role at the mitochondria. Mol Cell 2003; 11: 577–590.
35. Suzuki M, Youle RJ, Tjandra N. Structure of Bax: coregulation of dimer formation and intracellular localization. Cell 2000; 103: 645–654.
36. Scorrano L, Oakes SA, Opferman JT et al. BAX and BAK regulation of endoplasmic reticulum Ca2+: a control point for apoptosis. Science 2003; 300: 135–139.
37. Willis SN, Chen L, Dewson G et al. Proapoptotic Bak is sequestered by Mcl-1 and Bcl-xL, but not Bcl-2, until displaced by BH3-only proteins. Genes Dev 2005; 19: 1294–1305.
38. Du C, Fang M, Li Y et al. Smac, a mitochondrial protein that promotes cytochrome c-dependent caspase activation by eliminating IAP inhibition. Cell 2000; 102: 33–42.
39. Suzuki Y, Imai Y, Nakayama H et al. A serine protease, HtrA2, is released from the mitochondria and interacts with XIAP, inducing cell death. Mol Cell 2001; 8: 613–621.
40. Verhagen AM, Ekert PG, Pakusch M et al. Identification of DIABLO, a mammalian protein that promotes apoptosis by binding to and antagonizing IAP proteins. Cell 2000; 102: 43–53.
41. Hersh EM, Metch BS, Muggia FM et al. Phase II studies of recombinant human tumor necrosis factor alpha in patients with malignant disease: a summary of the Southwest Oncology Group experience. J Immunother 1991; 10: 426–431.
42. Ogasawara J, Watanabe-Fukunaga R, Adachi M et al. Lethal effect of the anti-Fas antibody in mice. Nature 1993; 364: 806–809.
43. Walczak H, Krammer PH. The CD95 (APO-1/Fas) and the TRAIL (APO-2L) apoptosis systems. Exp. Cell Res 2000; 256: 58–66.
44. Lienard D, Ewalenko P, Delmotte JJ et al. High-dose recombinant tumor necrosis factor alpha in combination with interferon gamma and melphalan in isolation perfusion of the limbs for melanoma and sarcoma. J Clin Oncol 1992; 10: 52–60.
45. Renard N, Lienard D, Lespagnard L et al. Early endothelium activation and polymorphonuclear cell invasion precede specific necrosis of human melanoma and sarcoma treated by intravascular high-dose tumour necrosis factor alpha (rTNF alpha). Int J Cancer 1994; 57: 656–663.
46. Ashkenazi A, Pai RC, Fong S, Leung S, Lawrence DA, Marsters SA et al. Safety and antitumor activity of recombinant soluble Apo2 ligand. J Clin Invest 1999; 104: 155–162.
47. Lawrence D, Shahrokh Z, Marsters SA et al. Differential hepatocyte toxicity of recombinant Apo2L/TRAIL versions. Nat Med 2001; 7: 383–385.
48. Pollack IF, Erff M, Ashkenazi A. Direct stimulation of apoptotic signaling by soluble Apo2l/tumor necrosis factor-related apoptosis-inducing ligand leads to selective killing of glioma cells. Clin Cancer Res. 2001; 7: 1362–1369.
49. Jo M, Kim TH, Seol DW et al. Apoptosis induced in normal human hepatocytes by tumor necrosis factor-related apoptosis-inducing ligand. Nat Med 2000; 6: 564–567.
50. Nitsch R, Bechmann I, Deisz RA et al. Human brain-cell death induced by tumour-necrosis-factor-related apoptosis-inducing ligand (TRAIL). Lancet 2000; 356: 827–828.
51. Chuntharapai A, Dodge K, Grimmer K et al. Isotype-dependent inhibition of tumor growth in vivo by monoclonal antibodies to death receptor 4. J Immunol 2001; 166: 4891–4898.
52. Ichikawa K, Liu W, Zhao L et al. Tumoricidal activity of a novel anti-human DR5 monoclonal antibody without hepatocyte toxicity. Nat Med 2001; 7: 954–960.
53. Shigeno M, Nakao K, Ichikawa T, Suzuki K, Kawakami A, Abiru S, Miyazoe S, Nakagawa Y, Ishikawa H, Hamasaki K et al. Interferon-alpha sensitizes human

hepatoma cells to TRAIL-induced apoptosis through DR5 upregulation and NF-kappa B inactivation. Oncogene 2003; 22: 1653–1662.
54. Miao L, Yi P, Wang Y, Wu M. Etoposide upregulates Bax-enhancing tumour necrosis factor-related apoptosis inducing ligand-mediated apoptosis in the human hepatocellular carcinoma cell line QGY-7703. Eur J Biochem 2003; 270: 2721–2731.
55. Hotta T, Suzuki H, Nagai S, Yamamoto K, Imakiire A, Takada E, Itoh M, Mizuguchi J. Chemotherapeutic agents sensitize sarcoma cell lines to tumor necrosis factor-related apoptosis-inducing ligand-induced caspase-8 activation, apoptosis and loss of mitochondrial membrane potential. J Orthop Res 2003; 21: 949–957.
56. Ramp U, Caliskan E, Mahotka C, Krieg A, Heikaus S, Gabbert HE, Gerharz CD. Apoptosis induction in renal cell carcinoma by TRAIL and gamma-radiation is impaired by deficient caspase-9 cleavage. Br J Cancer 2003; 88: 1800–1807.
57. Totzke G, Schultze-Osthoff K, Jänicke RU. Cyclooxygenase-2 (cox-2) inhibitors sensitize tumor cells specifically to death receptor-induced apoptosis independently of COX-2 inhibition. Oncogene 2003; 22: 8021–8030.
58. Meng RD, McDonald ER, Sheikh MS, Fornace AJ, El-Deiry WS. The TRAIL decoy receptor TRUNDD (DcR2, TRAIL-R4) is induced by adenovirus-p53 overexpression and can delay TRAIL-, p53-, and KILLER/DR5-dpendent colon cancer apoptosis. Mol Ther 2000; 1: 130–144.
59. Lacour S, Hammann A, Grazide S, Lagadic-Gossmann D, Athias A, Sergent O et al. Cisplatin-induced CD95 redistribution into membrane lipid rafts of HT29 human colon cancer cells. Cancer Res 2004; 64: 3593–3598.
60. Olsson A, Diaz T, Aguilar-Santelises M. Sensitization to TRAIL-induced apoptosis and modulation of FLICE-inhibitory protein in B chronic lymphocytic leukemia by actinomycin D. Leukemia 2001; 15: 1868–1877.
61. Micheau O, Hammann A, Solary E, Dimanche-boitrel MT. STAT-1-independent upregulation of FADD and procaspase-3 and -8 in cancer cells treated with cytotoxic drugs. Biophys Res Commun 1999; 256: 603–611.
62. Singh TR, Shankar S, Chen X, Asim M, Srivastava RK. Synergistic interactions of chemotherapeutic drugs and tumor necrosis factor-related apoptosis-inducing ligand/ Apo-2 ligand on apoptosis and on regression of breast carcinoma in vivo. Cancer Res. 2003; 63(17): 5390–5400.
63. Singh TR, Shankar S, Srivastava RK. HDAC inhibitors enhance the apoptosis-inducing potential of TRAIL in breast carcinoma. Oncogene 2005; 24(29): 4609–4623.
64. Fandy TE, Ross DD, Gore SD, Srivastava RK. Flavopiridol synergizes TRAIL cytotoxicity by downregulation of FLIPL. Cancer Chemother Pharmacol. 2007; 60(3): 313–319.
65. Fandy TE, Shankar S, Srivastava RK. Smac/DIABLO enhances the therapeutic potential of chemotherapeutic drugs and irradiation, and sensitizes TRAIL-resistant breast cancer cells. Mol Cancer 2008; 7: 60.
66. Fulda S, Meyer E, Debatin KM. Metabolic inhibitors sensitize for CD95 (APO-1/ Fas)-induced apoptosis by down-regulating Fas-associated death domain-like interleukin 1-converting enzyme inhibitory protein expression, Cancer Res 2000; 60: 3947–3956.
67. Kim Y, Suh N, Sporn M, Reed JC. An inducible pathway for degradation of FLIP protein sensitizes tumor cells to TRAIL-induced apoptosis. J Biol Chem 2002; 277: 22320–22329.
68. Sayers TJ, Brooks AD, Koh CY, Ma W, Seki N, Raziuddin A, Blazar BR, Zhang X, Elliott PJ, Murphy WJ. The proteasome inhibitor PS-341 sensitizes neoplastic cells to TRAIL-mediated apoptosis by reducing levels of c-FLIP. Blood 2003; 102: 303–310.
69. Hengartner MO. (1997) Programmed cell death. In: *C. elegans* II. Riddle, DL et al. (eds.), pp. 383–496. Cold Spring Harbor Laboratory Press, Plainview, NY.

70. Conradt B, Xue D. Programmed cell death. WormBook 2005; 6: 1–13.
71. Lamkanfi M, Declercq W, Kalai M et al. Alice in caspase land: a phylogenetic analysis of caspases from worm to man. Cell Death Differ 2002; 9: 358–361.
72. Riedl SJ, Shi Y. Molecular mechanisms of caspase regulation during apoptosis. Nat Rev Mol Cell Biol 2004; 5: 897–907.
73. Salvesen GS, Duckett CS. IAP proteins: blocking the road to death's door. Nat Rev Mol Cell Biol 2002; 3: 401–410.
74. Vaux DL, Silke J. IAPs, RINGs and ubiquitylation. Nat Rev Mol Cell Biol 2005; 6: 287–297.
75. Zhivotovsky B, Orrenius S. Carcinogenesis and apoptosis: paradigms and paradoxes. Carcinogenesis 2006; 27: 1939–1945.
76. Nakagawara A, Nakamura Y, Ikeda H et al. High levels of expression and nuclear localization of interleukin-1 beta converting enzyme (ICE) and CPP32 in favorable human neuroblastomas. Cancer Res 1997; 57: 4578–4584.
77. Fujikawa K, Shiraki K, Sugimoto K. Reduced expression of ICE/caspase1 and CPP32/caspase3 in human hepatocellular carcinoma. Anticancer Res 2000; 20: 1927–1932.
78. Satoh K, Kaneko K, Hirota M et al. The pattern of CPP32/caspase-3 expression reflects the biological behavior of the human pancreatic duct cell tumors. Pancreas 2000; 21: 352–357.
79. Volm M, Koomagi R. Prognostic relevance of c-Myc and caspase-3 for patients with non-small cell lung cancer. Oncol Rep 2000; 7: 95–98.
80. Koomagi R, Volm M. Relationship between the expression of caspase-3 and the clinical outcome of patients with non-small cell lung cancer. Anticancer Res 2000; 20: 493–496.
81. Jonges LE, Nagelkerke JF, Ensink NG et al. Caspase-3 activity as a prognostic factor in colorectal carcinoma. Lab Invest 2001; 81: 681–688.
82. Isobe N, Onodera H, Mori A et al. Caspase-3 expression in human gastric carcinoma and its clinical significance. Oncology 2004; 66: 201–209.
83. Joseph B, Ekedahl J, Sirzen F et al. Differences in expression of pro-caspases in small cell and non-small cell lung carcinoma. Biochem Biophys Res Commun 1999; 262: 381–387.
84. Teitz T, Wei T, Valentine MB et al. Caspase 8 is deleted or silenced preferentially in childhood neuroblastomas with amplification of MYCN. Nat Med 2000; 6: 529–535.
85. Fulda S, Kufer MU, Meyer E et al. Sensitization for death receptor- or drug-induced apoptosis by re-expression of caspase-8 through demethylation or gene transfer. Oncogene 2001; 20: 5865–5877.
86. Mandruzzato S, Brasseur F, Andry G et al. A CASP-8 mutation recognized by cytolytic T lymphocytes on a human head and neck carcinoma. J Exp Med 1997; 186: 785–793.
87. Takita J, Yang HW, Chen YY et al. Allelic imbalance on chromosome 2q and alterations of the caspase 8 gene in neuroblastoma. Oncogene 2001; 20: 4424–4432.
88. Liu B, Peng D, Lu Y et al. A novel single amino acid deletion caspase-8 mutant in cancer cells that lost proapoptotic activity. J Biol Chem 2002; 277: 30159–30164.
89. Fischer U, Schulze-Osthoff K. New approaches and therapeutic targeting apoptosis in disease. Pharmacol Rev 2005; 57: 187–215.
90. MacCorkle RA, Freeman KW, Spencer DM. Synthetic activation of caspases: artificial death switches. Proc Natl Acad Sci USA 1998; 95: 3655–3660.
91. Shariat SF, Desai S, Song W, Khan T, Zhao J, Nguyen C, Foster BA, Greenberg N, Spencer DM, Slavin KM. Adenovirus-mediated transfer of inducible caspases: a novel "death switch" gene therapeutic approach to prostate cancer. Cancer Res 2001; 61: 2562–2571.
92. Xie X, Zhao X, Liu Y, Zhang J, Matusik RJ, Slavin KM, Spencer DM. Adenovirus-mediated tissue-targeted expression of a caspase-9-based artificial death switch for the treatment of prostate cancer. Cancer Res 2001; 61: 6795–6804.
93. Nor JE, Hu Y, Song W, Spencer DM, Nunez G. Ablation of microvessels in vivo upon dimerization of icaspase-9. Gene Therap 2002; 9: 444–451.

94. Komata T, Kondo Y, Kanzawa T, Hirohata S, Koga S, Sumiyoshi H, Srinivasula SM, Barna BP, Germano IM, Takakura M et al. Treatment of malignant glioma cells with the transfer of constitutively active caspase-6 using the human telomerase catalytic subunit (human telomerase reverse transcriptase) gene promoter. Cancer Res 2001; 61: 5796–5802.
95. Jia JT, Zhang LH, Yu CJ, Zhao J, Xu YM, Gui JH, Jin M, Ji ZL, Wen WH, Wang CJ, et al. Specific tumoricidal activity of a secreted proapoptotic protein consisting of HER2 antibody and constitutively active caspase-3. Cancer Res 2003; 63: 3257–3262.
96. Xu YM, Wang LF, Jia JT, Qiu XC, Zhao J, Yu CJ, Zhang R, Zhu F, Wang CJ, Jin BQ et al. A caspase-6 and anti-human epidermal growth factor receptor-2 antibody chimeric molecule suppresses the growth of HER2-overexpressing tumors. J Immunol 2004; 173: 61–67.
97. Tse E, Rabbitts TH. Intracellular antibody-caspase-mediated cell killing: an approach for application in cancer therapy. Proc Natl Acad Sci USA 2000; 97: 12266–12271.
98. Buckley CD, Pilling D, Henriquez NV, Parsonage G, Threlfall K, Scheel-Tollner D, Simmons DL, Akbar AN, Lord JM, Salmon M. RGD peptide induces apoptosis by direct caspase-3 activation. Nature (London) 1999; 397: 534–539.
99. Jiang X, Kim HE, Shu H, Zhao Y, Zhang H, Kofron J, Donnelly J, Burns D, Ng SC, Rosenberg S, Wang X. Distinctive roles of PHAP proteins and prothymosin-alpha in a death regulatory pathway. Science (Washington, DC) 2003; 299: 223–226.
100. Nguyen JT, Wells JA. Direct activation of the apoptosis machinery as a mechanism to target cancer cells. Proc Natl Acad Sci USA 2003; 100: 7533–7538.
101. Zhang HZ, Kasibhatla S, Wang Y, Herich J, Guastella J, Tseng B, Drewe J, Cai SX. Discovery, characterization and SAR of gambogic acid as a potent apoptosis inducer by a HTS assay. Bioorg Med Chem 2004; 12: 309–317.
102. Clem RJ, Fechheimer M, Miller LK. Prevention of apoptosis by a baculovirus gene during infection of insect cells. Science 1991; 254: 1388–1390.
103. Deveraux QL, Reed JC. IAP family proteins-suppressors of apoptosis. Genes Dev 1999; 13: 239–252.
104. Ashhab Y, Alian A, Polliack A, Panet A, Yehuda DB. Two splicing variants of a new inhibitor of apoptosis gene with different biological properties and tissue distribution pattern. FEBS Lett 2001; 495: 56–60.
105. Vucic D, Stennicke HR, Pisabarro MT, Salvesen GS, Dixit VM. ML-IAP, a novel inhibitor of apoptosis that is preferentially expressed in human melanomas. Curr Biol 2000; 10: 1359–1366.
106. Yang YL, Li XM. The IAP family: endogenous caspase inhibitors with multiple biological activities. Cell Res 2000; 10: 169–177.
107. Verhagen AM, Coulson EJ, Vaux DL. Inhibitor of apoptosis proteins and their relatives: IAPs and other BIRPs. Genome Biol 2001; 2: 1–10.
108. Roy N, Mahadevan MS, McLean M, et al. The gene for neuronal apoptosis inhibitory protein is partially deleted in individuals with spinal muscular atrophy. Cell 1995; 80: 167–178.
109. Ambrosini G, Adida C, Altieri DC. A novel anti-apoptosis gene, survivin, expressed in cancer and lymphoma. Nat Med 1997; 3: 917–921.
110. Hinds MG, Norton RS, Vaux DL. Solution structure of a baculoviral inhibitor of apoptosis (IAP) repeat. Nat Struct Biol 1999; 6: 648–651.
111. Sun C, Cai M, Meadows RP. NMR structure and mutagenesis of the third Bir domain of the inhibitor of apoptosis protein XIAP. J Biol Chem 2000; 275: 33777–33781.
112. Sun C, Cai M, Gunasekera AH. NMR structure and mutagenesis of the inhibitor-of-apoptosis protein XIAP. Nature 1999; 401: 818–822.

113. Shi Y. Mechanisms of caspase activation and inhibition during apoptosis. Mol Cell 2002; 9: 459–470.
114. Scott FL, Denault JB, Riedl SJ, Shin H, Renatus M, Salvesen GS. XIAP inhibits caspase-3 and -7 using two binding sites: evolutionarily conserved mechanism of IAPs. EMBO J 2005; 24: 645–655.
115. Suzuki Y, Nakabayashi Y, Nakata K, Reed JC, Takahashi R. X-linked inhibitor of apoptosis protein (XIAP) inhibits caspase-3 and -7 in distinct modes. J Biol Chem 2001; 276: 27058–27063.
116. Zapata JM, Takahashi R, Salvesen GS, Reed JC. Granzyme release and caspase activation in activated human T-lymphocytes. J Biol Chem 1998; 273: 6916–6920.
117. Wu G, Chai J, Suber TL, et al. Structural basis of IAP recognition by Smac/DIABLO. Nature 2000; 408: 1008–1012.
118. Chai J, Du C, Wu JW, Kyin S, Wang X, Shi Y. Structural and biochemical basis of apoptotic activation by Smac/DIABLO. Nature 2000; 406: 855–862.
119. Eckelman BP, Salvesen GS, Scott FL. Human inhibitor of apoptosis proteins: why XIAP is the black sheep of the family. EMBO Rep 2006; 7: 988–994.
120. Shiozaki EN, Shi Y. Caspases, IAPs and Smac/DIABLO: mechanisms from structural biology. Trends Biochem Sci 2004; 29: 486–494.
121. Lu M, Lin SC, Huang Y. XIAP induces NF-kappaB activation via the BIR1/TAB1 interaction and BIR1 dimerization. Mol Cell 2007; 26: 689–702.
122. Duffy MJ, O'Donovan N, Brennan DJ. Survivin: a promising tumor biomarker. Cancer Lett 2007; 249: 49–60.
123. Altieri DC. Survivin, versatile modulation of cell division and apoptosis in cancer. Oncogene 2003; 22: 8581–8589.
124. Danson S, Dean E, Dive C. IAPs as a target for anticancer therapy. Curr Cancer Drug Targets 2007; 7: 785–794.
125. Sasaki H, Sheng Y, Kotsuji F et al. Down-regulation of X-linked inhibitor of apoptosis protein induces apoptosis in chemoresistant human ovarian cancer cells. Cancer Res 2000; 60: 5659–5666.
126. Holcik M, Yeh C, Korneluk RG et al. Translational upregulation of X-linked inhibitor of apoptosis (XIAP) increases resistance to radiation induced cell death. Oncogene 2000; 19: 4174–4177.
127. Chawla-Sarkar M, Bae SI, Reu FJ et al. Downregulation of Bcl-2, FLIP or IAPs (XIAP and survivin) by siRNAs sensitizes resistant melanoma cells to Apo2L/TRAIL-induced apoptosis. Cell Death Differ 2004; 11: 915–923.
128. McManus DC, Lefebvre CA, Cherton-Horvat G et al. Loss of XIAP protein expression by RNAi and antisense approaches sensitizes cancer cells to functionally diverse chemotherapeutics. Oncogene 2004; 23: 8105–8117.
129. Mesri M, Wall NR, Li J, Kim RW, Altieri DC. Cancer gene therapy using a survivin mutant adenovirus. J Clin Invest 2004; 108: 981–990.
130. Hu Y, Cherton-Horvat G, Dragowska V, et al. Antisense oligonucleotides targeting XIAP induce apoptosis and enhance chemotherapeutic activity against human lung cancer cells in vitro and in vivo. Clin Cancer Res 2003; 9: 2826–2836.
131. Bilim V, Kasahara T, Hara N, Takahashi K, Tomita Y. Role of XIAP in malignant phenotype of transitional cell cancer (TCC) and therapeutic activity of IAP antisense oligonucleotides against multidrug-resistant TCC in vitro. Int J Cancer 2003; 103: 29–37.
132. Patel B, Carrasco R, Stamm N et al. Antisense inhibition of survivin expression as a cancer therapeutic [abstract]. Clin Cancer Res 2003; 9: S16.
133. Izquierdo M. Short interfering RNAs as a tool for cancer gene therapy. Cancer Gene Ther 2005; 12: 217–227.
134. Pennati M, Folini M, Zaffaroni N. Targeting survivin in cancer therapy: fulfilled promises and open questions. Carcinogenesis 2007; 28: 1133–1139.

135. Oost TK, Sun C, Armstrong RC et al. Discovery of potent antagonists of the antiapoptotic protein XIAP for the treatment of cancer. J Med Chem 2004; 47: 4417–4426.
136. Sun H, Nikolovska-Coleska Z, Yang CY et al. Structure-based design, synthesis, and evaluation of conformationally constrained mimetics of the second mitochondria-derived activator of caspase that target the X-linked inhibitor of apoptosis protein/caspase-9 interaction site. J Med Chem 2004; 47: 4147–4150.
137. Li L, Thomas RM, Suzuki H et al. A small molecule Smac mimic potentiates TRAIL- and TNFalpha-mediated cell death. Science 2004; 305: 1471–1474.
138. Wu TY, Wagner KW, Bursulaya B, Schultz PG, Deveraux QL. Development and characterization of nonpeptidic small molecule inhibitors of the XIAP/caspase-3 interaction. Chem Biol 2003; 10: 759–767.
139. Nikolovska-Coleska Z, Xu L, Hu Z et al. Discovery of embelin as a cell-permeable, small-molecular weight inhibitor of XIAP through structure-based computational screening of a traditional herbal medicine three-dimensional structure database. J Med Chem 2004; 47: 2430–2440.
140. Schimmer AD, Welsh K, Pinilla C, Wang Z, Krajewska M, Bonneau MJ, Pedersen IM, Kitada S, Scott FL, Bailly-Maitre B et al. Small molecule antagonists of apoptosis suppressor XIAP exhibit broad antitumor activity. Cancer Cell 2004; 5: 25–35.
141. Nikolovska-Coleska Z, Meagher JL, Jiang S. Design and characterization of bivalent Smac-based peptides as antagonists of XIAP and development and validation of a fluorescence polarization assay for XIAP containing both BIR2 and BIR3 domains. Anal Biochem 2008; 374: 87–98.
142. Srinivasula SM, Datta P, Fan XJ. Molecular determinants of the caspase-promoting activity of Smac/DIABLO and its role in the death receptor pathway. J Biol Chem 2000; 275: 36152–36157.
143. Fulda S, Wick W, Weller M. Smac agonists sensitize for Apo2L/TRAIL- or anticancer drug-induced apoptosis and induce regression of malignant glioma in vivo. Nat Med 2002; 8: 808–815.
144. Grossman D, McNiff JM, Li F et al. Expression and targeting of the apoptosis inhibitor, survivin, in human melanoma. J Invest Dermatol 1999; 113: 1076–1081.
145. Yan H, Thomas J, Liu T et al. Induction of melanoma cell apoptosis and inhibition of tumor growth using a cell-permeable survivin antagonist. Oncogene 2006; 25: 6968–6974.
146. Chen JS, Liu JC, Shen L et al. Cancer-specific activation of the survivin promoter and its potential use in gene therapy. Cancer Gene Ther 2004; 11: 740–747.
147. Van Houdt WJ, Haviv YS, Lu B et al. The human survivin promoter: a novel transcriptional targeting strategy for treatment of glioma. J Neurosurg 2006; 104: 583–592.
148. Andersen MH, Thor SP. Survivin – a universal tumor antigen. Histol Histopathol 2002; 17: 669–675.
149. Rohayem J, Diestelkoetter P, Weigle B et al. Antibody response to the tumor-associated inhibitor of apoptosis protein in cancer patients. Cancer Res 2000; 60: 1815–1817.
150. Schmidt SM, Schag K, Müller MR et al. Survivin is a shared tumor-associated antigen expressed in a broad variety of malignancies and recognized by specific cytotoxic T cells. Blood 2003; 102: 571–576.
151. Schmitz M, Diestelkoetter P, Weigle B et al. Generation of survivin-specific CD8 + T effector cells by dendritic cells pulsed with protein or selected peptides. Cancer Res 2000; 60: 4845–4849.
152. Otto K, Andersen MH, Eggert A et al. Lack of toxicity of therapy-induced T cell responses against the universal tumour antigen survivin. Vaccine 2005; 23: 884–889.
153. Bakhshi A, Jensen JP, Goldman P et al. Cloning the chromosomal breakpoint of t(14;18) human lymphomas: clustering around JH on chromosome 14 and near a transcriptional unit on 18. Cell 1985; 41: 899–906.

154. Cleary ML, Sklar J. Nucleotide sequence of a t(14;18) chromosomal breakpoint in follicular lymphoma and demonstration of a breakpoint-cluster region near a transcriptionally active locus on chromosome 18. Proc Natl Acad Sci USA 1985; 82: 7439–7443.

155. Tsujimoto Y, Cossman J, Jaffe E et al. Involvement of the bcl-2 gene in human follicular lymphoma. Science 1985; 228: 1440–1443.

156. Vaux DL, Cory S, Adams JM. Bcl-2 gene promotes haemopoietic cell survival and cooperates with c-myc to immortalize pre-B cells. Nature 1988; 335: 440–442.

157. Vaux DL. CED-4–the third horseman of apoptosis. Cell 1997; 90: 389–390.

158. Hengartner MO, Horvitz HR. *C. elegans* cell survival gene ced-9 encodes a functional homolog of the mammalian proto-oncogene bcl-2. Cell 1994; 76: 665–676.

159. Huang CSD, Adams JM, Cory S. The conserved N-terminal BH4 domain of homologues is essential for inhibition of apoptosis and interaction with CED-4. EMBO J 1998; 17: 1029–1039.

160. Lee LC, Hunter JJ, Mujeeb A et al. Evidence for alpha helical conformation of an essential N-terminal region in the human Bcl-2 protein. J Biol Chem 1996; 271: 23284–23288.

161. Huang DC, Strasser A. BH3-only proteins – essential initiators of apoptotic cell death. Cell 2000; 103: 839–842.

162. Muchmore SW, Sattler M, Liang H, et al. X-ray and NMR structure of human Bcl-XL, an inhibitor of programmed cell death. Nature 1996; 381: 335–341.

163. Fesik SW. Insights into programmed cell death through structural biology. Cell 2000; 103: 273–282.

164. Minn AJ, Velez P, Schendel SL et al. Bcl-xL forms an ion channel in synthetic lipid membranes. Nature 1997; 385: 353–357.

165. Schendel SL, Xie Z, Montal MO et al. Channel formation by antiapoptotic protein Bcl-2. Proc Natl Acad Sci USA 1997; 94: 5113–5118.

166. Antonsson B, Conti F, Ciavatta A et al. Inhibition of Bax channel-forming activity by Bcl-2. Science 1997; 277: 370–372.

167. Vander Heiden MG, Chandel NS, Williamson EK et al. Thompson, Bcl-xL regulates the membrane potential and volume homeostasis of mitochondria. Cell 1997; 91: 627–637.

168. Zha J, Harada J, Yang E et al. Serine phosphorylation of death agonist BAD in response to survival factor results in binding to 14-3-3 not Bcl-xL. Cell 1996; 87: 619–628.

169. Gustafsson AB, Gottlieb RA. Bcl-2 family members and apoptosis, taken to heart. Am J Physiol Cell Physiol 2007; 292: C45–C51.

170. Finucane DM, Bossy-Wetzel E, Waterhouse NJ et al. Bax-induced caspase activation and apoptosis via cytochrome *c* release from mitochondria is inhibitable by Bcl-xL. J Biol Chem 1999; 274: 2225–2233.

171. Cartron PF, Gallenne T, Bougras G et al. The first α-helix of Bax plays a necessary role in its ligand-induced activation by the BH3-only proteins Bid and PUMA. Mol Cell 2004; 16: 807–818.

172. Cheng EH, Wei MC, Weiler S et al. BCL-2, BCL-X$_L$ sequester BH3 domain-only molecules preventing BAX- and BAK-mediated mitochondrial apoptosis. Mol Cell 2001; 8: 705–711.

173. Cheng EH, Kirsch DG, Clem RJ et al. Conversion of Bcl-2 to a Bax-like death effector by caspases. Science 1997; 278: 1966–1968.

174. Clem RJ, Cheng EH, Karp CL et al. Modulation of cell death by Bcl-XL through caspase interaction. Proc Natl Acad Sci USA 1998; 95: 554–559.

175. Lin B, Kolluri SK, Lin F et al. Conversion of Bcl-2 from protector to killer by interaction with nuclear orphan receptor Nurr77/R3. Cell 2004; 116: 527–540.

176. Rosse T, Olivier R, Monney L et al. Bcl-2 prolongs cell survival after Bax-induced release of cytochrome c. Nature 1998; 391: 496–499.
177. Pastorino JG, Chen ST, Tafani M et al. The overexpression of Bax produces cell death upon induction of the mitochondrial permeability transition. J Biol Chem 1998; 273: 7770–7775.
178. Liu X, Kim CN, Yang J et al. Induction of apoptotic program in cell-free extracts: requirement for dATP and cytochrome c. Cell 1996; 86: 147–157.
179. Zou H, Henzel WJ, Liu X et al. Apaf-1, a human protein homologous to *C. elegans* CED-4, participates in cytochrome c-dependent activation of caspase-3. Cell 1997; 90: 405–413.
180. Li P, Nijhawan D, Budihardjo I et al. Cytochrome c and dATP-dependent formation of Apaf-1/caspase-9 complex initiates an apoptotic protease cascade. Cell 1997; 91: 479–489.
181. Pan G, Humke EW, Dixit VM. Activation of caspases triggered by cytochrome c in vitro. FEBS Lett 1998; 426: 151–154.
182. Thomadaki H, Scorilas A. BCL2 family of apoptosis-related genes: functions and clinical implications in cancer. Crit Rev Clin Lab Sci 2006; 43: 1–67.
183. Letai A. Pharmacological manipulation of Bcl-2 family members to control cell death. J Clin Invest 2005; 115: 2648–2655.
184. Armstrong JS. Mitochondrial Medicine: Pharmacological targeting of mitochondria in disease. Br J Pharmacol 2007; 151: 1154–1165.
185. Zamzami N, Marzo I, Susin SA et al. The thiol crosslinking agent diamide overcomes the apoptosis-inhibitory effect of Bcl-2 by enforcing mitochondrial permeability transition. Oncogene 1998; 16: 1055–1063.
186. Armstrong JS, Jones DP. Glutathione depletion enforces the mitochondrial permeability transition and causes cell death in Bcl-2 overexpressing HL60 cells. FASEB J 2002; 16: 1263–1265.
187. Hirsch T, Decaudin D, Susin SA et al. PK11195, a ligand of the mitochondrial benzodiazepine receptor, facilitates the induction of apoptosis and reverses Bcl-2-mediated cytoprotection. Exp Cell Res 1998; 241: 426–434.
188. Ackermann EJ, Taylor JK, Narayana R et al. The role of antiapoptotic Bcl-2 family members in endothelial apoptosis elucidated with antisense oligonucleotides. J Biol Chem 1999; 274: 11245–11252.
189. O'Brien S, Moore JO, Boyd TE et al. Randomized phase III trial of fludarabine plus cyclophosphamide with or without oblimersen sodium (Bcl-2 antisense) in patients with relapsed or refractory chronic lymphocytic leukemia. J Clin Oncol 2007; 25: 1114–1120.
190. Zangemeister-Wittke U, Leech SH, Olie RA, Simoes-Wust AP, Gautschi O, Leudke GH, Natt F, Haner R, Martin P, Hall J et al. A novel bispecific antisense oligonucleotide inhibiting both bcl-2 and bcl-xL expression efficiently induces apoptosis in tumor cells. Clin Cancer Res 2000; 6: 2547–2555.
191. Taylor JK, Zhang QQ, Wyatt JR, Dean NM. Induction of endogenous Bcl-xS through the control of Bcl-x pre-mRNA splicing by antisense oligonucleotides. Nat Biotechnol 1999; 17: 1097–1100.
192. Bedikian AY, Millward M, Pehamberger H et al. Bcl-2 antisense (oblimersen sodium) plus dacarbazine in patients with advanced melanoma: The Oblimersen Melanoma Study. J Clin Oncol 2006; 24: 4738–4745.
193. Kagawa S, Pearson SA, Ji L et al. A binary adenoviral vector system for expressing high levels of the proapoptotic gene bax. Gene Ther 2000; 7: 75–79.
194. Xiang J, Gomez-navarro J, Arafat W et al. Pro-apoptotic treatment with an adenovirus encoding Bax enhances the effect of chemotherapy in ovarian cancer. J Gene Med 2000; 2: 97–106.
195. Li X, Marani M, Yu J et al. Adenovirus-mediated Bax overexpression for the induction of therapeutic apoptosis in prostate cancer. Cancer Res 2001; 61: 186–191.

196. Walensky LD, Kung AL, Escher I et al. Activation of apoptosis in vivo by a hydro-carbon-stapled BH3 helix. Science 2004; 305: 1466–1470.
197. Holinger EP, Chittenden T, Lutz RJ. Bak BH3 peptides antagonize Bcl-xL function and induce apoptosis through cytochrome c-independent activation of caspases. J Biol Chem 1999; 274: 13298–13304.
198. Wang JL, Zhang ZJ, Choski S, Shan S, Lu Z, Croce CM, Alnemri ES, Korngold R, Huang Z. Cell permeable Bcl-2 binding peptides: a chemical approach to apoptosis induction in tumor cells. Cancer Res 2000b; 60: 1498–1502.
199. Nakashima T, Miura M, Hara M. Tetrocarcin A inhibits mitochondrial functions of Bcl-2 and suppresses its anti-apoptotic activity. Cancer Res 2000; 60: 1229–1235.
200. Wang JL, Liu D, Zhang ZJ, Shan S, Han X, Srinivasula SM, Croce CM, Alnemri ES, Huang Z. Structure-based discovery of an organic compound that binds Bcl-2 protein and induces apoptosis of tumor cells. Proc Natl Acad Sci USA 2000a; 97: 7124–7129.
201. Tzung SP, Kim KM, Basanez G, Diedt CD, Simon J., Zimmerberg J., Zhang, KY, Hockenbery DM. Antimycin A mimics a cell-death-inducing Bcl-2 homology domain 3. Nat. Cell Biol. 2001; 3: 183–191.
202. Degterev A, Lugovskoy A, Cardone M, Mulley B, Wagner G, Mitchison T, Yuan J. Identification of small-molecule-inhibitors of interaction between the BH3 domain and Bcl-xL. Nat Cell Biol 2001; 3: 173–182.
203. Chan SL, Lee MC, Tan KO, Yang LK, Lee AS, Flotow H, Fu NY, Butler MS, Soejarto DD, Buss AD, Yu VC. Identification of Chelerythrine as an inhibitor of BclXL function. J Biol Chem 2003; 278: 20453–20456.
204. Meng XW, Sun-Hee L, Kaufmann SH. Apoptosis in the treatment of cancer: A promise kept? Curr Opin Cell Biol 2006; 18: 668–676.
205. Oltersdorf T, Elmore SW, Shoemaker AR et al. An inhibitor of Bcl-2 family proteins induces regression of solid tumours. Nature 2005; 435: 677–681.
206. Trudel S, Li ZH, Rauw J et al. Preclinical studies of the pan-Bcl inhibitor obatoclax (GX015-070) in multiple myeloma. Blood 2007; 109: 5430–5438.
207. Levine AJ, Momand J, Finley CA. The p53 tumour suppressor gene. Nature 1991; 351: 453–456.
208. Maurici D, Monti P, Campomenosi P et al. Amifostine (WR2721) restores transcrip-tional activity of specific p53 mutant proteins in a yeast functional assay. Oncogene 2001; 20: 3533–3540.
209. Selivanova G, Ryabchenko L, Jansson E, Iotsova V, Wiman KG. Reactivation of mutant p53 through interaction of a C-terminal peptide with the core domain. Mol Cell Biol 1999; 19: 3395–3402.
210. Kim AL, Raffo AJ, Brandt-Rauf PW, Pincus MR, Monaco R, Abarzua P, Fine RL. Conformational and molecular basis for induction of apoptosis by a p53 C-terminal peptide in human cancer cells. J Biol Chem 1999; 274: 34924–34931.
211. Ryu J, Lee HJ, Kim KA, et al. Intracellular delivery of p53 fused to the basic domain of HIV-1 Tat. Mol Cells 2004; 17: 353–359.
212. Takenobu T, Tomizawa K, Matsushita M, et al. Development of p53 protein transduc-tion therapy using membrane-permeable peptides and the application to oral cancer cells. Mol Cancer Ther 2002; 1: 1043–1049.
213. Weisbart RH, Hansen JE, Chan G, et al. Antibody-mediated transduction of p53 selectively kills cancer cells. Int J Oncol 2004; 25: 1867–1873.
214. Hansen JE, Fischer LK, Chan G, Chang SS, Baldwin SW, Aragon RJ, Carter JJ, Lilly M, Nishimura RN, Weisbart RH, Reeves ME. Antibody-mediated p53 protein therapy prevents liver metastasis in vivo. Cancer Res 2007; 67(4): 1769–1774.
215. Butz K, Denk C, Ullmann A, Scheffner M, Hoppe-Seyler F. Induction of apoptosis in human papillomaviruspositive cancer cells by peptide aptamers targeting the viral E6 oncoprotein. Proc Natl Acad Sci USA 2000; 97: 6693–6697.

216. Buolamwini JK, Addo J, Kamath S, Patil S, Mason D, Ores M. Small molecule antagonists of the MDM2 oncoprotein as anticancer agents. Curr Cancer Drug Targets 2005; 5: 57–68.
217. Chene P. Inhibition of p53–MDM2 interaction: Targeting a protein–protein interface. Mol Cancer Res 2004; 2: 20–28.
218. Vassilev LT, Vu BT, Graves B, Carvajal D, Podlaski F, Filipovic Z, Kong N, Kammlott U, Lukacs C, Klein C et al. In vivo activation of the p53 pathway by small-molecule antagonists of MDM2. Science 2004; 303: 844–848.
219. Tovar C, Rosinski J, Filipovic Z, Higgins B, Kolinsky K, Hilton H, Zhao X, Vu BT, Qing W, Packman K, Myklebost O, Heimbrook DC, Vassilev LT. Small-molecule MDM2 antagonists reveal aberrant p53 signaling in cancer: implications for therapy. Proc Natl Acad Sci USA 2006; 103(6): 1888–1893.
220. Grasberger BL, Lu T, Schubert C et al. Discovery and cocrystal structure of benzodiazepinedione HDM2 antagonists that activate p53 in cells. J Med Chem 2005; 48(4): 909–912.
221. Ding K, Lu Y, Nikolovska-Coleska Z et al. Structure-based design of potent nonpeptide MDM2 inhibitors. J Am Chem Soc 2005; 127(29): 10130–10131.
222. Issaeva N, Bozko P, Enge M, Protopopova M, Verhoef LG, Masucci M, Pramanik A, Selivanova G. Small molecule RITA binds to p53, blocks p53-HDM-2 interaction and activates p53 function in tumors. Nat Med 2004; 10: 1321–1328.
223. Hainaut P, Hollstein M. p53 and human cancer: the first ten thousand mutations. Adv Cancer Res 2000; 77: 81–137.
224. Moll UM, Marchenko N, Zhang X-K. p53 and Nur77/TR3-transcription factors that directly target mitochondria for cell death induction. Oncogene 2006; 25: 4725–4743.
225. Blagosklonny MV, Toretsky J, Neckers L. Geldanamycin selectively destabilizes and conformationally alters mutated p53. Oncogene 1995; 11(5): 933–939.
226. Kastan MB, Berkovich E. p53: A two-faced cancer gene. Nat Cell Biol 2007; 9: 489–491.
227. Kastner P, Mark M, Chambon, P. Nonsteroid nuclear receptors: What are genetic studies telling us about their role in real life? Cell 1995; 83: 859–869.
228. Mangelsdorf DJ, Thummel C, Beato M, Herrlich P, Schütz G, Umesono K, Blumberg B, Kastner P, Mark M, Chambon P, Evans RM. The nuclear receptor superfamily: The second decade. Cell 1995; 83: 835–839.
229. Baker KD, Shewchuk LM, Kozlova T et al. The Drosophila orphan nuclear receptor DHR38 mediates an atypical ecdysteroid signaling pathway. Cell 2003; 113(6): 731–742.
230. Wang Z, Benoit G, Liu J, Prasad S, Aarnisalo P, Liu X, Xu H, Walker NP, Perlmann T. Structure and function of Nurr1 identifies a class of ligand-independent nuclear receptors. Nature 2003; 423: 555–560.
231. Uemura H, Chang C. Antisense TR3 orphan receptor can increase prostate cancer cell viability with etoposide treatment. Endocrinology 1998; 139(5): 2329–2334.
232. Chen GQ, Lin B, Dawson MI, Zhang XK. Nicotine modulates the effects of retinoids on growth inhibition and RAR beta expression in lung cancer cells. Int J Cancer 2002; 99(2): 171–178.
233. Ke N, Claassen G, Yu DH, Albers A, Fan W, Tan P, Grifman M, Hu X, Defife K, Nguy V, Meyhack B, Brachat A, Wong-Staal F, Li QX. Nuclear hormone receptor NR4A2 is involved in cell transformation and apoptosis. Cancer Res 2004; 64(22): 8208–8212.
234. Woronicz JD, Calnan B, Ngo V, Winoto A. Requirement for the orphan steroid receptor Nur77 in apoptosis of T-cell hybridomas. Nature 1994; 367: 277–281.
235. Cheng LE, Chan FK, Cado D, Winoto A. Functional redundancy of the Nur77 and Nor-1 orphan steroid receptors in T-cell apoptosis. EMBO J 1997; 16(8): 1865–1875.
236. Kuang A, Cado D, Winoto A. Nur77 transcription activity correlates with its apoptotic function in vivo. Eur J Immunol 1999; 29: 3722–3728.
237. Li Y, Lin B, Agadir A et al. Molecular determinants of AHPN (CD437)-induced growth arrest and apoptosis in human lung cancer cell lines. Mol Cell Biol 1998; 18: 4719–4731.

238. Holmes WF, Soprano DR, Soprano KJ. Early events in the induction of apoptosis in ovarian carcinoma cells by CD437: activation of the p38 MAP kinase signal pathway. Oncogene 2003; 22: 6377–6386.
239. Chintharlapalli S, Burghardt R, Papineni S et al. Activation of Nur77 by selected 1,1-Bis(3'-indolyl)-1-(p-substituted phenyl)methanes induces apoptosis through nuclear pathways. J Biol Chem 2005; 280: 24903–24914.
240. Chinnaiyan P, Varambally S, Tomlins SA et al. Enhancing the antitumor activity of ErbB blockade with histone deacetylase (HDAC) inhibition. Int J Cancer 2006; 118: 1041–1050.
241. Shipp MA, Ross KN, Tamayo P, Weng AP, Kutok JL, Aguiar RC, Gaasenbeek M, Angelo M, Reich M, Pinkus GS, Ray TS, Koval MA, Last KW, Norton A, Lister TA, Mesirov J, Neuberg DS, Lander ES, Aster JC, Golub TR. Diffuse large B-cell lymphoma outcome prediction by gene-expression profiling and supervised machine learning. Nat Med 2002; 8: 68–74.
242. Li H, Kolluri SK, Gu J et al. Cytochrome c release and apoptosis induced by mitochondrial targeting of nuclear orphan receptor TR3. Science 2000; 289: 1159–1164.
243. Luciano F, Krajewska M, Oritz-Rubio P et al. Nur77 converts phenotype of Bcl-B, an anti-apoptotic protein expressed in plasm cells and myeloma. Blood 2007; 109(9): 3849–3855.
244. Wilson AJ, Arango D, Mariadason JM, Heerdt BG, Augenlicht LH. TR3/Nur77 in colon cancer cell apoptosis. Cancer Res 2003; 63: 5401–5407.
245. Jacobs CM, Boldingh KA, Slagsvold HH, Thoresen GH, Paulsen RE. ERK2 prohibits apoptosis-induced subcellular translocation of orphan nuclear receptor NGFI-B/TR3. J Biol Chem 2004; 279: 50097–50101.
246. Kolluri SK, Corr M, James SY et al. The R-enantiomer of the nonsteroidal antiinflammatory drug etodolac binds retinoid X receptor and induces tumor-selective apoptosis. Proc Natl Acad Sci USA 2005; 102: 2525–2530.
247. Lee KW, Ma L, Yan X, Liu B, Zhang XK, Cohen P. Rapid apoptosis induction by IGFBP-3 involves an insulin-like growth factor-independent nucleomitochondrial translocation of RXRalpha/Nur77. J Biol Chem 2005; 280: 16942–16948.
248. Yip KW, Godoi PH, Zhai D, Garcia X, Cellitti JF, Cuddy M, Gerlic M, Chen Y, Satterthwait A, Vasile S, Sergienko E, Reed JC. A TR3/Nur77 peptide-based high-throughput fluorescence polarization screen for small molecule Bcl-B inhibitors. J Biomol Screen 2008; 13: 665–673.
249. Rishi AK, Zhang L, Boyanapalli M, Wali A, Mohammad RM, Yu Y, Fontana JA, Hatfield JS, Dawson MI, Majumdar APN, Reichert U. Identification and characterization of a Cell-Cycle and Apoptosis Regulatory Protein (CARP)-1 as a novel mediator of apoptosis signaling by Retinoid CD437. J Biol Chem 2003; 278: 33422–33435.
250. Rishi AK, Zhang L, Yu Y, Jiang Y, Nautiyal J, Wali A, Fontana JA, Levi E, Majumdar APN. Cell cycle and apoptosis regulatory protein (CARP)-1 is involved in apoptosis signaling by epidermal growth factor receptor. J Biol Chem 2006; 281: 13188–13198.
251. Zhang L, Levi E, Majumder P, Yu Y, Aboukameel A, Du J, Xu H, Mohammad RM, Hatfield JS, Wali A, Adsay V, Majumdar APN, Rishi AK. Transactivator of transcription-tagged Cell Cycle and Apoptosis Regulatory Protein-1 peptides suppress growth of human breast cancer cells in vitro and in vivo. Mol Cancer Ther. 2007; 6: 1661–1672.
252. Yoo AS, Bais C, Greenwald I. Crosstalk between the EGFR and LIN-12/Notch pathways in C. elegans vulval development. Science 2004; 303: 663–666.
253. Beausoleil SA, Jedrychowski M, Schwartz D, Elias JE, Villen J, Li J, Cohn MA, Cantley LC, Gygi SP. Large-scale characterization of HeLa cell nuclear phosphoproteins. Proc Natl Acad Sci USA 2004; 101: 12130–12135.

254. Blagoev B, Kratchmarova I, Ong SE, Nielsen M, Foster LJ, Mann M. A proteomics strategy to elucidate functional protein–protein interactions applied to EGF signaling. Nat Biotechnol 2003; 21: 315–318.
255. Matsuoka S, Ballif BA, Smogorzewska A, McDonald ER 3rd, Hurov KE, Luo J, Bakalarski CE, Zhao Z, Solimini N, Lerenthal Y, Shiloh Y, Gygi SP, Elledge SJ. ATM and ATR substrate analysis reveals extensive protein networks responsive to DNA damage. Science 2007; 316: 1160–1166.
256. Bouwmeester T, Bauch A, Ruffner H et al. A physical and functional map of the human TNF-alpha/NF-kappa B signal transduction pathway. Nat Cell Biol 2004; 6: 97–105.
257. Kim JH, Yang CK, Heo K, Roeder RG, An W, Stallcup MR. CCAR1, a key regulator of mediator complex recruitment to nuclear receptor transcription complexes. Mol Cell 2008; 31: 510–519.

Role of Telomerase in Cancer Therapeutics

Kyung H. Choi and Michel M. Ouellette

1 Introduction

Telomerase is responsible for the maintenance of telomeres, specialized structures that cap the ends of chromosomes. Because most human cells lack
telomerase, telomeres shorten each time cells divide and this attrition acts as a
clock that limits their lifespan. During cancer development, this limited lifespan
is almost always bypassed by the reactivation of telomerase, the enzyme responsible for the synthesis of telomeres. This upregulation of telomerase provides
the cancer cells with cellular immortality or ability to proliferate for an unlimited number of cell divisions. Inhibitors of the enzyme telomerase have been
developed to reverse this immortal phenotype and limit the lifespan of cancer
cells. Following conventional chemotherapy, these inhibitors could be used to
prevent the regrowth of residual disease and reduce the incidence of recurrence.
In this chapter, we discuss the development of the first such inhibitor to enter
clinical trials, GRN163L. The inhibitor, a lipid-conjugated oligonucleotide
developed by Geron Corporation (Menlo Park, CA), inhibits telomerase in a
wide range of cancer cell lines. In mice bearing human tumor cells, GRN163L
can reduce tumor growth and metastasis. In this chapter, we discuss the development of GRN163L, its mechanism of action, and its potential value in the
treatment of cancer patients. In the second half, we discuss anticipated
challenges associated with the development of these new drugs, from the search
for new compounds to the testing and optimization of current inhibitors.

2 Human Telomeres Act as a Mitotic Clock

Telomeres are essential structures that cap the ends of linear chromosomes.
Human telomeres are made of a simple DNA repeat, $(TTAGGG)_n$ [1, 2]. These
repeats serve as anchor for the recruitment of sequence-specific DNA-binding

M.M. Ouellette (✉)
Eppley Institute for Research in Cancer, University of Nebraska Medical Center,
Omaha, NE 68198, USA
e-mail: mouellet@unmc.edu

Y. Lu, R.I. Mahato (eds.), *Pharmaceutical Perspectives of Cancer Therapeutics*,
DOI 10.1007/978-1-4419-0131-6_6, © Springer Science + Business Media, LLC 2009

factors TRF1, TRF2, and POT1. Through protein–protein interactions, these factors recruit several other proteins to telomeres, with which they form a large capping complex. This complex is needed to protect chromosomal ends from degradation, interchromosomal fusions, and other forms of inadequate recombination [1, 3]. A second vital function of telomeres is to hide chromosomal ends from DNA damage-sensing mechanisms, which would otherwise sense them as double-stranded (ds) DNA breaks [1]. In human cells, the presence of just one such break can activate DNA damage checkpoints and lead to either senescence or apoptosis. Telomeres end with G-rich single-stranded $3'$-overhang of 50–300 bases. Evidence suggests that this extension is sequestered into a large looping structure, termed a T-loop [1, 4]. Formation of this structure involves the looping of the telomere and the insertion of its $3'$-telomeric overhang into upstream duplex telomeric DNA [1, 5, 6]. It has been proposed that T-loops are especially well adapted to shield the ends of telomeres from DNA damage-sensing mechanisms and other biochemical activities.

Maintenance of telomeres requires telomerase, the enzyme responsible for the synthesis of telomeric DNA repeats. In cells that lack telomerase, telomeres shorten each time cells divide and this attrition acts as a mitotic clock that limits cellular lifespan [7–9]. Telomeres shorten because of a number of problems associated with the replication of linear DNA molecules (the so-called "end replication problems"). As replication forks approach the ends of linear DNA, problems are encountered with both the lagging and the leading strand synthesis. On the lagging strand, priming of the last Okazaki fragment can occur internally and removal of the RNA primer creates a gap, which cannot be filled for lack of an upstream primer. On the leading strand, postreplication processing is needed to regenerate a single-stranded $3'$-telomeric overhang that can be used as a substrate for T-loop formation and POT1 binding (an ssDNA-binding protein). The net result is the production of daughter chromatids that contain gaps of unreplicated DNA, causing telomeres to shorten each time cells divide [7, 9]. When the shortest telomere reaches a threshold size, it becomes uncapped and is recognized as a ds-DNA break. In primary human cells possessing functional DNA damage checkpoints, this presence of such an unrepairable break elicits one of two responses: senescence or apoptosis [10, 11]. Because they lack telomerase or have insufficient level of enzyme to maintain telomeres, somatic human cells lose telomeres with cell divisions and, as a consequence, have a limited lifespan. During cancer development, this limited lifespan poses an obstacle that the tumor cells have to overcome on their way to become malignant. In the great majority of cancers, overcoming this barrier is achieved by means of telomerase expression.

3 Telomerase Extends Cellular Lifespan

Telomerase can compensate the effects of the end replication problems and extend the lifespan of human cells. The enzyme solves these problems by the synthesis and addition of new telomeric repeats to its substrate, the $3'$-telomeric overhangs [12]. The enzyme has the ability to make DNA without primers or DNA templates. It solves this problem by carrying its own internal template in the form of an RNA component. The human enzyme contains two essential subunits: the protein hTERT (*human Telomerase Reverse Transcriptase*) and the small nuclear RNA hTR (*human Telomerase RNA*). The first provides catalytic activity and the second contains a short sequence (5'-CUAACC-CUAA-3') that serves as a template for the synthesis of telomeric repeats (Fig. 1). The enzyme functions as a reverse transcriptase and uses the RNA hTR as a template to add telomeric DNA repeats to the 3'-telomeric overhangs [12]. In cells that lack telomerase activity, the hTERT component is missing whereas hTR is ubiquitously expressed, irrespective of telomerase activity [13]. In primary human cells lacking telomerase activity, the forced expression of telomerase is sufficient to reconstitute telomerase activity and maintain telomeres [14]. In primary human cells, expression of hTERT can overcome senescence, extend cellular lifespan, and provide cells with immortality [15–17]. These hTERT-expressing cells are capable of indefinite cell divisions but tend to maintain their normal growth properties, chromosome number, and capacity to differentiate [18, 19].

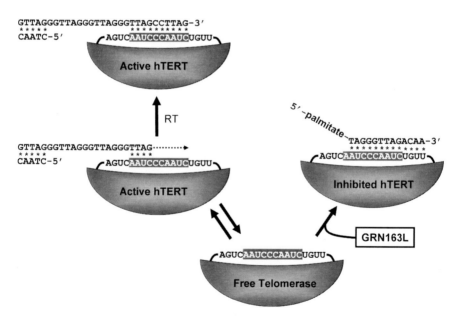

Fig. 1 Activity of telomerase and its inhibition by GRN163L. Telomerase is a reverse transcriptase that uses an internal RNA template (10 nucleotides; white letters over *dark gray box*) to synthesize (*dotted arrow*; RT) a 6-base telomeric DNA repeat. GRN163L hybridizes to the template region of telomerase and to surrounding nucleotides to block the activity of the enzyme

4 Telomerase Expression in Normal and Cancerous Tissues

Telomerase activity is typically measured using the Telomeric Repeat Amplification Protocol (TRAP) assay. In the TRAP assay, products of the telomerase reaction are quantified following their PCR amplification [20, 21]. The assay is exquisitely sensitive and incorporates an internal standard (ITAS) with which to normalize signals for differences in PCR efficiency. Telomerase activity is calculated as the ratio of the intensity of the telomeric products to that of the ITAS. With this assay, telomerase activity can be measured in a wide range of specimens, from tissue biopsies to cell pellets [22]. High throughput assays have been developed to adapt the telomerase assay to the clinical environment. Many of these new assays take advantage of fluorophores that alleviate the use of radioisotopes and facilitate the quantification of PCR products.

At the early stages of human development, telomerase activity is ubiquitously expressed throughout the embryo [23, 24]. At this stage, telomerase is needed to reset telomere length and allow for the massive numbers of cell divisions needed to complete embryogenesis. But by birth, telomerase activity becomes absent from most somatic tissues, with the exception of the blood, skin, and gastro-intestinal track [23, 24]. In these renewal tissues, tissue homeostasis is maintained by the continuous proliferation and differentiation of endogenous stem cells. To support this need for continued proliferation throughout life, active telomerase is needed. The enzyme is activated transiently during the differentiation of these normal stem cells [25]. This activation, however, is not sufficient to prevent the attrition of telomeres or lead to cellular immortality. As in all proliferative tissues, telomeres shorten with age in these renewal tissues [26].

Cancer is a notable exception to the universal shortening of telomeres in normal human tissues. Human cancer cells have in common that they possess mechanisms that block telomere attrition to give them immortality. In more than 85% of cancers, irrespective of the tumor type, this mechanism is the upregulation of telomerase activity [9, 27, 28]. Malignancies that develop from telomerase-negative tissues are almost always positive for the activity. Even in cancer cells originating from telomerase-positive precursors, telomerase is almost always upregulated. Yet, a small percent of cancer specimens has no detectable telomerase activity. In cancer cells that lack the activity, an alternate mechanism of telomere maintenance can be activated [29]. This other mechanism, termed ALT (alternate maintenance of telomeres), uses gene conversion events that use longer telomeres as template to elongate shorter ones. This ability to maintain telomeres is a fundamental property of cancer cells, which normal somatic human cells do not possess. This lack of telomere attrition gives cancer cells their cellular immortality or capacity for unlimited number of cell divisions. This transition to immortality is needed to allow the many stages of carcinogenesis to proceed unimpeded by senescence and to give the resulting cancer cells the ability to invade without being halted by the induction of senescence or crisis [9, 30]. Because most cancer cells are immortal as a result of telomerase reactivation, targeting telomerase is an attractive strategy for cancer therapy.

5 Telomerase Inhibitors in Cancer Therapy

5.1 Telomerase Inhibition and the Viability of Cancer Cells

Inhibiting telomerase in telomerase-expressing cancer cells causes the telomeres to shorten, and when sufficient telomeres have become uncapped, the cancer cells will experience one of two antiproliferative barriers – either senescence or crisis [31– 34]. The two barriers are different and whether cancer cell experience one or the other is dictated by the functionality of their DNA damage response and cell cycle checkpoints [2, 9]. Senescence is a viable but irreversible state of permanent cell cycle arrest. Crisis is a form of p53-independent apoptosis, which for the purpose of killing cancer cells, represents the preferred outcome. Cells that possess functional checkpoints, such as primary human cells, undergo senescence as soon as the shortest telomere has become uncapped. When uncapped, this short telomere will be recognized as a ds-DNA break by the DNA damage-sensing machinery, and this recognition will lead to the activation of the ATM kinase, phosphorylation of p53, and induction of cell cycle inhibitor p21^{WAF1} [2, 10]. A late response involving the induction of p16^{INK4a} and downstream activation of tumor suppressor pRB will also be observed [2, 9, 35]. The net result is an irreversible cell cycle arrest and establishment of the senescent state. Akin to terminal differentiation, senescence will be accompanied by changes in morphology and gene expression. In cells that lack functional checkpoints, senescence fails to be observed and the cells will continue to divide in spite of uncapped telomeres [9]. During this extended lifespan, however, the telomeres will continue to shorten for lack of active telomerase. When sufficient numbers of terminally shortened telomeres have accumulated, a state of crisis characterized by massive cell death is induced. Terminally shortened telomeres are highly reactive and will recombine with one another to produce sister chromatid fusions and dicentric chromosomes. At anaphase, these fusions fail to segregate and resolving the anaphase bridges that result leads to more chromosome breakage. The net result is a form of mitotic failure accompanied by the induction of p53-independent apoptosis [36]. Because they lack functional checkpoints as a result of mutations affecting the p53 and/or p16INK4a/pRB pathways, most cancer cells will undergo crisis rather than senescence after continuous telomerase inhibition [31– 34].

An important prediction is the expectation of a delay in the actions of telomerase inhibitors. Because sufficient telomere shortening needs to occur for senescence and crisis to be induced, the effects of telomerase inhibition will be observed only after the treated cancer cells have done sufficient number of cell divisions [2, 37]. Because of their delayed action, telomerase inhibitors are not going to be useful as a primary line of treatment. But to block the regrowth of residual disease after standard therapy, these inhibitors should be most valuable (Fig. 2). To produce recurrent tumors, surviving cancer cells need to undergo massive numbers of cell divisions. In the presence of a telomerase inhibitor, the

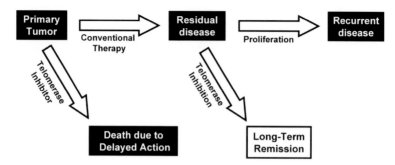

Fig. 2 Therapeutic potential of telomerase inhibitors GRN163L to block disease recurrence.
Because sufficient telomere attrition needs to occur before telomerase-inhibited cancer cells
reach crisis, the effects of telomerase inhibitors will be delayed until the target cells have done
sufficient numbers of cell divisions. This delay, which may preclude their use as a first line of
treatment, should not reduce the ability of these compounds to block the regrowth of residual
disease. After conventional therapy, telomerase inhibitors could be used to reduce the incidence of recurrences and promote long-term survival

several rounds of cell divisions needed for residual cancer cells to produce a
recurrent tumor will almost certainly lead to the accumulation of critically
short telomeres and the induction of crisis. Telomerase inhibitors are the first
new class of drug especially designed to reduce the incidence of recurrence when
used in combination with conventional cancer therapy.

5.2 GRN163L, a First Telomerase Inhibitor

For inhibiting telomerase, the template region of the human telomerase RNA
(hTR) presents an accessible target for oligonucleotide-based inhibitors
[38–41]. As shown previously, telomerase can be inhibited by oligonucleotides
that hybridize to the template region of its RNA component (Fig. 1). In one
study, telomerase in immortal human breast epithelial cells was inhibited with
peptide nucleic acid and 2′-methoxy oligomers [42]. Repeated transfection leads
to progressive telomere shortening and caused cells to undergo apoptosis with
increasing frequency until no cells remained. More recently, several N3′-P5′
thio-phosphoramidate oligonucleotides complementary to the template of hTR
have been used as potential telomerase inhibitors [43]. These compounds are
water soluble, acid stable, resistant to nucleases, and demonstrate high thermal
stability of duplexes formed with their complementary RNA strands [31,
43–46]. One compound GRN163 caused telomerase inhibition and subsequent
telomere shortening in many cancer cell lines [31, 46–50]. As with most anionic
oligonucleotides, repeated transfection of GRN163 with cationic lipophilic
carriers was required for efficient intracellular uptake, as naked oligonucleotides are poorly internalized. A second generation of GRN163 analogues,
modified by lipidation, was made to facilitate cellular uptake. One such

compound, GRN163L, is a GRN163 oligonucleotide modified to carry a 5'-terminal palmitoyl (C16) moiety conjugated to the N3'-P5'thio-phosphoramidate backbone (5'-palmitate-TAGGGTTAGACAA-NH$_2$-3'; Fig. 3) [49]. GRN163L is lipid soluble and does not rely on any membrane transporter for cellular uptake. When compared to GRN163, GRN163L displayed greatly improved cellular uptake, inhibition of telomerase, and rate of telomere shortening [46, 48, 49].

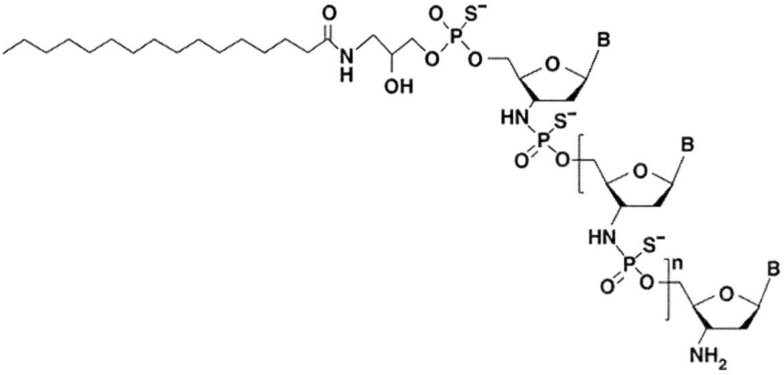

Fig. 3 Chemical structure of GRN163L. GRN163L is an N3'-P5' thio-phosphoramidate oligonucleotide complementary to the template of hTR. Three of the 13 nucleotides (5'-palmitate-TAGGGTTAGACAA-NH$_2$-3') are shown. Nucleotidic bases (A, C, G, or T) are shown as B. To facilitate cellular uptake, the 5'-end has been modified to carry a 5'-terminal palmitoyl (C16) moiety

5.3 Clinical and Preclinical Studies of GRN163L

The short- and long-term effects of GRN163L have been studied in both cultured cancer cells and mice bearing human tumor xenografts. With IC$_{50}$ in the nanomolar range, GRN163L was found to inhibit telomerase in a wide variety of cancer cell lines. Within 24 hours of its addition to the culture media, GRN163L inhibits telomerase [49]. In cancer cells chronically exposed to GRN163L, telomeres shorten with cell divisions [31]. After a delay, continuous exposure to the drug leads to crisis, as evidenced by the presence of chromosomal fusions, anaphase bridges, and widespread apoptosis. This capacity of GRN163L to limit lifespan was reported in cancer cell lines of diverse origins, including multiple myeloma and tumors of the bladder, breast, liver, lung, and stomach [31, 48, 51– 54]. In mice bearing human tumor xenografts, GRN163L was determined to be efficacious and well tolerated. The maximum tolerated dose was 1000 mg/kg and telomerase inhibition could already be detected with just 5 mg/kg [31]. In biodistribution studies, ^{35}S-labeled GRN163L spread to most, if not all, mouse tissues and was still present after 72 hours [31]. A week after a single dose of GRN163L at 30 mg/kg, 60% telomerase inhibition was still observed. In a xenograft model of lung cancer metastasis, administration of a single dose of GRN163L (15 mg/kg) could reduce the growth of lung metastases [31]. In mice carrying liver cancer xenografts, systemic administration of GRN163L inhibited tumor growth and sensitized tumor cells to chemotherapeutic agents [48]. On the basis of these preclinical results, GRN163L has now entered phase I and II clinical trials in patients with cancer. Phase I trials with dose escalation are underway in patients with solid tumors (ClinicalTrials.gov Identifier: NCT00310895) and chronic lymphocytic leukemia (NCT00124189). Other trials in patients with multiple myeloma (NCT00594126), lung (NCT00510445) and breast (NCT00732056) cancer have just recently begun to recruit patients. These trials are designed to assess safety, determine the maximum tolerated dose, and identify dose-limiting toxicities. Some are combined phase I/II trials, which have been designed to evaluate the ability of GRN163L to inhibit telomerase systemically, in both tumor specimens and normal surrogate tissues.

6 Challenges in the Clinical Application of Telomerase Inhibitors

Telomerase inhibitors are just beginning to find their way into human clinical trials. How efficacious and what side effects these inhibitors will have in real patients is difficult to predict. As with most new drugs, the transition from preclinical to clinical studies would be expected to come with its own set of new challenges. In the next sections, we discuss five areas that will necessitate further investigation to ensure the best possible results in patients.

6.1 Measuring the Effects on Recurrences After Conventional Therapy

Unlike conventional cancer drugs, telomerase inhibitors are not expected to produce an immediate response. Because sufficient telomere shortening needs to occur before these inhibitors can induce senescence or apoptosis, these effects should be observed only after the exposed cancer cells have done sufficient number of cell divisions [2, 37]. For this reason, telomerase inhibitors are expected to have a delayed action, and as a consequence, are unlikely to be efficacious as a fist line of treatment. These inhibitors, on the other hand, should be most useful to block the growth of locally advanced disease or to inhibit the regrowth of residual disease following conventional therapy. Clinical trials to assess the value of these inhibitors should be designed to reflect this mode of action. Rather than using RECIST (Response Evaluation Criteria in Solid Tumors) criteria to detect an immediate tumor response, these inhibitors should be tested for their ability to extend lifespan and reduce the incidence the recurrence. An ideal cohort would be patients with minimal disease for which a measurable chance of recurrent disease is anticipated. Long-term exposure of these patients to GRN163L would be expected to extend survival and progression-free survival as well as reduce the incidence of relapses. This need to follow patients over extended period to detect differences in survival and recurrence could impede progression toward determining the best dose and schedule and identifying the standard therapies that synergize with GRN163L. A second challenge will be to overcome the need to show evidence of efficacy in early clinical trials. Phase I/II trials tend to be conducted in patients with advanced disease, the worst possible cohort with which to test the value of telomerase inhibitors. Overcoming this obstacle might require the use of more sensitive methods to allow detection of weak responses in the context of short-term treatment.

6.2 Targeting the Cancer Stem Cells

Telomerase inhibitors will be especially valuable to block the regrowth of residual disease after conventional cancer therapy, as a means of reducing the incidence of recurrences. But for these inhibitors to be effective, they will need to target the specific subset of cancer cells that give rise to recurrent disease. Mounting evidence suggests that, in certain forms of cancer, recurrences are the products of the survival of residual cancer cells that possess properties of stem cells. The consensus definition of a cancer stem cell is a cell within a tumor that can self-renew and regenerate all of the heterogeneous lineages of cancer cells that comprise a tumor [55]. Rare cells that fall within this definition have been identified in a growing number of diseases, from hematological malignancies to brain, breast, and pancreatic cancer [56–58]. Conventional therapies have been optimized for the killing of bulk tumor cells, not necessarily for the targeting of the cancer stem cells. As the current literature suggests, cancer stem cells can express high levels of multidrug-resistant pumps, which can provide protection from the effects of certain chemotherapeutic drugs, such as gemcitabine [58, 59]. Therefore, an important question is whether GRN163L can target these cells efficiently. Alas, little is known of the effects of GRN163L on cancer stem cells, as past studies have all been focused on the effects of the drug on bulk tumor cells.

An important challenge will be to test the effects of telomerase inhibitors in cancer stem cells, especially those that may be present in solid tumors. As cancer stem cells are identified in growing numbers of malignancies, markers to isolate these cells are being identified (CD133, CD24, ESA1, CD44, and ALDH1). With the help of these markers, it will be possible to study the effect of GRN163L on cancer stem cells. To be able to reconstitute tumors, a critical property of these cells is their ability to self-renew. One prediction would be that if GRN163L inhibits telomerase in cancer stem cells, their telomeres will shorten and this attrition will interfere with their self-renewal. To measure the self-renewal of cancer stem cells, a serial transplantation assay is typically used [56–58]. Cancer stem cells are isolated and implanted into mice until tumor forms. For these tumors the same cancer stem cells are reisolated, which are then transferred to a second-generation mice. Cancer stem cells are often passaged for up to six such transplantations while maintaining their high tumorigenicity and capacity to reconstitute the histopathological complexity of the original tumor. Studies are in progress in several laboratories, including ours, that will use this assay to define the activities of GRN163L on cancer stem cells. These studies should determine whether cancer stem cells have detoxification mechanisms that may prevent the compounds from being able to target the cancer stem cells.

6.3 Impact of Telomerase Inhibitors on Normal Renewal Tissues

Telomerase activity is by no means limited to cancer cells. Low levels of telomerase activity are present in a limited number of normal tissues, including the skin, blood, lung, and gastrointestinal track. These renewal tissues require low-level telomerase activity to allow for the massive number of cell divisions needed to maintain tissue homeostasis throughout the life of an individual. We know little about how these normal telomerase-positive tissues will respond to antitelomerase therapies. In preclinical studies, GRN163L was tested in mice carrying human tumors cells but because laboratory mice have much longer telomeres than humans (40–60 kb instead of 2–20 kb) [25], these studies failed to delineate the side effects of the compound on the normal mouse tissues. Studies have been done in Rhesus monkeys, which share with humans a similar biology of telomeres and telomerase, but these studies have looked only at the short-term effects of GRN163L [60]. The effects of the lack of telomerase in renewal tissues are exemplified in the symptoms of patients that carry mutations in components of the telomerase complex, alternatively affecting hTR, hTERT, or dyskerin [12, 61]. These patients have 50% of normal telomerase level, and this haploinsufficiency accelerates the shortening of telomeres in renewal tissues. Short telomeres in these patients have been implicated in a variety of disorders, which include dyskeratosis congenita, aplastic anemia, and idiopathic pulmonary fibrosis [61– 65]. A first key feature of these diseases is the observation that they affect tissues that normally express telomerase. Bone marrow failure leading to premature death is a common characteristic of aplastic anemia and dyskeratosis congenital, with the latter disorder also presenting with mucocutaneous abnormalities. In patients with idiopathic pulmonary fibrosis, the bronchial epithelium fails to self-renew and is replaced gradually with connective tissue [65]. A second key feature of these diseases is the relatively long latency observed before symptoms develop, which varies from 6 to 60 years [61]. This latency suggests that years of uninterrupted telomerase inhibition may be required before declines in renewal tissue function are noted. The wide range of clinical presentations seen in patients with mutations in telomerase complex components provides an overview of the possible side effects arising from long-term exposure to telomerase inhibitors. In future clinical trials, this knowledge should help provide a framework with which to assess the risks of antitelomerase therapies.

To help predict the risk–benefit ratio of antitelomerase therapy, an important question is whether cancer cells will be more acutely targeted than the normal renewal tissues. Several key observations have been made that support the idea that these drugs will have the required specificity. First, telomerase in renewal tissues does not appear to be expressed by the most primitive stem cells [25]. In hair follicles and gastrointestinal crypts, for example, the activity is restricted to the transiently amplifying cells [25, 66]. These cells, which are born out of the asymmetric division of the more primitive stem cells, are lineage-restricted progenitors. It is the proliferation and differentiation of these progenitors that give rise to a functional tissue. Because they lack telomerase, the more primitive stem cells should not be affected directly by the presence of a telomerase inhibitor. If so, then renewal tissues should resist the effects of these drugs far better than most cancers would, as cancer specimens tend to be uniformly positive for the activity of telomerase. A second key observation is that cancer specimens, as a general rule, have shorter telomeres than normal tissues [67]. So why should cancer cells have short telomeres if they express telomerase? Cancer cells reactivate telomerase as a mean of escaping crisis, when their telomeres have become critically short, and it may be that once reactivated, telomerase is expressed at levels that are insufficient to re-elongate the telomeres. In cancer cells that divide rapidly, these short telomeres should first become uncapped after telomerase inhibition, much before the telomeres of normal telomerase-expressing cells. Even more promising is the recent discovery that certain cancer cells arbor T-stumps, a distinct class of extremely short telomeres with just a few telomeric repeats [68]. During GRN163L therapy, the almost immediate uncapping of these T-stumps would therefore be expected to provide a more selective and rapid response toward the killing of cancer cells.

However encouraging the preclinical studies may be, understanding the risks and benefits of antitelomerase therapy will need to await completion of the first clinical trials. These preclinical studies, performed in mice and with cultured human cells, did little to help predict the effects of telomerase inhibitors on renewal tissues. As a result, much remains to be learned and so many key questions are left to be answered. How will normal telomerase-expressing tissues respond to telomerase inhibition? How long will we be able to treat patients before causing irreversible damages to their renewal tissues? Could the use of these drugs lead to a premature aging of the renewal tissues, which may not be discernable until later in life? Will the adverse effects be more pronounced in older individuals who may have shorter telomeres? None of these problems can be modeled using laboratory mice. GRN163L is now entering clinical trials and an important challenge will be to design future trials to address all of these outstanding concerns. Future trials will need to monitor renewal tissues for signs of premature aging and provide for a long-term follow-up of cancer survivors.

6.4 Development of Resistance to Antitelomerase Therapy

There has been no report yet of acquired resistance from cultured cancer cells treated with GRN163L, and the drug was found to be active in a wide range of cancer cell lines [49]. Yet, it is fair to predict that if the compound is efficacious, a selection process will take place that will favor the emergence of resistant cells. Several mechanisms of resistance can be envisioned, some specific to GRN163L and others applicable to all forms of antitelomerase therapy. A first possible source of resistance will be the emergence of cells that take advantage of the ALT pathway (Alternative Lengthening of Telomeres). In cells that use the ALT pathway, telomeres are maintained through gene conversion events that take place between long and short telomeres [29]. A subset of human tumors has already been determined to use the ALT pathway rather than telomerase. In cultures of human cells experiencing crisis, clones of ALT cells can emerge spontaneously as a result of rare mutational events (at a frequency of less than $1/10^7$ cell or division). So the possibility of ALT cells arising as a consequence of long-term GRN163L exposure is a real possibility. A second possible source of resistance could come from alterations affecting the composition of the telomerase complex. Mutations in the template region of hTR could cause GRN163L to fail to hybridize and could do so without blocking telomere maintenance. Change in levels of expression of hTR and hTERT could flood cells with sufficient telomerase complexes to out-compete the effects of limited amounts of GRN163L. Changes in membrane composition could interfere with the uptake and transport of the drug. The heterogeneity in the composition of tumors might be a source of additional problems. Tumors could contain rare cells that may possess longer telomeres or that may remain dormant, or quiescent, during the course of antitelomerase therapy. After therapy is discontinued, once the bulk of the tumor cells have been killed, these cells could resume cell division to give rise to recurrent disease.

Identifying and cataloguing the different mechanisms of resistance to GRN163L and other telomerase inhibitors will be challenging. It may also be that mechanisms of resistance will differ whether they have been selected for in vitro, in animal models, or in real patients. Clearly, these efforts would best be pursued with samples from patients who have relapsed following long-term therapy with inhibitors of telomerase. If sources of resistance are identified in these patients, a second challenge will be to devise strategies to overcome the specific underlying mechanisms. Thus, it may be that new compounds will need to be developed to overcome as yet unforeseen mechanisms of detoxification that may limit the activities of the current telomerase inhibitors.

6.5 Development of New Antitelomerase Compounds

GRN163L is the first inhibitor of telomerase to enter clinical trials. As the first prototype to be tested, GRN163L will undoubtedly be followed by the development of new derivatives with improved potency and selectivity. Already in progress at Geron Corporation (Menlo Park, CA) are several new derivatives of GRN163L with different activity profiles. In a recent study, GRN163L was reported to have both antitelomerase and antiadhesive activities [69]. When added to trypsinized cells, the compound could block reattachment of these cells to the plastic dish. These effects were determined to be independent of telomerase activity or size of telomeres. To separate the antiadhesive and antitelomerase activities of GRN163L, Geron Corporation made several new derivatives of GRN163L. The antiadhesive effect was dependent on the molecular properties of the lipid moiety, the phosphorothioate backbone, and the presence of triplet-G sequences within the GRN163L structure [69]. Whether the antiadhesive properties of GRN163L add to its clinical value has not been determined, but Geron identified new compounds that could inhibit telomerase without blocking cell adhesion. Room for improvement exists for important aspects, dictating the activities of GRN163L. The lipid moiety, for example, could further be optimized to improve cellular uptake. Modifications to the oligonucleotide moiety could also be made to improve stability or increase the affinity of the compound for telomerase.

It is important to realize that the ongoing search for telomerase inhibitors is by no means limited to oligonucleotides. Several new classes of compounds have so far been identified as a result of drug screening efforts and other rational design schemes. Among these are molecules designed to stabilize the formation of G-quadruplexes and others that reduce the processivity of the enzyme. The native substrate of telomerase, the 3'-telomeric overhang, can fold into a G-quadruplex structure and formation of this structure blocks the activity of telomerase. Developed through rational design, many G-quadruplex stabilizers have been found to inhibit telomerase. A leading candidate, which should soon be entering phase I clinical trial, is the acridine compound BRACO-19 [70]. The effect of this drug on the structure of the 3'-telomeric overhang has been determined not only to inhibit telomerase but also to block the binding of POT1, an essential component of telomeres. Therefore, a major concern has been that these compounds could perturb the structure of telomeres in normal telomerase-negative cells, thereby causing widespread telomere dysfunction. Drug screening efforts have also led to the discovery of additional candidates. Two such candidates, BIBR1532 and BIBR1591, were found to inhibit the processivity of telomerase with IC_{50} in the nanomolar range [71]. BIBR1532 is a noncompetitive inhibitor that binds to a site distinct from the active center. Treating cancer cells with these compounds can lead to telomere dysfunction and to the induction of senescence [72, 73]. To discover promising new compounds and identify the most valuable ones, a concerted effort on the part of the public and private sectors will undoubtedly be needed.

7 Concluding Remarks

GRN163L is the first telomerase inhibitor to enter clinical trial. Being a first prototype, GRN163L will be instrumental in defining the range of activities associated with these new drugs. As a new class of drugs is aimed at reducing recurrence following conventional treatment, telomerase inhibitors are truly unique. If GRN163L is found to be beneficial to cancer patients, this would most certainly lead to the development of second-generation inhibitors, with improved potency and selectivity. In the clinics of the future, these inhibitors could become a ubiquitous component of the standard of care for most cancers. While much remains to be learned, the potential is there for these inhibitors to revolutionize the way we treat cancer patients.

References

1. de Lange T. Protection of mammalian telomeres. *Oncogene* 2002; **21**: 532–540.
2. Ouellette MM, Lee K. Telomerase: diagnostics, cancer therapeutics and tissue engineering. *Drug Discov Today* 2001; **6**: 1231–1237.
3. de Lange T. Shelterin: the protein complex that shapes and safeguards human telomeres. *Genes Dev* 2005; **19**: 2100–2110.
4. de Lange T. T-loops and the origin of telomeres. *Nat Rev Mol Cell Biol* 2004; **5**: 323–329.
5. Griffith JD *et al.* Mammalian telomeres end in a large duplex loop. *Cell* 1999; **97**: 503–514.
6. Stansel RM, de Lange T, Griffith JD. T-loop assembly in vitro involves binding of TRF2 near the 3' telomeric overhang. *Embo J* 2001; **20**: 5532–5540.
7. Harley CB. Telomere loss: mitotic clock or genetic time bomb? *Mutat Res* 1991; **256**: 271–282.
8. Harley CB, Futcher AB, Greider CW. Telomeres shorten during ageing of human fibroblasts. *Nature* 1990; **345**: 458–460.
9. Shay JW, Wright WE. Telomerase activity in human cancer. *Curr Opin Oncol* 1996; **8**: 66–71.
10. Karlseder J *et al.* p53- and ATM-dependent apoptosis induced by telomeres lacking TRF2. *Science* 1999; **283**: 1321–1325.
11. Robles SJ, Adami GR. Agents that cause DNA double strand breaks lead to p16INK4a enrichment and the premature senescence of normal fibroblasts. *Oncogene* 1998; **16**: 1113–1123.
12. Collins K, Mitchell JR. Telomerase in the human organism. *Oncogene* 2002; **21**: 564–579.
13. Meyerson M *et al.* hEST2, the putative human telomerase catalytic subunit gene, is up-regulated in tumor cells and during immortalization. *Cell* 1997; **90**: 785–795.
14. Weinrich SL *et al.* Reconstitution of human telomerase with the template RNA component hTR and the catalytic protein subunit hTRT. *Nat Genet* 1997; **17**: 498–502.
15. Bodnar AG *et al.* Extension of life-span by introduction of telomerase into normal human cells. *Science* 1998; **279**: 349–352.
16. Yang J *et al.* Human endothelial cell life extension by telomerase expression. *J Biol Chem* 1999; **274**: 26141–26148.
17. Herbert BS, Wright WE, Shay JW. p16(INK4a) inactivation is not required to immortalize human mammary epithelial cells. *Oncogene* 2002; **21**: 7897–7900.
18. Jiang XR *et al.* Telomerase expression in human somatic cells does not induce changes associated with a transformed phenotype. *Nat Genet* 1999; **21**: 111–114.
19. Morales CP *et al.* Absence of cancer-associated changes in human fibroblasts immortalized with telomerase. *Nat Genet* 1999; **21**: 115–118.
20. Herbert BS, Hochreiter AE, Wright WE, Shay JW. Nonradioactive detection of telomerase activity using the telomeric repeat amplification protocol. *Nat Protoc* 2006; **1**: 1583–1590.

21. Wright WE, Shay JW, Piatyszek MA. Modifications of a telomeric repeat amplification protocol (TRAP) result in increased reliability, linearity and sensitivity. *Nucleic Acids Res* 1995; **23**: 3794–3795.

22. Hess JL, Highsmith WE, Jr. Telomerase detection in body fluids. *Clin Chem* 2002; **48**: 18–24.

23. Wright WE *et al*. Telomerase activity in human germline and embryonic tissues and cells. *Dev Genet* 1996; **18**: 173–179.

24. Ulaner GA, Giudice LC. Developmental regulation of telomerase activity in human fetal tissues during gestation. *Mol Hum Reprod* 1997; **3**: 769–773.

25. Forsyth NR, Wright WE, Shay JW. Telomerase and differentiation in multicellular organisms: turn it off, turn it on, and turn it off again. *Differentiation* 2002; **69**: 188–197.

26. Vaziri H *et al*. Evidence for a mitotic clock in human hematopoietic stem cells: loss of telomeric DNA with age. *Proc Natl Acad Sci USA* 1994; **91**: 9857–9860.

27. Shay JW, Bacchetti S. A survey of telomerase activity in human cancer. *Eur J Cancer* 1997; **33**: 787–791.

28. Kim NW *et al*. Specific association of human telomerase activity with immortal cells and cancer. *Science* 1994; **266**: 2011–2015.

29. Henson JD, Neumann AA, Yeager TR, Reddel RR. Alternative lengthening of telomeres in mammalian cells. *Oncogene* 2002; **21**: 598–610.

30. Ouellette MM, Choi KH. Telomeres and telomerase in ageing and cancer. In: *Encyclopedia of Life Sciences* (*http://www.els.net/*). John Wiley & Sons Ltd: Chichester, UK, 2007.

31. Dikmen ZG *et al*. In vivo inhibition of lung cancer by GRN163L: a novel human telomerase inhibitor. *Cancer Res* 2005; **65**: 7866–7873.

32. Guo C *et al*. Inhibition of telomerase is related to the life span and tumorigenicity of human prostate cancer cells. *J Urol* 2001; **166**: 694–698.

33. Hahn WC *et al*. Inhibition of telomerase limits the growth of human cancer cells. *Nat Med* 1999; **5**: 1164–1170.

34. Zhang X *et al*. Telomere shortening and apoptosis in telomerase-inhibited human tumor cells. *Genes Dev* 1999; **13**: 2388–2399.

35. Shay JW, Pereira-Smith OM, Wright WE. A role for both RB and p53 in the regulation of human cellular senescence. *Exp Cell Res* 1991; **196**: 33–39.

36. Macera-Bloch L *et al*. Termination of lifespan of SV40-transformed human fibroblasts in crisis is due to apoptosis. *J Cell Physiol* 2002; **190**: 332–344.

37. Shay JW, Wright WE. Telomerase: a target for cancer therapeutics. *Cancer Cell* 2002; **2**: 257–265.

38. Shay JW, Wright WE. Mechanism-based combination telomerase inhibition therapy. *Cancer Cell* 2005; **7**: 1–2.

39. White LK, Wright WE, Shay JW. Telomerase inhibitors. *Trends Biotechnol* 2001; **19**: 114–120.

40. Hamilton SE *et al*. Identification of determinants for inhibitor binding within the RNA active site of human telomerase using PNA scanning. *Biochemistry* 1997; **36**: 11873–11880.

41. Norton JC *et al*. Inhibition of human telomerase activity by peptide nucleic acids. *Nat Biotechnol* 1996; **14**: 615–619.

42. Herbert B *et al*. Inhibition of human telomerase in immortal human cells leads to progressive telomere shortening and cell death. *Proc Natl Acad Sci USA* 1999; **96**: 14276–14281.

43. Herbert BS *et al*. Oligonucleotide N3'–>P5' phosphoramidates as efficient telomerase inhibitors. *Oncogene* 2002; **21**: 638–642.

44. Asai A *et al*. A novel telomerase template antagonist (GRN163) as a potential anticancer agent. *Cancer Res* 2003; **63**: 3931–3939.

45. Gryaznov S *et al*. Telomerase inhibitors – oligonucleotide phosphoramidates as potential therapeutic agents. *Nucleosides Nucleotides Nucleic Acids* 2001; **20**: 401–410.

46. Gellert GC *et al.* Effects of a novel telomerase inhibitor, GRN163L, in human breast cancer. *Breast Cancer Res Treat* 2006; **96**: 73–81.
47. Chen Z, Koeneman KS, Corey DR. Consequences of telomerase inhibition and combination treatments for the proliferation of cancer cells. *Cancer Res* 2003; **63**: 5917–5925.
48. Djojosubroto MW *et al.* Telomerase antagonists GRN163 and GRN163L inhibit tumor growth and increase chemosensitivity of human hepatoma. *Hepatology* 2005; **42**: 1127–1136.
49. Herbert BS *et al.* Lipid modification of GRN163, an N3'–>P5' thio-phosphoramidate oligonucleotide, enhances the potency of telomerase inhibition. *Oncogene* 2005; **24**: 5262–5268.
50. Perry PJ, Arnold JR, Jenkins TC. Telomerase inhibitors for the treatment of cancer: the current perspective. *Expert Opin Investig Drugs* 2001; **10**: 2141–2156.
51. Shammas MA *et al.* Telomere maintenance in laser capture microdissection-purified Barrett's adenocarcinoma cells and effect of telomerase inhibition in vivo. *Clin Cancer Res* 2008; **14**: 4971–4980.
52. Dikmen ZG, Wright WE, Shay JW, Gryaznov SM. Telomerase targeted oligonucleotide thio-phosphoramidates in T24-luc bladder cancer cells. *J Cell Biochem* 2008; **104**: 444–452.
53. Shammas MA *et al.* Telomerase inhibitor GRN163L inhibits myeloma cell growth in vitro and in vivo. *Leukemia* 2008; **22**: 1410–1418.
54. Hochreiter AE *et al.* Telomerase template antagonist GRN163L disrupts telomere maintenance, tumor growth, and metastasis of breast cancer. *Clin Cancer Res* 2006; **12**: 3184–3192.
55. Clarke MF *et al.* Cancer stem cells – perspectives on current status and future directions: AACR Workshop on cancer stem cells. *Cancer Res* 2006; **66**: 9339–9344.
56. Allan AL, Vantyghem SA, Tuck AB, Chambers AF. Tumor dormancy and cancer stem cells: implications for the biology and treatment of breast cancer metastasis. *Breast Dis* 2006; **26**: 87–98.
57. Farnie G, Clarke RB. Breast stem cells and cancer. *Ernst Schering Found Symp Proc* 2006; **5**: 141–153.
58. Hermann PC *et al.* Distinct populations of cancer stem cells determine tumor growth and metastatic activity in human pancreatic cancer. *Cell Stem Cell* 2007; **1**: 313–323.
59. Li C *et al.* Identification of pancreatic cancer stem cells. *Cancer Res* 2007; **67**: 1030–1037.
60. Tressler RJ *et al.* pGRN163L, a potent and specific inhibitor of telomerase: integrated pharmacokinetics, pharmacodynamic, and safety data guide design of practical treatment for targeting inhibitory levels. *Blood* 2006; **108**: Abstract 2595.
61. Garcia CK, Wright WE, Shay JW. Human diseases of telomerase dysfunction: insights into tissue aging. *Nucleic Acids Res* 2007; **35**: 7406–7416.
62. Vulliamy T, Marrone A, Dokal I, Mason PJ. Association between aplastic anaemia and mutations in telomerase RNA. *Lancet* 2002; **359**: 2168–2170.
63. Marrone A *et al.* Heterozygous telomerase RNA mutations found in dyskeratosis congenita and aplastic anemia reduce telomerase activity via haploinsufficiency. *Blood* 2004; **104**: 3936–3942.
64. Armanios M *et al.* Haploinsufficiency of telomerase reverse transcriptase leads to anticipation in autosomal dominant dyskeratosis congenita. *Proc Natl Acad Sci USA* 2005; **102**: 15960–15964.
65. Armanios MY *et al.* Telomerase mutations in families with idiopathic pulmonary fibrosis. *N Engl J Med* 2007; **356**: 1317–1326.
66. Ramirez RD, Wright WE, Shay JW, Taylor RS. Telomerase activity concentrates in the mitotically active segments of human hair follicles. *J Invest Dermatol* 1997; **108**: 113–117.
67. Broccoli D, Godwin AK. Telomere length changes in human cancer. *Methods Mol Med* 2002; **68**: 271–278.
68. Xu L, Blackburn EH. Human cancer cells harbor T-stumps, a distinct class of extremely short telomeres. *Mol Cell* 2007; **28**: 315–327.

69. Jackson SR *et al.* Antiadhesive effects of GRN163L – an oligonucleotide N3'->P5' thio-phosphoramidate targeting telomerase. *Cancer Res* 2007; **67**: 1121–1129.
70. Gunaratnam M *et al.* Mechanism of acridine-based telomerase inhibition and telomere shortening. *Biochem Pharmacol* 2007; **74**: 679–689.
71. Barma DK, Elayadi A, Falck JR, Corey DR. Inhibition of telomerase by BIBR 1532 and related analogues. *Bioorg Med Chem Lett* 2003; **13**: 1333–1336.
72. El Daly H, Martens UM. Telomerase inhibition and telomere targeting in hematopoietic cancer cell lines with small non-nucleosidic synthetic compounds (BIBR1532). *Methods Mol Biol* 2007; **405**: 47–60.
73. Parsch D, Brassat U, Brummendorf TH, Fellenberg J. Consequences of telomerase inhibition by BIBR1532 on proliferation and chemosensitivity of chondrosarcoma cell lines. *Cancer Invest* 2008; **26**: 590–596.

Polymeric Carriers for Anticancer Drugs

Dongin Kim and You Han Bae

1 Introduction

Chemotherapy together with debulking surgery is a major treatment for cancer. There are, however, major limitations of conventional cytotoxic drugs that result from their nonspecific toxicity (e.g., the lack of selectivity) in the body and the intrinsic or acquired multidrug resistance (MDR) of cancer cells. To this end, polymeric drug carriers have been developed to address this nonspecificity and MDR [1]. It is believed that these drug carriers alter the biodistribution and increase the bioavailability of incorporated anticancer agents to the target cells [2].

Polymers are the most common materials that are used as drug carriers due to their diverse chemistry and safety characteristics in the body [1]. A polymer can be used to carry drugs in different manners (or forms), such as conjugates [3], dendrimers [4], nanoparticles [5], micelles [6, 7], nanogels [7], or polymersomes [8], using a variety of delivery mechanisms. Figure 1 shows the structures of common polymer carriers.

This chapter briefly reviews polymer delivery systems for anticancer drugs and is followed by a discussion of concerns about conventional anticancer drugs such as solubility, biodistribution, cytosolic drug delivery, and MDR.

2 Polymeric Drug Carriers

2.1 Conjugates

Polymer–drug conjugates comprise drug molecules that are covalently linked to a polymer backbone as side groups or end groups [3]. A representative system has at least three components: a water-soluble polymer, bioactive anticancer agents, and a biodegradable spacer between the polymer and the drug [9].

Y.H. Bae (✉)
Department of Pharmaceutics and Pharmaceutical Chemistry, University of Utah,
Suite 315, Salt Lake City, Utah 84108, USA
e-mail: you.bae@utah.edu

Y. Lu, R.I. Mahato (eds.), *Pharmaceutical Perspectives of Cancer Therapeutics*,
DOI 10.1007/978-1-4419-0131-6_7, © Springer Science+Business Media, LLC 2009

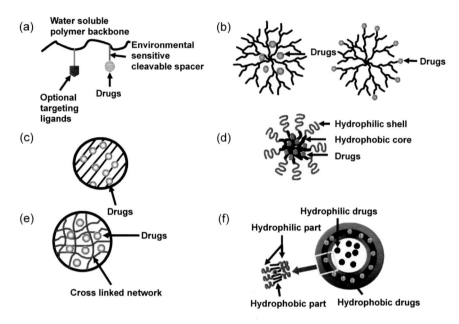

Fig. 1 Various polymeric drug carriers: (**a**) conjugates, (**b**) dendrimers, (**c**) nanoparticles, (**d**) micelles, (**e**) nanogels, (**f**) polymersomes

The polymer chemistry makes the conjugate unique and also provides diversity [3]. The system can be tailored by selecting the appropriate polymer and drug molecules, by changing the polymer's molecular weight, by altering the number of drug molecules that is conjugated per polymer chain, and by introducing targeting moieties and bioresponsive elements. The conjugates are then regarded as new chemical entities (NCEs) [10]. N-(2-Hydroxypropyl) methacrylamide (HPMA) copolymer-doxorubicin (PK1; FCE28068), involved in phase I/II clinical trials, showed a significant decrease in anthracycline-related toxicity and no cardiotoxicity despite cumulative doses of up to 1680 mg/m^2 (doxorubicin equivalent) [11]. More than 10 anticancer drug polymer conjugates are now in various phases of clinical trials.

2.2 Dendrimers and Hyperbranched Polymers

A dendrimer is a hyperbranched polymer molecule that has a well-defined molecular weight. It has a globular architecture with several dendrons (dendron: a tree-like polymer molecule with a trunk) that are connected to a central core. Its distinctive features include a controlled size (15 nm in diameter), multivalency, and the surface charge of ionizable dendrimer terminal groups, which can vary in the generation number [4].

One example of a dendrimer as an anticancer drug carrier is the covalent attachment of drug molecules to the dendrimer periphery, which is in a conjugated form. The generation number of the dendrimer determines the drug content. The degradable linkages between the drug and the dendrimer control the release of the drug [4].

Duncan and colleagues [12] have investigated the conjugates of a polyamidoamine (PAMAM) dendrimer with cisplatin. The dendrimer–drug conjugates showed increased drug solubility, decreased systemic toxicity of the drug, and selective accumulation in solid tumors. Their results using dendrimer–platinum conjugates showed increased efficacy when compared with free cisplatin in the treatment of subcutaneous B16F10 melanoma.

In addition, Zhuo et al. [13] prepared PAMAM dendrimers from a cyclic tetraamine core and subsequently attached 5-fluorouracil to the dendrimer periphery. These conjugates released free 5-fluorouracil on incubation in phosphate-buffered saline. The drug molecules can also be physically entrapped with a limited loading capacity in the dendrimer core (a few drug molecules per dendrimer).

2.3 Micelles

Polymeric micelles, which were first introduced by Ringsdorf in 1984 [14], are an assembly of amphiphilic block copolymers in an aqueous environment. Primary polymeric micelles have a well-defined core–shell structure – a hydrophobic inner core and a hydrophilic shell. Micelles can incorporate water-insoluble drugs into the cores through chemical, physical, or electrostatic interactions [15], such as in micelles that are composed of a block copolymer of poly(ethylene glycol) and polyaspartate (Fig. 2) [16–18]. A phase II study of a paclitaxel (PTX)-incorporated micelle, NK105, that is used in the treatment of stomach cancer, has begun [19].

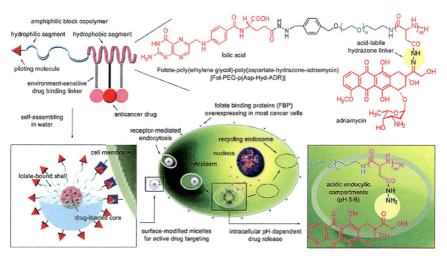

Fig. 2 Multifunctional polymeric micelles composed of a block copolymer of poly(ethylene glycol) and polyaspartate with tumor selectivity for active drug targeting and pH sensitivity for intracellular site-specific drug transport. Folic acid with high tumor affinity due to the overexpression of its receptors was conjugated onto the surface of the micelle (adapted from Ref. [114] with permission)

2.4 Nanoparticles

There has been considerable interest in developing biodegradable nanoparticles (NPs) for drug delivery due to their stability and controlled release properties. The size of NPs ranges from 10 to 1000 nm. NPs can be a solid sphere or a hollow capsule, depending on the fabrication methods. Nanocapsules are vesicular systems in which a drug is enclosed in a polymer cavity, while nanospheres are matrix systems in which the drug molecules are dissolved or dispersed. Typical degradable polymers that are used for NPs are poly(D,L-lactide), poly(D,L-glycolide), poly(lactide-*co*-glycolide), polyanhydride, and poly(alkyl cyanoacrylate), among others [5, 20–22].

2.5 Nanogels

A nanogel is a nanosized hydrogel made of physically or chemically cross-linked polymers that are water-soluble. A nanogel that is composed of responsive polymers may change volume depending on the external environment [23].

Vinogradov et al. prepared a poly(ethylene glycol)-*cl*-polyethyleneimine nanogel using a modified emulsification-solvent evaporation method. The size distribution of the nanogels ranged between 40 and 300 nm. The nanogels formed complexes with negatively charged oligonucleotides, which enhanced the uptake of oligonucleotides by cells in culture [24].

Bae recently reported a virus-mimetic (VM) nanogel that consisted of a hydrophobic core composed of poly(histidine-*co*-phenylalanine)(poly(His-*co*-Phe)) and two layers of hydrophilic shells [PEG and bovine serum albumin (BSA)] (Fig. 3) [25]. The PEG is linked to the core-forming block and to BSA, which forms a capsid-like outer shell through an oil-in-water emulsion method. At high pHs, the core of this nanogel is hydrophobic and becomes rigid; the core swells, however, due to hydrophilicity from the ionization of polyHis at low pHs. As a result, when the nanogels were exposed to an early endosomal pH of 6.4, the gel grew from 55 nm to 355 nm. This pH-dependent size change between pH 7.4 and 6.4 was reversible (Fig. 3) and was closely linked to the release rate of incorporated doxorubicin (DOX). The nanogels released a significant amount of DOX at endosomal pHs (~6.4) while reducing the DOX release rate at cytosolic or extracellular pHs (e.g., pH 6.8–7.4).

Furthermore, nanogels can disrupt the endosomal membrane through the proton-buffering effect of polyHis and the observed nanogel volume expansion within cell endosomes. This allows VM nanogels and the anticancer drug (that is released from the nanogels) to transfer from the endosomes to the cytosol, where the VM nanogels rapidly shrink to their original size as a result of the more neutral local pH, and thereby reduce the drug release rate. Release of the drug as triggered by endosomal pH would be in the cytosol. The drug would then diffuse into the nucleus, which is the pharmacological target site. The

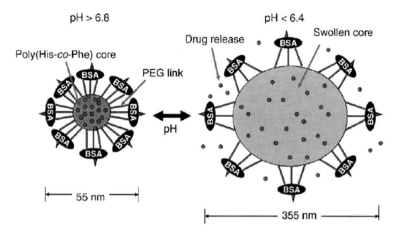

Fig. 3 Schematic picture of pH-sensitive, virus-mimetic (VM) nanogel and its in vitro swelling/deswelling property by particle size results between pH 7.4 and 6.5 (adapted from Ref. [25] with permission)

drug's action on the cells would induce apoptosis, which in turn would release the nanogels for subsequent infection and activity in neighboring cells. This infectious cycle has been demonstrated in cultures of drug-resistant tumor cells and is thought to have a high potential for maximizing drug efficacy in treating tumors, inflamed tissues, and other diseases due to sequential cytotoxic action.

2.6 Polymersomes

Polymersomes are self-assembled polymeric vesicles, analogs of liposomes, that are formed from a diverse array of synthetic amphiphilic block copolymers [26, 27]. Their advantages over liposomes are improved stability in storage [28–30] and prolonged circulation time [31]. While the hydrophilic aqueous core accommodates water-soluble drugs, the thick hydrophobic wall membrane of the polymersome provides room for hydrophobic drugs [32]. In addition, multifunctional polymersomes can be designed from functional block copolymers [8]. Most polymersomes contain poly(ethylene glycol) (PEG) as a hydrophilic outer shell, providing a stealth-like character to the drug, which increases circulation times and biocompatibility [28].

Polymersomes offer advantages for clinical therapeutic and diagnostic imaging applications. The ratio of the hydrophilic-to-hydrophobic volume fraction is the key in determining the mesoscopic formulations among micelles (spherical, prolate, or oblate) or vesicles (polymersomes) in aqueous solution [33–35]. In general, a proportion of hydrophilic block-to-total polymer from 25 to 45% favors polymersome formation, while block copolymers that have proportions greater than 45% favors micelle formation [36].

Hydrophobic blocks that are used for polymersome fabrication are inert polyethylethylene, polybutadiene, polystyrene, polydimethylsiloxane, degradable poly(lactic acid) (PLA), and poly(ε-caprolactone) (PCL). Hydrophilic blocks include negatively charged poly(acrylic acid) and cross-linkable polymethyloxazoline. Neutral PEG is more common for bioapplications. Among block copolymers, PEO–PLA and PEO–PCL are becoming widely adopted [26].

2.7 Depot Systems

Depot systems are usually formulated as implants. Their application focuses on either limiting high drug concentrations to the immediate area that surrounds the pathologic site or providing patients with sustained drug release for systemic therapy [37, 38]. Clinical implant systems have been used in hormone replacement therapy and in the treatment of prostate cancer [39]. The implants can be formulated into highly viscous liquids or semisolids [40, 41]. Degradable polymeric materials are used as implants, including polysaccharides, poly(lactic acid-*co*-glycolic acid) (PLGA), and nonbiodegradable methacrylates [42, 40, 37]. Biodegradable polymers are more favorable because they do not need to be surgically removed later.

Implants with anticancer agents confine potentially toxic anticancer drugs within tumors with sustained drug release. A viscous gelatin solution or a galactoxyloglucan gel of mitomycin C that is administered intraperitoneally has been used [40]. A 5-fluorouracil poly(ortho ester) implant increased the benefit of the drug, although the high dose of the drug was associated with related toxicity [43]. Biodegradable copolymers of PLA, poly(mandelic acid), and poly(hydroxyphenylacetic acid) provided therapeutic anticancer drug levels for 10 weeks [44].

Low-molecular-weight biodegradable ABA- or BAB-type triblock copolymers have been investigated as thermogelling depots [45–47], where A is PEG and B is PLGA. Their aqueous polymer solutions have reverse gelation properties, enabling them to be soluble in water at or below room temperature or allowing them to become hydrogels at the injection site. Such depots slowly degrade over 4–6 weeks [48]. The copolymers can solubilize poorly soluble paclitaxel (PTX), can stabilize liable protein drugs, and can provide a sustained release of drugs for 1–6 weeks [49].

3 Solubility

An intrinsic challenge for most anticancer drugs in clinical applications is low solubility in water [50]. This is one of the major issues in drug formulations. For intracellular delivery, a drug molecule must have a certain degree of hydrophobicity, enabling it to cross the cell membrane [51, 52]. The binding affinity to target cells is often associated with the lipophilicity of the drug molecules. Consequently, most potent drug candidates often present poor water solubility, which leads to poor absorption and bioavailability [53] and causes aggregation on intravenous administration and embolization in the blood vessels [50]. The aggregates can induce side effects as severe as respiratory system failure, can increase local toxicity, and can lower systemic bioavailability because of high local concentrations at the sites of deposition [54].

A large fraction (40%) of potential drug candidates fail to enter formulation development due to problems with solubility [55]. Conventional approaches to increase solubility include using excipients such as ethanol and other organic solvents, Cremophor EL (polyethoxylated castor oil), and surfactants [54]. Applying salts or adjusting pH can increase the aqueous solubility if drug molecules contain ionizable groups [56]. Reprecipitation on dilution of the solubilized drug with aqueous solutions (such as physiological fluids by parenteral administration) should be addressed.

The toxicity and side effects of cosolvents or surfactants are also problems in formulations [57]. Drug carriers, such as nanoparticles [58], conjugates [3], and micelles [6], have shown promising results with significantly improved solubility. Their capacity to solubilize varies, depending on the incorporated drugs. For example, PTX can be incorporated into PEO–PLA micelles. The solubility of PTX can be up to 50 mg/mL [59], while the solubility of PTX in water has been shown to be as low as 0.5 μg/mL [60]. In addition, the aqueous solubility of PTX that was conjugated to PEG and a polyamidoamine (PAMAM) dendrimer increased dramatically to 2.5 mg/mL and 3.2 mg/mL, respectively [61].

4 Biodistribution

With intravenous administration, conventional low-molecular-weight anticancer drugs are distributed throughout the body via the bloodstream and affect both malignant and normal cells. The goal of chemotherapy is to concentrate a drug to the target site as much as possible and to minimize side effects.

4.1 Long Circulation

To increase the residence time of drug carriers in the blood, the carriers are modified with hydrophilic synthetic polymers, such as PEG [62–64]. Coating nanoparticles with PEG sterically disrupts the interactions of blood components with the carrier surface and subsequently decreases the binding of plasma proteins. This minimizes opsonin adsorption onto the carrier and carrier uptake rates by the reticuloendothelial system (RES) [65–67]. Repulsive interactions [68] and poor permeability of proteins through PEG coating [69] may contribute to this observation.

The following are various appealing properties of PEG as a protecting polymer: excellent solubility in aqueous solutions, high flexibility of its polymer chain, low toxicity, low immunogenicity, low antigenicity, lack of accumulation in the RES, and minimal influence on specific biological properties of modified pharmaceuticals [70–72]. PEG does not create any toxic metabolites because PEG is not biodegradable. PEG molecules that have a molecular weight below 40 kDa are readily excreted from the body through the kidneys [73].

Currently, there exist many chemical approaches to synthesize activated derivatives of PEG and to conjugate these derivatives to a variety of drugs and drug carriers [70–74]. Other polymers have been used as alternatives to PEG [75]. They must have biocompatibility, hydrophilicity, and a highly flexible main chain. Examples are single-end, lipid-modified poly(acryl amide), poly(vinyl pyrrolidone) [66, 76], poly(acryloyl morpholine), [77] phospholipid-modified poly(2-methyl-2-oxazoline) or poly(2-ethyl-2-oxazoline), [78] phosphatidyl polyglycerols [79], and polyvinyl alcohol [80]. Surface modification of poly-meric carriers can be carried out by physical adsorption of a protecting polymer on the carrier surface or by chemical grafting of polymer chains onto the carriers.

The concentration of DOX in plasma after injection of free DOX in animal models ranges from several micrograms per milliliter to ~20 µg/mL after 5–10 min at a dose of 10 mg/kg [81–83]. One study reported a DOX half-life of 26 min [81]. As compared with the values of free DOX, DOX that was carried by PEG–po-ly[Asp(ADR)] micelles demonstrated a high initial concentration in the blood (and plasma), with a long half-life of 70 min. This result indicates that the PEG chains in the outer shell play a crucial role in the extended circulation of PEG–P[Asp(ADR)] micelles in the blood and promote less absorption of DOX-loaded micelles into living tissues and less metabolic activity by the tissues than free DOX [84].

4.2 Distribution Volume

The process of drug deposition depends on the distribution volume. When a drug is associated with a carrier, the rate of drug clearance is decreased (the half-life increases), and the volume of distribution is decreased. Consequently, it pro-motes tumor uptake [85]. The size of the carrier (normally 5–200 nm) minimizes penetration of the drugs into the organs and renal clearance. The volume dis-tribution of the carrier is similar to the plasma volume when the blood circulation of the drug carrier is increased and the drug release rate from the carriers is slow [2]. Therefore, this limited distribution volume increases the maximum tolerated dose (MTD), as in the case of HPMA copolymer-linked doxorubicin [86].

4.3 Toxicity Profile

Ideal chemotherapeutics should target only tumor cells and should decrease tumor burden by inducing cytostatic or cytotoxic effects. Their lack of specifi-city, however, allows most chemotherapeutic drugs to have an adverse effect on normal cells and organs, leading to various side effects, including nephrotoxi-city, hematotoxicity, cardiotoxicity, neurotoxicity, and impairment of other functions [87–89].

In vitro toxicology using cell cultures has been used as an alternative method for early toxicity in in vivo tests. Alteration of cultured cell lines, however, compared with their tissues of origin, as well as the contrasting sensitivities of these cells and original normal tissues to chemical agents, has revealed a discrepancy in toxicity profiles between in vitro cell cultures and in vivo animal studies. Several studies have reported that human primary cells are good models for toxicity analysis and provide a promising alternative to animal models [90–92].

Nephrotoxicity is a major side effect of chemotherapy. Evaluating renal toxicity from anticancer drugs uses renal slices and isolated cell suspensions of renal proximal tubules [93]. Cisplatin, *cis*-diamminedichloroplatinum II (CDDP), is an inorganic platinum anticancer agent that offers broad-spectrum antitumor activity against various types of animal and human tumors [94]. CDDP-induced nephrotoxicity is the most important dose-limiting factor in chemotherapy [87, 95]. Earlier studies have reported that CDDP therapy is related to cardiotoxicity [89].

In one study, polymeric micelles that incorporated CDDP were prepared as a polymer–metal complex between CDDP and poly(ethylene glycol)–poly(glutamic acid) block copolymers. Four of 10 mice that were treated with CDDP micelles (4 mg/kg; five doses at 2-day intervals) showed complete tumor regression with no significant body weight loss, whereas free CDDP treatment at the same drug dose and regimen resulted in tumor survival and 20% body weight loss. It appears that CDDP-incorporated micelles are less toxic than free CDDP, in addition to its improved therapeutic efficacy [96, 97].

4.4 EPR Effect

Recent studies have reported that polymer–drug conjugates and nanoparticulates experience prolonged circulation in the blood and more passive accumulation in tumors, even in the absence of targeting moieties [10], suggesting the existence of a passive retention mechanism. Tumor blood vessels have abnormal qualities, such as a high proportion of proliferating endothelial cells, open pores, increased tortuosity, pericyte deficiency, and aberrant basement membrane formation. This defective vascular structure is due to rapid vascularization, providing tumor cells with oxygen and nutrients for rapid growth and rendering the vessels permeable to macromolecules and nanoparticles.

Decreased lymphatic drainage keeps the carriers in the tumor. This passive targeting mechanism has been called the "enhanced permeation and retention (EPR) effect" and was first identified by Maeda et al. [98, 99]. Numerous studies have shown that the EPR effect results in passive accumulation of macromolecules and nanosized particulates (e.g., polymer conjugates, polymeric micelles, dendrimers, and liposomes) in solid tumor tissues, increasing the therapeutic index while decreasing side effects. Figure 4 describes the concept of passive tumor targeting by EPR effects.

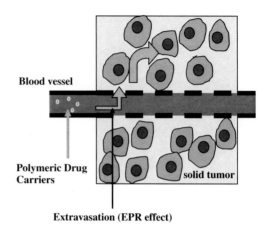

Fig. 4 Schematic picture of EPR effect. Tumor targeting of long-circulating polymer drug carrier occurs passively by the "enhanced permeability and retention" (EPR) effect. The inset is the chemical structure of folic acid

Although the optimal size of nanoparticles that accumulate in a tumor by the EPR effect is unknown, studies that have used liposomes and nanoparticles have reported that the cutoff size of the pores in tumor vessels is 200 nm–1.2 μm [84]. A tumor-dependent pore cutoff size of 200 nm–2 μm was proven by direct observation of tumor vasculature [100, 101]. These results suggest that drug-loaded nanosized carriers accumulate in malignant tumor cells [102].

DOX-incorporating polymer-based nanoparticles circulate in the blood for more than 3 days and gradually accumulate in tumors via the EPR effect [103]. Although a wide variety of polymer-based drug carriers may be used for tumor targeting of anticancer drugs via the EPR effect, it should be noted that vessel permeability, which forms a cornerstone of the EPR effect, varies during tumor progression. In addition, extravasation of polymeric carriers depends on tumor type and anatomical location, as well as the physicochemical properties of the utilized polymer [104].

5 Triggered Release

Despite various advantages of nanosized drug carriers, such as extended circulation [62], passive accumulation in solid tumors [103], improved stability [104], tumor targeting via conjugation to a specific ligand [105], and biodegradability in vivo [106], the kinetics of release of an incorporated drug is another critical factor in determining the success of the design and development of carriers. If the drug releases prematurely in the blood during a lengthy circulation, it may cause systemic side effects and fail to meet the sufficient therapeutic window of drug concentration at acting sites, while the delay of drug release in tumors could contribute to the development of MDR in tumor cells [107].

Recently, there have been various attempts to develop responsive systems for release to specific signals. For example, thermoresponsive polymeric carriers that respond to hyperthermic conditions [108] and pH-sensitive systems that activate in tumor-acidic pHs [109] have been investigated.

5.1 pH-Responsive Delivery

The use of acidic pH has been a common strategy for the development of various pH-sensitive systems for modulated drug delivery. In particular, most extracellular pHs (pH_e) of solid tumors are more acidic (pH, 6.5–7.2) than normal tissues [110, 111]. A major cause of acidic tumor pH is the high rate of glycolysis in tumor cells under aerobic or anaerobic conditions [99, 112]. The acidic environment may benefit tumor invasion (metastasis) by disturbing the extracellular matrix of the surrounding normal tissues [113] Thus, triggering drug release at this tumor pH_e may induce localized high-dose therapy that is effective for tumor treatment. Another distinct acidic pH is found in subcellular organelles, such as endosomes and lysosomes.

Two major design approaches have been implemented in designing pH-responsive release systems: the use of degradable chemical bonds between drugs and carriers [114, 115] that are cleaved by acidic endolysosomal pH (<6.5) [116] and structural destabilization of self-assembled carriers [117–120]. An example of pH-induced chain cleavage in drug delivery applications is the acetal bond. 5-Fluorouridine release from 5-fluorouridine–PEG conjugate was shown to be due to the pH-sensitive acetal bond, which is cleaved at pH 5.0 through hydrolysis with minimal release at pH 7.4 [121].

pH-sensitive micelles composed of polymer–DOX conjugates via a hydrazone bond also have been investigated. In one study, DOX was conjugated to PEG/polyaspartate-folate, and the conjugate block copolymers formed a micelle. The micelles were assessed for endosomal pH sensitivity. They were stable during blood circulation with minimal drug leakage, successfully accumulated in solid tumors, and internalized into cancer cells by folate receptor-mediated endocytosis, followed by DOX release after endosomal pH (pH<6.5)-induced cleavage of the hydrazone linkage [122].

Acidic pH can also change the structure of the polymeric carrier, resulting in drug release from the destabilized carriers. One example is tumor extracellular pH (pH_e)-sensitive polymeric micelles that are composed of poly(L-histidine) (polyHis) (Mw 5000)/PEG (Mw 2000) diblock copolymers [117, 118, 120]. These micelles are stable at pH 7.4 but unstable at pH_e. They are associated with the ability of polyHis to switch by protonation below pK_b. Unprotonated polyHis above its pK_b becomes hydrophobic. Protonation below pK_b renders polyHis hydrophilic due to the ionization of its imidazole ring, resulting in gradual disintegration of the micelle into monomers.

In one study, polyHis/PEG micelles were prepared at pH 8.0 via dialysis. DOX-encapsulated polyHis/PEG micelles, however, showed relative instability at pH 7.4. To overcome this limitation, a mixed micelle system composed of polyHis/PEG (75 wt%) and PLLA/PEG-folate (25 wt%) was prepared. The incorporation of a nonionizable block copolymer (PLLA/PEG) in the micellar structure of polyHis/PEG endowed it with improved stability at pH 7.4 due to increased hydrophobicity of the micelle core. The pH-sensitive mixed micelles (PHSMs) started to disintegrate below pH 7.0.

The results from in vivo tests that have used DOX-loaded PHSMs (equivalent DOX = 10 mg/kg) showed significant inhibition ($P<0.05$ compared with free DOX or saline solution) of the growth of subcutaneous s.c. MCF-7 xenografts, as presented in Fig. 5. The tumor volume of mice that were treated with PHSMs ($P<0.05$ compared with free DOX) was 4.5 or 3.6 times smaller than those compared with saline solution or free DOX treatment after 6 weeks.

Fig. 5 Tumor growth inhibition of s.c. human breast MCF-7 carcinoma xenografts in BALB/c nude mice. Mice were injected i.v. with 10 mg/kg DOX equivalent dose: DOX-loaded PHSM (€), PHSM/f (▲), PHIM (∇), PHIM/f (◇), and DOX (●). Two i.v. injections on days 0 and 3 were made. (a) Tumor volume change and (b) body weight change ($n = 5$). Values are the means of the standard deviations (SD) (adapted from Ref. [120] with permission)

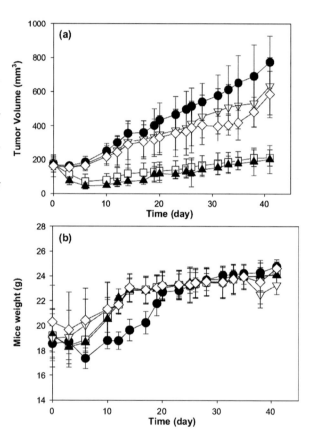

The combination of the EPR effect and triggered release of DOX by tumor pH_e may be synergistic in tumor chemotherapy, leading to higher local concentrations of the drug at tumor sites (targeted high-dose tumor therapy) with a minimal release of the drug from the micelles during circulation in the blood (pH 7.4). The volume of tumors that were treated with PHSMs was 3.0 times smaller than that of tumors that were treated with ordinary, pH-insensitive micelles (Fig. 5A). Stable body weight in the experimental groups, except for free DOX, indicated a minimum toxicity of the micellar systems (Fig. 5B).

For PTX delivery, the micellar system of a pH-sensitive diblock copolymer was investigated. The block copolymer consisted of a hydrophilic block of 2-(methacryloyloxy)ethyl phosphorylcholine (MPC) and a pH-sensitive hydrophobic block of 2-(diisopropylamino)ethyl methacrylate (DPA) [123]. The results showed complete PTX release after 20 hours at pH 5.0 and 70% of the initial PTX release after 50 hours at pH 7.4.

5.2 Temperature-Responsive Delivery

The principal mechanism of temperature-sensitive polymers is the sharp transition from coil to globule in water on heating, indicating a change from a hydrophilic state (coil) below the lower critical solution temperature (LCST) to a hydrophobic state (globule) above the LCST. Representative temperature-sensitive polymers include N-isopropylacrylamide (NIPAAm), its copolymers (LCST: 30–50°C) [108, 124–127], polyester block copolymers (20–100°C) [97, 128], and elastin-like polypeptides (27–40°C) [129–131]. To achieve both spatial and temporal control in conjunction with local temperature increases (2–5°C), the LCST of a given polymer can be tailored through its comonomer composition, hydrophilic–hydrophobic balance, stereochemistry [125–127, 132], and the addition of salts and surfactants [133]. These thermosensitive polymers with controlled LCSTs (around body temperature) can be applied to specific applications (e.g., tumor treatment).

An example is the fabrication of micelles that are composed of inert hydrophobic cores with an outer shell of polyNIPAAm, which have shown phase transitions that are slightly above 32°C [125]. This change in the outer shell above the LCST from hydrophilic to hydrophobic results in micelle aggregation, self-reorganization, accelerated drug release, and enhanced interactions with cells. The hydrophobic blocks that are used to form the core of PNIPAAm-based micelles are: methacrylic acid stearoyl ester (MASE), stearoyl chloride (SC) [126], poly(N-butyl methacrylate) (PBMA) [125, 126, 134], polystyrene (PS) [124], and poly(D,L-lactide-co-glycolide) (PLGA) [135, 136].

Drug release from polyNIPAAm/PBMA micelles shows temperature dependence. The initial drug was released up to 10% below 37°C and accelerated up to 90% at 37°C [127]. This change was caused by structural deformation of PNIPAAm/PBMA micelles on heating. Interestingly, similar behaviors have been shown in studies using poly(NIPAAm-co-N,N-dimethylacrylamide)/PLGA block copolymers (LCST 39.1°C) [135, 136]. The drug-loaded micelles, with an average size below 200 nm, were stable at 37°C, while the micelles became deformed and induced triggered drug release at 39.5°C (above normal body temperature).

In vitro cytotoxicity studies with drug-loaded micelles have also shown greater cytotoxicity above the LCST, resulting from thermally induced drug release. These results suggest that combination therapy can be implemented, using both thermosensitive systems and local hyperthermic treatment of tumors, primarily at 42°C. The coupled treatment may prove to be more effective as a result of passive drug accumulation in tumors by the EPR effect [99] and increased tumoral drug concentration by externally modulated hyperthermic conditions.

Despite successful results from in vitro studies, however, the clinical applications of systems that are based on polyNIPAAm may be limited, because polyNIPAAm is nondegradable and insoluble. In addition, a major problem of polyNIPAAm-based drug delivery systems is that thermal treatment is required for controlled destabilization of the micelles and concurrent drug release, which is not always feasible in clinical situations. Therefore, to overcome the disadvantages of polyNIPAAm, controlled biodegradable systems that use polyester block copolymers as thermosensitive polymers have been investigated.

Biodegradable and temperature-sensitive nanoparticles from alternating multiblock copolymers (PLLA/PEG/PLLA) were synthesized by coupling dicarboxylated PEG (Mw 2000) with PLLA [128]. The antitumor drug DOX was incorporated into the nanoparticles through dialysis. The results from in vitro studies that used Lewis lung carcinoma (LLC) cells indicated that DOX-loaded micelles showed more cytotoxicity against LLC cells at 42°C than at 37°C. The treatment of tumors using this nanoparticle is induced from a synergistic effect, such as combined biodegradation and thermal sensitivity at 42°C when coupled with local hypothermia.

Elastin-like polypeptides (ELPs) that have a pentapeptide (Val-Pro-Gly-Val-Gly) repeat have a similar LCST to PNIPAAm and also have hydrophobic folding and assembly transitions at ∼40°C [130, 137]. The hydrophobicity of ELPs can determine their LCST and is dependent on the fourth amino acid. For example, substituting Ala or Gly with Val in the fourth position of the ELP sequence increases the LCST of ELP from 27°C to 40°C [138]. ELP accumulates in solid tumors on heating to 42°C, as compared with tumors that are heated to 34°C [139]. In addition, ELPs that are conjugated with DOX using a pH-sensitive hydrazone bond [140] increase cellular DOX uptake two- to threefold in hyperthermal tumor cells over control cells [141]. Based on these results, ELP–drug conjugates are a promising carrier for tumor targeting under hyperthermic conditions [142]. Upcoming clinical trials will determine the antitumoral efficacy of thermal-sensitive systems that are based on ELP as well as systems that are based on polyesters or PNIPAAm.

5.3 Ultrasound-Responsive Drug Delivery

Ultrasonography has various advantages for drug delivery because its noninvasive energy through the skin can be limited to specific locations and can trigger drug release at that site. Liposome formulation for anticancer drugs initially was studied using ultrasonography [143, 144]. Ultrasonography generates thermal energy to cause hyperthermic conditions, as described previously.

A recent and novel application of ultrasonography in drug delivery showed the ability to produce cavitation activity, a process by which gas bubbles are created and oscillate in the membrane [145, 146]. There are two major mechanisms in ultrasound-triggered drug release [147]. The first contribution is the disruption of drug carriers. Drug-loaded vesicles (or micelles) that are denser than the surrounding liquid will be ruptured and will release their contents if the shear stress (e.g., strength from ultrasonography) exceeds the strength of the drug carrier. The second mechanism is promoted by the low frequency of high-intensity ultrasonography, resulting in collapse cavitation. When drugs are bound to a polymeric carrier, the backbone of the polymers can be pulled apart by viscous shear stresses that are generated from collapse cavitation, and the drug may be released from the polymer backbone. Other mechanisms have also been discussed [147].

Ultrasound-activated drug release using Pluronic (PEG/poly(propylene oxide) (PPO)/PEG) micelle solutions has been studied by Rapoport and Pitt [148–151]. Marin et al. proposed two mechanisms that control acoustic activation of drug release and uptake from Pluronic micelles [152, 153]. The first mechanism indicated that acoustically triggered micelles release the drug, leading to higher concentrations of free drug in the medium. The other mechanism involves uptake of micelle-encapsulated drugs into cells based on the perturbation of cell membranes by ultrasonography. Both mechanisms were noted to function cooperatively.

Recently, several in vivo studies have supported acoustically activated drug delivery [148, 149]. Nelson et al. [151] showed that applying low-frequency ultrasonography (20 and 70 kHz) significantly reduced tumor size when compared with noninsonated controls in rats using encapsulated DOX in Pluronic micelles. Gao et al. evaluated the effects of ultrasonography on drug targeting and release using Pluronic P-105 micelles [148, 149]. They stabilized micelles using PEG–diacylphospholipid and tested DOX-loaded micelles. Micelles accumulated in the tumor effected reduced tumor growth using local ultrasonic irradiation (1 or 3 MHz for 30 seconds) at the tumor site in ovarian tumor-bearing mice.

5.4 Enzyme-Responsive Delivery

Over the past few decades, enzyme-triggered drug release has been attractive because it uses linkers or bonds that are cleavable by certain enzymes. These carriers reach the target area by the EPR effect and by active targeting. The destabilization of carriers due to the enzymes at the target site induces drug release from carriers that contain enzyme-sensitive linkers. The primary advantage of this system is that carrier destabilization and consequent drug release can be controlled by modifying the cleavable bonds or linkers to be specific to enzymes that are present at the target sites.

Various PEG–DOX conjugates have been formed micelles in aqueous solution and prepared using different peptide linkers (GFLG, GLFG, GLG, GGRR, and RGLG) for covalent attachment of DOX to the carriers. Their particle sizes have ranged from 13 to 46 nm [154]. PEGs of linear or branched architecture (MW 5000–20000) have been used. The release of DOX in vitro indicated that the micelle was destabilized by linker degradation from lysosomal enzymes, triggering drug release.

Oishi et al. prepared polyion complex (PIC) micelles to deliver antisense oligodeoxynucleotides (asODN) to cells. They were formed by conjugating PEG with ODN using a disulfide linkage (PEG-SS-asODN) and assembling them into branched poly(ethylenimine) (PEI) [155]. Cleavage of the disulfide linkage induced release of the active asODN molecules into the cellular interior, leading to a high glutathione concentration in the cytoplasm.

Recently, biodegradable and disassembled dendritic molecules have been introduced for anticancer drug delivery. Several anticancer prodrugs have been developed to be activated selectively in malignant tissues by a specific enzyme, which is targeted [156] or secreted [157] near the tumor cells. The release of the free drug occurs through cleavage of a prodrug from a protecting group.

Recently, a polyamidoamine (PAMAM) dendrimer–succinic acid–PXT conjugate was prepared with a hydrolysable ester bond that is cleaved by esterase-hydrolyzing enzyme [61]. The conjugate formulation showed 10-fold higher in vitro cytotoxicity than did the unconjugated drug.

Self-immolative dendrimers have been developed as a novel prodrug platform [158, 159]. These dendrimers have a unique structure that can release all of their tail units through self-immolative chain fragmentation, which is initiated by a single cleavage event at the dendrimer core. The drug is incorporated into the tail units, and a multiprodrug unit is released from the dendrimers by a single enzymatic cleavage.

One study focused on a heterotrimeric system with the anticancer drugs camptothecin (CPT), DOX, and etoposide using retroaldol, a retro-Michael trigger that is activated by antibody 38C2 [158]. In vitro studies using cell growth inhibition assays reported that cell growth was inhibited 15-fold when using the heterotrimeric prodrug over the control group due to activation by antibody 38C2. In a recent study, a series of dendritic prodrugs with four molecules, including the anticancer agent CPT, have been studied. A drug has also been shown to be released by penicillin-G-amidase activation under physiological conditions [160]. Cell growth inhibition results showed increased toxicity of the dendritic prodrug on incubation with the enzyme.

6 Cytosolic Delivery

6.1 Active Targeting

Research has focused on developing a drug delivery system that uses active targeting, because cancer cells often overexpress surface (glyco)proteins (tumor-associated antigens or tumor-specific antigens) that may be found at low levels on normal cells. The chemical attachment of a targeting moiety on drug carriers induces cellular uptake of the drug carriers and drug by active endocytosis.

Monoclonal antibodies (mAbs) are most often used for active targeting [161]. Drug carriers are conjugated with a whole mAb or binding fragments of an mAb for active intracellular delivery of anticancer drugs. There are reviews on mAb-based active targeting [161–163], but the stability and economic issues of mAbs, however, should not be ignored.

Folic acid is one member of the vitamin B family. Folate receptor targeting presents several advantages over antigen targeting. Folic acid is a simple, low-molecular-weight compound, and it is stable and economic. Folate conjugates offer flexible conjugation chemistry. As a result, its conjugates have been used to deliver a variety of drugs and imaging agents [164–166]. In addition, various tumors of colon, lung, prostate, ovaries, mammary glands, and brain over-express folate receptor (FR) [167–170].

Folate-conjugated drugs [162] or folate-conjugated nanoparticles [171] use receptor-mediated endocytosis for cellular internalization and can bypass cancer cell drug efflux pumps and overcome MDR [172]. The receptor-mediated uptake of folate conjugates proceeds through distinct steps (Fig. 6). The folate conjugates initiate by binding to FRs on the cell surface. After invagination of

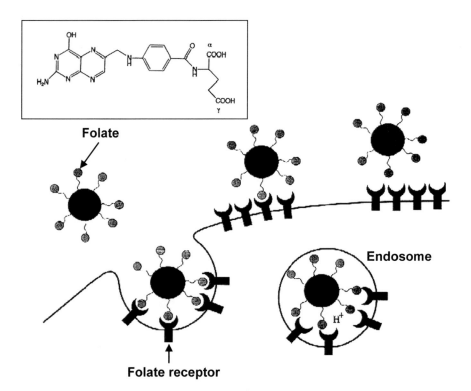

Fig. 6 The chemical structure of folic acid and the series of distinct steps of the folate receptor-mediated endocytosis (adapted from Ref. [187] with permission)

the plasma membrane, they form unique endocytic vesicles (endosomes). The acidic pH in endosomes enables FR–carrier complexes to disassemble FR from the complexes. The disassembled and membrane-bound FRs are directed back to the cell surface to mediate the delivery of additional folate conjugates. Concurrently, the folate conjugates that are released from FRs escape the endosome if there is any endosomal membrane disruption [173], resulting in drug deposition in the cytoplasm. To date, a number of conjugates (including protein toxins [174], immune stimulants, chemotherapeutic agents, liposomes, nanoparticles, and imaging agents) have been developed with folic acid and have been delivered to FR-expressing cells [175].

Transferrin, an 80-kDa glycoprotein, is also an appropriate ligand for tumor targeting because its receptors are overexpressed on cancer cells [176, 177]. In biological terms, the liver synthesizes transferrin, which is secreted into the plasma. In blood, transferrin binds to endogenous iron, forming the iron–transferrin chelate, which is an important physiological source of iron for cells in the body. Transferrin receptors on cell surfaces recognize the chelate and mediate its endocytosis into acidic compartments. Sahoo and Labhasetwar [178] prepared PXT-loaded PLGA nanoparticles, wherein transferrin was conjugated to them via epoxy linkages. There in vitro results using transferrin-conjugated nanoparticles showed greater cellular uptake and reduced exocytosis, leading to greater antiproliferative activity and more sustained effects compared with the free drug or unconjugated nanoparticles.

Another example of targeting moieties includes luteinizing hormone-releasing hormone (LHRH). The surfaces of healthy human cells have little LHRH receptor, while it is overexpressed on ovarian and other cancer cells [179]. Recently, an LHRH–PEG–camptothecin conjugate was developed as a targeted anticancer drug delivery system [180]. The validity of LHRH receptor targeting was evidenced by higher cytotoxicity against cancer cells using the targeted conjugate compared with the nontargeted PEG–camptothecin conjugate or the free drug in vivo.

Other active targeting systems include specific peptides to target cells and organs that are selected from a phase display method [181–182] and aptamers, which are short molecules of double-stranded DNA or single-stranded RNA that bind to specific molecular targets [183].

6.2 Endosomolysis

Drug carriers localize to acidic endosomes (pH 5.0–6.5) after internalization into cells via an endocytic process and can reach the lysosome, where they face harsh conditions, such as extreme lower pHs and enzymatic degradation. Therefore, therapeutic agents should be released from the endosomes into the cytoplasm before reaching the lysosomes to avoid degradation and inactivation. Drug carriers circumvent these challenges by facilitating drug transport into the cytoplasm, which leads to increased bioavailability in the cytosol and nucleus [184]. Several systems have been proposed, including supplementation of fusogenic peptides [185] and the use of polymers that have intrinsic abilities to escape endosomolysis [186–188]. Another approach is the use of cell-penetrating peptides (CPPs) to facilitate uptake of various molecules.

Fusogenic peptides of natural (e.g., N-terminus of hemagglutinin subunit HA-2 of influenza virus) or synthetic [e.g., WEAALAEALAEALAEHLAEA-LAEALEALAA (GALA) or WEAKLAKALAKALAKHLAKALAKALK-ACEA (KALA)] origin have been applied to the endo- and lysosomal escape of several drug delivery systems [185]. The conformational transition of peptides by pH enables them to interact with the phospholipid membranes, resulting in pore formation, membrane fusion, or lysis. As a consequence, incorporation of synthetic membrane-active peptides into delivery systems can enhance intracellular delivery of drugs. The efficiency and the cost, however, prevent the use of synthetic peptides to enhance cellular delivery of various compounds.

Endolysosomal escape has also been demonstrated by various endosomolytic polymers [186–188] using the "proton sponge hypothesis," which is based on osmotic swelling of the vesicle via buffering of the endosomal environment. Under these conditions, the endosomal membrane will rupture, leading to the release of drugs into the cytoplasm.

pH-sensitive micelles (PHSMs) that are composed of poly(L-histidine)/PEG and PLLA/PEG are strong candidates for cytoplasmic drug delivery by active intracellular translocation of the drug carriers via specific interactions combined with triggered release at endosomal pH (pH<6.5). Micelles have been conjugated with folic acid (PHSM/f) for folate receptor-mediated tumor targeting [117]. From the results of an in vitro cell experiment, DOX-loaded PHSM/f showed enhanced cytotoxicity (cell viability ~16% at DOX 10 µg/mL) at pH 7.4 after folate receptor-mediated endocytosis, while pH-insensitive micelles composed of PLLA/PEG-folate (PHIM/f) exhibited reduced cytotoxicity (cell viability ~80% at DOX 10 µg/mL) at the same pH.

Interestingly, the confocal results using DOX-loaded PHSM/f revealed the widespread presence of drug or micelles in the cytosol and nucleus in MCF-7 cells. PHSM/f is able to deliver a drug into the cytosol efficiently. On the other hand, PLLA/PEG-folate micelles targeted drugs or micelles to endosomes instead of the cytosol [117]. This difference verifies the endosomal escape of the folate-conjugated PHSM, which is underlied by two possible mechanisms. One is the proton-sponge effect of polyHis that is caused by the protonation of imidazole groups at endosomal pH, and the other is the interaction of protonated polyHis with the negatively charged phospholipid membrane.

Similarly, N-acetyl histidine-conjugated glycol chitosan was used to trigger cytoplasmic drug release [189]. Histidine was conjugated with poly(2-hydroxyethyl aspartamide) (PHEA) and octadecylamine-grafted PHEA via an ester linkage to induce pH sensitivity. The results showed endosomal destabilization by histidine and endosomal pH-triggered drug release [190]. These observations clarify the role of polyHis in antitumor activity by destabilization in drug release using the pH sensitivity of polyHis and fusogenicity.

"Cell-penetrating peptides" (CPPs) or "protein transduction domains" (PTDs) were introduced as a novel approach to deliver drug carriers into intracellular compartments. One advantage is that they are able to maintain the bioactivity of the transported drug. Among the most frequently used peptides are TAT [191], Antennapedia (Antp) [192], poly-arginine peptides [193], Tp10 [194], a variant of transportan [195], YTA2 [196], and penetratin [197]. Although the mechanism by which they internalize is unclear, the intracellular access of the drug is increased. Nevertheless, the mechanism is not determined by the cell type but by the different peptides [198]. Tat-mediated delivery uses energy for macropinocytosis for subsequent escape from the endosome into the cytoplasm, eventually for transport into the nucleus. Other CPPs penetrate cells via electrostatic interactions and hydrogen bonding [198].

The following is an example of a novel drug-targeting system for cellular internalization using TAT. The delivery system consists of two components: (1) a polymeric micelle that has a hydrophobic core of poly(L-lactic acid) (PLLA) and a hydrophilic shell of PEG conjugated to TAT (TAT micelle); (2) an ultra-pH-sensitive diblock copolymer of poly(methacryloyl sulfadimethoxine) (PSD) and PEG (PSD/PEG) [199]. The final carrier system is formulated by complexation of the anionic PSD with the cationic TAT of the micelles. The complex formulation and TAT peptide can be systemically shielded. However, TAT is exposed to slightly acidic tumor pH levels due to disassembly of the complexed micelle.

Figure 7 describes the TAT-complexed micelle. In one study, TAT micelles had particle sizes between 20 and 45 nm, and their critical micellar concentrations were 3.5 mg/L–5.5 mg/L. The complex formulation showed increased particle size at pH 8.0 compared with the particle size at pH 6.8, indicating complex formation. pH sensitivity of PSD–PEG induced this difference on mixing with TAT micelles. At low pHs (pH 6.6–6.0), the particle sizes showed bimodal distribution, one indicating normal TAT micelles (45 nm) and the other forming from the aggregation of hydrophobic PSD-*b*-PEG. Zeta potential results confirmed the shielding/deshielding process. Flow cytometry and confocal microscopy demonstrated higher uptake of TAT micelles at pH 6.6 compared with pH 7.4, explaining the shielding of TAT peptides at physiological pH due to complexation of the micelle and deshielding at tumoral pH due to disassembly. Interestingly, flow cytometry demonstrated that TAT peptide was detected on the surface of the nucleus, indicating that the TAT peptide facilitates micelle transport to near the nucleus. These results indicate that TAT-containing drug-loaded micelles target hydrophobic drugs to the nucleus.

7 Multidrug Resistance

The resistance of tumor cells to multiple structurally unrelated chemotherapeutic drugs has been termed as multidrug resistance (MDR) [200]. Clinical resistance of certain tumors to cytotoxic agents has been observed in early

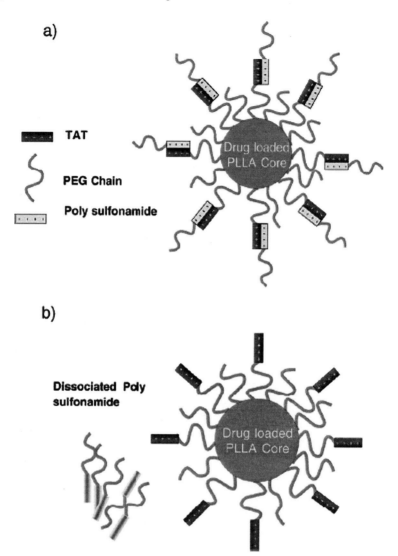

Fig. 7 Schematic model for the proposed drug delivery system consists of two components, a PLLA-*b*-PEG micelle conjugated to TAT and a pH-sensitive diblock polymer PSD-*b*-PEG. (**a**) At normal blood pH, the sulfonamide is negatively charged, and when mixed with the TAT micelle, it shields the TAT by electrostatic interaction. Only PEG is exposed to the outside, which could make the carrier long circulating; (**b**) when the system experiences a decrease in pH (near tumor), sulfonamide loses charge and detaches, thus exposing TAT for interaction with tumor cells (adapted from Ref. [199] with permission)

chemotherapy or after exposure to drugs. The degree of resistance depends on the type of tumor and the history of chemotherapy [201].

In the past, various mechanisms of MDR, as described in Fig. 8, have been studied, such as the expression of multidrug efflux pumps (P-glycoprotein (Pgp)

Fig. 8 Clinical settings of
MDR mechanisms:
enhanced drug transport
(Pgp, MRP, LRP, BCRP),
reduced or altered drug
target (Topo II), exocytosis,
and resistance to
programmed cell death

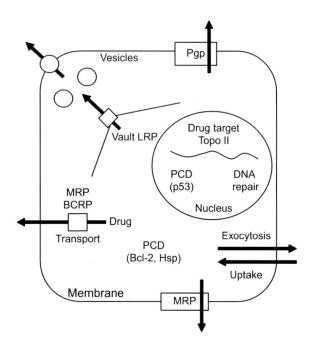

or multidrug resistance-associated proteins) [202–204], altered glutathione metabolism [205], reduced activity of topoisomerase II [206], and various changes in cellular proteins and mechanisms [207–209]. These MDR mechanisms recognize antitumor drugs and decrease intracellular drug concentration.

In addition, acidic intracellular organelles, endosomes, and lysosomes also participate in resistance to chemotherapeutic drugs [210]. Because most antitumor drugs are in an ionizable form, weakly basic drugs accumulate to a greater extent in an acidic phase (such as endosomes and lysosomes). An ionized drug is quarantined due to the impermeability of an ionized drug through cellular or subcellular membranes. Drug extrusion into the external medium (exocytosis) after drug sequestration is another mechanism of MDR for weakly acidic drugs [211, 212]. A combination of an efflux pump, drug sequestration that is induced by a pH gradient, and exocytosis are the most influential factors in MDR. The combination of several mechanisms of drug resistance makes chemotherapy difficult. The development of novel drugs and drug formulations that are effective against drug-resistant cancers is necessary.

After identifying Pgp as a major cause of MDR in in vitro cell studies and discovering that verapamil (a blocker) modulates Pgp activity, researchers have devoted a tremendous effort to discovering other Pgp modulators (inhibitors) that have high binding affinity to Pgp without other biological activities and also have minimal pharmacokinetic interactions with anticancer drugs [213].

Numerous pharmaceutical companies have created Pgp modulators by modifying existing drugs such as verapamil, cyclosporine A, glibenclamide, and others from certain related chemical structures. These research efforts are in various phase I, II, and III clinical studies [214]. No single chemical structure has proven to be effective in phase III studies to date.

As mentioned previously, Pgp plays a critical role in experimental MDR, and Pgp modulators block Pgp. MDR in clinical settings is multifaceted, and Pgp inhibition does not seem to be as effective as anticipated [215]. In addition, tumor-specific Pgp modulators have not been reported as yet. Thus, Pgp modulators interact with Pgp in healthy organs, such as placenta, kidney, blood–brain barrier (BBB), liver, and kidney. PK interactions (particularly slow elimination kinetics) seem intrinsic, resulting in greater toxic effects of an anticancer drug.

Simply modulating Pgp appears to be an extreme challenge in overcoming MDR in a clinical setting. As an alternative to Pgp modulators alone, various nanosized drug carriers have been tested to circumvent MDR in vitro and in vivo. Carriers include liposomes [216], alkylcyanoacrylate [217], nanoparticles [218], polymeric micelles of Pluronics [219] and other amphiphilic block copolymers [220], and PLGA nanoparticles [221].

Pluronic formulations below their CMC with anticancer drugs have been effective in treating MDR tumors [222], whereby these positive results are linked to the functions of Pluronic (PEO/PPO/PEO) block copolymers in crossing the plasma membrane, suppressing ATP production, and to gene modulation. The formulation seems to be effective with MDR tumors but less so with sensitive tumors. This approach lacks tumor specificity, and little is known about its influence on normal cells that express Pgp. On the other hand, Pluronic micelles under ultrasound stimulation have been effective in treating MDR cells [219].

Some nanovehicles carry the drug alone and contain a targeting moiety, while some carry both an anticancer drug and a Pgp modulator [220]. Delivering agents that can silence the *Pgp* genes, such as siRNA and ODN, which are often carried together with an anticancer drug, have also been examined [223]. Many of these approaches have demonstrated a potential to overcome MDR under certain experimental conditions. However, they primarily target a single mechanism of MDR, and no approach has been proven to be effective in clinical MDR tumor treatments.

With regard to MDR mechanisms that are linked to microenvironments that allow poor access to drugs, soluble factors, and cell–cell contacts, Au's group tested a bFGF inhibitor [224] and a method of priming anticancer drugs prior to drug treatment carried by nanosized PLGA particles. This induced partial apoptosis [225] and reduction in tumor tissue size [226]. Improved nanoparticle distribution and MDR reduction were achieved. This approach seems to be promising, although only local administration was used [224–226].

Endosomal pH-sensitive micelles can be internalized into cancer cells that overexpress FR by folate receptor (FR)-mediated endocytosis, such as in

ovarian and breast tumors. After endocytosis of micelles, simultaneously triggered release in early endosomes (~pH 6) and endosomal disruption for drug
escape provide high concentrations of the drug in the cytosol and nucleus
(potential drug-acting sites) and provide effective anticancer drug delivery,
particularly for MDR cells.

This approach has been tested by Bae's group [227] using micelles that are a
mixed micellar system that consists of poly(histidine-*co*-phenylalanine)/PEG
and PLLA/PEG-folate. They do not distinguish between sensitive and MDR

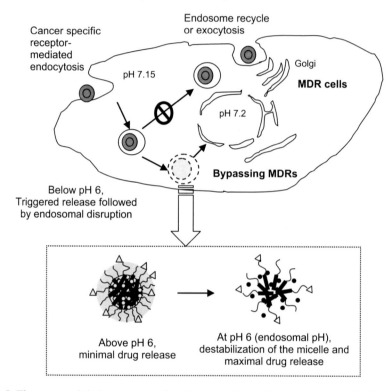

Fig. 9 The proposed design concept of endosomal pH-sensitive micelles for effective anticancer drug delivery to MDR cells with receptor-mediated endocytosis, switching release rate
and endosomal escape activity of polymeric micelle components

cells that use various MDR mechanisms, as shown in cytotoxicity tests in vitro.
In addition, ovarian cancer MDR xenografts in mice were effectively treated
and showed lower toxicity than the control groups that received free DOX
treatment or pH-insensitive micelles/DOX treatment. The scheme of these
endosomal pH-sensitive micelles is described in Fig. 9.

This unique cancer nanotechnology, based on pH-sensitive micelles, boasts
four important features for chemotherapy treatment: (1) it is equally cytotoxic
to wild-type and MDR cancer cells; (2) it is cytotoxic to MDR cells, regardless
of unicellular MDR mechanisms; (3) it is effective in in vivo models; and (4) it

causes no apparent polymer cytotoxicity and systemic toxicity in mice. Significant progress in chemotherapy is anticipated by this novel cancer nano-technology using clear mechanisms in treating MDR tumors.

This application targets MDR breast and ovarian cancers because of their high expression levels of FR. The technology can be expanded to most tumors by tailoring anticancer drugs and molecular tools for active internalization into cancer cells, potentially becoming a general platform for cancer chemotherapy.

8 Challenges

Most studies in this area have highlighted "cell specificity" by discussing short-range interactions between pairs of antigen–mAb, ligand–receptor, aptamer–counterpart, and phase display peptide–counterpart. Specific interactions imply "target cell-unique expression" or "overexpression" when compared with other organs and cells. Quantitative analyses of such specific interactions, however, have been under-reported for active endocytosis in clinical settings. There are issues in these regards, including the fraction of tumor cells from patients that express a specific antigen or receptor, the expression level in each individual cell, the binding affinity between a carrier and a target cell for effective internalization, and the rates of endocytosis and exocytosis.

Tumor cells are known for their diversity with regard to cell type, genomics, and proteomics [228]. They are in a dynamic developmental state. Accumulating evidence supports the side population of stem-like cells from cancer cells. They are recognized by different surface markers from the bulk of cancer cells, although cancer stem cells are quiescent under normal conditions. It has been known that the stem-like cells are the underlying cause of MDR and are primarily responsible for metastasis and recurrence. Considering these factors, the extent and the interaction of specific antigens or receptors in active endocytosis of active targeting approaches may be the primary keys in removing tumors and cancer stem cells.

In breast cancer patients, less than 30% is diagnosed positive for the Her-2/*neu* antigen. Immunostaining can indicate the extent of antigen expression. "Positive" is determined by the staining level above a standard (but never 100%) and does not guarantee Herceptin therapy [229]. Recently, the use of Her-2 targeting has been investigated. The investigation of folate receptor expression by immunoas-say on clinical breast tumors has also been challenging [230]. This obstacle has raised the issue of whether results from in vitro or in vivo animal studies using active targeting approaches can be used in clinical settings. Despite various past and current studies, these challenges remain unsolved.

One of the most commonly used terms to explain drug targeting is the EPR effect. The porosity and pore size of tumor blood vessels has been amenable to nanocarriers for tumor-targeting therapy, imaging, and diagnosis. The porosity facilitates the supply of adequate nutrients to the developing area in tumors. When tumor growth is inhibited or when the tumor size is decreased by any therapy, however, does the porosity keep its conformational structure and allow continuous EPR effects with nanocarriers? We hypothesize that the conformational structure of the blood vessel shifts from a wide pore size to a narrow pore size for a normal supply [100]. In this case, what will be the role of nanocarriers?

9 Conclusion

Polymeric anticancer drug carriers are versatile drug delivery systems that have tremendous potential for treatment of cancers in humans. Studies to date offer a variety of polymeric carriers that facilitate proper design of highly efficient anticancer drugs. Incorporation of hydrophobic anticancer drugs leads to increased solubility in an aqueous environment. Polymeric carriers also enable delivery of more drugs to cancer sites by extending circulation through steric stabilization, EPR effects from leaky tumor blood vessels, active internalization, and efficient cytoplasmic drug delivery from environment-responsive properties. Using these advantages, drug efficacy to tumors can be increased, and the side effects on normal cells can be decreased by limiting biodistribution. MDR, one of the major challenges in tumor chemotherapy, may be addressed by carrier design.

The heterogeneity of tumor cells and tumor physiology, metastasis of tumor, and cancer stem-like cells restricts research on polymeric carriers. These hurdles still remain as challenges for the development of multifunctional and custom-made polymeric carriers. Nonetheless, the combined findings from polymer chemistry and tumor biology provide researchers with the potential tools to overcome such barriers in the future.

References

1. Peer D, Karp JM, Hong S, Farokhzad OC, Margalit R, Langer R. Nanocarriers as an emerging platform for cancer therapy. *Nat Nanotechnol* 2007; **2**: 751–760.
2. Allen TM, Cullis PR. Drug delivery systems: Entering the mainstream. *Science* 2004; **303**: 1818–1822.
3. Minko T. Soluble polymer conjugates for drug delivery. *Drug Discov Today* 2005; **2**: 15–20.
4. Gillies ER, Frechet JMJ. Dendrimers and dendritic polymers in drug delivery. *Drug Discov Today* 2005; **10**: 35–43.
5. Soppimath KS, Aminabhavi TM, Kulkarni AR, Rudzinski WE. Biodegradable polymeric nanoparticles as drug delivery devices. *J Control Release* 2001; **70**: 1–20.
6. Kataoka K, Harada A, Nagasaki Y. Block copolymer micelles for drug delivery: Design, characterization and biological significance. *Adv Drug Deliver Rev* 2001; **47**: 113–131.
7. Lee ES, Gao Z, Bae YH. Recent progress in tumor pH targeting nanotechnology. *J Control Release* 2008, doi:10.1016/j.jconrel.2008.05.003
8. Levine DH, Ghoroghchian PP, Freudenberg J, Zhang G, Therien MJ, Greene MI, Hammer DA, Murali R. Polymersomes: A new multi-functional tool for cancer diagnosis and therapy. *Methods* 2008, doi:10.1016/j.ymeth.2008.05.006

9. Khandare J, Minko T. Polymer – drug conjugates: Progress in polymeric prodrugs. *Prog Polym Sci* 2006; **31**: 359–397.
10. Duncan R. The dawning era of polymer therapeutics. *Nat Rev Drug Discov* 2003; **2**: 347–360.
11. Duncan R, Vicent MJ, Greco F, Nicholson RI. Polymer–drug conjugates: Towards a novel approach for the treatment of endrocine-related cancer. *Endocr-Relat Cancer* 2005; **12**: S189–S199.
12. Malik N, Evagorou EG, Duncan R. Dendrimer–platinate: A novel approach to cancer chemotherapy. *Anti-Cancer Drugs* 1999; **10**: 767–776.
13. Zhuo RX, Du B, Lu ZR. *In vitro* release of 5-fluorouracil with cyclic core dendritic polymer. *J Control Release* 1999; **57**: 249–257.
14. Bader H, Ringsdorf H, Schmidt B. Water soluble polymers in medicine. *Angew Makromol Chem* 1984; **123/124**: 457–485.
15. Jones MC, Leroux JC. Polymeric micelles – a new generation of colloidal drug carriers. *Eur J Pharm Biopharm* 1999; **48**:101–111.
16. Kataoka K, Kwon GS, Yokoyama M, Okano T, Sakurai Y. Block copolymer micelles as vehicles for drug delivery. *J Control Release* 1993; **24**:119–132.
17. Yokoyama M, Okano T, Sakurai Y, Ekimoto H, Shibazaki C, Kataoka K. Toxicity and antitumor activity against solid tumors of micelle forming polymeric anticancer drug and its extremely long circulation in blood. *Cancer Res* 1991; **51**: 3229–3236.
18. Yokoyama M, Miyauchi M, Yamada N, Okano T, Sakurai Y, Kataoka K, Inoue S. Polymer micelles as novel drug carrier: Adriamycin conjugated poly(ethylene glycol)-poly(aspartic acid) block copolymer. *J Control Release* 1990; **11**: 269–278.
19. Matsumura Y. Poly (amino acid) micelle nanocarriers in preclinical and clinical studies. *Adv Drug Deliver Rev* 2008; **60**: 899–914.
20. Peppas LB. Recent advances on the use of biodegradable microparticles and nanoparticles in the controlled drug delivery. *Int J Pharm* 1995; **116**: 1–9.
21. Zimmer A, Kreuter J. Microspheres and nanoparticles used in ocular drug delivery systems. *Adv Drug Deliver Rev* 1995; **16**: 61–73.
22. Uhrich KE, Cannizzaro SM, Langer RS, Shakessheff KM. Polymeric systems for controlled drug release. *Chem Rev* 1999; **99**: 3181–3198.
23. Vinogradov SV, Bronich TK, Kabanov AV. Nanosized cationic hydrogels for drug delivery: Preparation, properties and interactions with cells. *Adv Drug Deliver Rev* 2002; **54**: 135–147.
24. Vinogradov SV, Zeman AD, Batrakova EV, Kabanov AV. Polyplex Nanogel formulations for drug delivery of cytotoxic nucleoside analogs. *J Control Release* 2005; **107**: 143–157.
25. Lee ES, Kim D, Youn YS, Oh KT, Bae YH. A novel virus-mimetic nanogel vehicle. *Angew Chem Int Edit* 2008; **47**: 2418–2421.
26. Dischera DE, Ortiz V, Srinivas G, Klein ML, Kim Y, Christian D, Photos SCP, Ahmed F. Emerging applications of polymersomes in delivery: From molecular dynamics to shrinkage of tumors. *Prog Polym Sci* 2007; **32**: 838–857.
27. Discher BM, Won YY, Ege DS, Lee JCM, Bates FS, Discher DE, Hammer DA. Polymersomes: Tough vesicles made from diblock copolymers. *Science* 1999; **284**: 1143–1146.
28. Lee JCM, Bermu-dez H, Discher BM, Sheehan MA, Won YY, Bates FS, Discher DE. Preparation, stability, and in vitro performance of vesicles made with diblock copolymers. *Biotechnol Bioeng* 2001; **73**: 135–145.
29. Meng F, Engbers GHM, Feijen J. Biodegradable polymersomes as a basis for artificial cells: encapsulation, release and targeting. *J Control Release* 2005; **101**: 187–198.
30. Bermu-dez H, Brannan AK, Hammer DA, Bates FS, Discher DE. Molecular weight dependence of polymersome membrane structure, elasticity, and stability. *Macromolecules* 2002; **35**: 8203–8208.
31. Photos PJ, Bacakova L, Discher B, Bates FS, Discher DE. Polymer vesicles in vivo: correlations with PEG molecular weight. *J Control Release* 2003; **90**: 323–334.

32. Ghoroghchian PP, Frail PR, Su-sumu K, Blessington D, Brannan AK, Bates FS, Chance B, Hammer DA, Therien MJ. Near-infrared-emissive polymersomes: Self-assembled soft matter for *in vivo* optical imaging. *P Natl Acad Sci USA* 2005; **102**: 2922–2927.
33. Antonietti M, Forster S. Vesicles and liposomes: A self-assembly principle beyond lipids. *Adv Mater* 2003; **15**: 1323–1333.
34. Zu-pancich JA, Bates FS, Hillmyer MA. Design and synthesis of a low band gap conjugated macroinitiator: Toward rod-coil donor-acceptor block copolymers *Macromolecules* 2006; **39**: 4286–4288.
35. Hillmyer MA, Bates FS. Synthesis and characterization of model polyalkane–poly(ethylene oxide) block copolymers. *Macromolecules* 1996; **29**: 6994–7002.
36. Discher DE, Ahmed F. POLYMERSOMES. *Annu Rev Biomed Eng* 2006; **8**: 323–341.
37. Garvin KL, Miyano JA, Robinson D, Giger D, Novak J, Radio S. Polylactide/polyglycolide antibiotic implants in the treatment of osteomyelitis. A canine model. *J Bone Joint Surg Am* 1994; **76**: 1500–1506.
38. Lesser GJ, Grossman SA, Leong KW, Lo HN, Eller S. *In vitro* and *in vivo* studies of subcutaneous hydromorphone implants designed for the treatment of cancer pain. *Pain* 1996; **65**: 265–272.
39. Suhonen SP, Allonen HO, Lahteenmaki P. Gynecology: Sustained-release estradiol implants and a levonorgestrel-releasing intrauterine device in hormone replacement therapy. *Am J Obstet Gynecol* 1995; **172**: 562–567.
40. Fujita T, Tamura T, Yamada H, Yamamoto A, Muranishi S. Pharmacokinetics of mitomycin C (MMC) after intraperitoneal administration of MMC-gelatin gel and its anti-tumor effects against sarcoma-180 bearing mice. *J Drug Target* 1997; **4**: 289–296.
41. Bernatchez SF, Merkli A, Tabatabay C, Gurny R, Zhao QH, Anderson JM. Biotolerance of a semisolid hydrophobic biodegradable poly(ortho ester) for controlled drug delivery. *J Biomed Mater Res* 1993; **27**: 677–681.
42. Chen J, Jo S, Park K. Polysaccharide hydrogels for protein drug delivery. *Carbohyd Polym* 1995; **28**: 69–76.
43. Seymour LW, Duncan R, Duffy J, Ng SY, Heller J. Poly(ortho ester) matrices for controlled-release of the antitumor agent 5-fluorouracil. *J Control Release* 1994; **31**: 201–206.
44. Imasaka K, Yoshida M, Fukuzaki H, Asano M, Kumakura M, Mashimo T. New biodegradable polymers of L-lactic acid and aromatic hydroxy-acids and their applications in drug delivery systems. *Int J Pharm* 1992; **81**: 31–38.
45. Cha Y, Choi YK, Bae YH. 1997. Thermosensitive biodegradable polymers based on poly(ether-ester) block copolymers. US Patent 5 702-717.
46. Jeong B, Bae YH, Lee DS, Kim SW. Biodegradable block copolymers as injectable drug delivery system. *Nature* 1997; **388**: 860–862.
47. Rathi R, Zentner GM, Jeong B. 2000. Biodegradable low molecular weight triblock poly(lactide-co-glycolide) polyethylene glycol copolymers having reverse thermal gelation properties. US Patent 6 117 949.
48. Jeong B, Choi YK, Bae YH, Zentner G, Kim SW. New biodegradable polymers for injectable drug delivery systems. *J Control Release* 1999; **62**: 109–114.
49. Qiao M, Chen D, Ma X, Liu Y. Injectable biodegradable temperature-responsive PLGA–PEG–PLGA copolymers: Synthesis and effect of copolymer composition on the drug release from the copolymer-based hydrogels. *Int J Pharm* 2005; **294**: 103–112.
50. Lukyanov AN, Torchilin VP. Micelles from lipid derivatives of water-soluble polymers as delivery systems for poorly soluble drugs. *Adv Drug Deliver Rev* 2004; **56**: 1273–1289.
51. Yokogawa K, Nakashima E, Ishizaki J, Maeda H, Nagano T, Ichimura F. Relationships in the structure – tissue distribution of basic drugs in the rabbit, *Pharm Res* 1990; **7**: 691–696.
52. Hageluken A, Grunbaum L, Nurnberg B, Harhammer R, Schunack W, Seifert R. Lipophilic beta-adrenoceptor antagonists and local anesthetics are effective direct activators of G-proteins. *Biochem Pharmacol* 1994; **47**: 1789–1795.

53. Lipinski CA, Lombardo F, Dominy BW, Feeney PJ. Experimental and computational approaches to estimate solubility and permeability in drug discovery and development settings. *Adv Drug Deliver Rev* 2001; **46**: 3–26.
54. Torchilin VP. Targeted polymeric micelles for delivery of poorly soluble drugs. *Cell Mol Life Sci* 2004; **61**: 2549–2559.
55. Thompson D, Chaubal MV. Cyclodextrins (CDS)-excipients by definition, drug delivery systems by function (part I: injectable applications), *Drug Deliver Technol* 2000; **2**: 34–38.
56. Ansel HC, Allen LV, Popovich NG. *Pharmaceutical Dosage Forms and Drug Delivery Systems*. Kluwer, Philadelphia, Baltimore, New York, London, 1999.
57. Ray R, Kibbe AH, Rowe R, Shleskey P, Weller P. *Handbook of Pharmaceutical Excipients*, APhA Publications, Washington, 2003.
58. Mu L, Feng SS. A novel controlled release formulation for the anticancer drug paclitaxel (Taxol[R]): PLGA nanoparticles containing vitamin E TPGS. *J Control Release* 2003; **86**: 33–48.
59. Zhang X, Burt HM. Diblock copolymers of poly(dl-lactide-block-methoxy polyethylene glycol) as micellar carriers of taxol. *Pharm Res* 1995; **12**: S-265.
60. Swindell CS, Krauss NE. Biologically active taxol analogues with deleted A-ring side chain substituents and variable C-2' configurations. *J Med Chem* 1991; **34**: 1176–1184.
61. Khandare JJ, Jayant S, Singh A, Chandna P, Wang Y, Vorsa N, Minko T. Dendrimer versus linear conjugate: Influence of polymeric architecture on the delivery and anticancer effect of paclitaxel. *Bioconjugate Chem* 2006; **17**: 1464–1472.
62. Klibanov AL, Maruyama K, Torchilin VP, Huang L. Amphipathic polyethyleneglycols effectively prolong the circulation time of liposomes. *FEBS Lett* 1990; **268**: 235–238.
63. Senior J, Delgado C, Fisher D, Tilcock C, Gregoriadis G. Influence of surface hydrophilicity of liposomes on their interaction with plasma protein and clearance from the circulation: studies with poly(ethylene glycol)-coated vesicles. *Biochim Biophys Acta* 1991; **1062**: 77–82.
64. Allen TM, Hansen C, Martin F, Redemann C, Young YA. Liposomes containing synthetic lipid derivatives of poly (ethylene glycol) show prolonged circulation half-lives in vivo. *Biochim Biophys Acta* 1991; **1066**: 29–36.
65. Naper DH. *Polymeric Stabilization of Colloidal Dispersions*. Academic Press, New York, 1983.
66. Chonn A, Semple SC, Cullis PR. Association of blood proteins with large unilamellar liposomes in vivo: relation to circulation lifetimes. *J Biol Chem* 1992; **267**: 18759–18765.
67. Senior JH. Fate and behavior of liposomes in vivo: a review of controlling factors. *Crit Rev Ther Drug* 1987; **3**: 123–193.
68. Needham D, McIntosh TJ, Lasic DD. Repulsive interactions and mechanical stability of polymer-grafted lipid membranes. *Biochim Biophys Acta* 1992; **1108**: 40–48.
69. Torchilin VP, Omelyanenko VG, Papisov MI, Bogdanov Jr AA, Trubetskoy VS, Herron JN, Gentry CA. Poly(ethylene glycol) on the liposome surface: On the mechanism of polymer-coated liposome longevity. *Biochim Biophys Acta* 1994; **1195**: 11–20.
70. Zalipsky S. Chemistry of polyethylene glycol conjugates with biologically active molecules. *Adv Drug Deliver Rev* 1995; **16**: 157–182.
71. Powell GM. Polyethylene glycol. In: RL Davidson (Ed.), *Handbook of Water Soluble Gums and Resins*. McGraw-Hill, New York, 1980.
72. Yamaoka T, Tabata T, Ikada Y. Distribution and tissue uptake of poly(ethylene glycol) with different molecular weights after intravenous administration to mice. *J Pharm Sci* 1994; **83**: 601–606.
73. Torchilin VP. Multifunctional nanocarriers. *Adv Drug Deliver Rev* 2006; **58**: 1532–1555.
74. Veronese FM. Peptide and protein PEGylation: A review of problems and solutions. *Biomaterials* 2001; **22**: 405–417.
75. Torchilin VP, Trubetskoy VS. Which polymers can make nanoparticulate drug carriers long-circulating? *Adv Drug Deliver Rev* 1995; **16**: 141–155.

76. Torchilin VP, Levchenko TS, Whiteman KR, Yaroslavov AA, Tsatsakis AM, Rizos AK, Michailova EV, Shtilman MI. Amphiphilic poly-N-vinylpyrrolidones: Synthesis, properties and liposome surface modification. *Biomaterials* 2001; **22**: 3035–3044.
77. Monfardini C, Schiavon O, Caliceti P, Morpurgo M, Harris JM, Veronese FM. A branched monomethoxypoly(ethylene glycol) for protein modification, *Bioconjugate Chem* 1995; **6**: 62–69.
78. Woodle MC, Engbers CM, Zalipsky S. New amphipathic polymer-lipid conjugates forming long-circulating reticuloendothelial system-evading liposomes, *Bioconjugate Chem* 1994; **5**: 493–496.
79. Maruyama K, Okuizumi S, Ishida O, Yamauchi H, Kikuchi H, Iwatsuru M. Phosphatidyl polyglycerols prolong liposome circulation in vivo. *Int J Pharm* 1994; **111**: 103–107.
80. Takeuchi H, Kojima H, Toyoda T, Yamamoto H, Hino T, Kawashima Y. Prolonged circulation time of doxorubicin loaded liposomes coated with a modified polyvinyl alcohol after intravenous injection in rats. *Eur J Pharm Biopharm* 1999; **48**: 123–129.
81. Yesair DW, Schwartzbach E, Shuck D, Denine EP, Asbell MA. Comparative pharmacokinetics of daunomycin and Adriamycin in several animal species. *Cancer Res* 1972; **32**: 1177–1183.
82. Formelli F, C'arsana R, Pollini C. Pharmacokinetics of 4'-deoxy-4'-iodo-doxorubicin in plasma and tissues of tumor-bearing mice compared with doxorubicin. *Cancer Res* 1987; **47**: 5401–5406.
83. Cummings J, Merry S, Willmott N. Disposition kinetics of adriamycin, adriamycinol and their 7-deoxyglycones in AKR mice bearing a subcutaneously growing ridgway osteogenic sarcoma (ROS). *Eur J Cancer Clin Oncol* 1986; **22**: 451–460.
84. Yokoyama M, Okaiio T, Sakurai Y, Ekimoto H, Shibazaki C, Kataoka K. Toxicity and antitumor activity against solid tumors of micelle-forming polymeric anticancer drug and its extremely long circulation in blood, *Cancer Res* 1991; **51**: 3229–3236.
85. Gabizon A, Shmeeda H, Barenholz Y. Pharmacokinetics of pegylated liposomal doxorubicin: Review of animal and human studies. *Clin Pharmacokinet* 2003; **42**: 419–436.
86. Vasey PA, Kaye SB, Morrison R, Twelves C, Wilson P, Duncan R, Thomson AH, Murray LS, Hilditch TE, Murray T, Burtles S, Fraier D, Frigerio E, Cassidy J. Phase I clinical and pharmacokinetic study of PK1 [N-(2-Hydroxypropyl)methacrylamide copolymer Doxorubicin]:First member of a new class of chemotherapeutic agents – drug-polymer conjugates, *Clin Cancer Res* 1999; **5**: 83–94.
87. Kintzel PE. Anticancer drug-induced kidney disorders: Incidence, prevention and management. *Drug Safety* 2001; **24**: 19–38.
88. Viale MA, Minetti SB, Ottone MA. Preclinical in vitro evaluation of hematotoxicity of the cisplatin-procaine complex DPR. *Anticancer Drugs* 2003; **14**: 163–166.
89. Pai VB, Nahata MC. Cardiotoxicity of chemotherapeutic agents: Incidence, treatment and prevention. *Drug Safety* 2000; **22**: 263–302.
90. Cummings BS, Lash LH. Metabolism and toxicity of trichloroethylene and S-(1,2-dichlorovinyl)-L-cysteine in freshly isolated human proximal tubular cells. *Toxicol Sci* 2000; **53**: 458–466.
91. Dvorak Z, Kosina P, Walterova D, Simanek V, Bachleda P, Ulrichova J. Primary cultures of human hepatocytes as a tool in cytotoxicity studies: Cell protection against model toxins by flavonolignans obtained from *Silybum marianum*. *Toxicol Lett* 2003; **137**: 201–212.
92. David ME, Berndt WO. Renal methods for toxicology. In: Wallace Hayes, A. (Ed.), *Principles and Methods of Toxicology*, 4th ed. Taylor and Francis Publisher, Philadelphia, 2001.
93. Li C, Wallace S. Polymer-drug conjugates: Recent development in clinical oncology. *Adv Drug Deliver Rev* 2008; **60**: 886–898.
94. Loehrer PJ, Einhom LH. Cisplatin. *Ann Intern Med* 1984; **100**: 704–713.
95. Lieberthal W, Triaca V, Levine J. Mechanisms of death induced by cisplatin in proximal tubular epithelial cells: Apoptosis vs. necrosis. *Am J Physiol* 1996; **240**: F700–F708.

96. Mizumura Y, Matsumura Y, Hamaguchi T, Nishiyama N, Kataoka K, Kawaguchi T, Hrushesky WJM, Moriyasu F, Kakizoe T. Cisplatin-incorporated polymeric micelles eliminate nephrotoxicity, while maintaining antitumor activity. *Jpn J Cancer Res* 2001; **92**: 328–336.

97. Nishiyama N, Okazaki S, Cabral H, Miyamoto M, Kato Y, Sugiyama Y, Nishio K, Matsumura Y, Kataoka K. Novel cisplatin-incorporated polymeric micelles can eradicate solid tumors in mice. *Cancer Res* 2003; **63**: 8977–8983.

98. Matsumura Y, Maeda HA. A new concept for macromolecular therapeutics in cancer chemotherapy: Mechanism of tumoritropic accumulation of proteins and the antitumor agent smancs. *Cancer Res* 1986; **46**: 6387–6392.

99. Maeda HA. The enhanced permeability and retention (EPR) effect in tumor vasculature: the key role of tumor-selective macromolecular drug targeting. *Adv Enzyme Regul* 2001; **41**: 189–207.

100. Hobbs SK, Monsky WL, Yuan F, Roberts WG, Griffith L, Torchilin VP. Regulation of transport pathways in tumor vessels: role of tumor type and microenvironment. *P Natl Acad Sci USA* 1998; **95**: 4607–4612.

101. Hashizume H, Baluk P, Morikawa S, McLean JW, Thurston G, Roberge S. Openings between defective endothelial cells explain tumor vessel leakiness. *Am J Pathol* 2000; **156**: 1363–1380.

102. Moghimi SM, Hunter AC, Murray JC. Nanomedicine: Current status and future prospects. *FASEB J* 2005; **19**: 311–330.

103. Park JH, Kwon S, Lee M, Chung H, Kim JH, Kim YS. Self-assembled nanoparticles based on glycol chitosan bearing hydrophobic moieties as carriers for doxorubicin: In vivo biodistribution and anti-tumor activity. *Biomaterials* 2006; **27**: 119–126.

104. Vega-Villa KR, Takemoto JK, Yáñez JA, Remsberg CM, Forrest ML, Davies NM. Clinical toxicities of nanocarrier systems. *Adv Drug Deliver Rev* 2008; **60**: 929–938.

105. Peppas LB, Blanchette JO. Nanoparticle and targeted systems for cancer therapy. *Adv Drug Deliver Rev* 2004; **56**: 1649–1659.

106. Avgoustakisa K, Beletsia A, Panagia Z, Klepetsanisa P, Karydasb AG, Ithakissios DS. PLGA–mPEG nanoparticles of cisplatin: in vitro nanoparticle degradation, in vitro drug release and in vivo drug residence in blood properties. *J Control Release* 2002; **79**: 123–135.

107. Fenga SS, Chien S. Chemotherapeutic engineering: Application and further development of chemical engineering principles for chemotherapy of cancer and other diseases. *Chem Eng Sci* 2003; **58**: 4087–4114.

108. Fang JY, Chen JP, Leu YL, Hu JW. Temperature-sensitive hydrogels composed of chitosan and hyaluronic acid as injectable carriers for drug delivery. *Eur J Pharm Biopharm* 2008; **68**: 626–636.

109. Ulbrich K, Subr V. Polymeric anticancer drugs with pH-controlled activation. *Adv Drug Deliver Rev* 2004; **56**: 1023–1050.

110. Engin K, Leeper DB, Cater JR, Thistlethwaite AJ, Tupchong L, McFarlane JD. Extracellular pH distribution in human tumours. *Int J Hyperther* 1995; **11**: 211–216.

111. Volk T, Jahde E, Fortmeyer HP, Glusenkamp KH, Rajewsky MR. pH in human tumour xenografts: effect of intravenous administration of glucose. *Brit J Cancer* 1993; **68**: 492–500.

112. Tannockand IF, Rotin D. Acid pH in tumors and its potential for therapeutic exploitation. *Cancer Res* 1989; **49**: 4373–4384.

113. Yamagata M, Hasuda K, Stamato T, Tannock IF. The contribution of lactic acid to acidification of tumours: studies of variant cells lacking lactate dehydrogenase. *Brit J Cancer* 1998; **77**: 1726–1731.

114. Bae Y, Jang WD, Nishiyama N, Fukushima S, Kataoka K. Multifunctional polymeric micelles with folate-mediated cancer cell targeting and pH-triggered drug releasing properties for active intracellular drug delivery. *Mol Biosyst* 2005; **1**: 242–250.

115. Bae Y, Nishiyama N, Fukushima S, Koyama H, Yasuhiro M, Kataoka K. Preparation and biological characterization of polymeric micelle drug carriers with intracellular pH-triggered drug release property: Tumor permeability, controlled subcellular drug distribution, and enhanced in vivo antitumor efficacy. *Bioconjugate Chem* 2005; **16**: 122–130.

116. Nori A, Kopecek J. Intracellular targeting of polymer-bound drugs for cancer chemotherapy. *Adv Drug Deliver Rev* 2005; **57**: 609–636.

117. Lee ES, Na K, Bae YH. Polymeric micelle for tumor pH and folate-mediated targeting. *J Control Release* 2003; **91**: 103–113.

118. Lee ES, Shin HJ, Na K, Bae YH. Poly(L-histidine)–PEG block copolymer micelles and pH-induced destabilization. *J Control Release* 2003; **90**: 363–374.

119. Gerasimov OV, Boomer JA, Qualls MM, Thompson DH. Cytosolic drug delivery using pH- and light-sensitive liposomes. *Adv Drug Deliver Rev* 1999; **38**: 317–338.

120. Lee ES, Na K, Bae YH. Doxorubicin loaded pH-sensitive polymeric micelles for reversal of resistant MCF-7 tumor. *J Control Release* 2005; **103**: 405–418.

121. Gillies ER, Goodwin AP, Frechet JM. Acetals as pH-sensitive linkages for drug delivery. *Bioconjugate Chem* 2004; **15**: 1254–1263.

122. Bae Y, Fukushima S, Harada A, Kataoka K. Design of environment-sensitive supramolecular assemblies for intracellular drug delivery: Polymeric micelles that are responsive to intracellular pH change. *Angew Chem Int Ed Engl* 2003; **42**: 4640–4643.

123. Licciardi M, Giammona G, Du J, Armes SP, Tang Y, Lewis AL. New folate-functionalized biocompatible block copolymer micelles as potential anti-cancer drug delivery systems. *Polymer* 2006; **47**: 2946–2955.

124. Cammas S, Suzuki K, Sone C, Sakurai Y, Kataoka K, Okano T. Thermo-responsive polymer nanoparticles with a core-shell micelle structure as site-specific drug carriers. *J Control Release* 1997; **48**: 157–164.

125. Chung JE, Yokoyama M, Okano T. Inner core segment design for drug delivery control of thermo-responsive polymeric micelles. *J Control Release* 2000; **65**: 93–103.

126. Chung JE, Yokoyama M, Aoyagi T, Sakurai Y, Okano T. Effect of molecular architecture of hydrophobically modified poly(*N*-isopropylacrylamide) on the formation of thermoresponsive core-shell micellar drug carriers. *J Control Release* 1998; **53**: 119–130.

127. Chung JE, Yokoyama M, Yamato M, Aoyagi T, Sakurai Y, Okano T. Thermo-responsive drug delivery from polymeric micelles constructed using block copolymers of poly(*N*-isopropylacrylamide) and poly(butylmethacrylate). *J Control Release* 1999; **62**: 115–127.

128. Jeong B, Bae YH, Kim SW. Biodegradable thermosensitive micelles of PEG-PLGA-PEG triblock copolymers. *Colloid Surface B* 1999; **16**: 185–193.

129. Na K, Lee KH, Lee DH, Bae YH. Biodegradable thermo-sensitive nanoparticles from poly(l-lactic acid)/poly(ethylene glycol) alternating multi-block copolymer for potential anti-cancer drug carrier. *Eur J Pharm Sci* 2006; **27**: 115–122.

130. Chilkoti A, Dreher MD, Meyer DE, Raucher D. Targeted drug delivery by thermally responsive polymers. *Adv Drug Deliver Rev* 2002; **54**: 613–630.

131. Dreher MR, Raucher D, Balu N, Colvin OM, Ludeman SM, Chilkoti A. Evaluation of an elastin-like polypeptide–doxorubicin conjugate for cancer therapy. *J Control Release* 2003; **91**: 31–43.

132. Kikuchi A, Okano T. Intelligent thermoresponsive polymeric stationary phases for aqueous chromatography of biological compounds. *Prog Polym Sci* 2002; **27**: 1165–1193.

133. Makhaeva EE, Tenhu H, Khokhlov AR. Conformational changes of poly(vinylcaprolactam) macromolecules and their complexes with ionic surfactants in aqueous solution. *Macromolecules* 1998; **31**: 6112–6118.

134. Rodriguez-Cabello JC, Reguera J, Girotti A, Alonso M, Testera AM. Developing functionality in elastin-like polymers by increasing their molecular complexity: the power of the genetic engineering approach. *Prog Polym Sci* 2005; **30**: 1119–1145.

135. Liu SQ, Tong YW, Yang YY. Incorporation and in vitro release of doxorubicin in thermally sensitive micelles made from poly(*N*-isopropylacrylamide-*co*-*N*,*N*-dimethylacrylamide)-*b*-poly(d,l-lactide-*co*-glycolide) with varying compositions. *Biomaterials* 2005; **26**: 5064–5074.

136. Liu SQ, Tong YW, Yang YY. Thermally sensitive micelles self-assembled from poly(*N*-isopropylacrylamide-*co*-*N*,*N*-dimethylacrylamide)-*b*-poly(D,L-lactide-*co*-glycolide) for controlled delivery of paclitaxel. *Mol Biosyst* 2005; **1**: 158–165.

137. Dewhirst M. *Principles and Practice of Thermoradiotherapy and Thermochemotherapy.* Springer-Verlag, Berlin, Edition, 1995.

138. Urry DW, Luan CH, Parker TM, Gowda DC, Prasad KU, Reid MC, Safavy A. Temperature of polypeptide inverse temperature transition depends on mean residue hydrophobicity. *J Am Chem Soc* 1991; **113**: 4346–4348.

139. Meyer DE, Shin BC, Kong GA, Dewhirst MW, Chilkoti A. Drug targeting using thermally responsive polymers and local hyperthermia. *J Control Release* 2001; **74**: 213–224.

140. Kaneko T, Willner D, Monkovic I, Knipe JO, Braslawsky GR, Greenfield RS, Vyas DM. New hydrazone derivatives of adriamycin and their immunoconjugates – a correlation between acid stability and cytotoxicity. *Bioconjugate Chem* 1991; **2**: 133–141.

141. Raucher D, Chilkoti A. Enhanced uptake of a thermally responsive polypeptide by tumor cells in response to its hyperthermia-mediated phase transition. *Cancer Res* 2001; **61**: 7163–7170.

142. Kong G, Dewhirst MW. Hyperthermia and liposomes. *Int J Hyperther* 1999; **15**: 345–370.

143. Ning S, Macleod K, Abra RM, Huang AH, Hahn GM. Hyperthermia induces doxorubicin release from long-circulating liposomes and enhances their anti-tumor efficacy. *Int J Radiat Oncol Biol Phys* 1994; **29**: 827–834.

144. Tacker JR, Anderson RU. Delivery of anti-tumor drug to bladder cancer by use of phase transition liposome and hypothermia. *J Urology* 1982; **127**: 1211–1214.

145. Mitragotri S, Blankschtein D, Langer R. Ultrasound-mediated transdermal protein delivery. *Science* 1995; **269**: 850–853.

146. Lauer U, Burgelt E, Squire Z, Messmer K, Hofschneider PH, Gregor M, Delius M. Shock wave permeabilization as a new gene transfer method. *Gene Ther* 1997; **4**: 710–715.

147. Pitt WG, Husseini GA, Staples BJ. Ultrasonic drug delivery – a general review. *Expert Opin Drug Deliv* 2004; **1**: 37–56.

148. Gao Z, Fain HD, Rapoport N. Ultrasound-enhanced tumor targeting of polymeric micellar drug carriers. *Mol Pharm* 2004; **1**: 317–330.

149. Gao Z, Fain HD, Rapoport N. Controlled and targeted tumor chemotherapy by micellar-encapsulated drug and ultrasound. *J Control Release* 2005; **102**: 203–222.

150. Husseini GA, El-Fayoumi RI, O'Neill KL, Rapoport NY, Pitt WG. DNA damage induced by micellar-delivered Doxorubicin and ultrasound: a Comet Assay Study. *Cancer Lett* 2000; **154**: 211–216.

151. Nelson JL, Roeder BL, Carmen JC, Roloff F, Pitt WG. Ultrasonically activated chemotherapeutic drug delivery in a rat model. *Cancer Res* 2002; **62**: 7280–7283.

152. Marin A, Muniruzzaman M, Rapoport N. Acoustic activation of drug delivery from polymeric micelles: Effect of pulsed ultrasound. *J Control Release* 2001; **71**: 239–249.

153. Marin A, Muniruzzaman M, Rapoport N. Mechanism of the ultrasonic activation of micellar drug delivery. *J Control Release* 2001; **75**: 69–81.

154. Veronese FM, Schiavon O, Pasut G, Mendichi R, Andersson L, Tsirk A, Ford J, Wu G, Kneller S, Davies J, Duncan R. PEG-Doxorubicin conjugates: Influence of polymer structure on drug release, in vitro cytotoxicity, biodistribution, and antitumor activity. *Bioconjug Chem* 2005; **16**: 775–784.

155. Oishi M, Hayama T, Akiyama Y, Takae S, Harada A, Yamasaki Y, Nagatsugi F, Sasaki S, Nagasaki Y, Kataoka K. Supramolecular assemblies for the cytoplasmic delivery of antisense oligodeoxynucleotide: Polyion complex (PIC) micelles based on poly(ethylene glycol)-SS-oligodeoxynucleotide conjugate. *Biomacromolecules* 2005; **6**: 2449–2454.
156. Bagshawe KD, Springer CJ, Searle F, Antoniw P, Sharma SK, Melton RG, Sherwood RF. A cytotoxic agent can be generated selectively at cancer sites. *Brit J Cancer* 1988; **58**: 700–703.
157. de Groot FM, Damen EW, Scheeren HW. Anticancer prodrugs for application in monotherapy: targeting hypoxia, tumor-associated enzymes, and receptors. *Curr Med Chem* 2001; **8**: 1093–1122.
158. Haba K, Popkov M, Shamis M, Lerner RA, Barbas CF, Shabat D. Single-triggered trimeric prodrugs. *Angew Chem Int Ed Engl* 2005; **44**: 716–720.
159. Shamis M, Lode HN, Shabat D. Bioactivation of self-immolative dendritic prodrugs by catalytic antibody 38C2. *J Am Chem Soc* 2004; **126**: 1726–1731.
160. Gopin A, Ebner S, Attali B, Shabat D. Enzymatic activation of second-generation dendritic prodrugs: Conjugation of self-immolative dendrimers with poly(ethylene glycol) via click chemistry. *Bioconjugate Chem* 2006; **17**: 1432–1440.
161. Carter P. Improving the efficacy of antibody-based cancer therapies. *Nat Rev Cancer* 2001; **1**: 118–129.
162. Schrama D, Reisfeld RA, Becker JC. Antibody targeted drugs as cancer therapeutics. *Nat Rev Drug Discov* 2006; **5**: 147–159.
163. Okamoto OK, Perez JF. Targeting cancer stem cells with monoclonal antibodies: A new perspective in cancer therapy and diagnosis. *Expert Rev Mol Diagn* 2008; **8**: 387–393.
164. Destito G, Yeh R, Rae CS, Finn MG, Manchester M. Folic acid-mediated targeting of cowpea mosaic virus particles to tumor cells. *Chem Biol* 2007; **14**: 1152–1162.
165. Lu Y, Low PS. Folate-mediated delivery of macromolecular anticancer therapeutic agents. *Adv Drug Deliver Rev* 2002; **54**: 675–693.
166. Hilgenbrink AR, Low PS. Folate receptor-mediated drug targeting: From therapeutics to diagnostics. *J Pharm Sci* 2005; **94**: 2135–2146.
167. Lu Y, Low PS. Immunotherapy of folate receptor-expressing tumors: review of recent advances and future prospects. *J Control Release* 2003; **91**: 17–29.
168. Weitman SD, Lark RH, Coney LR, Fort DW, Frasca V, Zurawski VR, Kamen BA. Distribution of the folate receptor GP38 in normal and malignant cell lines and tissues. *Cancer Res* 1992; **52**: 3396–3401.
169. Reddy JA, Low PS. Folate-mediated targeting of therapeutic and imaging agents to cancers. *Crit Rev Ther Drug* 1998; **15**: 586–627.
170. Leamon CP, Low PS. Folate-mediated targeting: from diagnostics to drug and gene delivery. *Drug Discovery Today* 2001; **6**: 44–51.
171. Satyam A. Design and synthesis of releasable folate–drug conjugates using a novel heterobifunctional disulfide-containing linker. *Bioorg Med Chem Lett* 2008; **18**: 3196–3199.
172. Stella B, Appicco S, Peracchia MT, Desmaele D, Hoebeke J, Renoir M, D'angelo J, Cattel L, Couvreur P. Design of folic acid-conjugated nanoparticles for drug targeting. *J Pharm Sci* 2000; **89**: 1452–1464.
173. Brigger I, Dubernet C, Couvreur P. Nanoparticles in cancer therapy and diagnosis, *Adv Drug Deliver Rev* 2002; **54**: 631–651.
174. Leamon CP, Pastan I, Low PS. Cytotoxicity of folate-pseudomonas exotoxin conjugates toward tumor cells: contribution of translocation domain. *J Biol Chem* 1993; **268**: 24847–24854.
175. Sudimack J, Lee RJ. Targeted drug delivery via the folate receptor. *Adv Drug Deliver Rev* 2000; **41**: 147–162.
176. Qian ZM, Li H, Sun H, Ho K. Targeted drug delivery via the transferrin receptor-mediated endocytosis pathway. *Pharmacol Rev* 2002; **54**: 561–587.

177. Zenke M, Steinlein P, Wagner E, Cotton M, Beug H, Birnstiel ML. Receptor-mediated endocytosis of transferrin-polycation conjugates: An efficient way to introduce DNA into hematopoietic cells. *P Natl Acad Sci USA* 1990; **87**: 3655–3659.

178. Sahoo SK, Labhasetwar V. Enhanced antiproliferative activity of transferrin-conjugated paclitaxel-loaded nanoparticles is mediated via sustained intracellular drug retention. *Mol Pharm* 2005; **2**: 373–383.

179. Grundker C, Gunthert AR, Millar RP, Emons G. Expression of gonadotropin-releasing hormone II (GnRH-II) receptor in human endometrial and ovarian cancer cells and effects of GnRH-II on tumor cell proliferation. *J Clin Endocrinol Metab* 2002; **87**: 1427–1430.

180. Dharap SS, Qiu B, Williams GC, Sinko P, Stein S, Minko T. Molecular targeting of drug delivery systems to ovarian cancer by BH3 and LHRH peptides. *J Control Release* 2003; **91**: 61–73.

181. Ruoslahti E. Targeting tumor vasculature with homing peptides from phage display. *Cancer Biol* 2000; **10**: 435–442.

182. Nilsson F, Tarli L, Viti F, Neri D. The use of phage display for the development of tumour targeting agents. *Adv Drug Deliver Rev* 2000; **43**: 165–196.

183. Farokhzad OC, Karp JM, Langer R. Nanoparticle–aptamer bioconjugates for cancer targeting. *Expert Opin Drug Deliver* 2006; **3**: 311–324.

184. Leroux JC. pH-responsive carriers for enhancing the cytoplasmic delivery of macromolecular drugs. *Adv Drug Deliver Rev* 2004; **56**: 925–926.

185. Plank C, Zauner W, Wagner E. Application of membrane-active peptides for drug and gene delivery across cellular membranes. *Adv Drug Deliver Rev* 1998; **34**: 21–35.

186. Richardson SCW, Pattrick NG, Man YKS, Ferruti P, Duncan R. Poly(amidoamine)s as potential nonviral vectors: ability to form interpolyelectrolyte complexes and to mediate transfection in vitro. *Biomacromolecules* 2001; **2**: 1023–1028.

187. Putnam D, Zelikin AN, Izumrudov VA, Langer R. Polyhistidine-PEG:DNA nanocomposites for gene delivery. *Biomaterials* 2003; **24**: 4425–4433.

188. Wang CY, Huang L. Polyhistidine mediates an acid dependent fusion of negatively charged liposomes. *Biochemistry* 1984; **23**: 4409–4416.

189. Park JS, Han TH, Lee KY, Han SS, Hwang JJ, Moon DH, Kim SY, Cho YW. N-acetyl histidine-conjugated glycol chitosan self-assembled nanoparticles for intracytoplasmic delivery of drugs: Endocytosis, exocytosis and drug release. *J Control Release* 2006; **115**: 37–45.

190. Yang SR, Lee HJ, Kim JD. Histidine-conjugated poly(amino acid) derivatives for the novel endosomolytic delivery carrier of doxorubicin. *J Control Release* 2006; **114**: 60–68.

191. Fawell S, Seery J, Daikh Y, Moore C, Chen LL, Pepinsky B, Barsoum J. Tat-mediated delivery of heterologous proteins into cells. *P Natl Acad Sci USA* 1994; **91**: 664–668.

192. Joliot A, Pernelle C, Deagostini-Bazin H, Prochiantz A. Antennapedia homeobox peptide regulates neural morphogenesis. *P Natl Acad Sci USA* 1991; **88**: 1864–1868.

193. Wu HY, Tomizawa K, Matsushita M, Lu YF, Li ST, Matsui H. Poly-arginine-fused calpastatin peptide, a living cell membrane-permeable and specific inhibitor for calpain. *Neurosci Res* 2003; **47**: 131–135.

194. Nekhotiaeva N, Elmquist A, Rajarao GK, Hallbrink M, Langel U, Good L. Cell entry and antimicrobial properties of eukaryotic cell-penetrating peptides. *FASEB J* 2004; **18**: 394–396.

195. Pooga M, Hallbrink M, Zorko M, Langel U. Cell penetration by transportan. *FASEB J* 1998; **12**: 67–77.

196. Myrberg H, Lindgren M, Langel U. Protein delivery by the cell-penetrating peptide YTA2. *Bioconjugate Chem* 2007; **18**: 170–174.

197. Derossi D, Chassaing G, Prochiantz A. Trojan peptides: the penetratin system for intracellular delivery. *Trends Cell Biol* 1998; **8**: 84–87.

198. Vives E. Present and future of cell-penetrating peptide mediated delivery systems: "Is the Trojan horse too wild to go only to Troy?" *J Control Release* 2005; **109**: 77–85.

199. Sethuraman VA, Bae YH. TAT peptide-based micelle system for potential active targeting of anti-cancer agents to acidic solid tumors. *J Control Release* 2007; **118**: 216–224.
200. Thomas H, Coley HM. Overcoming multidrug resistance in cancer: An update on the clinical strategy of inhibiting p-glycoprotein. *Cancer Control* 2003; **10**: 159–165.
201. Choi CH. Abc transporters as multidrug resistance mechanisms and the development of chemosensitizers for their reversal. *Cancer Cell Inter* 2005, doi:10.1186/1475-2867-5-30.
202. Gottesman MM, Fojo T, Bates SE. Multidrug resistance in cancer: Role of atp-dependent transporters. *Nat Rev Cancer* 2002; **2**: 48–58.
203. Gottesman MM. Mechanisms of cancer drug resistance. *Annu Rev Med* 2002; **53**: 615–627.
204. Szakacs G, Paterson JK, Ludwig JA, Booth-Genthe C, Gottesman MM. Targeting multidrug resistance in cancer. *Nat Rev Drug Discov* 2006; **5**: 219–234.
205. Grech KV, Davey RA, Davey MW. The relationship between modulation of MDR and glutathione in MRP-overexpressing human leukemia cells. *Biochem Pharmacol* 1998; **55**: 1283–1289.
206. Matsuo K, Kohno K, Takano H, Sato S, Kiue A, Kuwano M. Reduction of drug accumulation and DNA topoisomerase II activity in acquired teniposide-resistant human cancer KB cell lines. *Cancer Res* 1990; **50**: 5819–5824.
207. Sugawara I, Akiyama S, Scheper RJ, Itoyama S. Lung resistance protein (LRP) expression in human normal tissues in comparison with that of MDR1 and MRP. *Cancer Lett* 1997; **112**: 23–31.
208. Pohl G, Filipits M, Suchomel RW, Stranzl T, Depisch D, Pirker R. Expression of the lung resistance protein (LRP) in primary breast cancer. *Anticancer Res* 1999; **19**: 5051–5056.
209. Gonçlaves A, Braguer D, Kamath K, Martello L, Briand C, Horwitz S, Wilson L, Jordan MA. Resistance to taxol in lung cancer cells associated with increased microtubule dynamics. *P Natl Acad Sci USA* 2001; **98**: 11737–11741.
210. Simon SM, Schindler M. Cell biological mechanisms of multidrug resistance in tumors. *P Natl Acad Sci USA* 1994; **91**: 3497–3504.
211. Simon SM. Role of organelle pH in tumor cell biology and drug resistance. *Drug Discovery Today* 1999; **4**: 32–38.
212. Belhoussine R, Morjani H, Millot JM, Sharonov S, Manfait M. Confocal scanning microspectrofluorometry reveals specific anthracycline accumulation in cytoplasmic organelles of multidrug-resistant cancer cells. *J Histochem Cytochem* 1998; **46**: 1369–1376.
213. Mahadevan D, List AF. Targeting the multidrug resistance-1 transporter in aml: Molecular regulation and therapeutic strategies. *Blood* 2004; **104**: 1940–1951.
214. Golstein PE, Boom A, van Geffel J, Jacobs P, Masereel B, Beauwens R. P-glycoprotein inhibition by glibenclamide and related compounds. *Pflugers Arch* 1999; **437**: 652–660.
215. Pierre A, Dunn TA, Kraus-Berthier L, Leonce S, Saint-Dizier D, Regnier G, Dhainaut A, Berlion M, Bizzari JP, Atassi G. *In vitro* and *in vivo* circumvention of multidrug resistance by Servier 9788, a novel triazinoaminopiperidine derivative. *Invest New Drug* 1992; **10**: 137–148.
216. Kobayashi T, Ishida T, Okada Y, Ise S, Harashima H, Kiwada H. Effect of transferrin receptor-targeted liposomal doxorubicin in p-glycoprotein-mediated drug resistant tumor cells. *Int J Pharm* 2007; **329**: 94–102.
217. Soma CE, Dubernet C, Bentolila D, Benita S, Couvreur P. Reversion of multidrug resistance by co-encapsulation of doxorubicin and cyclosporin a in polyalkylcyanoacrylate nanoparticles. *Biomaterials* 2000; **21**: 1–7.
218. van Vlerken LE, Duan Z, Seiden MV, Amiji MM. Modulation of intracellular ceramide using polymeric nanoparticles to overcome multidrug resistance in cancer. *Cancer Res* 2007; **67**: 4843–4850.

219. Kabanov AV, Alakhov VY. Pluronic block copolymers in drug delivery: From micellar nanocontainers to biological response modifiers. *Crit Rev Ther Drug* 2002; **19**: 1–73.
220. Deng WJ, Yang XQ, Liang YJ, Chen LM, Yan YY, Shuai XT, Fu LW. FG020326-loaded nanoparticle with PEG and PDLLA improved pharmacodynamics of reversing multidrug resistance in vitro and in vivo. *Acta Pharmacol Sin* 2007; **28**: 913–920.
221. Chavanpatil MD, Patil Y, Panyam J. Susceptibility of nanoparticle-encapsulated paclitaxel to p-glycoprotein-mediated drug efflux. *Int J Pharm* 2006; **320**: 150–156.
222. Batrakova E, Lee S, Li S, Venne A, Alakhov V, Kabanov A. Fundamental relationships between the composition of pluronic block copolymers and their hypersensitization effect in MDR cancer cells. *Pharm Res* 1999; **16**: 1373–1379.
223. Advani R, Lum BL, Fisher GA, Halsey J, Chin DL, Jacobs CD, Sikic BI. A phase I trial of liposomal doxorubicin, paclitaxel and valspodar (psc-833), an inhibitor of multidrug resistance. *Ann Oncol* 2005; **16**: 1968–1973.
224. Song S, Yu B, Wei Y, Wientjes MG, Au JL. Low-dose suramin enhanced paclitaxel activity in chemotherapy-naive and paclitaxel-pretreated human breast xenograft tumors. *Clin Cancer Res* 2004; **10**: 6058–6065.
225. Song S, Wientjes MG, Gan Y, Au JL. Fibroblast growth factors: An epigenetic mechanism of broad spectrum resistance to anticancer drugs. *P Natl Acad Sci USA* 2000; **97**: 8658–8663.
226. Lu D, Wientjes MG, Lu Z, Au JL, Tumor priming enhances delivery and efficacy of nanomedicines. *J Pharmacol Exp Ther* 2007; **322**: 80–88.
227. Kim D, Lee ES, Oh KT, Gao Z, Bae YH. Doxorubicin-loaded polymeric micelle overcomes multidrug resistance of cancer by double-targeting folate receptor and early endosomal pH. *Small* 2008 (in press).
228. Greller LD, Tobin FL, Poste G. Tumor heterogeneity and progression: Conceptual foundations for modeling. *Invas Metast* 1996; **16**: 177–208.
229. http://www.medscape.com/viewarticle/424719
230. Hartmann LC, Keeney GL, Lingle WL, Christianson TJ, Varghese B, Hillman D, Oberg AL, Low PS. Folate receptor overexpression is associated with poor outcome in breast cancer. *Int J Cancer* 2007; **121**: 938–942.

Application of Nanobiotechnology in Cancer Therapeutics

K.K. Jain

1 Introduction

Nanotechnology is the creation and utilization of materials, devices, and systems through the control of matter on the nanometer-length scale, i.e., at the level of atoms, molecules, and supramolecular structures. Nanotechnology, as defined by the National Nanotechnology Initiative (http://www.nano.gov/), is the understanding and control of matter at dimensions of roughly 1–100 nm, where unique phenomena enable novel applications. During the past few years, considerable progress has been made in the application of nanobiotechnology in cancer, i.e. nanooncology, which is currently the most important chapter of nanomedicine [1,2]. Other publications have covered applications of nanobiotechnology in diagnostics [3], drug discovery [4], and drug delivery [5]. Several drugs in development for cancer are based on nanotechnology and a few of these are already approved. Nanotechnology-based devices are in development as aids to cancer surgery. Some of the recent development in nanotechnologies and their applications in diagnosing and developing cancer therapies are reviewed in this chapter. The impact of nanobiotechnology on oncology is shown schematically in Fig. 1.

2 Nanotechnology for Detection of Cancer Biomarkers

2.1 Basics of Cancer Biomarkers

Any measurable specific molecular alteration of a cancer cell either on DNA, RNA, protein, or metabolite level can be referred to as a cancer biomarker [6]. The expression of a distinct gene can enable its identification in a tissue with none of the surrounding cells expressing the specific biomarker. Cancer cells themselves may be difficult to detect at an early stage but they leave a

K.K. Jain (✉)
Jain PharmaBiotech, Blaesiring 7, CH-4057 Basel, Switzerland
e-mail: jain@pharmabiotech.ch

Y. Lu, R.I. Mahato (eds.), *Pharmaceutical Perspectives of Cancer Therapeutics*,
DOI 10.1007/978-1-4419-0131-6_8, © Springer Science+Business Media, LLC 2009

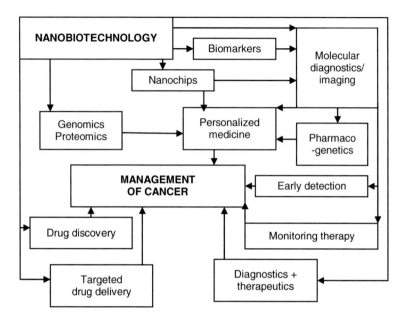

Fig. 1 Role of nanobiotechnology in the management of cancer. Various nanobiotechnologies have a direct as well as indirect effect on the diagnosis and management of cancer. Many of these technologies interact with each other

fingerprint, i.e., a pattern of change in biomarker proteins that circulate in the blood. There may be 20–25 biomarkers, which may require as many as 500 measurements, all of which should be made from a drop of blood obtained by pinprick. Miniaturized techniques such as nanotechnology are useful for the discovery of cancer biomarkers.

Silicon nanowires incorporated into arrays provide label-free, multiplexed electrical detection of cancer protein biomarkers such as prostate-specific antigen at femtomolar concentrations with high sensitivity in clinically relevant serum samples [7]. Real-time assays of the binding, activity, and small-molecule inhibition of telomerase could be performed with this technique using unamplified extracts from as few as 10 tumor cells. This opens up substantial possibilities for diagnosis and treatment of cancer.

2.2 Nucleoprotein Nanodevices for Detection of Cancer Biomarkers

DNA Y-junctions have been used as fluorescent scaffolds for EcoRII methyltransferase–thioredoxin (M●EcoRII–Trx) fusion proteins and covalent links were formed between the DNA scaffold and the methyltransferase at preselected sites on the scaffold containing 5FdC [8]. The resulting thioredoxin-targeted nanodevice was found to bind selectively to certain cell lines but not to others. The fusion protein was constructed so as to permit proteolytic cleavage of the thioredoxin peptide from the nanodevice. Proteolysis with thrombin or enterokinase effectively removed the thioredoxin peptide from the nanodevice and extinguished cell line-specific binding measured by fluorescence. Potential applications for devices of this type include the ability of the fused protein to selectively target the nanodevice to certain tumor cell lines and not others, suggesting that this approach can be used to probe cell surface receptors as biomarkers of cancer and may serve as an adjunct to immunohistochemical methods in tumor classification.

3 Nanoparticles for Combined Cancer Diagnosis and Therapy

Nanoparticles have refined molecular diagnostics and enabled early detection of tumors and discovery of biomarkers of cancer. Nanoparticles are also therapeutic agents as well as carriers for targeted drug delivery. Main advantage of using nanoparticles in cancer is combining diagnosis with therapy. Important among the several nanoparticles used for this purpose are quantum dots (QDs), dendrimers, nanotubes, and gold or silver nanoparticles. Details of the basic characteristics and comparative advantages as well as drawbacks are discussed elsewhere [9].

3.1 Gold Nanoparticles

Photoacoustic flow cytometry has been used for real-time detection of circulating cells labeled with gold nanorods and the threshold sensitivity is estimated as one cancer cell in the background of 107 normal blood cells. An additional application of this technique is selective nanophotothermolysis of metastatic squamous cells [10]. Gold nanoparticles could play an important role in efficient drug delivery and biomarking of drug-resistant leukemia cells [11]. This could be explored as a novel strategy to inhibit multidrug resistance in targeted tumor cells and as a sensitive method for the early diagnosis of certain cancers. Interaction between the functionalized gold nanoparticles and biologically active molecules on the surface of leukemia cells may also contribute to the observed enhancement in cellular drug uptake. The strong plasmon resonance absorption and photothermal conversion of gold nanoparticles has been exploited in cancer therapy through the selective localized photothermal heating of cancer cells [12].

3.2 Silver Nanoparticles

Silver nanoparticles are bright enough to be seen by eye using optical microscopy but unlike fluorophores, fluorescent proteins, or quantum dots, silver nanoparticles do not photodecompose during extended illumination. Therefore, they can be used as a probe to continuously monitor dynamic events in living cells during studies that last for weeks or even months and detect early changes in malignancy. Further development of silver nanoparticle-based probes and assays may enable detection and diagnosis of cancer using only a single cell from the patient.

Size-tunable and water-soluble silver nanoparticles have been successfully synthesized with the assistance of glutathione. The optical properties of surface-modifiable silver nanoparticles depend on their size and the surface modification. Silver nanoparticles with an average diameter of 6 nm effectively suppress the proliferation of human leukemia cells in the dose- and time-dependent manners, suggesting their promising application in cancer therapy [13].

3.3 Quantum Dots

Quantum dots (QDs) are crystalline semiconductors composed of a few hundred or a few thousand atoms that emit different colors of light when illuminated by a laser. Stable QDs are made from cadmium selenide and zinc sulfide. Because these probes are stable, they have the ability to remain in a cell's cytoplasm and nucleus without fading out much longer than conventional fluorescent labels. Their longevity has also made QDs a molecular label, allowing scientists to study the earliest signs of cancer and track the effectiveness of pharmaceuticals that target the cellular underpinnings of disease. Conjugation of QDs with biomolecules, including peptides and antibodies, could be used to target tumors in vivo.

The specificity and sensitivity of a QD–aptamer–doxorubicin (QD–Apt–DOX) conjugate as a targeted cancer imaging, therapy, and sensing system has been demonstrated in vitro [14]. By functionalizing the surface of fluorescent QD with an RNA aptamer, which recognizes the extracellular domain of the prostate-specific membrane antigen (PSMA), the system is capable of differential uptake and imaging of prostate cancer cells that express the PSMA. The intercalation of DOX, an anticancer drug with fluorescent properties, in the double-stranded stem of the aptamer results in a targeted conjugate with reversible self-quenching properties based on a Bi-FRET mechanism. A donor–acceptor model FRET between QD and DOX and a donor–quencher model FRET between DOX and aptamer result when DOX is intercalated within the aptamer. This simple multifunctional nanoparticle system can deliver DOX to the targeted prostate cancer cells and sense the delivery of DOX by activating the fluorescence of QD, which concurrently images the cancer cells.

3.4 Nanotubes

Single-wall carbon nanotubes (SWCNT) are highly sensitive to single protein-binding events and can be massively multiplexed with millions of tubes per chip for proteomic profiling. The tubes have extraordinary strength, unique electronic properties, and the ability to tag cancer-specific proteins to their surface. With diameter of 1 nm and length of 1 μm, these tubes are smaller than a single strand of DNA. In other words, each tube is an atomic arrangement of one layer of carbon atoms, which are on the surface. Protein-binding events occurring on the surface of these nanotubes produce a measurable change in the mechanical and electrical properties. By coating the surfaces of nanotubes with MAbs, it is possible to detect cancer cells circulating in the blood. Combination of electrochemical immunosensors using SWCNT and multilabel secondary antibody–nanotube bioconjugates can be used for highly sensitive detection of a cancer biomarker in serum and other body fluids [15]. SWCNT immunosensors are promising for clinical screening of cancer biomarkers and point-of-care diagnostics.

Two main strategies are used for using carbon nanotubes with anticancer molecules: they can be either covalently or noncovalently modified to facilitate their manipulation and render them biocompatible [16]. Such soluble/dispersible nano-objects in physiological conditions are then able to penetrate into the cells or they can be administered in vivo to deliver their cargo molecules. Nanotubes are feasible carriers for carboplatin, a therapeutic agent for cancer treatment. The drug has been introduced into nanotubes to demonstrate that they are suited as nanocontainers and nanocarriers and can release the drug for therapeutic effect [17].

3.5 Multifunctional Nanoparticles

Two promising approaches for diagnosing and treating cancer have been combined in a targeted multifunctional polymer nanoparticle that successfully images and kills brain tumors in laboratory animals [18]. A 40-nm-diameter polyacrylamide nanoparticle was loaded with Photofrin, a photosensitizing agent, and iron oxide. When irradiated with laser light, Photofrin triggers the production of reactive oxygen species that destroy a wide variety of molecules within a cell. The iron oxide nanoparticles function as an MRI contrast agent and a 31-amino-acid-long peptide targets an unknown receptor found on the surface of new blood vessels growing around tumors as well as triggers cell uptake of nanoparticles attached to it. Because of the targeted delivery of nanoparticles to the tumor, there is enhanced Photofrin exposure within the tumor but less exposure throughout the rest of the body. This allows a larger window for activating the drug with light, which is accomplished by threading a fiber optic laser into the brain. In humans, this approach could reduce or eliminate a common side effect of photodynamic therapy, in which healthy skin becomes sensitive to light.

Nanoparticle-based diagnostics and therapeutics hold great promise because multiple functions can be built into the particles. One such function is an ability to home to specific sites in the body. Biomimetic particles that not only home to tumors but also amplify their own homing have been described [19]. The system is based on a peptide that recognizes clotted plasma proteins and selectively homes to tumors, where it binds to vessel walls and tumor stroma. Iron oxide nanoparticles and liposomes coated with this tumor-homing peptide accumulate in tumor vessels, where they induce additional local clotting, thereby producing new binding sites for more particles. The system mimics platelets, which also circulate freely but accumulate at a diseased site and amplify their own accumulation at that site. The self-amplifying homing is a novel function of nanoparticles. The clotting-based amplification greatly enhances tumor imaging, and the addition of a drug carrier function to the particles is envisioned.

4 Nanotechnology-Based Imaging for Management of Cancer

Nanobiotechnology plays an important role in diagnostic molecular imaging of cancer, particularly magnetic resonance imaging (MRI) and computed tomography (CT). Nanotechnology-based cancer imaging will lead to early detection of cancer and also help accurate delivery of cancer therapy. Newer generations of nanoparticles have been targeted to specific cell types and molecular targets via affinity ligands.

4.1 Nanoparticle CT Scan

Current computer tomography (CT) contrast agents are based on small iodinated molecules. They are effective in absorbing X-rays, but nonspecific distribution and rapid pharmacokinetics have rather limited their microvascular and targeting performance. While most of the nanoparticles are designed to be used in conjunction with MRI, bismuth sulfide (Bi2S3) nanoparticles naturally accumulate in lymph nodes containing metastases and show up as bright white spots in CT images [20]. A polymer-coated Bi2S3 nanoparticle preparation has been proposed as an injectable CT imaging agent. This preparation demonstrates excellent stability at high concentrations, high X-ray absorption (fivefold better than iodine), very long circulation times (>2 h) in vivo, and an efficacy/safety profile comparable to or better than iodinated imaging agents. The utility of these polymer-coated Bi2S3 nanoparticles for enhanced in vivo imaging of the vasculature, the liver, and lymph nodes has been demonstrated in mice. These nanoparticles and their bioconjugates are expected to become an important adjunct to in vivo imaging of molecular targets and pathological conditions. Tumor-targeting agents are now being added to the surfaces of these polymer-coated Bi2S3 nanoparticles.

4.2 Nanoparticles Designed for Dual-Mode Imaging of Cancer

The unique optical and electronic properties of QDs such as size-tunable light emission, improved signal brightness, resistance against photobleaching, and simultaneous excitation of multiple fluorescence colors are promising for improving the sensitivity of molecular imaging and quantitative cellular analysis by 1–2 orders of magnitude [21]. The best characteristics of QDs and magnetic iron oxide nanoparticles have been combined to create a single nanoparticle probe that can yield clinically useful images of both tumors and the molecules involved in cancer [22]. On average, 10 magnetic iron oxide particles link to a single dye-containing silica nanoparticle, and the resulting construct is approximately 45 nm in diameter. The combination nanoparticle performed better in both MRI and fluorescent imaging tests than did the individual components. In MRI experiments, the combination nanoparticle generated an MRI signal that was over threefold more intense than did the same number of iron oxide nanoparticles. Similarly, the fluorescent signal from the dual-mode nanoparticle was almost twice as bright as that produced by dye molecules linked directly to iron oxide nanoparticles. The dual-mode nanoparticles have been labeled with an antibody that binds to molecules known as polysialic acids, which are found on the surface of certain nerve cell and lung tumors. These targeted nanoparticles are quickly taken up by cultured tumor cells and are readily visible using fluorescence microscopy.

A novel PAMAM dendrimer-based nanoprobe, G6-(Cy5.5)(1.25)(1B4M-Gd)(145), has been synthesized for dual magnetic resonance and fluorescence imaging modalities [23]. The potential of this nanoprobe was demonstrated in vivo by the efficient visualization of sentinel lymph nodes in mice by both MRI and fluorescence imaging modalities.

5 Nanobiotechnology-Based Anticancer Drug Development

Nanoparticles have unique properties for potential use in drug discovery and have been used to study the mechanism of anticancer drug action. Some nanoparticles are anticancer agents by themselves. Several nanoparticles described in the section on drug delivery in cancer are conjugates of nanoparticles with known anticancer agents. Nanotechnology has also helped to elucidate the mechanism of action of some anticancer drugs. Using single-molecule nanomanipulation by magnetic tweezers has revealed that anticancer drug topotecan, a camptothecin, kills cancer cells by preventing the enzyme DNA topoisomerase I from uncoiling double-stranded DNA in those cells [24]. The DNA becomes locked in tight twists, called supercoils, which bulge out from the side of the overwound DNA molecule. If these supercoils accumulate and persist while the cell is trying to separate the two strands of DNA to make exact copies of the chromosomes during cell division, the cells will die. In vivo experiments in the budding yeast verified the resulting prediction that positive supercoils would accumulate during transcription and replication as a consequence of camptothecin poisoning of topoisomerase I. Based on the results of these studies, the supercoil theory was developed to explain camptothecins' cytotoxic effect, which could help in the clinical development of these agents.

Examples of nanoscale drug candidates include nanobodies, which are variable domains of camelid heavy chain-only antibodies. These have advantages compared with classical antibodies in that they are small, very stable, easy to produce in large quantities, and easy to reformat into multivalent or multispecific proteins. In vivo studies have demonstrated that nanobody conjugates have an excellent biodistribution profile and induced regression and cure of established tumor xenografts. The easy generation and manufacturing yield of nanobody-based conjugates together with their potent antitumor activity makes nanobodies promising vehicles for new generation cancer therapeutics.

Nanobodies can be specifically selected for a desired function by phage antibody display. Nanobodies selected by this method were found to efficiently inhibit EGF binding to the EGFR without acting as receptor agonists themselves [25]. In addition, they blocked EGF-mediated signaling and EGF-induced cell proliferation.

6 Nanobiotechnology-Based Drug Delivery in Cancer

Drug delivery in cancer is important for optimizing the effect of drugs and reducing toxic side effects. Several nanobiotechnologies, mostly based on nanoparticles, have been described to facilitate drug delivery in cancer. Some innovative nanoparticle formulations for drug delivery include encapsulating drugs in nanoparticles (Table 1).

The main advantage of various nanotechnology-based formulation is to overcome poor solubility of most anticancer drugs. Polymer micelles are becoming a powerful nanotherapeutic platform that affords several advantages for targeted drug delivery in cancer, including increased drug solubility, prolonged circulation half-life, selective accumulation at tumor sites, and a decrease in toxicity. However, the technology still lacks tumor specificity and controlled release of the entrapped agents. Therefore, the focus has gradually shifted from passive targeting micelles to active targeting and responsive systems that carry additional mechanisms for site-specific release. Ligand-targeted, pH-sensitive formulations are examples of how versatility of micelles can lead to a fusion of chemical customization with biological insight to achieve targeted drug delivery.

Table 1 Examples of nanobiotechnology-based formulations for drug delivery in cancer

Technology	Description	Application	References
Encapsulating drugs in hydrogel nanoparticles	2-nm-diameter polyacrylamide nanoparticles lacking charge on their surfaces, which prevents blood proteins from sticking to their surfaces	For delivery of photosensitizer meta-tetra(hydroxyphenyl) chlorin for head and neck cancer	26
Block copolymer micelles	The core is a loading space for hydrophobic drugs, and the shell is a hydrophilic corona that makes the micelle water soluble, thereby allowing delivery of the poorly soluble contents	For delivery of camptothecin, a topoisomerase I inhibitor that is effective against cancer but insoluble	27
Filomicelles: polymer micelle	Persisted in the circulation up to 1 W after intravenous injection – 10 times longer than their spherical counterparts.	For delivery of paclitaxel and shown to shrink human-derived tumors in mice	28
Stealth micelles	Have stabilizing PEG coronas to minimize opsonization of the micelles and maximize blood circulation times	Clinical data have been reported on three stealth micelle systems: SP1049C, NK911, and Genexol-PM	29
Silica-based nanoparticles	Incorporation of a hydrophobic anticancer drug into the pores of fluorescent mesoporous silica nanoparticles	For delivery of camptothecin and other water-insoluble drugs into human cancer cells	30
Nanocells (400 nm)	Encapsulates drugs of differing charge, hydrophobicity, and solubility, which results in endocytosis, intracellular degradation, and drug release at target site	Targeted delivery of poorly soluble anticancer drugs via bispecific antibodies to receptors on cancer cell membranes	31

© Jain PharmaBiotech

7 Nanoparticles for Targeted Delivery of Drugs in Cancer

Nanosystems that may be very useful for tumor-targeted drug delivery are emerging: novel nanoparticles are preprogrammed to alter their structure and properties during the drug delivery process to make them most effective for the different extra- and intracellular delivery steps [32]. This is achieved by the incorporation of molecular sensors that are able to respond to physical or biological stimuli, including changes in pH, redox potential, or enzymes. Tumor-targeting principles include systemic passive targeting and active receptor targeting. Physical forces (e.g., electric or magnetic fields, ultrasound, hyperthermia or light) may contribute to focusing and triggered activation of nanosystems. Biological drugs delivered with programmed nanosystems also include plasmid DNA, siRNA, and other therapeutic nucleic acids.

A drug delivery system has been developed to destroy tumors more effectively by using synthesized smart nanoparticles that target and kill cancer cells while sparing healthy cells [33]. The system is intended to improve the efficiency of cancer treatment. These particles are injected intravenously into the blood circulation. Each of the particles can recognize the cancer cell, anchor itself to it, and diffuse inside the cell. Once inside, the particle disintegrates causing a nearly instantaneous release of the drug precisely where it is needed. Nanoparticles are chemically programmed to have an affinity for the cell wall of tumors. To be effective, the particles must evade being recognized by the body's reticuloendothelial system, penetrate into the cancer cells, and discharge the drugs before being recognized by the cancer cells. Advantages of this system are the following:

- This system can fool cancer cells, which are very good at detecting and rejecting drugs.
- It provides very rapid drug delivery at sufficiently high concentration that can overwhelm the cancer cell's resistance mechanisms.
- It should reduce side effects because it targets only the cancer cells.

7.1 Innovations in Dendrimers for Anticancer Drug Delivery

Earlier studies of dendrimers in drug delivery systems focused on their use for encapsulating drug molecules. However, it was difficult to control the release of the drug. New developments in polymer and dendrimer chemistry have provided a new class of molecules called "dendronized polymer," i.e., linear polymer that bears dendrons at each repeat unit. Their behavior differs from that of linear polymers and provides drug delivery advantages because of their longer circulation time. Another approach is to attach the drug to the periphery of the dendrimer so that the release of the drug can be controlled by incorporating a degradable linkage between the drug and the dendrimer.

Doxorubicin (DOX) has been conjugated to a biodegradable dendrimer with optimized blood circulation time through size and molecular architecture, drug loading through multiple attachment sites, solubility through PEGylation, and drug release through the use of pH-sensitive hydrazone linkages [34]. In culture, dendrimer–DOX was >10 times less toxic than free DOX toward colon carcinoma cells. Upon intravenous administration to tumor-bearing mice, tumor uptake of dendrimer–DOX was ninefold higher than intravenous free DOX. In efficacy studies it caused complete tumor regression and 100% survival of the mice over the 60-day experiment. No cures were achieved in tumor-implanted mice treated with free DOX, drug-free dendrimer, or dendrimer–DOX in which the DOX was attached by means of a stable carbamate bond. The antitumor effect of dendrimer–DOX was similar to that of an equimolar dose of liposomal DOX (Doxil). The remarkable antitumor activity of dendrimer–DOX results from the ability of the dendrimer to favorably modulate the pharmacokinetics of attached DOX.

7.2 Nanoparticles for Enhancing Tumor Targeting by Antibodies

Although it was previously possible to attach drug molecules directly to antibodies, attaching more than a handful of drug molecules to an antibody significantly limits its targeting ability because the chemical bonds that are used to attach the drugs tend to block the targeting centers on the antibody's surface. A number of nanoparticles have been investigated to overcome this limitation. Tumor-targeting SWCNT constructs have been synthesized by covalently attaching multiple copies of tumor-specific MAbs, radiometal–ion chelates, and fluorescent probes [35]. A new class of anticancer compounds have been created that contain both tumor-targeting antibodies and nanoparticles called fullerenes (C60), which can be loaded with several molecules of anticancer drugs like Taxol® [36]. It is possible to load as many as 40 fullerenes into a single skin cancer antibody called ZME-018, which can be used to deliver drugs directly into melanoma tumors. Certain binding sites on the antibody are hydrophobic (water repelling) and attract the hydrophobic fullerenes in large numbers, so multiple drugs can be loaded into a single antibody in a spontaneous manner. No covalent bonds are required, so the increased payload does not significantly change the targeting ability of the antibody. The real advantage of fullerene immunotherapy over other targeted therapeutic agents is likely the fullerene's potential to carry multiple drug payloads, such as Taxol plus other chemotherapeutic drugs. Cancer cells can become drug resistant, and one can cut down on the possibility of their escaping treatment by attacking them with more than one kind of drug at a time. The first fullerene immunoconjugates have been prepared and characterized as an initial step toward the development of fullerene immunotherapy.

7.3 Nanocarriers to Improve Cancer-Targeting Therapy

Various nanomaterials have been used to deliver anticancer drugs and are simply referred to as nanocarriers. This can be passive delivery but other strategies can be combined to use nanocarriers for targeted drug delivery in cancer. One example of this is transforming growth factor (TGF)-β, which plays a pivotal role in the regulation of progression of cancer through effects on tumor microenvironment as well as on cancer cells. TGF-β inhibitors have recently been shown to prevent the growth and metastasis of certain cancers. However, there may be adverse effects caused by TGF-β signaling inhibition, including the induction of cancers by the repression of TGF-β-mediated growth inhibition. A short-acting, small-molecule TGF-β type I receptor (TR-I) inhibitor has been used at a low dose in treating several experimental intractable solid tumors, including pancreatic adenocarcinoma and diffuse-type gastric cancer, characterized by hypovascularity and thick fibrosis in tumor microenvironments [37]. Low-dose TR-I inhibitor altered neither TGF-β signaling in cancer cells nor the amount of fibrotic components. However, it decreased pericyte coverage of the endothelium without reducing endothelial area specifically in tumor neovasculature and promoted accumulation of macromolecules, including anticancer nanocarriers, in the tumors. Compared with the absence of TGF-β-I inhibitor, anticancer nanocarriers exhibited potent growth-inhibitory effects on these cancers in the presence of TR-I inhibitor. The use of TR-I inhibitor combined with nanocarriers may thus be of significant clinical and practical importance in treating intractable solid cancers.

7.4 Gold Nanoparticles for Targeted Drug Delivery in Cancer

The unique chemical properties of colloidal gold make it a promising targeted delivery approach for drugs or genes to specific cells. The physical and chemical properties of colloidal gold permit more than one protein molecule to bind to a single particle of colloidal gold. Tumor necrosis factor (TNF)-α can be bound to gold nanocrystals and targeted effectively to tumors in experimental animals following intravenous delivery. The cytotoxicity of TNF-α is confined to the tumor and normal tissues are spared. Anticancer drugs based on this technology are in preclinical development.

Biocompatible and nontoxic pegylated gold nanoparticles with surface-enhanced Raman scattering (SERS) have been used for in vivo tumor targeting and detection [38]. These pegylated SERS nanoparticles are considerably brighter than semiconductor QDs with light emission in the near-infrared window. When conjugated to tumor-targeting ligands such as single-chain variable fragment antibodies, the conjugated nanoparticles are able to target tumor biomarkers such as epithelial growth factor receptors (EGFRs) on human cancer cells and in xenograft tumor models.

7.5 Carbon Nanotubes for Targeted Drug Delivery to Cancer Cells

An improved delivery scheme for intracellular tracking and anticancer therapy uses a novel double functionalization of a carbon nanotube delivery system containing antisense oligodeoxynucleotides as a therapeutic gene and CdTe QDs as fluorescent labeling probes via electrostatically layer-by-layer assembling [39].

Chemically functionalized single-wall carbon nanotubes (SWCNTs) have shown promise in tumor-targeted accumulation in mice and exhibit biocompatibility, excretion, and little toxicity. The anticancer drug paclitaxel (PTX) has been conjugated to branched PEG chains on SWCNTs via a cleavable ester bond to obtain a water-soluble SWCNT–PTX conjugate [40]. SWCNT–PTX is more efficient than Taxol in suppressing tumor growth in a murine 4T1 breast cancer model, owing to prolonged blood circulation and 10-fold higher tumor PTX uptake by SWCNT delivery, likely through enhanced permeability and retention. Drug molecules carried into the reticuloendothelial system are released from SWCNTs and excreted via biliary pathway without toxic effects on normal organs. Thus, nanotube drug delivery is promising for enhancing treatment efficacy and minimizing side effects of cancer therapy with low drug doses. Water-dispersed carbon nanohorns (similar to nanotubes), prepared by adsorption of polyethylene glycol–doxorubicin conjugate (PEG–DOX) onto oxidized single-wall carbon nanohorns, have been shown to be effective anticancer drug delivery carriers when administered intratumorally to human non-small cell lung cancer-bearing mice [41]. There was significant retardation of tumor growth associated with prolonged DOX retention in the tumor.

Although considerable further work is required before any new drugs based on carbon nanotubes are developed, it is hoped that it will eventually lead to more effective treatments for cancer. However, it is too early to claim whether carbon-based nanomaterials will become clinically viable tools to combat cancer, although there is definitely room for them to complement existing technologies.

7.6 Polymersomes for Targeted Cancer Drug Delivery

Polymersomes, hollow-shell nanoparticles, have unique properties that allow them to deliver two distinct drugs, paclitaxel and doxorubicin, directly to tumors implanted in mice [42]. Loading, delivery, and cytosolic uptake of drug mixtures from degradable polymersomes are shown to exploit both the thick membrane of these block copolymer vesicles and their aqueous lumen as well as pH-triggered release within endolysosomes. Drug-delivering polymersomes break down in the acidic environment of the cancer cells resulting in targeted release of these drugs within tumor cells. While cell membranes and liposomes (vesicles often used for drug delivery) are created from a double layer of fatty molecules called phospholipids, a polymersome is composed of two layers of synthetic polymers.

The individual polymers are degradable and considerably larger than individual phospholipids but have many of the same chemical features. The large polymers making up the shell allow paclitaxel, which is water insoluble, to embed within the shell. Doxorubicin, which is water soluble, stays within the interior of the polymersome until it degrades. The polymersome and drug combination is self-assembling as the structure spontaneously forms when all of the components are suitably mixed together. Recent studies have shown that cocktails of paclitaxel and doxorubicin lead to better tumor regression than either drug alone, but previously there was no carrier system that could carry both drugs efficiently to a tumor. Polymersomes get around those limitations.

Another approach is by assembling diverse bioactive agents, such as DNA, proteins, and drug molecules, into core–shell multifunctional polymeric nano-particles (PNPs) that can be internalized in human breast cancer cells [43]. Using ring-opening metathesis polymerization, block copolymers containing small-molecule drug segments and tosylated hexaethylene glycol segments were prepared and assembled into PNPs that allowed for the surface conjugation of single-stranded DNA sequences and/or tumor-targeting antibodies. The result-ing antibody-functionalized particles were readily uptaken by breast cancer cells that overexpressed the corresponding antigens.

7.7 Polymer Nanoparticles for Targeted Drug Delivery in Prostate Cancer

A prostate-specific, locally delivered gene therapy has been developed for the targeted killing of prostate cells using C32/DT-A, a degradable polymer nano-particulate system, to deliver a diphtheria toxin suicide gene (DT-A) driven by a prostate-specific promoter to cells [44]. These nanoparticles were directly injected to the normal prostate and to prostate tumors in mice. Nearly 50% of normal prostates showed a significant reduction in size, attributable to cellular apopto-sis, whereas injection with naked DT-A-encoding DNA had little effect. A single injection of C32/DT-A nanoparticles triggered apoptosis in 80% of tumor cells present in the tissue. It is expected that multiple nanoparticle injections would trigger a greater percentage of prostate tumor cells to undergo apoptosis. These results suggest that local delivery of polymer/DT-A nanoparticles may have application in the treatment of benign prostatic hypertrophy and prostate can-cer. Nonviral gene delivery using nanoparticles avoids the undesirable effects of viral vectors and has a higher transfection rate of tumor cells.

7.8 Use of Nanoparticles for Drug Delivery in Glioblastoma Multiforme

Treatment of glioblastoma multiforme (GBM), a primary malignant tumor of the brain, is one of the most challenging problems as no currently available treatment is curative. The currently available anticancer therapeutics have less than optimal usefulness for GBM mainly because of delivery problems to the tumor. Nanotechnology-based methods have been shown to enhance the delivery of therapeutic substances to GBM by improving targeting, passage across BBB, controlled release, and by reducing the amount of anticancer drugs required for effectiveness with resulting reduction in toxic adverse effects [45]. Several types of nanoparticles have been used to enhance drug delivery to GBM but liposome-based methods are considered to be among the promising methods. Superparamagnetic iron oxide particles can be used in conjunction with MRI to localize the tumor as well as for subsequent thermoablation. Further research in nanobiotechnology-based delivery methods will be required as innovative methods for treatment of GBM are in development.

7.9 Nanoparticle-Based Anticancer Drug Delivery to Overcome MDR

Although multidrug resistance (MDR) is known to develop through a variety of molecular mechanisms within the tumor cell, many tend to converge toward the alteration of apoptotic signaling. The enzyme glucosylceramide synthase (GCS), responsible for bioactivation of the proapoptotic mediator ceramide to a nonfunctional moiety glucosylceramide, is overexpressed in many MDR tumor types and has been implicated in cell survival in the presence of chemotherapy.

A study has investigated the therapeutic strategy of coadministering ceramide with paclitaxel in an attempt to restore apoptotic signaling and overcome MDR in the human ovarian cancer cell line using modified poly(ϵ-caprolactone) (PEO–PCL) nanoparticles to encapsulate and deliver the therapeutic agents for enhanced efficacy [46]. Results show that indeed the complete population of MDR cancer cells can be eradicated by this approach. Moreover, with nanoparticle drug delivery, the MDR cells can be resensitized to a dose of paclitaxel near the IC50 of non-MDR (drug sensitive) cells, indicating a 100-fold increase in chemosensitization via this approach. Molecular analysis of activity verified the hypothesis that the efficacy of this therapeutic approach is due to a restoration in apoptotic signaling, although the beneficial properties of PEO–PCL nanoparticle delivery enhanced the therapeutic success even further, showing the promising potential for the clinical use of this therapeutic strategy to overcome MDR.

8 Nanoparticles Adjuncts to Physical Methods of Cancer Therapy

Several physical methods of therapy are used in cancer besides radiotherapy. These include photodynamic therapy, lasers, ultrasound, and thermotherapy.

8.1 Nanoparticles as Adjuncts to Photodynamic Therapy of Cancer

Photodynamic therapy (PDT) uses light-activated drugs called photosensitizers to treat a range of diseases characterized by rapidly growing tissues, including the formation of abnormal blood vessels, such as cancer, and age-related macular degeneration. Some new developments in the use of nanoparticles in PDT are described in this section.

A nanocarrier consisting of polymeric micelles of diacylphospholipid–poly(ethylene glycol) (PE–PEG) coloaded with the photosensitizer drug 2-[1-hexyloxyethyl]-2-devinyl pyropheophorbide-a (HPPH) and magnetic Fe_3O_4 nanoparticles has been used for guided drug delivery together with light-activated photodynamic therapy for cancer [47]. The nanocarrier shows excellent stability and activity over several weeks. The loading efficiency of HPPH is practically unaffected upon coloading with the magnetic nanoparticles, and its phototoxicity is retained. The magnetic response of the nanocarriers was demonstrated by their magnetically directed delivery to tumor cells in vitro. The magnetophoretic control on the cellular uptake provides enhanced imaging and phototoxicity. These multifunctional nanocarriers demonstrate the exciting prospect offered by nanochemistry for targeting photodynamic therapy.

In a novel nanoformulation for PDT of cancer, the photosensitizer molecules are covalently incorporated into organically modified silica (ORMOSIL) nanoparticles [48]. The incorporated photosensitizer molecules retain their spectroscopic and functional properties and can robustly generate cytotoxic singlet oxygen molecules upon photoirradiation. The synthesized nanoparticles are of ultralow size (approximately 20 nm) and are highly monodispersed and stable in aqueous suspension. The advantage offered by this covalently linked nanofabrication is that the drug is not released during systemic circulation, which is often a problem with physical encapsulation. These nanoparticles are also avidly taken up by tumor cells in vitro and demonstrate phototoxic action, thereby improving the diagnosis as well as PDT of cancer.

8.2 Ultrasonic Tumor Imaging and Targeted Chemotherapy by Nanobubbles

Drug delivery in polymeric micelles combined with tumor irradiation by ultrasound results in effective drug targeting, but this technique requires prior tumor imaging. A new targeted drug delivery method uses ultrasound to image tumors, while also releasing the drug from nanobubbles into the tumor [49]. Mixtures of drug-loaded polymeric micelles and perfluoropentane (PFP) nanobubbles stabilized by the same biodegradable block copolymer were prepared. Size distribution of nanoparticles was measured by dynamic light scattering. Cavitation activity (oscillation, growth, and collapse of microbubbles) under ultrasound was assessed based on the changes in micelle/nanobubble volume ratios. The effect of the nanobubbles on the ultrasound-mediated cellular uptake of doxorubicin (DOX) in MDA MB231 breast tumors in vitro and in vivo (in mice bearing xenograft tumors) was determined by flow cytometry. Phase state and nanoparticle sizes were sensitive to the copolymer/perfluoro-carbon volume ratio. At physiological temperatures, nanodroplets converted into nanobubbles. Doxorubicin was localized in the nanobubble walls formed by the block copolymer. Upon intravenous injection into mice, DOX-loaded micelles and nanobubbles extravasated selectively into the tumor interstitium, where the nanobubbles coalesced to produce microbubbles. When exposed to ultrasound, the bubbles generated echoes, which made it possible to image the tumor. The sound energy from the ultrasound popped the bubbles, releasing DOX, which enhanced intracellular uptake by tumor cells in vitro to a statisti-cally significant extent relative to that observed with unsonicated nanobubbles and unsonicated micelles and resulted in tumor regression in the mouse model. In conclusion, multifunctional nanoparticles that are tumor-targeted drug carriers, long-lasting ultrasound contrast agents, and enhancers of ultrasound-mediated drug delivery have been developed and deserve further exploration as cancer therapeutics.

8.3 Nanobomb for Cancer

Nanobombs are tiny bombs on nanoscale, which are selective, localized, and minimally invasive. Like cluster bombs, they start exploding one after another once they are exposed to light and the resulting heat. The nanobomb holds great promise as a therapeutic agent for killing cancer cells, particularly breast cancer cells, because its shock wave kills the cancerous cells as well as the biological pathways that carry instructions to generate additional cancerous cells and the small blood vessels that nourish the tumor. Its effect can be spread over a wide area to create structural damage to the surrounding cancer cells. In another approach, Nanoclusters (gold nanobombs) can be activated in cancer cells only by confining near-infrared laser pulse energy within the critical mass of the nanoparticles in the nanocluster [10]. Once the nanobombs are exploded and kill cancer cells, macrophages can effectively clear the cell debris and the exploded nanotube along with it.

8.4 Thermotherapy of Prostate Cancer Using Magnetic Nanoparticles

Thermotherapy using biocompatible superparamagnetic nanoparticles has been evaluated in a phase 1 trial patients with locally recurrent prostate cancer [50]. The magnetic fluid was injected transperineally into the prostates and hyperthermic to thermoablative temperatures were achieved in the prostates at 25% of the available magnetic field strength, indicating a significant potential for higher temperatures. Another study has used monoclonal antibody-linked iron oxide magnetic nanoparticles to evaluate nanoparticle thermotherapy of human prostate cancer cell line by heating the magnetic component of the probes through an externally applied alternating magnetic field [51]. The study also explored the potential enhancement of the anticancer effect through added external beam radiation therapy because both forms of treatment have a different, and potentially complementary, mechanism of causing cell death. Results showed that nanoparticle thermotherapy applied as a single modality caused cell death that correlated with total heat dose estimation. Because complete cell death occurred with this approach alone, enhancement of the effect through the addition of external beam radiation therapy could not be addressed.

In vitro studies have demonstrated that gold nanorods are novel contrast agents for both molecular imaging and photothermal cancer therapy [52]. Nanorods are synthesized and conjugated to anti-EGFR monoclonal antibodies (MAbs) and incubated in cancer cell cultures. The anti-EGFR antibody-conjugated nanorods bind specifically to the surface of the malignant-type cells with a much higher affinity due to the overexpressed EGFR on the cytoplasmic membrane of the malignant cells. As a result of the strongly scattered red light from gold nanorods in dark field, observed using a laboratory microscope, the malignant cells are clearly visualized and diagnosed from the nonmalignant cells. It is found that, after exposure to continuous red laser at 800 nm, malignant cells require about half the laser energy to be photothermally destroyed than the nonmalignant cells. Thus, both efficient cancer cell diagnostics and selective photothermal therapy are realized at the same time. To ensure accumulation of nanoparticles in neoplastic tissue, targeting ligands such as antibodies and targeted gene therapy vectors are being incorporated into the nanoparticles, which act as thermal scalpels upon laser irradiation and destroy tumor tissue [53].

8.5 Application of Nanoparticles in Boron Neutron Capture Therapy

Boron neutron capture therapy (BNCT) offers a potential method for localized destruction of tumor cells. The technology is based on the nuclear reaction between thermal neutrons and boron-10 (10B) to yield alpha particles and lithium-7 nuclei. The destructive effect of this reaction is limited to a range of about the diameter of a single cell. In order for BNCT to be effective in cancer therapy, there must be selective delivery of an adequate concentration of 10B to tumors. Various types of antibodies as well as epidermal growth factor have been utilized to investigate receptor-mediated boron delivery; however, in vivo studies have demonstrated that only a small percentage of the total administered dose actually accumulates in tumors, while high concentrations end up in the liver. Interest in classical BCNT faded because of the lack of efficacy but new strategies have been employed to enhance the effect of BNCT including the use of nanoparticles. The use of dendrimers as boron carriers for antibody conjugation is based on their well-defined structure and multivalency. Boronated PAMAM dendrimers have been designed to target the epidermal growth factor receptor, a cell surface receptor that is frequently overexpressed in brain tumor cells. Preclinical evaluation has been described of a multipurpose STARBURST PAMAM (polyamidoamine) dendrimer prototype (Dendritic Nanotechnologies Inc.) that exhibits properties suitable (i) for use as targeted, diagnostic MRI/near-infrared contrast agents and/or (ii) for controlled delivery of cancer therapies [54]. The lead candidate is 1,4-diaminobutane, a dendritic nanostructure ~5 nm in diameter, which was selected on the basis of a very favorable biocompatibility profile on in vitro studies, i.e., benign and nonimmunogenic.

9 Nanobiotechnology-Based Aids to Cancer Surgery

Several applications of nanobiotechnology in cancer surgery include the use of nanoparticles to visualize tumor during surgery as aid to proper removal.

9.1 Lymph Node Mapping in Cancer

Sentinel lymph node (SLN) mapping is a common procedure used to identify the presence of cancer in a single, "sentinel" lymph node, thus avoiding the removal of a patient's entire lymph system. Effective and rapid (few minutes) detection of SLN using fluorescent imaging of QDs has been demonstrated in experimental animals and is relevant to axillary lymph node dissection during surgery of breast cancer [55]. The use of QD imaging is a significant improvement over the dye/radioactivity method currently used to perform SLN mapping, enabling the surgeon to see not only the lymph nodes but also the underlying anatomy. The imaging system and QDs allow the pathologist to focus on specific parts of the SLN that would be most likely to contain malignant cells, if cancer were present. The imaging system and QDs minimize inaccuracies and permit real-time confirmation of the total removal of the target lymph nodes, drastically reducing the potential for repeated procedures.

SLN mapping has already revolutionized cancer surgery. Near-infrared QDs have the potential to improve this important technique even further. Because the QDs in the study are composed of heavy metals, which can be toxic, they have not yet been approved for use in humans. The next step is to develop QDs that can be used safely in human trials.

9.2 Nanotechnology-Based Devices as Aids to the Detection of Cancer During Surgery

Cancer surgeons are faced with the difficult task of knowing where to stop cutting when removing cancer cells in the body. Sensor nanodevices for detection can attain resolution of ~ 20 μm or even less. As this dimension is comparable to single cell dimension, it may be possible to see a single cancer cell in a tissue. High-resolution thermal imaging devices and ultrasound detector might provide a much better image resolution to enable detection of malignant tumors at early stages.

10 Nanobiotechnology for the Management of Metastatic Cancer

Early detection of metastases plays an important role in the management of metastatic cancer. In patients with prostate cancer who undergo surgical lymph node resection or biopsy, MRI with lymphotropic superparamagnetic nanoparticles can correctly identify all patients with nodal metastases. This diagnosis is not possible with conventional MRI alone and has implications for the management of men with metastatic prostate cancer, in whom adjuvant androgen-deprivation therapy with radiation is the mainstay of management.

Nanoparticle formulations of anticancer drugs may be more effective against cancer metastases. Oral administration of α-TEA formulated in liposome or biodegradable poly(D, L-lactide-co-glycolide) nanoparticle has been shown to significantly reduce tumor burden in a mammary cancer mouse model [56]. Both formulations reduced lymph node and lung micrometastatic tumor foci, but nanoparticle formulation was more effective in reducing metastases. Tumor targeting with nanoparticles facilitates systemic delivery of immunomodulatory cytokine genes to remote sites of cancer metastasis. Targeted delivery and localized expression of the intravenously administered nanoparticles bearing the gene encoding granulocyte/macrophage colony-stimulating factor was confirmed in a patient with metastatic cancer, as was the recruitment of significant tumor-infiltrating lymphocytes [57].

11 Role of Nanobiotechnology in Personalized Cancer Therapy

Personalized medicine simply means the prescription of specific therapeutics best suited for an individual. It is usually based on pharmacogenetic, pharmacogenomic, and pharmacoproteomic information but other individual variations in patients are also taken into consideration. In case of cancer, the variation in behavior of cancer of the same histological type from one patient to another is also taken into consideration. Nanodiagnostics have also improved diagnosis of cancer, which is an important basis of personalized treatment.

Nanobiotechnology is facilitating the discovery of molecular biomarkers that are used to predict disease development, prognosis, and monitoring of treatment in individual patients. Personalized oncology is based on a better understanding of the cancer at the molecular level and nanotechnology will play an important role in this area [58]. An example is QDs conjugated with monoclonal anti-HER2 antibody (Trastuzumab), which can be used for single molecular in vivo imaging of breast cancer cells in a 3D microscopic system [59]. Cancer cells expressing HER2 protein can be visualized by the nanoparticles in vivo at subcellular resolution, enabling personalized decision on chemotherapy based on HER2-positive or HER2-negative status of the tumor.

Nanoparticle-based diagnosis combined with targeted delivery of appropriate anticancer therapy enables personalized treatment of a tumor sparing the patient of systemic toxicity and obviating the need for pharmacogenetic testing. With numerous nanotechnologies available for drug delivery, computational mathematical tools are recommended for selection of nanovectors, surface modifications, therapeutic agents, and penetration enhancers for optimal use in a multistage-targeted drug delivery of chemotherapeutic drugs to a tumor leading to significant improvements in therapy efficacy and reduced systemic toxicity [60]. Such an approach can be optimized for personalized oncology.

12 Concluding Remarks and Future Prospects

The basic rationale for using nanobiotechnology in oncology is that nanoparticles have optical, magnetic, or structural properties that are not available from larger molecules or bulk solids. When linked with tumor-targeting ligands such as MAbs, peptides, or small molecules, these nanoparticles can be used to target tumor antigens (biomarkers) as well as tumor vasculatures with high affinity and specificity [61]. In the size range of 5–100 nm diameter, nanoparticles have large surface areas and functional groups for conjugating to multiple diagnostic and therapeutic anticancer agents.

Recent advances have led to bioaffinity nanoparticle probes for molecular and cellular imaging, targeted nanoparticle drugs for cancer therapy, and integrated nanodevices for early cancer detection and screening. Another important role of nanoparticles is in integrating diagnosis and treatment of cancer. These developments have provided opportunities for personalized oncology in which biomarkers are used to diagnose and treat cancer based on the molecular profiles of individual patients. Nanobiotechnology has also provided refinements in aids to surgery of cancer and for guidance of thorough extirpation of cancer.

Further improvements in QD technology will refine identification of metastatic cancer cells, enable quantification of the level of specific molecular targets, and guide targeted cancer therapy by providing biodynamic biomarkers for target inhibition [62].

References

1. Jain KK. *A Handbook of Nanomedicine*. Humana/Springer, Totowa, NJ, 2008.
2. Jain KK. Recent Advances in Nanooncology. *Technol Cancer Res Treat* 2008; **7**: 1–13.
3. Jain KK. Applications of Nanobiotechnology in Clinical Diagnostics. *Clin Chem* 2007; **53**: 2002–2009.
4. Jain KK. Role of nanobiotechnology in drug discovery. In: Guzman CA, Feuerstein G (eds) *Pharmaceutical Biotechnology*. Austin, TX, Landes Press, 2009.
5. Jain KK. Nanotechnology-based drug delivery for cancer. *Technol Cancer Res Treat* 2005; **4**: 407–416.
6. Jain KK. Cancer Biomarkers: Current issues and future directions. *Curr Opin Mol Ther* 2007; **9**: 563–571.
7. Zheng G, Patolsky F, Cui Y, et al. Multiplexed electrical detection of cancer markers with nanowire sensor arrays. *Nat Biotechnol* 2005; **23**: 1294–1301.
8. Singer EM, Smith SS. Nucleoprotein Assemblies for Cellular Biomarker Detection. *Nano Lett* 2006; **6**: 1184–1189.
9. Jain KK. *Nanobiotechnology: Applications, Markets and Companies*. Basel, Jain Pharma-Biotech, 2009.
10. Zharov VP, Galitovskaya EN, Johnson C, Kelly T. Synergistic enhancement of selective nanophotothermolysis with gold nanoclusters: Potential for cancer therapy. *Lasers Surg Med* 2005; **37**: 219–226.
11. Li J, Wang X, Wang C, et al. The enhancement effect of gold nanoparticles in drug delivery and as biomarkers of drug-resistant cancer cells. *ChemMedChem* 2007; **2**: 374–378.
12. Jain PK, Huang X, El-Sayed IH, El-Sayed MA. Noble metals on the nanoscale: Optical and photothermal properties and some applications in imaging, sensing, biology, and medicine. *Acc Chem Res* 2008c May 1; doi:10.1021/ar7002804.
13. Wu Q, Cao H, Luan Q, et al. Biomolecule-assisted synthesis of water-soluble silver nanoparticles and their biomedical applications. *Inorg Chem* 2008; **47**: 5882–5888.
14. Bagalkot V, Zhang L, Levy-Nissenbaum E, et al. Quantum Dot-Aptamer Conjugates for Synchronous Cancer Imaging, Therapy, and Sensing of Drug Delivery Based on Bi-Fluorescence Resonance Energy Transfer. *Nano Lett* 2007; **7**: 3065–3070.
15. Yu X, Munge B, Patel V, et al. Carbon nanotube amplification strategies for highly sensitive immunodetection of cancer biomarkers. *J Am Chem Soc* 2006; **128**: 11199–11205.
16. Bianco A, Kostarelos K, Prato M. Opportunities and challenges of carbon-based nano-materials for cancer therapy. *Expert Opin Drug Deliv* 2008; **5**: 331–342.
17. Hampel S, Kunze D, Haase D, et al. Carbon nanotubes filled with a chemotherapeutic agent: a nanocarrier mediates inhibition of tumor cell growth. *Nanomedicine* 2008; **3**: 175–182.
18. Reddy GR, Bhojani MS, McConville P, et al. Vascular targeted nanoparticles for imaging and treatment of brain tumors. *Clin Cancer Res* 2006; **12**: 6677–6686.
19. Simberg D, Duza T, Park JH, et al. Biomimetic amplification of nanoparticle homing to tumors. *Proc Natl Acad Sci* 2007; **104**: 932–936.
20. Rabin O, Manuel Perez J, Grimm J. An X-ray computed tomography imaging agent based on long-circulating bismuth sulphide nanoparticles. *Nat Mater* 2006; **5**: 118–122.
21. Gao D, Xu H, Philbert MA, et al. Ultrafine Hydrogel Nanoparticles: Synthetic Approach and Therapeutic Application in Living Cells. *Angew Chem Int Ed Engl* 2007; **46**: 2224–2227.
22. Choi J, Jun Y, Yeon S, et al. Biocompatible Heterostructured Nanoparticles for Multi-modal Biological Detection. *JACS* 2006; **128**: 5982–15983.
23. Talanov VS, Regino CA, Kobayashi H, et al. Dendrimer-based nanoprobe for dual modality magnetic resonance and fluorescence imaging. *Nano Lett* 2006; **6**: 1459–1463.
24. Koster DA, Palle K, Bot ES, et al. Antitumour drugs impede DNA uncoiling by topoisomerase I. *Nature* 2007; **448**: 213–217.

25. Roovers RC, Laeremans T, Huang L, et al. Efficient inhibition of EGFR signaling and of tumour growth by antagonistic anti-EFGR Nanobodies. *Cancer Immunol Immunother* 2007; 56: 303–317.

26. Gao X, Dave SR. Quantum dots for cancer molecular imaging. *Adv Exp Med Biol* 2007; **620**: 57–73.

27. Koo OM, Rubinstein I, Onyuksel H. Camptothecin in sterically stabilized phospholipid nano-micelles: A novel solvent pH change solubilization method. *J Nanosci Nanotechnol* 2006; **6**: 2996–3000.

28. Geng Y, Dalhaimer P, Cai S, et al. Shape effects of filaments versus spherical particles in flow and drug delivery. *Nat Nanotech* 2007; **2**: 249–255.

29. Sutton D, Nasongkla N, Blanco E, Gao J. Functionalized Micellar Systems for Cancer Targeted Drug Delivery. *Pharmaceutical Res* 2007; **24**: 1029–1046.

30. Lu J, Liong M, Zink JI, Tamanoi F. Mesoporous silica nanoparticles as a delivery system for hydrophobic anticancer drugs. *Small* 2007; **3**: 1341–1346.

31. MacDiarmid JA, Mugridge NB, Weiss JC, et al. Bacterially Derived 400 nm Particles for Encapsulation and Cancer Cell Targeting of Chemotherapeutics. *Cancer Cell* 2007; 11: 431–445.

32. Wagner E. Programmed drug delivery: Nanosystems for tumor targeting. *Expert Opin Biol Ther* 2007; **7**: 587–593.

33. Radosz M, Shen Y, Tang H. *Nanoparticles for Cytoplasmic Drug Delivery to Cancer Cells.* Patent #WO/2007/001356, Publication Date 4 January 2007.

34. Lee CC, Gillies ER, Fox ME. A single dose of doxorubicin-functionalized bow-tie dendrimer cures mice bearing C-26 colon carcinomas. *Proc Natl Acad Sci* 2006; **103**: 16649–16654.

35. McDevitt MR, Chattopadhyay D, Kappel BJ, et al. Tumor targeting with antibody-functionalized, radiolabeled carbon nanotubes. *J Nucl Med* 2007; **48**: 1180–1189.

36. Ashcroft JM, Tsyboulski DA, Hartman KB, et al. Fullerene (C60) immunoconjugates: Interaction of water-soluble C60 derivatives with the murine anti-gp240 melanoma antibody. *Chem Commun* 2006; **28**: 3004–3006.

37. Kano MR, Bae Y, Iwata C, et al. Improvement of cancer-targeting therapy, using nanocarriers for intractable solid tumors by inhibition of TGF-{beta} signaling. *Proc Natl Acad Sci* 2007; **104**: 3460–3465.

38. Qian X, Peng XH, Ansari DO, et al. In vivo tumor targeting and spectroscopic detection with surface-enhanced Raman nanoparticle tags. *Nat Biotech* 2008; **26**: 83–90.

39. Jia N, Lian Q, Shen H, et al. Intracellular delivery of quantum dots tagged antisense oligodeoxynucleotides by functionalized multiwalled carbon nanotubes. *Nano Lett* 2007; **7**: 2976–2980.

40. Liu Z, Chen K, Davis C, et al. Drug delivery with carbon nanotubes for in vivo cancer treatment. *Cancer Res* 2008; **68**: 6652–6660.

41. Murakami T, Sawada H, Tamura G, et al. Water-dispersed single-wall carbon nanohorns as drug carriers for local cancer chemotherapy. *Nanomed* 2008; **3**: 453–463.

42. Ahmed F, Pakunlu RI, Srinivas G, et al. Shrinkage of a rapidly growing tumor by drug-loaded polymersomes: pH-triggered release through copolymer degradation. *Mol Pharm* 2006; **3**: 340–350.

43. Bertin PA, Gibbs JM, Shen CK, et al. Multifunctional polymeric nanoparticles from diverse bioactive agents. *J Am Chem Soc* 2006; **128**: 4168–4169.

44. Peng W, Anderson DG, Bao Y, et al. Nanoparticulate delivery of suicide DNA to murine prostate and prostate tumors. *Prostate* 2007; **67**: 855–862.

45. Jain KK. Use of nanoparticles for drug delivery in glioblastoma multiforme. *Expert Rev Neurother* 2007; **7**: 363–372.

46. van Vlerken LE, Duan Z, Seiden MV, Amiji MM. Modulation of intracellular ceramide using polymeric nanoparticles to overcome multidrug resistance in cancer. *Cancer Res* 2007; **67**: 4843–4850.

47. Cinteza LO, Ohulchanskyy TY, Sahoo Y, et al. Diacyllipid Micelle-Based Nanocarrier for Magnetically Guided Delivery of Drugs in Photodynamic Therapy. *Mol Pharm* 2006; **3**: 415–423.
48. Ohulchanskyy TY, Roy I, Goswami LN, Organically modified silica nanoparticles with covalently incorporated photosensitizer for photodynamic therapy of cancer. *Nano Lett* 2007; **7**: 2835–2842.
49. Rapoport N, Gao Z, Kennedy A. Multifunctional Nanoparticles for Combining Ultrasonic Tumor Imaging and Targeted Chemotherapy. *J Natl Cancer Inst* 2007; **99**: 1095–1106.
50. Johannsen M, Gneveckow U, Thiesen B, et al. Thermotherapy of prostate cancer using magnetic nanoparticles: Feasibility, imaging, and three-dimensional temperature distribution. *Eur Urol* 2007; **52**: 1653–1661.
51. Lehmann J, Natarajan A, Denardo GL, et al. Short communication: nanoparticle thermotherapy and external beam radiation therapy for human prostate cancer cells. *Cancer Biother Radiopharm* 2008; **23**: 265–271.
52. Huang X, El-Sayed IH, Qian W, El-Sayed MA. Cancer cell imaging and photothermal therapy in the near-infrared region by using gold nanorods. *J Am Chem Soc* 2006; **128**: 2115–2120.
53. Everts M. Thermal scalpel to target cancer. *Expert Rev Med Devices* 2007; **4**: 131–136.
54. Tomalia DA, Reyna LA, Svenson S. Dendrimers as multi-purpose nanodevices for oncology drug delivery and diagnostic imaging. *Biochem Soc Trans* 2007; **35**: 61–67.
55. Robe A, Pic E, Lassalle HP, et al. Quantum dots in axillary lymph node mapping: Biodistribution study in healthy mice. *BMC Cancer* 2008; **8**: 111.
56. Wang P, Jia L, Sanders BG, Kline K. Liposomal or nanoparticle alpha-TEA reduced 66 cl-4 murine mammary cancer burden and metastasis. *Drug Deliv* 2007; **14**: 497–505.
57. Gordon EM, Levy JP, Reed RA, et al. Targeting metastatic cancer from the inside: A new generation of targeted gene delivery vectors enables personalized cancer vaccination in situ. *Int J Oncol* 2008; **33**: 665–675.
58. Jain KK. Role of nanobiotechnology in developing personalized medicine for cancer. *Technol Cancer Res Treat* 2005; **4**: 645–650.
59. Takeda M, Tada H, Higuchi H, et al. In vivo single molecular imaging and sentinel node navigation by nanotechnology for molecular targeting drug-delivery systems and tailor-made medicine. *Breast Cancer* 2008; **15**: 145–152.
60. Sakamoto J, Annapragada A, Decuzzi P, Ferrari M. Antibiological barrier nanovector technology for cancer applications. *Expert Opin Drug Deliv* 2007; **4**: 359–369.
61. Nie S, Xing Y, Kim GJ, Simons JW. Nanotechnology Applications in Cancer. *Annu Rev Biomed Eng* 2007; **9**: 12.1–12.32.
62. Zhang H, Yee D, Wang C. Quantum dots for cancer diagnosis and therapy: Biological and clinical perspectives. *Nanomedicine* 2008; **3**: 83–91.

Receptor-Mediated Delivery of Proteins and Peptides to Tumors

Christian Dohmen and Manfred Ogris

1 Introduction

In the last decades, many approaches have been tried for the treatment of cancers. The most common therapies so far are surgery, radiation and chemotherapy or combination thereof. Despite significant improvements, these therapies still lack tumor specificity and can cause severe side effects. Therefore, developing new therapies and methods for cancer treatment is a demanding issue in medical science.

A promising approach is the delivery of proteins and peptides to tumor cells with the aim of reprogramming or their destruction. This method has the advantage of being a well-controllable system: proteins can be modulated to be more stable, less toxic, more specific, and resistant against proteases or in case of enzymes optimized in terms of activity. Due to the controllable half-life of a protein inside a cell, the therapeutic effect can be regulated. State-of-the-art protein chemistry and analysis allows molecular modeling to optimize the protein structure prior to delivery. Due to the advantages of direct protein delivery to tumors, this field gained significant importance as a new approach in tumor therapy. Here, we will discuss all aspects of targeted protein delivery to tumors, including protein/peptide design, general delivery strategies, targeting aspects, and intracellular hurdles for protein delivery. An overview is given for proteins and peptides currently used in preclinical studies; ongoing clinical studies and applications in the clinics are discussed.

2 Protein Expression and Chemical Modifications, Cleavability

To develop a targeted protein delivery system, a functional domain (the therapeutically active protein) has to be connected to a targeting domain, which directs the therapeutic protein to the site of desired action, i.e., tumor tissue. In

M. Ogris (✉)
Pharmaceutical Biology-Biotechnology, Ludwig-Maximilians Universität, München, Germany
e-mail: manfred.ogris@cup.uni-muenchen.de

Y. Lu, R.I. Mahato (eds.), *Pharmaceutical Perspectives of Cancer Therapeutics*, DOI 10.1007/978-1-4419-0131-6_9, © Springer Science+Business Media, LLC 2009

principle, these protein systems can be produced in two ways: either by production and subsequent isolation of recombinant fusion proteins or by covalent coupling of targeting and function domain by means of chemical protein conjugation techniques.

2.1 Recombinant Fusion Proteins

Target proteins can be generated by expressing fusion protein containing the targeting and the effector domain. Depending on the protein expressed and the necessary posttranslational modifications (e.g., glycosylation), this can be accomplished either in bacteria, yeast, or mammalian cells [1]. Potential problems due to protein insolubility and formation of inclusion bodies have to be kept in mind. Attaching a polypeptide fusion partner, termed affinity tag, allows specific purification by affinity chromatography [2]. To minimize the influence of protein fusion on the structure of the two domains and to enable a possible cleavage (see below), a peptidic spacer can be engineered to separate the two fusion partners. A disadvantage of producing fusion proteins is the limited alternative to modulate the system: the two domains can be interconnected only via their N- or C-terminus.

2.2 Chemical Conjugates

An alternative to the molecular biological approach is the chemical conjugation of functional domains. The major advantage is the high flexibility of the system: in principle, any molecule can be attached to a therapeutic protein (for an excellent overview on coupling chemistry, see [3]). The only features required are functional groups suitable for coupling, for example, free N- or C-terminus containing primary amine or carboxy function, respectively. Within the molecule, the epsilon amino group of lysine, free sulfhydryl from cysteine, or specific glycosylation sites can be used for site-specific modification. A plethora of linker molecules exist (reviewed in [4]).

Cross-linking can be achieved either via homo- or heterobifunctional cross-linking. With a symmetric, bifunctional cross-linker, two similar reactive groups present on targeting and effector molecule are linked, e.g., two amines or two sulfhydryl groups. The advantage of this approach is having only one reaction step being necessary for synthesis. The main disadvantage is the occurrence of a mixture of homodimeric (e.g., two targeting molecules) and the desired heterodimeric (targeting and effector function) conjugates. With a heterobifunctional asymmetric linker, two different functional moieties can be linked. For example, 1-ethyl-3- [3-dimethylaminopropyl]carbodiimide hydrochloride (EDC) is a coupling reagent frequently used for coupling effector domains to antibodies forming a stable amide bond between a carboxy group and a primary amine. The reaction is usually carried out in the presence of an activating agent, such as *N*-hydroxysulfosuccinimide (Sulfo-NHS) [5]. *N*-Succinimidyl 3-(2-pyridyldithio)-propionate (SPDP) is a heterobifunctional cross-linker bearing an amine-reactive succinimidyl ester on one end and a protected and activated thiol group (thiopyridyl) on the distal end [6]. With the help of SPDP, free thiol groups (e.g., cysteine residues) can be directly coupled to primary amines via a reducible disulfide bond. A related heterobifunctional linker is sulfosuccinimidyl-4-(*N*-maleimidomethyl)cyclo-hexane-1-carboxylate (Sulfo-SMCC) containing an amine-reactive sulfosuccinimidyl- and a sulfhydryl-reactive maleimide group, which forms a stable thioether bond. When utilizing glycosylated proteins like antibodies or the serum protein transferrin, sugar residues can be oxidized by adding periodate and the resulting aldehyde function reacts with primary amines forming a Schiff base. This bond can be reduced to a more stable amine bond by adding sodium cyanoborohydride. The selectivity of this coupling procedure is insofar of advantage as proteins are specifically coupled via glycosylation sites. Many more coupling strategies have been developed in the recent years and the cross-linking molecules are commercially available [4].

2.3 Designing the Bond

When targeting therapeutic proteins to tumors, bifunctional molecules containing a targeting and a functional domain are generated. Depending on the intracellular function of the protein, cleavability between these two domains is often necessary to enable full functionality of the effector domain. Intracellular cleavage can be achieved in different ways. After receptor-mediated endocytosis, endosomes become acidified to pH below 6. In this case, pH-labile bonds, for example, based on acetals can be utilized [7]. Another approach is harnessing the intracellular redox potential leading to the cleavage of disulfide bonds. Several linker molecules exist, which can be specifically cleaved by ubiquitously present enzymes [8]. Furin, an intracellular peptidase, recognizes the cleavage-site sequence Arg-Xaa-Lys/Arg-Arg [9]. Targeting *Pseudomonas* exotoxin A domain via a Her2 antibody to Her2/neu-overexpressing tumors led to specific cell killing when antibody and toxin were interconnected via a furin-cleavable peptide sequence [10]. Alternative to intracellular cleavage, the toxin can also be released within the tumor matrix to gain full activity: matrix metalloproteinases (MMP) are often overexpressed by tumor cells and responsible for their invasiveness [11]. Generating protein conjugates containing an MMP-cleavable peptide sequence can now lead to tumor site-specific activation of such a conjugate, as it has been shown for PEG-modified liposomes [12]. In any case it has to be kept in mind that, for example, diester and disulfide bonds can also be cleaved in the bloodstream in case of systemic application. This is especially of importance when using long circulating formulation.

3 Delivery Strategies

Reaching tumor tissue can in principle be achieved by two routes of administration: either direct application (intratumoral or topical) or systemic application via the bloodstream. Local application is an issue in case of localized, accessible tumors, like superficial skin melanoma. Delivery of therapeutic proteins in case of metastasized disease or inaccessible tumors can be only achieved via the systemic route. In principle, every solid tumor can be reached via the bloodstream, as above a size of several millimeters, support by the bloodstream with nutrients and oxygen is inevitable and diffusion processes become the limiting factor for further growth. The so-called angiogenic switch induces the formation of blood vessels connecting the tumor tissue to the blood circulation [13]. The main problems are to achieve a certain circulation of proteins in the bloodstream and the necessity of targeting while reducing the nonspecific delivery to other cell types to prevent negative side effects. Within the harsh environment in the bloodstream, proteins and peptides have to be protected against premature degradation. Several delivery concepts have been developed for this purpose. Making the proteins more stable against proteolytic degradation by selectively changing the peptide sequence is one strategy. Alternatively or additionally, proteins and peptides can be covalently modified with hydrophilic polymers to prevent opsonization and subsequent clearance by the reticuloendothelial system (RES). The third option is to generate particulate delivery systems, i.e., where proteins or peptides are encapsulated in micro- or nanometer-sized structures.

3.1 Direct Delivery

The most common way for targeted protein delivery to tumors remains systemic application via the bloodstream. For this purpose, the protein has to withstand the harsh environment in the bloodstream, i.e., attacks by proteases. Approaches to increase the conformational stability of proteins can be applied [14]. Changing the physiological L-amino acids to D-amino acids can prevent proteolytic degradation and hence improve plasma half-life: octreotide, a 14-amino-acid peptide derived from somatostatin, inhibits pancreatic secretion and is used in the treatment of gastrointestinal tumors. Due to rapid degradation in the bloodstream, systemic application was limited and required continuous infusion. When shortening the peptide and changing the amino acid conformation from L- to D- enantiomers, a plasma half-life of 1.5 hours was achieved [15].

3.2 PEGylation

Main reasons for a short blood circulation of proteins are renal filtration and excretion by liver and kidney, aggregation with blood components, enzymatic degradation, and opsonization with subsequent RES clearance. Renal filtration and excretion is size dependent: molecules with a molecular weight of less then

60 kDa are cleared via kidney [16]. To prevent small proteins from filtration and clearance, the simplest way is to increase the molecular weight of the protein/peptide. For this purpose, polymers are covalently coupled to the protein surface. The most frequently used polymer is polyethylene glycol (PEG) [17], a highly water-soluble polymer available within a broad range of molecular weight and different distal reactive groups allowing convenient coupling to proteins and peptides [18]. Conjugation of PEG (also termed PEGylation) strongly improves the pharmacokinetic of attached proteins [16, 19]. Beside the advantages of preventing clearance, PEG also improves the water solubility of the drug to be delivered and protects from proteolytic degradation and aggregation (for review: [20, 21]). Besides N- and C-terminal modification, disulfide bridges can also be used as specific site of PEGylation [22]. When coupling PEG via amine-reactive or thiol-reactive linker, primary amines within the polypeptide chain (ε-amino group in lysine) resp. the terminal sulfhydryl group in cysteine can be modified. This in turn can lead to loss of function due to impaired ligand binding or enzymatic function. To prevent such effects, PEG is attached at a specific site or via a bioreversible cleavable linker. Recombinant interferon-α has been successfully used for treating viral infection and also shows promising antitumoral properties [23, 24]. After systemic application, interferon is rapidly cleared from the bloodstream, whereas the PEGylated version shows significantly improved pharmacokinetic and improved bioactivity in patients [25]. PEG–interferon is now commercialized for hepatitis treatment (Pegasys[®] from Roche). In the latter case, PEGylation is carried out with an amine-reactive PEG molecule also potentially modifying lysine in the peptide chain. Bell and coworkers generated a PEGylated interferon where the PEG chain was specifically attached via a maleinimide group to a genetically modified interferon carrying a cysteine with a free thiol group [26]. Experiments on nude mice xenografted with a subcutaneous human tumor clearly showed that site-specific PEGylated interferon exhibited elevated circulation times in blood (Fig. 1) and stronger antitumoral activity compared to randomly PEGylated interferon.

3.3 Polymers, Scaffolds, Nanoparticles

Therapeutic proteins can be coupled to scaffolds bearing several functional groups. Molecules that can be used as scaffold are, for example, polyamines like polyethylenimine or polyamidoamine (PAMAM) dendrimers, which bear several primary amino groups. This allows coupling of several functional molecules in addition to the therapeutically active protein including shielding, targeting, and endosomal release functions. Alternatively, polymers can be attached to a protein with a negative surface charge by simply mixing in water. Due to its positive surface charge, this leads to cationic particles containing both protein and polycation, which in turn promotes cellular internalization

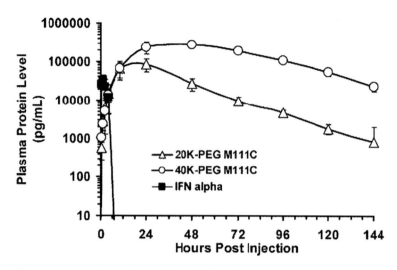

Fig. 1 Plasma concentrations of recombinant IFN-α after subcutaneous injection in rats. Each animal received 100 μg/kg unmodified (*full rectangle*) or PEGylated (20-kDa PEG, *open triangles*, 40-kDa PEG, *open circles*) recombinant IFN-α. Plasma levels of proteins were measured by ELISA (mean±std dev shown for three rats per group). With permission from Ref. [25]

via heparan sulfates (see below). It was recently shown that glutathione S-transferase (GST)-fused proteins could be coupled to polyethylenimine (PEI) carrying several glutathione molecules, which in turn led to efficient transfer of the payload into cells in vitro [27]. Covalent attachment of PEI via 1-ethyl-3-(3-dimethylaminopropyl) carbodiimide hydrochloride (EDC) linker to avidin, streptavidin, and protein G enhanced cellular protein internalization in vitro [28]; in a similar way, PEI-modified fluorescent proteins and antibodies were efficiently internalized [29]. Binding proteins to nondegradable polyamines like PEI also bears the advantage of protecting the protein from degradation.

4 Targeting Strategies

Tumor targeting is based on the principle to distinguish between healthy tissue and malignant tumor tissue. In case of systemic delivery, protein formulations exhibiting a certain blood circulation can efficiently reach tumor tissue and extravasate through the leaky tumor vasculature: Maeda et al. first described this passive accumulation as the enhanced permeability and retention (EPR) effect [30]. Molecules with a molecular weight exceeding the threshold for renal excretion and exhibiting a certain circulation time in blood will passively accumulate in tumor tissue over time. This first phase of tumor targeting is independent of tumor-specific expression of certain tumor markers, and rather due to the tumor architecture. When a solid tumor exceeds a size of 1–2 mm, supply with oxygen and nutrients cannot be accomplished by simple diffusion. At this stage, the so-called angiogenic switch occurs, i.e., tumor cells start to express angiogenic factors resulting in the recruiting of new blood vessels and capillaries to satisfy the increasing demand for nutrients and oxygen [13]. In contrast to normal vasculature, these blood vessels exhibit a leaky architecture and are mosaic like, with endothelial cells and tumor cells forming vessel-like structures [31]. Additionally, solid tumors lack a network of functional lymphatic drainage. For this reason, compounds exceeding a certain molecular weight can enter the tumor through the leaky vasculature but cannot be removed by lymphatic drainage or diffuse out of the tumor like low molecular drugs. This implicates that, if a macromolecular drug is delivered systemically, the concentration inside the tumor rises as long as the blood concentration of the drug is high. When the drug is cleared from circulation, high-molecular-weight particles remain in the tumor [32].

After their accumulation in tumor tissue the macromolecular drugs delivered have to be internalized by the target cells. Besides endothelial and stroma cells, tumor cells are the major target for delivery of therapeutically active proteins and peptides. Targeting internalizing receptors does not always increase the total amount of macromolecular drugs accumulated in the tumor but rather potentiates their biological activity due to internalization into the desired target cells. Internalization can appear by direct transduction or by receptor-mediated endocytosis as shown in Fig. 2.

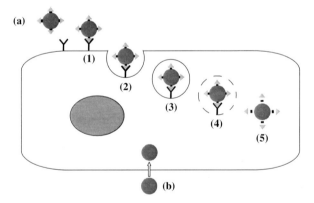

Fig. 2 **Steps in cellular protein delivery**. (a) Receptor-mediated endocytosis; binding of the cell surface receptor (1) is followed by invagination of the plasma membrane (2) and subsequent inclusion into endosomes (3); specific mechanism leading to rupture of the endosome (4) and access to the cytoplasm (5). (b) Protein transduction can also occur in a receptor-independent fashion

4.1 Proteoglycans and Cationic Ligands

Proteoglycans are abundantly expressed on adherent cells and are natural receptors for viruses like adeno-associated virus [33] or pathogenic bacteria [34]. Formulations with a net positive charge based on either polycations or cationic lipids have been mostly used for nucleic acid delivery but are in principle also suitable for protein delivery. It was shown that tumor endothelium has a high preference for binding cationic liposomes [35], whereas with neutral or anionic liposomes, no differences were found between normal and tumor endothelium [36]. It is speculated that a higher density of negative charge on tumor endothelial cells is responsible for such a targeting effect. Proteins can be cationized also by direct chemical modification of their surface: Futami and coworkers cationized negatively charged carboxy groups on the surface of a ribonuclease, which led to subsequent adsorptive endocytosis into target cells [37]. Cationizing the cargo allows to efficiently deliver proteins into a broad range of different adherent cells but can lack specificity in vivo, as systemic application of cationized proteins or particles leads to their opsonization and/or aggregation with blood components and entrapment in the first vascular bed encountered in the lung [38].

4.2 Integrins and Other Targets on Tumor Endothelium

Integrins are a group of transmembrane adhesion proteins expressed in all cell types (except erythrocytes) and act as important mediators of intercellular communication. Exhibiting a heterodimeric structure (usually one alpha sub-unit and one beta subunit) they also play an important role in tumor angiogenesis also [39]. αvβ3 integrin is the natural ligand for vitronectin and upregulated in tumor endothelium. By phage display technique (see below) a short peptide structure, arginine-glycine-aspartic acid (RGD), was found to be highly selective for tumor vasculature [40]. Zavorni and colleagues expressed the highly potent cytokine TNF-α as a fusion protein containing the RGD sequence after intramuscular injection of plasmid DNA into tumor bearing mice [41]. RGD–TNF-α was released into the bloodstream and efficiently targeted to tumor endothelium. In combination with chemotherapy a clear antitumoral effect was observed (Fig. 3). Similarly, NGR–TNF-α was generated to target aminopeptidase-N that is also upregulated in tumor endothelium and certain tumors. Kessler and colleagues generated RGD- or NGR-containing fusion proteins with tissue factor (tF) [42]. Tissue factor, naturally being present on subendothelial cells, leukocytes, and platelets, is a key protein in the initiation of coagulation. When applying recombinant tF as fusion protein with NGR or RGD peptide, thrombotic occlusion of tumor blood vessels was achieved. Only the targeted versions of tF led a therapeutically relevant reduction of tumor growth in nude mice bearing subcutaneous human xenografts.

4.3 Transferrin Receptor

The transferrin receptor (TfR) is ubiquitously expressed in tissues like liver and brain but also upregulated in many solid cancers that have high metabolic

Fig. 3 Effect of melphalan alone or in combination with pTNF or pRGD–TNF on tumor growth in a subcutaneous RMA-T lymphoma model. Tumor-bearing animals were treated with 240 µg of plasmid DNA (intramuscularly) 3 days after tumor implantation. Two days later, mice were treated intraperitoneally with 50 µg of melphalan. Results are presented as means of five animals per group ± std dev. Modified from Ref. [41]

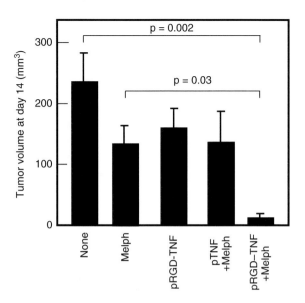

activity and hence the need for iron [43]. Its natural ligand, the plasma protein transferrin (Tf) with a molecular weight of ~79 kDa, belongs to a superfamily of iron-binding glycoproteins and is located in blood, lymph, and cerebrospinal fluid and mainly responsible for iron transport within the organism [44]. The tertiary structure of the peptide chains consists of two homologues subdomains, each one having binding sites for Fe^{3+}. The iron-free apo-Tf forms a large opening, easy to be reached by Fe^{3+}. Binding of two Fe^{3+} ions to the binding pockets leads to a conformational change and strongly increases affinity for Fe^{3+}. The release of Fe^{3+} inside the cell is due to the fast pH drop during endocytosis. Protonation of the amino acids leads to conformational changes and the release of the iron molecule [45]. Following the release of iron, receptor-bound apotransferrin recycles to the cell surface rather than being degraded in lysosomes. The transferrin receptor has been extensively used for targeted drug delivery to tumors, including chemotherapeutics, genes, and proteins [43]. As Tf is a well-soluble plasma protein, drugs coupling to Tf can be advantageous in terms of circulation properties (endogenous Tf has a plasma half-life of 7–10 days) and lack of immune responses against this targeting moiety. In contrast to Tf conjugates, aTfR antibody conjugate does not compete with free Tf for receptor binding and internalization [46]. Applying Tf conjugates containing Tf from the same species will prevent a humoral immune response by the formation of antibodies against Tf, whereas when using aTfR antibodies or Tf from different species, immunogenicity can occur after multiple applications as shown, for example, in a nonhuman primate model using human Tf for targeting [47].

4.4 EGF Receptor

Epidermal growth factor (EGF) is a globular protein of 6.2 kDa consisting of 53 amino acids that binds specifically and with high affinity to the EGF receptor (EGFR) [48]. EGFR, also known as HER1 or ErbB1, belongs to the four members of the ErbB receptor family of receptor tyrosine kinases consisting of an N-terminal extracellular ligand-binding domain, a hydrophobic trans-membrane region, and a cytoplasmic domain that carries tyrosine kinase activity [49]. Proliferation, differentiation, and cell survival of a wide range of cell types are regulated via EGFR. EGF binding induces dimerization of EGFR [50] and the trans-autophosphorylation of tyrosine residues in the cytoplasmic domain of EGFRs, which in turn leads to subsequent internalization of the activated EGFR complex via clathrin-dependent endocytosis [51]. After internalization, receptors can be sorted to recycling endosomes from which they travel back to the cell surface. Alternatively, they can be directed to lysosomes where they are degraded [52]. EGFR is highly upregulated in many solid tumors including glioblastoma, hepatoma, colon and breast carcinoma [53] and is hence a promising target for tumor-directed therapies. Monoclonal antibodies that bind to EGFR and inhibit EGF-EGFR signaling have been developed and are already in clinical use (see below). Targeting of immunostimulatory- and apoptosis-inducing RNA to EGFR-overexpressing glioblastoma cells led to complete tumor eradication in an orthotopic mouse model [54]. Treatment of EGFR-overexpressing tumors in mice with a systemically applied fusion protein consisting of EGF and the plant-derived toxin saporin led specific anti-tumoral activity [55]; in contrast, when applying toxin without EGF domain or fusion toxin in EGFR-nonoverexpressing tumors, the effect was only moderate.

4.5 Folate Receptor

Folate (vitamin B_9) is a low-molecular-weight (441 Da) compound essential in cell proliferation and for the biosynthesis of methionine, serine, deoxythymine acid, and purine. Folate is internalized via two independent pathways: either by transport of folate by the folate receptor or as 5-methyl-tetrahydrofolate by the reduced folate carrier. The expression of folate receptor (FR) in healthy tissue is limited to activated macrophages, placental cells, and the apical surface of polarized epithelia, where it is present in different isoforms [56]. The overexpression of FR on a broad range of solid tumors (ovary, lung, breast, kidney, brain, endometrium, and colon) makes it a suitable target for selective tumor drug delivery (for review, see [57]).

4.6 Other Targeting Strategies

Tumor targeting can be achieved via known, overexpressed surface receptors being more or less specific for tumor tissue or tumor endothelium. Nevertheless, there is still a plethora of potential targets in different tumor types, which could be utilized for drug and protein targeting. A powerful method to discover such potential targets is the phage display technique (for a comprehensive description, see [58]). Phage display libraries consist of 10^9 or more bacteriophages displaying permutated short peptide structures on their surface. Proteins or cells are immobilized to a plastic surface and incubated with the phage library. After removing unbound phages, bound phages are extracted and amplified in host bacteria, hereafter enriched and amplified phages are again incubated with the target and further selected. High-affinity phages are identified after several rounds of selection and their expressed cell-binding peptide sequences identified within the separate phage clones. One of the best known examples is the RGD peptide (see above) being identified by this method, which allows to target drugs to inflamed and tumor endothelium by interacting with integrin $\alpha v\beta 3$.

Aptamers are single-stranded nucleotides, which bind with high affinity and specificity to molecular targets. The technology for aptamer selection is termed SELEX (systematic evolution of ligands by exponential enrichment), where combinatorial libraries of synthetic nucleic acids are exponentially enriched in an iterative process in vitro [59]. A nucleic acid library obtained via combinatorial chemistry contains at least $10^{14}-10^{15}$ different DNA or RNA molecules with a random region flanked on both sides with fixed primer sequences for amplification. As for phage display library, the nucleic acid library is incubated with the target, unbound nucleic acids are removed, bound ones are reisolated, and the selection process is repeated for at least 10 times. After enrichment the library is cloned and sequenced, and individual sequences are investigated for their ability to bind to the target to confirm their specificity. Most recently it was shown that a lysosomal enzyme conjugated to a TfR-specific aptamer was selectively internalized via the TfR [60], pointing out the great potential of this technology for protein targeting to tumors [61]. In addition to nucleotide-based aptamers, peptide aptamers have been developed to target extracellular and intracellular targets in cancer cells (for review, see [62]). Peptide aptamers consist of up to 20 amino acids and are selected from a random peptide library based on phage display technique (see above). Most peptide aptamers are developed against intracellular targets but can in principle also be designed to target surface molecules expressed on tumor cells. For example, designing a peptide aptamer against matrix metalloproteinase 9 (MMP-9) led to specific binding and inactivation of MMP-9, which in turn blocked tumor cell migration and invasion [63]. Nakamura and colleagues developed a 9-amino-acid peptide binding to the EGFR and at the same time inhibiting EGFR-mediated tyrosine phosphorylation [64].

5 Intracellular Fate

Except for direct membrane passage by protein transduction domains (see section below), payload internalized via endocytic pathways still remains entrapped within intracellular vesicle. However, most therapeutically active proteins and peptides have to be released into the cytoplasm and/or have access to the nucleus to gain full functional activity. Viruses and bacteria have developed different peptide-based strategies to evade from endosomes with the help of membrane-active peptide sequences [65] and other "biomimetical" processes.

5.1 Direct Membrane Passage (Protein Transduction)

A natural structure showing direct protein transduction is found in a class of peptides called protein transduction domains (PTD). PTDs are subunits of proteins that naturally transduce cells, i.e., the TAT protein of human immunodeficiency virus 1 (HIV-1) [66], the PTD of VP22, a structural protein of the herpes simplex virus [67], or the antennapedia domain of a Drosophila protein [68]. The transport of peptides and proteins bearing such peptides was reported to be an energy- and temperature-independent process, which led to the theory that such PTDs enable delivery directly into the cell by membrane penetration. Schwarze et al. showed that a protein linked to the TAT domain resulted in cellular delivery in almost all tissues in vivo [69]. Proposing a direct membrane passage of such proteins led to discussions within the scientific community concerning the possibility of artifacts, especially in the case of TAT [70]. It is now a mostly accepted view that cationic PTDs bind the cell surface by electrostatic interaction and are subsequently internalized by lipid raft-dependent macropinocytosis in a temperature- and energy-dependent manner [71]. However, when utilizing cationic amphipathic sequences noncovalently attached to cargo proteins, a direct membrane transition is still discussed [72].

5.2 Endosomal Release

After endocytosis and acidification of endosomes by ATP-dependent proton pumps and fusion with lysosomes, proteins are prone to proteolytic degradation. Hence, release from the endosome into the cytoplasm is still a major bottleneck in the delivery of macromolecular drugs including proteins. Viruses have developed mechanisms to escape the endosome utilizing microenvironmental changes, for example, influenza virus: the N-terminus of hemagglutinin exhibits a random coil structure at physiological pH, whereas after acidification to pH 5, acidic amino acid residues become protonated and form a membrane-lytic helical structure [65]. Different approaches have been made in the field of macromolecular drug delivery mimicking such processes: cointernalizing membrane-active peptides with cationized ribonucleases efficiently assisted in endosomal release of the protein delivered [37]. Another approach is to chemically modify the peptide side chain with pH-sensing molecules; such peptide derivatives are not membrane lytic at neutral pH but regain full lytic activity after endosomal acidification and cleavage of the pH-sensing modification [73, 74]. Several polymers suitable for delivery of proteins bear intrinsic endosomolytic properties. Polyethylenimine (PEI), an organic molecule with the highest density of protonable amines, has so far mostly been used for delivery of nucleic acids into cells [75]. Branched PEI bears a mixture of primary, secondary, and tertiary amines with only a fraction of them being protonated at neutral pH. When PEI is internalized into endosomes, protons pumped into the endosome by ATP-dependent proton pumps are absorbed by PEI, leading to swelling of the polymer and further protonation of amino groups. This proton-buffering effect in turn leads to influx of chloride counter ions, the osmotic imbalance leads to diffusion of water into the endosome, leading to osmotic pressure and subsequent lysis of the endosome [76]. This makes PEI and other polyamines suitable candidates for efficient protein delivery.

6 Protein/Peptide Therapeutics

A broad range of biologically active peptides and proteins exist being potentially suitable for targeted tumor therapies. In the following section a selection of peptides and proteins are described, including their natural biological function, antitumoral activity, and application in tumor targeting.

6.1 Membrane-Lytic Peptides

Membrane-lytic peptides are natural defense molecules expressed in different species including insects, invertebrates, and vertebrates. In humans they are part of the innate immune system (for review, see [77, 78]). Due to their membrane-lytic activity they have been initially utilized as antimicrobial agents, but they also have the potential to act as cytotoxic agents in tumor therapy [79]. The mechanism of their action is often based on their cationic and amphipathic nature, which allows efficient cell binding and/or membrane lysis (see also Sections 4.1 and 5.1). After charge-mediated membrane binding, the amphipathic part of the peptide interacts with the cell membrane, which leads to insertion into the bilayer and subsequent membrane lysis. Targeting them to tumor tissue is vital to prevent side effects on healthy tissue. Being macromolecular drugs they are less prone to become inactive due to resistance mechanisms based on the upregulation of efflux pumps [80], a major resistance mechanism in tumor cells against low molecular drugs [81, 82]. The luteinizing hormone/choriogonadotropin receptor (LH/CR) is expressed in ovaries, testis, and the uterus but also upregulated in different tumors, making it a suitable candidate for targeted tumor therapies [83]. Melittin is a cationic, 25-amino-acid peptide found in bee venom that causes membrane lysis [84]. To achieve targeting of a melittin derivative to cancer cells, a peptide sequence targeting the luteinizing hormone receptor was attached [85]. After multiple administrations of the construct via the bloodstream, even tumor metastases could be selectively destroyed. Similar approaches targeting LH/CR that is overexpressed in hepatocellular carcinoma [86], prostate [87], and gastric carcinoma [88] led to clear antitumoral activity on murine xenograft models. Rege and colleagues attached a monoclonal antibody targeting the prostate-specific membrane antigen (PSMA) to a cationic peptide sequence and achieved two orders of magnitude higher cell killing in vitro compared to the nontargeted peptide [89].

6.2 Peptides Influencing Intracellular Functions of Tumor Cells

Tumor cells are also characterized by deregulated cellular pathways in signal transduction and growth regulation leading to proliferation, metastasis, and invasion. Peptide sequences can be utilized to specifically interfere with these pathways by binding to proteins, thus leading to their selective inactivation and subsequent induction of apoptosis or redifferentiation (for review, see [90]). The de novo designed basic peptide sequence KLAKLAK has been initially described for its antimicrobial function but exhibiting low toxicity toward mammalian cells [91]. When attaching a protein transduction domain to the peptide in order to promote its uptake into mammalian cells, apoptosis was observed after intratumoral injection of the conjugate into murine sarcoma tumors [92]. In another case, intratumoral application of KLAKLAK peptide attached to an integrin-targeted RGD sequence led to reduced tumor growth in a murine melanoma tumor model [93].

6.3 Ribosome-Inactivating Proteins (RIP)

Ribosome-inactivating proteins (RIPs) belong to the superfamily of N-glycosidases and are mainly found in plants, fungi, and bacteria (for review, see [94]). RIPs are able to irreversibly damage ribosomes [95]: the N-glycosidic activity leads to removal of a highly conserved adenine residue from 28S rRNA. This alteration blocks its GTPase activities involved in the binding of elongation factor-2 (EF-2); due to loss of EF-2, binding translation is inhibited. RIPs can be separated into three main classes: Type 1 RIPs consist of a single, basic peptide chain of approximately 30 kDa having in common that they share highly conserved residues as well as the secondary structure within their active side [96]. Type 2 RIPs consist of two chains: the enzymatically active A chain (comparable to type 1 RIPs) and a B chain ($\sim$35 kDa), which exhibits a lectin structure. The latter binds to galactosyl moieties like glycoproteins or glycolipids that can be found on the surface of most eukaryotic cells [97]. Binding to the cell surface triggers endocytosis and transport into the cytoplasm, where the A chain can unfold its enzymatic activity. Type 3 RIPs represent the smallest group, which are translated as precursor molecules and have to be processed by proteases to gain full activity [98, 99].

Gelonin, a single-chain type I RIP, is virtually nontoxic toward mammalian cells, as it lacks an internalization function [100]. When chemically coupling gelonin to transferrin or an anti-TfR antibody, Yazdi and colleagues observed potent cell killing or TfR overexpressing tumor cells [101]. Hsu and colleagues applied a fusion toxin consisting of gelonin and a VEGF isoform binding to the VEGF receptor [102]. Tumor proliferation was significantly decreased and histological studies revealed that the tumor endothelium was damaged due to the targeted treatment with gelonin. The type I RIP saporin (first isolated from the plant *Saponaria officinalis*) expressed as a fusion protein with EGF led to specific antitumoral activity on EGF receptor-overexpressing tumors [55]. Coupling folate to saporin via carbohydrate residues allowed targeted delivery into FR-overexpressing tumor cells [103]. The high-molecular-weight melanoma-associated antigen (HMW-MAA) is expressed on most melanoma tissues, whereas it cannot be found in normal tissues or other tumors. Coupling of an HMW-MAA-specific antibody to gelonin specifically inhibited protein synthesis in melanoma cells [104].

Ricin, a type II RIP found in the bean of the castor plant, has been extensively used for targeted tumor therapies: replacing the lectin B chain, which binds to almost all mammalian cells, with peptides, antibodies, or proteins targeting cancer cells leads to selective target toxicity [105]. Several clinical trials by this approach have been conducted (see Section 7).

6.4 Ribonucleases

Ribonucleases are regulating the RNA half-life in the cytoplasm and hence leading to posttranscriptional control of gene expression. Several toxins found in plants and animals show ribonuclease activity and are evaluated for tumor-targeted therapies [106]. Ranpirnase (Onconase) is a secreted ribonuclease isolated from *Rana pipiens* and belongs to the pancreatic RNAse A superfamily of ribonucleases [107]. Several in vitro and in vivo studies have shown its cytotoxic and antiproliferative anticancer activity: due to degradation of tRNA, which in turn interferes with protein production, apoptotic cell death occurs. Meanwhile ranpirnase is already applied in several clinical trials including a phase III trial for unresectable mesothelioma [108]. Ranpirnase covalently linked to an anti-CD22 antibody showed promising activity against Daudi Burkitt lymphoma both in vitro and in a xenograft model in SCID mice [109]. To achieve targeted delivery, Rybak and colleagues coupled bovine pancreatic ribonuclease A to a TfR-directed, single-chain antibody (scFv) [110]. The rationale of utilizing a mammalian ribonuclease was to reduce the immunogenicity of the conjugate. In humans the ribonuclease eosinophil-derived neurotoxin is found in cytotoxic granules of eosinophils but also in liver tissue and plays an important role in the defense against viral infections [111]. When expressing eosinophil-derived neurotoxin as a fusion protein with a TfR-directed scFv, specific cell killing was observed in leukemia cells, whereas TfR-negative cells were not affected [112]. In a similar way, Menzel and colleagues used an scFv directed against CD30-positive lymphoma cells [113].

6.5 Bacterial Toxins

Bacterial toxins such as diphtheria toxin (DT), *Pseudomonas* exotoxin A (PE), and *Clostridium perfringens* enterotoxin (CPE) are potential candidates for selective tumor cell killing [114]. Both DT from *Corynebacterium diphtheriae* and PE from *Pseudomonas aeruginosa* irreversibly inhibit protein synthesis by catalyzing the ADP ribosylation of EF-2 leading to cell lysis or apoptosis; CPE is a pore forming toxin, leading directly to rapid cell lysis [115]. DT is a single-chain protein consisting of three domains: the B domain binds to heparin-binding epidermal growth factor receptor, which leads to endocytosis. After internalization into clathrin-coated vesicles, DT is cleaved by the endosomal enzyme furin, and the lowered endosomal pH induces conformational changes, which lead to insertion of the translocation domain into the endosomal membrane. After reductive cleavage of an intramolecular disulfide bridge, the catalytic domain A is unfolded and translates the toxin to the cytoplasm. By replacing the cell-binding B domain with tumor-specific ligands, DT can be specifically directed to tumor tissue. Replacing the B domain with human EGF, specific toxicity was observed in EGFR-overexpressing tumors [116]. Covalent attachment of transferrin to DT containing a mutated, inactive B domain redirected the conjugate to TfR-overexpressing cells and showed effective killing of glioblastoma tumors after intratumoral injection of the conjugate in an orthotopic xenograft model in nude mice [117]. The conjugate, termed Tf-CRM 107, was also tested later in clinical trials (see Section 7). Similar to DT, *Pseudomonas* exotoxin (PE) is a single-chain peptide with three domains for binding the cellular PE receptor (domain 1), the translocation across membranes (domain 2), and the ADP ribosylating activity (domain 3). When PE with truncated domain 1 fused to a TfR-binding antibody, the fusion protein showed selective killing of TfR-overexpressing tumor cells after systemic injection in a metastatic colon carcinoma tumor model, whereas no effect was found with the nontargeted truncated PE [118]. More recently, PE fusion proteins with the cytokine IL-13 as targeting moiety were used for treating IL-13 receptor-positive xenografted human tumors in nude mice, leading to eradication of head and neck cancer [119], renal cell carcinoma, and glioma [120]. The PE–IL-13 fusion protein is currently evaluated in clinical trials (Section 7).

6.6 Therapeutic Antibodies

Besides being used for site-specific delivery of chemotherapeutic drugs, peptides, proteins, or radionuclides in cancer therapy, monoclonal antibodies have been generated to interfere with the tumor cells' metabolism, leading to growth arrest, apoptosis, or inhibition of invasion and metastasis. Several therapeutic antibodies have been developed to interfere with the signaling involved in the overexpression of members of the EGFR family. Cetuximab (C225) binds to EGFR (Her 1), blocks activation of receptor tyrosine kinase, and finally leads to cell cycle arrest [121]. A fully humanized version of an EGFR-binding antibody has been shown to be effective in the treatment of metastasized colon carcinoma [122]. Trastuzumab (Herceptin) is a fully humanized antibody binding to the extracellular domain of the tyrosine kinase receptor Her 2 and is already applied clinically for the treatment of metastatic breast carcinoma (for review, see [123]). A proposed mechanism of action is the reduction of Her 2 signaling, leading to apoptosis or cell cycle arrest, but also the downregulation of Her 2/neu, and reduction in neoangiogenesis is discussed. Besides Her 1 and Her 2, also aberrant Her 3 signaling is thought to be involved in malignant growth of tumors. For this purpose, Robinson and colleagues developed a bispecific single-chain Fv antibody, which targets both ErbB2 and ErbB3 [124]. The antibody selectively homed to subcutaneously implanted ErbB2- and ErbB3-expressing tumors and led to concomitant cell cycle arrest and reduced tumor growth.

The vascular endothelial growth factor receptor tyrosine kinases (VEGFR1, VEGFR2, and VEGFR3) are the key regulators leading to the development of a functional circulation system (vasculogenesis) during embryonic development and to the formation of tumor blood vessels from existing blood vessels (angiogenesis) [125]. VEGFR activities are regulated by their natural ligands (VEGF (VEGF-A), VEGF-B, VEGF-C, VEGF-D), which leads to angiogenesis. Interfering with this pathway offers the possibility to cut off the blood supply of solid tumors by downregulation of tumor angiogenesis [126]. Bevacizumab (Avastin) is a clinically approved, fully humanized monoclonal antibody binding and neutralizing VEGF [127]. The antibody is approved for a broad range of solid cancers and often used in conjunction with classical chemotherapeutic agents like paclitaxel in breast cancer [128].

Monoclonal antibodies have also been developed for the treatment of leukemia: the leukocyte marker CD20 is expressed during B-cell development and its expression disappears during terminal differentiation [129]. In non-Hodgkin B-cell lymphoma, CD20 is upregulated and thus a valid tumor marker [130]. The monoclonal antibody rituximab, which binds to CD20, has been approved by FDA for the treatment of non-Hodgkin lymphoma and rheumatoid arthritis. After binding to CD20-positive cells, the exposed distal Fc part of the antibody leads to subsequent complement activation, antibody-dependent cell-mediated cytotoxicity, activation of natural killer cells, and finally cell lysis [131]. Recently, multivalent CD20 antibodies have been developed that comprise six binding sites for the antigen and one Fc part [132]. Such multivalent antibodies will cause clustering of several CD20 molecules on the cell surface, thus leading to inhibition of cell growth.

7 Clinical Applications and Challenges of Protein and Peptide Therapeutics

Several targeted peptide- and protein-based therapies have been in clinical trials or approved in the clinic (for a summary of targeted toxins, see Table 1). Targeted toxins (diphtheria toxin and *Pseudomonas* exotoxin) have been mostly applied locally in recurrent glioblastoma. As glioblastoma does not metastasize to other organs except within the brain, localized therapies for glioblastomas are promising. Therapy using DT targeting to the TfR (Tf-CRM107, Trans-MID) has been successfully applied in clinical phase II trial and is now in a phase III trial [133]. TP-38 is a fusion protein consisting of PE with a truncated cell-binding domain and transforming growth factor-α (TGF-α), which is related to EGF and also binds to EGFR [134]. No adverse systemic side effects were observed after intracranial application, and a partial response was observed in 2 out of 15 patients. Efficiency was limited due to inefficient distribution of the toxin within the brain [135]. Gliomas overexpressing inter-leukin-13 receptor were treated with a PE–IL-13 fusion protein by intracranial infusion in conjunction with chemotherapy and radiation [136]. The treatment was well tolerated and further clinical testing is planned. NBI-3001 (PE coupled to IL-4) was systemically applied in patients with IL-4 receptor-positive renal cell and nonsmall cell lung carcinoma [137]. Among 14 patients who received a total of 36 cycles of treatment, dose limiting toxicity and high levels of neutralizing antibodies were observed, whereas tumor growth was not significantly affected. ONTAK (denileukin diftitox), a DT fusion protein with IL-2 approved by FDA in 1999 for the treatment of T-cell lymphoma, was successfully applied in the treatment of chronic lymphocytic leukemia [138].

Like for all anticancer agents, the major limitations in their use are toxicity, or unwanted side effects, and the development of resistance mechanism. Proteins and peptides are potential immunogens, especially when derived from different species. Hence, repeated systemic application can lead to the induction of humoral immune response, which leads to either inactivation of the drug or even severe side effects. Strategies to overcome these limitations include: (1) simple localized application: in the case of glioblastoma, which does not metastasize outside the brain, this strategy can lead to a positive clinical outcome. In case systemic application is necessary, the protein or the peptide can be modified to be less immunogenic. (2) Covalent attachment of PEG decreases immunogenicity, and in case of synthetic peptides replacing L-amino acids with their D-enantiomers, antigen processing and immunogenic responses can be prevented. (3) Also decreasing the peptide length has been shown to reduce immunogenicity at least in a murine model [145]. Patients receiving toxins have developed antibodies with epitopes directed against the toxin [146]. Vascular leak syndrome (VLS) leads to decreased albumin blood levels, accumulation of fluid in the interstitial space, endema, and in severe cases to fluid accumulation in lung. Therefore, the appearance of VLS limits the dose being applied for most

Table 1 Targeted toxins for tumor treatment being in clinical trials or approved medication

Compound	Effector molecule	Targeting protein	Target	Application	Clinical status	References
Tf-CRM 107	Diphtheria toxin	Transferrin	TfR	Glioblastoma	Phase III	139
TP-38	Pseudomonas exotoxin	EGF	EGFR	Glioblastoma	Phase I	140
IL-13–PE38QQR	Pseudomonas exotoxin	IL-23	IL-13-R α2	Glioblastoma	Phase I/II Phase III (enrolled)	141
NBI-3001	Pseudomonas exotoxin	IL-4	IL-4-R	Renal cell carcinoma, NSLC, glioblastoma	Phase I	142,143
IL2-R-DAB (389)IL-2 (ONTAK)	Diphtheria toxin	IL-2	IL-2-R	Chronic lymphocytic leukemia	In clinic	144

targeted immunotoxins [147]. Pretreatment with immunosuppressive drugs showed success in rodent models, but failed in primates [148]. The use of humanized peptide sequences, i.e., utilizing human versions of toxins or humanized antibodies, has been shown to be successful in preventing the induction of neutralizing antibodies [149]. Nevertheless, immunogenicity of targeted toxins can also be beneficial for tumor therapy, as they can act as potent inducers of antitumor immunity [150]. Therapeutic antibodies face similar problems, i.e., the induction of so-called idiotype–anti-idiotype interactions [151]. Even when having a fully humanized sequence, antibodies can be induced binding to the paratope of the therapeutic antibody applied. When applying therapeutic antibody blocking, e.g., certain signaling pathways, a resistance mechanism also observed with other chemotherapeutic utilizing alternative signaling pathways can occur [152]. Combination therapies or simultaneous targeting of more than one pathway has the potential to overcome these shortcomings.

8 Conclusions and Future Directions

Targeted delivery of proteins and peptides to tumors is a very promising field for the treatment of cancer and several formulations have already been approved as drugs in cancer therapy. Their high molecular weight, which circumvents the appearance of resistance mechanisms based on elevated efflux of low molecular drugs, also limits antitumoral activity due to limited diffusion within tumor tissue. Novel technologies enabling the screening of short peptide sequences for receptor binding or intracellular target interaction (for example, peptide aptamers) will help to overcome such shortcomings and lead to the development of peptide drugs with elevated levels of specificity and efficiency. Delivery technologies based on chemical modification or formulation of peptides will further help to overcome current shortcomings. A major drawback of systemically applied therapeutic proteins is their potential immunogenicity, especially in the case of repeated systemic dosing, and such immunogenic responses were often dose-limiting side effects in several clinical trials (see Section 7). Increasing the specificity will allow to decrease the dose applied to achieve a clinically relevant effect and direct modification of the protein, e.g., by PEGylation or changes in the protein structure, will further help to reduce immunogenic reactions. Direct modification of the protein/peptide drug is the development of fully humanized antibodies and stability-optimized proteins and peptides containing nonproteogenic amino acids. Novel techniques, such as specific knockdown of protein expression by small interfering RNA or different protein–protein interaction techniques, will help to gain more knowledge about tumor development and lead to new approaches for cancer treatment.

References

1. Gellissen G (2008) Production of Recombinant Proteins: Novel Microbial and Eukaryotic Expression Systems. Wiley, Hoboken, NJ, USA
2. Terpe K (2003) Overview of tag protein fusions: from molecular and biochemical fundamentals to commercial systems. Appl Microbiol Biotechnol 60:523–533
3. Gauthier MA, Klok HA (2008) Peptide/protein–polymer conjugates: synthetic strategies and design concepts. Chem Commun (Camb) 2591–2611
4. Hermanson GT (2008) Bioconjugate Techniques. Academic Press, Inc.
5. Grabarek Z, Gergely J (1990) Zero-length crosslinking procedure with the use of active esters. Anal Biochem 185:131–135
6. Carlsson J, Drevin H, Axen R (1978) Protein thiolation and reversible protein-protein conjugation. N-Succinimidyl 3-(2-pyridyldithio)propionate, a new heterobifunctional reagent. Biochem J 173:723–737
7. Gillies ER, Goodwin AP, Frechet JM (2004) Acetals as pH-sensitive linkages for drug delivery. Bioconjug Chem 15:1254–1263
8. Reents R, Jeyaraj DA, Waldmann H (2002) Enzymatically cleavable linker groups in polymer-supported synthesis. Drug Discov Today 7:71–76
9. Nakayama K (1997) Furin: A mammalian subtilisin/Kex2p-like endoprotease involved in processing of a wide variety of precursor proteins. Biochem J 327(Pt 3):625–635
10. Zhang L, Zhao J, Wang T et al. (2008) HER2-targeting recombinant protein with truncated pseudomonas exotoxin A translocation domain efficiently kills breast cancer cells. Cancer Biol Ther 7:1226–1231
11. Deryugina EI, Quigley JP (2006) Matrix metalloproteinases and tumor metastasis. Cancer Metastasis Rev 25:9–34
12. Terada T, Iwai M, Kawakami S et al. (2006) Novel PEG-matrix metalloproteinase-2 cleavable peptide-lipid containing galactosylated liposomes for hepatocellular carcinoma-selective targeting. J Control Release 111:333–342
13. Folkman J (1995) Angiogenesis in cancer, vascular, rheumatoid and other disease. Nat Med 1:27–31
14. Torrent G, Benito A, Castro J et al. (2008) Contribution of the C30/C75 disulfide bond to the biological properties of onconase. Biol Chem Aug 8. [Epub ahead of print]
15. Harris AG (1994) Somatostatin and Somatostatin Analogs – Pharmacokinetics and Pharmacodynamic effects. Gut 35:S1–S4
16. Werle M, Bernkop-Schnurch A (2006) Strategies to improve plasma half life time of peptide and protein drugs. Amino Acids 30:351–367
17. Abuchowski A, McCoy JR, Palczuk NC et al. (1977) Effect of covalent attachment of polyethylene glycol on immunogenicity and circulating life of bovine liver catalase. J Biol Chem 252:3582–3586
18. Roberts MJ, Bentley MD, Harris JM (2002) Chemistry for peptide and protein PEGylation. Adv Drug Deliv Rev 54:459–476
19. Hamidi M, Azadi A, Rafiei P (2006) Pharmacokinetic consequences of pegylation. Drug Deliv 13:399–409
20. Torchilin VP, Lukyanov AN (2003) Peptide and protein drug delivery to and into tumors: challenges and solutions. Drug Discov Today 8:259–266
21. Veronese FM, Pasut G (2005) PEGylation, successful approach to drug delivery. Drug Discov Today 10:1451–1458
22. Brocchini S, Godwin A, Balan S et al. (2008) Disulfide bridge based PEGylation of proteins. Adv Drug Deliv Rev 60:3–12
23. Wiegand J, Jackel E, Cornberg M et al. (2004) Long-term follow-up after successful interferon therapy of acute hepatitis C. Hepatology 40:98–107

24. Schechter BA, Koreishi AF, Karp CL et al. (2008) Long-term follow-up of conjunctival and corneal intraepithelial neoplasia treated with topical interferon alfa-2b. Ophthalmology 115:1291–1296
25. Zeuzem S, Feinman SV, Rasenack J et al. (2000) Peginterferon alfa-2a in patients with chronic hepatitis C. N Engl J Med 343:1666–1672
26. Bell SJ, Fam CM, Chlipala EA et al. (2008) Enhanced circulating half-life and antitumor activity of a site-specific pegylated interferon-alpha protein therapeutic. Bioconjug Chem 19:299–305
27. Murata H, Futami J, Kitazoe M et al. (2008) Intracellular Delivery of Glutathione S-transferase-fused Proteins into Mammalian Cells by Polyethylenimine-Glutathione Conjugates. J Biochem 144:447–455
28. Kitazoe M, Murata H, Futami J et al. (2005) Protein transduction assisted by polyethylenimine-cationized carrier proteins. J Biochem 137:693–701
29. Didenko VV, Ngo H, Baskin DS (2005) Polyethyleneimine as a transmembrane carrier of fluorescently labeled proteins and antibodies. Anal Biochem 344:168–173
30. Matsumura Y, Maeda H (1986) A new concept for macromolecular therapeutics in cancer chemotherapy: mechanism of tumoritropic accumulation of proteins and the antitumor agent smancs. Cancer Res 46:6387–6392
31. Skinner SA, Tutton PJ, O'Brien PE (1990) Microvascular architecture of experimental colon tumors in the rat. Cancer Res 50:2411–2417
32. Seymour LW, Miyamoto Y, Maeda H et al. (1995) Influence of molecular weight on passive tumour accumulation of a soluble macromolecular drug carrier. Eur J Cancer 31A:766–770
33. Summerford C, Samulski RJ (1998) Membrane-associated heparan sulfate proteoglycan is a receptor for adeno-associated virus type 2 virions. J Virol 72:1438–1445
34. Finlay BB, Cossart P (1997) Exploitation of mammalian host cell functions by bacterial pathogens. Science 276:718–725
35. Thurston G, McLean JW, Rizen M et al. (1998) Cationic liposomes target angiogenic endothelial cells in tumors and chronic inflammation in mice. J Clin Invest 101:1401–1413
36. Krasnici S, Werner A, Eichhorn ME et al. (2003) Effect of the surface charge of liposomes on their uptake by angiogenic tumor vessels. Int J Cancer 105:561–567
37. Futami J, Yamada H (2008) Design of cytotoxic ribonucleases by cationization to enhance intracellular protein delivery. Curr Pharm Biotechnol 9:180–184
38. McLean JW, Fox EA, Baluk P et al. (1997) Organ-specific endothelial cell uptake of cationic liposome-DNA complexes in mice. Am J Physiol 273:H387–H404
39. Silva R, D'Amico G, Hodivala-Dilke KM et al. (2008) Integrins: the keys to unlocking angiogenesis. Arterioscler Thromb Vasc Biol 28:1703–1713
40. Arap W, Pasqualini R, Ruoslahti E (1998) Cancer treatment by targeted drug delivery to tumor vasculature in a mouse model. Science 279:377–380
41. Zarovni N, Monaco L, Corti A (2004) Inhibition of tumor growth by intramuscular injection of cDNA encoding tumor necrosis factor alpha coupled to NGR and RGD tumor-homing peptides. Hum Gene Ther 15:373–382
42. Kessler T, Schwoppe C, Liersch R et al. (2008) Generation of fusion proteins for selective occlusion of tumor vessels. Curr Drug Discov Technol 5:1–8
43. Qian ZM, Li H, Sun H et al. (2002) Targeted drug delivery via the transferrin receptor-mediated endocytosis pathway. Pharmacol Rev 54:561–587
44. Gomme PT, McCann KB, Bertolini J (2005) Transferrin: structure, function and potential therapeutic actions. Drug Discov Today 10:267–273
45. He QY, Mason AB, Nguyen V et al. (2000) The chloride effect is related to anion binding in determining the rate of iron release from the human transferrin N-lobe. Biochem J 350(Pt 3):909–915
46. Gosselaar PH, van Dijk AJ, de Gast GC et al. (2002) Transferrin toxin but not transferrin receptor immunotoxin is influenced by free transferrin and iron saturation. Eur J Clin Invest 32(Suppl 1):61–69

47. Heidel JD, Yu Z, Liu JY et al. (2007) Administration in non-human primates of escalating intravenous doses of targeted nanoparticles containing ribonucleotide reductase subunit M2 siRNA. Proc Natl Acad Sci USA 104:5715–5721
48. Kwok TT, Sutherland RM (1991) Differences in EGF related radiosensitisation of human squamous carcinoma cells with high and low numbers of EGF receptors. Br J Cancer 64:251–254
49. Wells A (1999) EGF receptor. Int J Biochem Cell Biol 31:637–643
50. Schlessinger J (2002) Ligand-induced, receptor-mediated dimerization and activation of EGF receptor. Cell 110:669–672
51. Wilde A, Beattie EC, Lem L et al. (1999) EGF receptor signaling stimulates SRC kinase phosphorylation of clathrin, influencing clathrin redistribution and EGF uptake. Cell 96:677–687
52. Katzmann DJ, Odorizzi G, Emr SD (2002) Receptor downregulation and multivesicular-body sorting. Nat Rev Mol Cell Biol 3:893–905
53. Khalil MY, Grandis JR, Shin DM (2003) Targeting epidermal growth factor receptor: novel therapeutics in the management of cancer. Expert Rev Anticancer Ther 3:367–380
54. Shir A, Ogris M, Wagner E et al. (2006) EGF receptor-targeted synthetic double-stranded RNA eliminates glioblastoma, breast cancer, and adenocarcinoma tumors in mice. PLoS Med 3:e6
55. Fuchs H, Bachran C, Li T et al. (2007) A cleavable molecular adapter reduces side effects and concomitantly enhances efficacy in tumor treatment by targeted toxins in mice. J Control Release 117:342–350
56. Elnakat H, Ratnam M (2004) Distribution, functionality and gene regulation of folate receptor isoforms: implications in targeted therapy. Adv Drug Deliv Rev 56:1067–1084
57. Hilgenbrink AR, Low PS (2005) Folate receptor-mediated drug targeting: from therapeutics to diagnostics. J Pharm Sci 94:2135–2146
58. Newton J, Deutscher SL (2008) Phage peptide display. Handb Exp Pharmacol 145–163
59. Stoltenburg R, Reinemann C, Strehlitz B (2007) SELEX–a (r)evolutionary method to generate high-affinity nucleic acid ligands. Biomol Eng 24:381–403
60. Chen CH, Dellamaggiore KR, Ouellette CP et al. (2008) Aptamer-based endocytosis of a lysosomal enzyme. Proc Natl Acad Sci USA 105:15908–15913
61. Perkins AC, Missailidis S (2007) Radiolabelled aptamers for tumour imaging and therapy. Q J Nucl Med Mol Imaging 51:292–296
62. Borghouts C, Kunz C, Groner B (2005) Peptide aptamers: recent developments for cancer therapy. Expert Opin Biol Ther 5:783–797
63. Bjorklund M, Heikkila P, Koivunen E (2004) Peptide inhibition of catalytic and non-catalytic activities of matrix metalloproteinase-9 blocks tumor cell migration and invasion. J Biol Chem 279:29589–29597
64. Nakamura T, Takasugi H, Aizawa T et al. (2005) Peptide mimics of epidermal growth factor (EGF) with antagonistic activity. J Biotechnol 116:211–219
65. Plank C, Zauner W, Wagner E (1998) Application of membrane-active peptides for drug and gene delivery across cellular membranes. Adv Drug Deliv Rev 34:21–35
66. Vives E, Brodin P, Lebleu B (1997) A truncated HIV-1 Tat protein basic domain rapidly translocates through the plasma membrane and accumulates in the cell nucleus. J Biol Chem 272:16010–16017
67. Elliott G, O'Hare P (1997) Intercellular trafficking and protein delivery by a herpes virus structural protein. Cell 88:223–233
68. Derossi D, Calvet S, Trembleau A et al. (1996) Cell internalization of the third helix of the Antennapedia homeodomain is receptor-independent. J Biol Chem 271:18188–18193
69. Schwarze SR, Ho A, Vocero-Akbani A et al. (1999) In vivo protein transduction: delivery of a biologically active protein into the mouse. Science 285:1569–1572
70. Brooks H, Lebleu B, Vives E (2005) Tat peptide-mediated cellular delivery: back to basics. Adv Drug Deliv Rev 57:559–577

71. Brooks H, Lebleu B, Vives E (2005) Tat peptide-mediated cellular delivery: back to basics. Adv Drug Deliv Rev 57:559–577
72. Deshayes S, Morris M, Heitz F et al. (2008) Delivery of proteins and nucleic acids using a non-covalent peptide-based strategy. Adv Drug Deliv Rev 60:537–547
73. Wolff JA, Rozema DB (2008) Breaking the bonds: non-viral vectors become chemically dynamic. Mol Ther 16:8–15
74. Meyer M, Philipp A, Oskuee R et al. (2008) Breathing life into polycations: functionalization with pH-responsive endosomolytic peptides and polyethylene glycol enables siRNA delivery. J Am Chem Soc 130:3272–3273
75. Demeneix B, Behr JP (2005) Polyethylenimine (PEI). Adv Genet 53:217–230
76. Sonawane ND, Szoka Jr FC, Verkman AS (2003) Chloride accumulation and swelling in endosomes enhances DNA transfer by polyamine-DNA polyplexes. J Biol Chem 278:44826–44831
77. Kourie JI, Shorthouse AA (2000) Properties of cytotoxic peptide-formed ion channels. Am J Physiol Cell Physiol 278:C1063–C1087
78. Clarke DJ, Campopiano DJ (2006) Structural and functional studies of defensin-inspired peptides. Biochem Soc Trans 34:251–256
79. Mader JS, Hoskin DW (2006) Cationic antimicrobial peptides as novel cytotoxic agents for cancer treatment. Expert Opin Investig Drugs 15:933–946
80. Leuschner C, Hansel W (2004) Membrane disrupting lytic peptides for cancer treatments. Curr Pharm Des 10:2299–2310
81. O'Connor R (2007) The pharmacology of cancer resistance. Anticancer Res 27:1267–1272
82. Sharom FJ (2008) ABC multidrug transporters: structure, function and role in chemoresistance. Pharmacogenomics 9:105–127
83. Ziecik AJ, Kaczmarek MM, Blitek A et al. (2007) Novel biological and possible applicable roles of LH/hCG receptor. Mol Cell Endocrinol 269:51–60
84. Raghuraman H, Chattopadhyay A (2007) Melittin: a membrane-active peptide with diverse functions. Biosci Rep 27:189–223
85. Hansel W, Enright F, Leuschner C (2007) Destruction of breast cancers and their metastases by lytic peptide conjugates in vitro and in vivo. Mol Cell Endocrinol 260–262:183–189
86. Szepeshazi K, Schally AV, Treszl A et al. (2008) Therapy of experimental hepatic cancers with cytotoxic peptide analogs targeted to receptors for luteinizing hormone-releasing hormone, somatostatin or bombesin. Anticancer Drugs 19:349–358
87. Stangelberger A, Schally AV, Nagy A et al. (2006) Inhibition of human experimental prostate cancers by a targeted cytotoxic luteinizing hormone-releasing hormone analog AN-207. Prostate 66:200–210
88. Szepeshazi K, Schally AV, Nagy A et al. (2003) Preclinical evaluation of therapeutic effects of targeted cytotoxic analogs of somatostatin and bombesin on human gastric carcinomas. Cancer 98:1401–1410
89. Rege K, Patel SJ, Megeed Z et al. (2007) Amphipathic peptide-based fusion peptides and immunoconjugates for the targeted ablation of prostate cancer cells. Cancer Res 67:6368–6375
90. Borghouts C, Kunz C, Groner B (2005) Current strategies for the development of peptide-based anti-cancer therapeutics. J Pept Sci 11:713–726
91. Javadpour MM, Juban MM, Lo WC et al. (1996) De novo antimicrobial peptides with low mammalian cell toxicity. J Med Chem 39:3107–3113
92. Mai JC, Mi Z, Kim SH et al. (2001) A proapoptotic peptide for the treatment of solid tumors. Cancer Res 61:7709–7712
93. Smolarczyk R, Cichon T, Graja K et al. (2006) Antitumor effect of RGD-4C-GG-D(KLAKLAK)2 peptide in mouse B16(F10) melanoma model. Acta Biochim Pol 53:801–805

94. Stirpe F, Battelli MG (2006) Ribosome-inactivating proteins: progress and problems. Cell Mol Life Sci 63:1850–1866
95. Endo Y, Mitsui K, Motizuki M et al. (1987) The mechanism of action of ricin and related toxic lectins on eukaryotic ribosomes. The site and the characteristics of the modification in 28 S ribosomal RNA caused by the toxins. J Biol Chem 262:5908–5912
96. Nielsen K, Boston RS (2001) RIBOSOME-INACTIVATING PROTEINS: A Plant Perspective. Annu Rev Plant Physiol Plant Mol Biol 52:785–816
97. Lord JM, Roberts LM, Robertus JD (1994) Ricin: structure, mode of action, and some current applications. FASEB J 8:201–208
98. Reinbothe S, Reinbothe C, Lehmann J et al. (1994) JIP60, a methyl jasmonate-induced ribosome-inactivating protein involved in plant stress reactions. Proc Natl Acad Sci USA 91:7012–7016
99. Walsh TA, Morgan AE, Hey TD (1991) Characterization and molecular cloning of a proenzyme form of a ribosome-inactivating protein from maize. Novel mechanism of proenzyme activation by proteolytic removal of a 2.8-kilodalton internal peptide segment. J Biol Chem 266:23422–23427
100. Sandvig K, van Deurs B (2005) Delivery into cells: lessons learned from plant and bacterial toxins. Gene Ther 12:865–872
101. Yazdi PT, Murphy RM (1994) Quantitative analysis of protein synthesis inhibition by transferrin-toxin conjugates. Cancer Res 54:6387–6394
102. Hsu AR, Cai W, Veeravagu A et al. (2007) Multimodality molecular imaging of glioblastoma growth inhibition with vasculature-targeting fusion toxin VEGF121/rGel. J Nucl Med 48:445–454
103. Atkinson SF, Bettinger T, Seymour LW et al. (2001) Conjugation of folate via gelonin carbohydrate residues retains ribosomal-inactivating properties of the toxin and permits targeting to folate receptor positive cells. J Biol Chem 276:27930–27935
104. Chan MC, Murphy RM (1999) Kinetics of cellular trafficking and cytotoxicity of 9.2.27-gelonin immunotoxins targeted against the high-molecular-weight melanoma-associated antigen. Cancer Immunol Immunother 47:321–329
105. Lord JM, Roberts LM, Robertus JD (1994) Ricin: structure, mode of action, and some current applications. FASEB J 8:201–208
106. Arnold U, Ulbrich-Hofmann R (2006) Natural and engineered ribonucleases as potential cancer therapeutics. Biotechnol Lett 28:1615–1622
107. Ardelt W, Shogen K, Darzynkiewicz Z (2008) Onconase and amphinase, the antitumor ribonucleases from Rana pipiens oocytes. Curr Pharm Biotechnol 9:215–225
108. Lee I (2008) Ranpirnase (Onconase), a cytotoxic amphibian ribonuclease, manipulates tumour physiological parameters as a selective killer and a potential enhancer for chemotherapy and radiation in cancer therapy. Expert Opin Biol Ther 8:813–827
109. Newton DL, Hansen HJ, Mikulski SM et al. (2001) Potent and specific antitumor effects of an anti-CD22-targeted cytotoxic ribonuclease: potential for the treatment of non-Hodgkin lymphoma. Blood 97:528–535
110. Rybak SM, Hoogenboom HR, Newton DL et al. (1992) Rational immunotherapy with ribonuclease chimeras. An approach toward humanizing immunotoxins. Cell Biophys 21:121–138
111. Rosenberg HF (2008) Eosinophil-derived neurotoxin/RNase 2: connecting the past, the present and the future. Curr Pharm Biotechnol 9:135–140
112. Zewe M, Rybak SM, Dubel S et al. (1997) Cloning and cytotoxicity of a human pancreatic RNase immunofusion. Immunotechnology 3:127–136
113. Menzel C, Schirrmann T, Konthur Z et al. (2008) Human antibody RNase fusion protein targeting CD30+ lymphomas. Blood 111:3830–3837
114. Michl P, Gress TM (2004) Bacteria and bacterial toxins as therapeutic agents for solid tumors. Curr Cancer Drug Targets 4:689–702

115. Caserta JA, Hale ML, Popoff MR et al. (2008) Evidence that membrane rafts are not required for the action of clostridium perfringens enterotoxin. Infect Immun 76:5677–5685
116. Shaw JP, Akiyoshi DE, Arrigo DA et al. (1991) Cytotoxic properties of DAB486EGF and DAB389EGF, epidermal growth factor (EGF) receptor-targeted fusion toxins. J Biol Chem 266:21118–21124
117. Laske DW, Ilercil O, Akbasak A et al. (1994) Efficacy of direct intratumoral therapy with targeted protein toxins for solid human gliomas in nude mice. J Neurosurg 80:520–526
118. Shinohara H, Fan D, Ozawa S et al. (2000) Site-specific expression of transferrin receptor by human colon cancer cells directly correlates with eradication by antitransferrin recombinant immunotoxin. Int J Oncol 17:643–651
119. Kawakami K, Husain SR, Kawakami M et al. (2002) Improved anti-tumor activity and safety of interleukin-13 receptor targeted cytotoxin by systemic continuous administration in head and neck cancer xenograft model. Mol Med 8:487–494
120. Kioi M, Seetharam S, Puri RK (2008) Targeting IL-13Ralpha2-positive cancer with a novel recombinant immunotoxin composed of a single-chain antibody and mutated Pseudomonas exotoxin. Mol Cancer Ther 7:1579–1587
121. Mendelsohn J (1997) Epidermal growth factor receptor inhibition by a monoclonal antibody as anticancer therapy. Clin Cancer Res 3:2703–2707
122. Gibson TB, Ranganathan A, Grothey A (2006) Randomized phase III trial results of panitumumab, a fully human anti-epidermal growth factor receptor monoclonal antibody, in metastatic colorectal cancer. Clin Colorectal Cancer 6:29–31
123. Valabrega G, Montemurro F, Aglietta M (2007) Trastuzumab: mechanism of action, resistance and future perspectives in HER2-overexpressing breast cancer. Ann Oncol 18:977–984
124. Robinson MK, Hodge KM, Horak E et al. (2008) Targeting ErbB2 and ErbB3 with a bispecific single-chain Fv enhances targeting selectivity and induces a therapeutic effect in vitro. Br J Cancer 99:1415–1425
125. Roskoski Jr R (2008) VEGF receptor protein-tyrosine kinases: structure and regulation. Biochem Biophys Res Commun 375:287–291
126. Kowanetz M, Ferrara N (2006) Vascular endothelial growth factor signaling pathways: therapeutic perspective. Clin Cancer Res 12:5018–5022
127. Gordon MS, Margolin K, Talpaz M et al. (2001) Phase I safety and pharmacokinetic study of recombinant human anti-vascular endothelial growth factor in patients with advanced cancer. J Clin Oncol 19:843–850
128. Sirohi B, Smith K (2008) Bevacizumab in the treatment of breast cancer. Expert Rev Anticancer Ther 8:1559–1568
129. Quintanilla-Martinez L, Preffer F, Rubin D et al. (1994) CD20+ T-cell lymphoma. Neoplastic transformation of a normal T-cell subset. Am J Clin Pathol 102:483–489
130. Cheson BD, Leonard JP (2008) Monoclonal antibody therapy for B-cell non-Hodgkin's lymphoma. N Engl J Med 359:613–626
131. Cerny T, Borisch B, Introna M et al. (2002) Mechanism of action of rituximab. Anticancer Drugs 13(Suppl 2):S3–S10
132. Rossi EA, Goldenberg DM, Cardillo TM et al. (2008) Novel designs of multivalent anti-CD20 humanized antibodies as improved lymphoma therapeutics. Cancer Res 68:8384–8392
133. Rainov NG, Soling A (2005) Technology evaluation: TransMID, KS Biomedix/Nycomed/Sosei/PharmaEngine. Curr Opin Mol Ther 7:483–492
134. Sampson JH, Akabani G, Archer GE et al. (2003) Progress report of a Phase I study of the intracerebral microinfusion of a recombinant chimeric protein composed of transforming growth factor (TGF)-alpha and a mutated form of the Pseudomonas exotoxin termed PE-38 (TP-38) for the treatment of malignant brain tumors. J Neurooncol 65:27–35

135. Sampson JH, Akabani G, Archer GE et al. (2008) Intracerebral infusion of an EGFR-targeted toxin in recurrent malignant brain tumors. Neuro Oncol 10:320–329
136. Vogelbaum MA, Sampson JH, Kunwar S et al. (2007) Convection-enhanced delivery of cintredekin besudotox (interleukin-13-PE38QQR) followed by radiation therapy with and without temozolomide in newly diagnosed malignant gliomas: phase 1 study of final safety results. Neurosurgery 61:1031–1037
137. Garland L, Gitlitz B, Ebbinghaus S et al. (2005) Phase I trial of intravenous IL-4 pseudomonas exotoxin protein (NBI-3001) in patients with advanced solid tumors that express the IL-4 receptor. J Immunother 28:376–381
138. Frankel AE, Fleming DR, Powell BL et al. (2003) DAB389IL2 (ONTAK) fusion protein therapy of chronic lymphocytic leukaemia. Expert Opin Biol Ther 3:179–186
139. Rainov NG, Soling A (2005) Technology evaluation: TransMID, KS Biomedix/Nycomed/Sosei/PharmaEngine. Curr Opin Mol Ther 7:483–492
140. Sampson JH, Akabani G, Archer GE et al. (2008) Intracerebral infusion of an EGFR-targeted toxin in recurrent malignant brain tumors. Neuro Oncol 10:320–329
141. Vogelbaum MA, Sampson JH, Kunwar S et al. (2007) Convection-enhanced delivery of cintredekin besudotox (interleukin-13-PE38QQR) followed by radiation therapy with and without temozolomide in newly diagnosed malignant gliomas: phase 1 study of final safety results. Neurosurgery 61:1031–1037
142. Garland L, Gitlitz B, Ebbinghaus S et al. (2005) Phase I trial of intravenous IL-4 pseudomonas exotoxin protein (NBI-3001) in patients with advanced solid tumors that express the IL-4 receptor. J Immunother 28:376–381
143. Weber F, Asher A, Bucholz R et al. (2003) Safety, tolerability, and tumor response of IL4-Pseudomonas exotoxin (NBI-3001) in patients with recurrent malignant glioma. J Neurooncol 64:125–137
144. Frankel AE, Fleming DR, Powell BL et al. (2003) DAB389IL2 (ONTAK) fusion protein therapy of chronic lymphocytic leukaemia. Expert Opin Biol Ther 3:179–186
145. Bogacki M, Enright FM, Todd WJ et al. (2008) Immune response to lytic peptides conjugated to a betaCG fragment in treated BALB/C mice. Reprod Biol 8:135–147
146. Roscoe DM, Pai LH, Pastan I (1997) Identification of epitopes on a mutant form of Pseudomonas exotoxin using serum from humans treated with Pseudomonas exotoxin containing immunotoxins. Eur J Immunol 27:1459–1468
147. Kuan CT, Pai LH, Pastan I (1995) Immunotoxins containing Pseudomonas exotoxin that target LeY damage human endothelial cells in an antibody-specific mode: relevance to vascular leak syndrome. Clin Cancer Res 1:1589–1594
148. Hubbard WJ, Moore JK, Contreras JL et al. (2001) Phenotypic and functional analysis of T-cell recovery after anti-CD3 immunotoxin treatment for tolerance induction in rhesus macaques. Hum Immunol 62:479–487
149. Frankel AE (2004) Reducing the immune response to immunotoxin. Clin Cancer Res 10:13–15
150. Ochiai H, Archer GE, Herndon JE et al. (2008) EGFRvIII-targeted immunotoxin induces antitumor immunity that is inhibited in the absence of CD4+ and CD8+ T cells. Cancer Immunol Immunother 57:115–121
151. Reinsberg J (2007) Detection of human antibodies generated against therapeutic antibodies used in tumor therapy. Methods Mol Biol 378:195–204
152. Piccart M (2008) Circumventing de novo and acquired resistance to trastuzumab: new hope for the care of ErbB2-positive breast cancer. Clin Breast Cancer 8(Suppl 3):S100–S113

Protein Transduction Domain-Mediated Delivery of Anticancer Proteins

Hiroshi Harada and Masahiro Hiraoka

1 Introduction

Advances in molecular and cellular biological techniques and genomic information obtained through the human genome project have been accelerating the elucidation of the molecular mechanisms underlying cancer. Both genetic mutations and epigenetic alterations have been associated with cancer [1]. The former include deletions, point mutations, or amplification of genes, chromosomal translocations, and gain or loss of entire chromosomes. The latter are modifications of genomic DNA, such as methylation and acetylation. All of these alterations lead to a gain of function of oncogenes or loss of function of tumor suppressor genes and have been recognized as effective targets for cancer therapy. Not only small chemicals but also various high-molecular weight biomacromolecules, such as oligonucleotides, antisense nucleotides, antisense peptide nucleic acids, small interference RNA, DNA (cDNA), peptides, proteins, and antibodies, have proven useful for regulating the function of these target genes. However, the plasma membrane of the cell surface forms an effective barrier and limits the internalization of such macromolecules into cells; therefore, the application of these information-rich macromolecules to cancer therapy has long been restricted. Although various methods to internalize macromolecules into living cells in vivo have been proposed, most of them resulted in inefficient delivery. Additionally, other problems such as complex manipulation, toxicity, and immunogenicity have prevented the routine therapeutic use of macromolecules.

Over the past decade, the unique activity of oligopeptides, known as protein transduction domains (PTDs) or cell penetrating peptides (CPPs), has made it possible to transduce biologically active macromolecules into living cells [2, 3]. It was accomplished by conjugating a PTD to the desired macromolecule. Various kinds of macromolecules have been successfully internalized into living

H. Harada (✉)
Department of Radiation Oncology and Image-applied Therapy, Graduate School of Medicine, Kyoto University, Sakyo-ku, Kyoto, 606-8507, Japan
e-mail: hharada@kuhp.kyoto-u.ac.jp

Y. Lu, R.I. Mahato (eds.), *Pharmaceutical Perspectives of Cancer Therapeutics*,
DOI 10.1007/978-1-4419-0131-6_10, © Springer Science+Business Media, LLC 2009

cells and confirmed to show the expected activity in the cells. Moreover, several groups have already applied this strategy in vivo and confirmed anticancer activity in preclinical experiments using tumor-bearing animals [4–17].

In this chapter, we focus on recent progress in PTD-mediated anticancer strategies. In addition, we review the characteristics of PTD polypeptides, mechanism of PTD-mediated internalization, problems and perspectives of PTD-mediated anticancer strategies, and history of this research field.

2 PTD as a Transducer of Macromolecules into Living Cells

In 1988, two groups, Green and Loewenstein, and Frankel and Pabo, independently reported that the transcriptional activator of transcription (Tat) protein of human immunodeficiency virus-1 (HIV-1) has the unique potential to enter cultured cells (Table 1) [18, 19]. Green and Loewenstein found that a chemically synthesized partial Tat protein (first 86 amino acids of the protein) entered HeLa cells when added to the culture medium and transactivated the expression of a Tat-responsive reporter gene pretransfected in the cells. Frankel and Pabo also demonstrated that the addition of a recombinant Tat protein to the culture medium was sufficient to induce the expression of a HIV-1 LTR-dependent reporter gene which was pretransfected in HeLa cells. Although the physiological importance of this internalization still remains to be elucidated, the reports marked an important first milestone in the development of a PTD-mediated anticancer strategy.

Table 1 Milestones for the development of PTD-mediated delivery of bioactive protein in vivo

Year	Finding	References
1988	Internalization of chemically synthesized partial Tat protein (first 86 a.a.) into living cells and its bioactivity	18
	Internalization of recombinant Tat protein into living cells and its bioactivity	19
1994	Tat-mediated internalization of heterologous protein into living cells	20
	Identification of the "tat protein transduction domain"	
1999	Tat-mediated delivery of biologically active protein in vivo	39

In 1994, Fawell et al. marked a second milestone, that the Tat protein can mediate the internalization of a heterologous protein into cells by chemical conjugation (Table 1) [20]. They chemically cross-linked Tat peptides (residues 1–72 or 37–72) to β-galactosidase, horseradish peroxidase, RNase A, and domain III of pseudomonas exotoxin A (PE) and monitored their uptake. Interestingly, all the cells in the culture dish were transduced with the Tat protein. In addition, the internalization was achieved in all cell types tested, such as HeLa, COS-1, CHO, H9, NIH3T3, primary human keratinocytes, and umbilical endothelial cells. The domain responsible for this translocation was identified in the short basic region (47–57 of the Tat protein) and termed the "Tat protein transduction domain (PTD)" [21–23]. Subsequent studies have further demonstrated that Tat-PTD facilitates the internalization of conjugated proteins into living cells in vitro [24]. Likewise, a number of other cationic peptides, e.g., a peptide from the third α–helix of the antennapedia homeodomain [25–28], and a peptide from the VP22 protein from the herpes simplex virus [29] have been reported as PTDs showing the same attractive activity as Tat-PTD [30]. Using these PTDs, various physiologically and therapeutically active macromolecules, such as peptides, proteins [20], antisense peptide nucleic acid [31, 32], DNA [33], super magnet beads [34], liposomes [35], λ phages [36], and antibodies [37] have been successfully transduced into living cells. The intracellular delivery of these macromolecules modulates the functions of various genes [30] related to the cell cycle [22] and apoptosis [38] in vitro. Moreover, in 1999, Schwarze et al. demonstrated that the intraperitoneal injection of a Tat-PTD-fused 120 kDa β-galactosidase (β-Gal) protein resulted in the delivery of the biologically active fusion protein to all tissues in mice, including the brain (Table 1) [39]. Their results revealed new possibilities for the direct delivery of macromolecules into patients.

3 Characteristics and Categories of PTD

Peptides capable of delivering macromolecules into living cells can be categorized as either "protein derived" or "designed" (Table 2) [40, 41]. Protein-derived peptides are short polypeptides encoded in natural proteins of various organisms and responsible for the penetration of proteins into cells. Tat-PTD derived from the HIV-1 Tat protein [23], penetratin from the homeodomain of *Drosophila* Antennapedia [28], pVEC from murine vascular endothelial cadherin [42], and signal sequence-based peptides from various cytokines [43] are categorized in this group. All the protein-derived PTDs share a "positive charge" caused by basic amino acids such as arginine and lysine residues. Such information has helped to the development of several potent synthetic peptides such as polyarginine and polylysine, which show potential for penetration [44]. Amphipathic polypeptides

Table 2 Peptide sequences of representative PTDs

Category	Peptide	Peptide sequence
Protein-derived peptides	HIV-1 Tat peptide	YGRKKRRQRRR
	Penetratin (Ant)	RQIKIWFQNRRMKWKK
	pVEC	LLIILRRRIRKQAHAHSK
Designed peptides	R8 (Octaarginine)	RRRRRRRR
	K8 (Octalysine)	KKKKKKKK
	Transportan	GWTLNSAGYLLGKINLKALAALAKKIL
	MPG	GALFLGFLGAAGSTMGAWSQPKKKRKV

are composed of hydrophobic and hydrophilic domains from different sources, such as transportan, comprising galanin fused to mastoparan [45], and MPG, comprising HIV-1 gp41 protein fused to a peptide from the nuclear localization signal of SV40 large T-antigen [46].

4 Mechanism of PTD-Mediated Protein Transduction into Living Cells

More than 100 reports concerning PTDs have appeared this decade, and significant progress has been achieved especially with regard to the molecular mechanisms underlying the internalization of both PTD peptides and PTD-conjugated macromolecules into living cells. It is widely accepted that electrostatic interaction of positively charged PTD with negatively charged cellular membrane is followed by three energy- and temperature-dependent processes, clathrin-mediated endocytosis, lipid raft-mediated caveolae endocytosis, or macropinocytosis (Fig. 1).

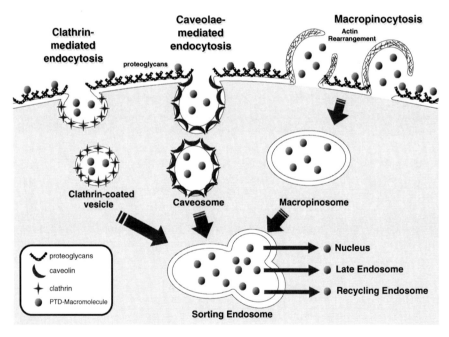

Fig. 1 Proposed model for the internalization of PTD-conjugated macromolecules into cells. Interaction of positively charged PTDs with negatively charged proteoglycans and glycosaminoglycans plays an important role in the internalization. The electrostatic interaction is followed by energy- and temperature-dependent endocytotic pathways. This involves phagocytotic and pinocytotic pathways: clathrin-mediated endocytosis, caveolae-mediated endocytosis, and macropinocytosis

Early on, it was reported that the internalization of Tat protein occurred even at 4°C [23], and similar observations were reported for the basic amino acid-rich peptide derived from the antennapedia homeodomain [47]. Therefore, it had been widely assumed that the PTD-mediated internalization occurs in an energy- and receptor-independent manner and is alternatively based on direct transport through the lipid bilayer. However, it has been reported that the energy independence and receptor independence resulted from experimental artifacts in the process of cell fixation prior to microscopic observation and also were due to the inadequate removal of PTD conjugates bound to the cell surface [48, 49]. Moreover, it has been reported that the internalization is almost completely suppressed at 4°C in unfixed conditions [49, 50]. All of these recent results, together with the observation that heparan sulfate and an inhibitor of low-density lipoprotein receptor-related protein precluded the cellular uptake of PTD peptides and PTD-fused macromolecules [50, 51], suggest that the interaction of positively charged PTDs with negatively charged cell surface constituents, such as proteoglycans and glycosaminoglycans (heparan sulfate, heparin), plays an important role in the internalization (Fig. 1) [51–54]. Also, the electrostatic interaction is followed by the three energy- and temperature-dependent processes [48].

A characteristic of clathrin-mediated endocytosis is the formation of clathrin-coated membrane pits that pinch off the cellular membrane to generate vesicles [49]. The involvement of clathrin-mediated endocytosis in the internalization of PTDs was suggested by the finding that an FITC-labeled avidin–Tat-PTD complex colocalized with transferrin, a classical endocytic marker [55]. The importance of the classical endocytotic pathway and the temperature sensitivity of PTD internalization was confirmed further [48].

A typical feature of caveola-mediated endocytosis is the formation of non-coated invaginations composed of detergent-resistant membrane components rich in cholesterol and sphingolipids, known as lipid rafts [56]. The importance of the caveola-mediated mechanism in the PTD-mediated internalization was confirmed in an experiment where the cellular uptake of Tat peptide was affected by drugs that either disrupt lipid rafts or alter caveolar trafficking [57]. Moreover, Tat-PTD-fused protein showed colocalization with a marker of caveolar uptake, caveolin, further strengthening the importance of the mechanism in the PTD-mediated internalization [57].

The importance of macropinocytosis in the PTD-mediated internalization of macromolecules was reported recently [58, 59]. Macropinocytosis defines a series of sequential events: (1) a dramatic reorganization and ruffling of the plasma membrane by actin filaments, (2) the formation of an external macropinocytic structure, and (3) the inclusion and internalization of large vesicles, known as macropinosomes, into the cytoplasm [60]. Using a permeable Tat-Cre recombinase reporter and living cells, Wadia et al. demonstrated that Tat-fusion proteins are rapidly internalized by the macropinocytic pathway after the initial ionic cell–surface interaction, confirming the importance of macropinocytosis for the internalization of macromolecules [58].

It is generally accepted that the mechanism responsible for the internalization depends on the size of the PTD conjugate. Namely, the macropinocytic pathway seems to be responsible for the internalization of macromolecules. In addition, caveolae-mediated pathway has also been reported to play an important role in it [57]. On the other hand, the caveolae-mediated or clathrin-mediated endocytic pathways seem to function in the internalization of PTD itself or PTD-conjugated small molecules.

5 Kinetics and Tissue Distribution of PTD-Fused Protein in Living Animals

Kinetics and tissue distribution of PTD-fused protein drugs in vivo are important information for the development of novel PTD-mediated anticancer therapeutics and for the optimization of therapeutic regimens. Schwarze et al. demonstrated that biologically active proteins could be delivered to many tissues including the liver, kidney, heart, muscle, lung, spleen, and brain of mice after intraperitoneal injection of 200–500 μg of Tat–β-Gal fusion protein [39]. Polyakov et al. reported a preliminary but important information that intravenous injection of Tat-PTD labeled with Technetium-99m (^{99m}Tc) showed a rapid distribution to whole body [61]. The level of Tat-^{99m}Tc in organs reached peak within 5 min after injection and showed modestly rapid blood clearance. The Tat-^{99m}Tc was rapidly cleared by both renal and hepatobiliary excretion over the subsequent 2 h with activity appearing in the urinary and bladder and bowel. In addition, Cai et al. analyzed in detail when Tat–β-Gal fusion protein is distributed in different organs, such as liver, kidney, spleen, lung, bowel, and brain, through four different routes, such as portal vein, intravenous, intraperitoneal, and oral administration [62]. Tissues were harvested 15 min, 1 h, 6 h, 10 h, and 24 h after the administration and subjected to enzymatic activity assay. β-Gal activity peaked at 15 min in most tissues after portal vein, intravenous, and intraperitoneal administration and at 1 h after oral dosing in all tissues (Fig. 2). β-Gal activity in the liver at 15 min after portal vein injection was higher than after intravenous, intraperitoneal, and oral dosing. The median initial half-life for activity was 2.2 h, ranging from 1.2 h to 3.4 h (Table 3). All of these pharmacokinetic data allow rational optimization of delivery route and schedules for therapeutic PTD-fused proteins.

6 Development of PTD-Mediated Anticancer Protein Drugs

Research on protein transduction has dramatically expanded from in vitro to in vivo in the last decade. The advantage of this application is that one can accomplish the rapid and equal distribution of PTD-conjugated macromolecules to all tissues and cells in vivo [39]. However, as medications, PTD-fused

Fig. 2 Quantitative analysis of Tat–β-Gal activity in organs. Tat–β-Gal fusion protein was injected through four routes (portal vein, intravenous, intraperitoneal, oral), and β-Gal activity of homogenates was normalized to the protein concentration in the sample. This figure was derived from Ref. [62]; therefore, see Ref. [62] for details

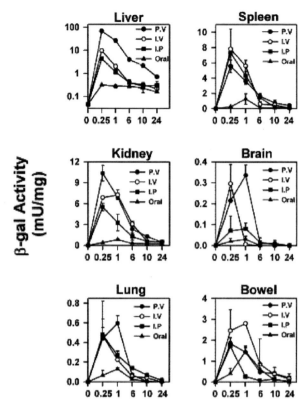

Hours after Treatment

Table 3 Half-life of β-galactosidase activity in the liver, kidney, and spleen of a mouse after administration

Route of administration	Half-life of β-Gal in each tissue after administration (500 μg/mouse)		
	Liver (h)	Kidney (h)	Spleen (h)
Portal vein	1.4	2.9	2.9
Intravenous	1.2	3.4	1.9
Intraperitoneal	1.7	2.9	2.3

The table was derived from Ref. [62]; therefore, see Ref. [62] for details.

anticancer macromolecules should have target specificity and act locally; otherwise damage to normal tissues and side effects may occur. In the following sections, we focus on the use of PTDs to develop anticancer macromolecules and introduce several representative strategies to distinguish between tumors and normal tissues to increase specificity but decrease side effects (Table 4).

Table 4 PTD-mediated anticancer strategies

Cargo	Effect	PTD	References
ODD-procaspase3	Tumor growth delay, radiosensitization	Tat	4–6, 78
p53 C-terminal region (p53C)	p53-dependent apoptosis	pAntp	7
p53C′ (modified p53C)	Tumor growth delay, 6 times extension in lifespan	Tat	8
p53 N-terminal region (p53N)	Activation of apoptotic genes, cytotoxicity for cancer cells, regression of human retinoblastoma cells in a rabbit eye	Tat	9
SmacN7	Enhancement of TRAIL in a tumor xenograft	Tat	10
SmacN7	Reversion of apoptosis resistance, synergistic effect with a chemotherapy	R8	11
Surv–T34A (Survivin T34A)	DNA fragmentation, aberrant nuclei formation, tumor cell apoptosis, tumor growth delay, 40–50% reduction in tumor mass	Tat	12
BH3 domain of Bak	Apoptosis of cancer cells	pAntp	13
BH3 domain of Bim	Apoptosis of cancer cells, tumor growth delay	Tat	14
$VHL_{104-123}$	Inhibition of thymidine incorporation into RCC cells, inhibition of MAP kinase pathway, inhibition of RCC proliferation in vitro, growth delay of RCC xenografts, regression of tumor volume, inhibition of invasion of RCC tumor	Tat	15
ESX	Reduction in ErbB2 protein level, induction of apoptosis retardation of growth of ErbB2-overexpressing breast cancer cells,	Tat	16
Tumor-associated antigen: OVA	Antigen presentation to CD4 T-cells, tumor regression in mice	Tat	17

6.1 Application of a HIF-1α ODD Domain; Development of Hypoxia-Targeting Protein Drugs

Genetic alterations directly cause the deregulated proliferation and high metabolic demands of tumor cells, which in turn lead to the imbalance of tumor
growth and the development of a tumor vasculature. These phenomena consequently cause hypoxic areas in solid tumors, to which the supply of oxygen from
tumor capillaries is inadequate [63, 64]. Hypoxia has been recognized as a
tumor-specific microenvironment; in other words, healthy adults probably
have few hypoxic tissues. Under hypoxic conditions, a transcription factor,
hypoxia-inducible factor-1 (HIF-1), induces the expression of various genes

related to angiogenesis [65] and glycolysis [66] and leads to invasive and meta-static properties of tumor cells [67]. Moreover, HIF-1 activity is associated with the resistance of tumor cells to conventional radiotherapy and chemotherapy [68, 69] and with patient mortality in clinical studies [70–72]. Therefore, extensive efforts have been devoted to the development of novel therapies, which specifically damage hypoxic/HIF-1-activating tumor cells [69, 73].

HIF-1 is a heterodimeric transcription factor composed of an alpha subunit (HIF-1α) and a constitutively expressed beta subunit (HIF-1β) [74]. HIF-1 activity is mainly dependent on the level of HIF-1α protein [74, 75]. Under hypoxic conditions, HIF-1α interacts with HIF-1β and functions as a transcription factor. Under normoxic conditions, the oxygen-dependent degradation (ODD) domain of HIF-1α is hydroxylated by prolyl hydroxylases (PHDs) and ubiquitinated by the von Hippel–Lindau (VHL) tumor suppressor protein-containing E3 ubiquitin ligase, resulting in rapid degradation of the HIF-1α protein [76, 77].

We took advantage of this unique property of the ODD domain to develop a novel hypoxia-targeting protein drug [4–6, 78]. First of all, we identified the minimum region of the ODD domain responsible for the oxygen-dependent degradation of arbitrary proteins fused to it [4]. We confirmed the hypoxia-dependent β-Gal and luciferase activity of ODD–β-Gal fusion protein [4] and ODD–luciferase fusion protein [79], respectively, in cultured cells. To apply the ODD-fusion protein to an in vivo study, we fused Tat-PTD to the N-terminal of the ODD–β-Gal protein and created a Tat–ODD–β-Gal triple-fusion protein [4]. After i.p. injection with the Tat–ODD–β-Gal fusion protein into subcutaneous tumor-bearing mice, β-Gal activity was detected only in the hypoxic regions of the solid tumor, not in normal tissue [4]. These results demonstrate that biologically active proteins can be exogenously delivered to hypoxic tumor cells by the Tat–ODD peptide in vivo. This was the first example of the target specificity of Tat-mediated protein delivery. To examine whether the Tat–ODD fusion protein with cytotoxicity shows a hypoxia-targeting effect, the Tat–ODD peptide was fused to a proapoptotic protein [4–6, 78]. We intentionally chose a precursor of caspase-3, procaspase-3, because it is activated in response to hypoxic stress, which was thought to reduce the possibility of side effects in the well-oxygenated normal tissues (Fig. 3A) [4, 78]. Systemic administration with the resultant fusion protein, Tat–ODD–procaspase-3 (TOP3), dramatically induced apoptosis of tumor cells in the border area between well-oxygenated viable cells and necrotic cells (Fig. 3B) [5]. TOP3 reduced volume of hypoxic tumor cells and entire tumor itself, as well as suppressed tumor growth without any obvious side effects (Fig. 3C) [4–6]. The hypoxia-targeting effect of TOP3 was proven using a rat ascites model, in which the intraperitoneal injection of MM1 cells results in highly hypoxic ascetic fluid [80]. Inoue et al. demonstrated that the intraperitoneal injection of TOP3 resulted in a significant increase in the lifespan of rats with malignant ascites, and furthermore, 60% of the treated animals were cured without the recurrence of ascites.

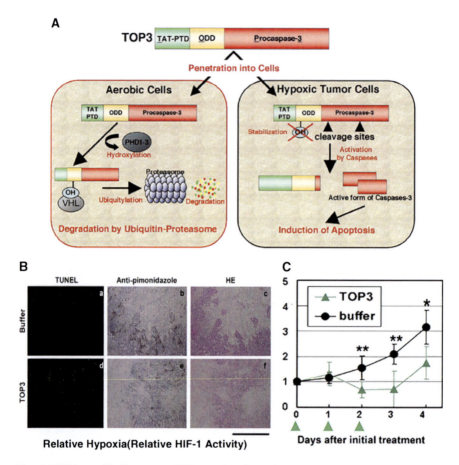

Fig. 3 TOP3 specifically targets HIF-1-active (hypoxic) tumor cells. (**A**) PTD facilitates internalization of TOP3 into tumor cells. In normoxic tumor cells, TOP3 is hydroxylated and ubiquitinated through the same regulation as HIF-1α protein, and resultantly degraded by 26S proteasome. Meanwhile, in hypoxic tumor cells, TOP3 is activated and induces apoptosis. See Ref. [78] for details. (**B**) TOP3 increased TUNNEL-positive apoptotic cells in border area between normoxic and necrotic areas. See Ref. [5] for details. (**C**) TOP3 significantly reduces HIF-1-positive (hypoxic) tumor cells. See Ref. [6] for details. This figure was modified from Ref. [5, 6, 78]

6.2 Restoration and Activation of p53 Function

Genetic alterations of oncogenes and/or tumor suppressor genes cause deregulated proliferation and the evasion of apoptosis and consequently make cells more malignant [1]. In the development of novel cancer therapy strategies, extensive efforts have been devoted to restoring the lesions preventing the implementation of the apoptotic response and leading to the death of malignant cells. Such treatments are expected to be much less toxic to normal tissue than the conventional genotoxic agents currently in clinical use.

The gene encoding the tumor suppressor p53 is the most common antiapoptotic lesion in cancer cells [81], and more than 50% of human cancers have been reported to harbor *p53* gene mutations. In most remaining cases, p53 activity is impaired by alternative molecular mechanisms, such as an elevated level of a p53 inhibitor, Mdm2 [82], and the E6 protein of HPV [83], or silencing of a p53 coactivator, ARF [84, 85]. One of the most important functions of p53 is "cell cycle arrest," in which p53 disturbs the replication of damaged genomic DNA and the fixation of mutations, allowing for DNA repair. Another important function is the "induction of apoptosis," which occurs when the damage to the genomic DNA is too severe to be repaired. Both of these functions are essential for the regulation of cell proliferation in multicellular organisms [85], and their loss frequently leads to cellular neoplastic transformation and increases the resistance of cancer cells to anticancer therapies [86]. Therefore, restoring p53 function in tumor cells has been recognized as an effective way to induce cancer cell death in a large population of cancer patients. Gene therapy strategies with viral or nonviral vectors have been used to introduce a functional p53 gene into experimental tumor xenografts; however, the transfer efficacy did not meet our demands [87]. Additionally, a problem associated with immunogenicity was inevitable with this drug delivery system [88]. To overcome these difficulties, Tat-mediated approaches were carried out as follows.

Selivanova et al. fused the Antennapedia transduction domain to a p53 C-terminal peptide (p53C), which was previously reported to activate the function of both wt p53 and several mutant forms of p53, and it confirmed that the fusion protein induced p53-dependent apoptosis in several tumor cell lines [7]. On the other hand, the fusion protein had no apparent apoptosis-inducing effect on normal cells with a functional *p53* gene. Snyder et al. then introduced a structural modification into the C-terminal to increase the stability of the protein, fused the resultant p53C' to Tat-PTD, and introduced the fusion protein (Tat-p53C') into tumor-bearing mice [8]. After an efficient delivery of Tat-p53C' to all the cells in mice, the protein was activated in the tumor xenograft but not in normal tissue. Moreover, intraperitoneal injection of the protein for 12 consecutive days caused a significant reduction in tumor growth and a 6-fold extension of lifespan.

Harbour et al. reported another strategy targeting *p53* lesion. They also aimed to restore endogenous p53 activity by using a permeable peptide [9]. HDM2 is known to decrease the ability of p53 to function as a positive transcription factor and facilitate proteolytic degradation of the protein through direct interaction with its N-terminal region [89]. Indeed, the over-expression of HDM2 has been reported in many clinically recognized tumors, which contain the wild-type *p53* gene and is associated with the functional inactivation of the p53 protein [90–92]. Therefore, the disruption of the inhibitory effect of HDM2 on p53 activity would be expected to yield therapeutic benefits in tumor cells that overexpress the HDM2 protein. Consequently, the N-terminal region of the p53 protein was fused to

Tat-PTD. The resultant Tat-p53N peptide induced the rapid accumulation of p53 and the activation of apoptotic genes, and it resulted in the preferential killing of tumor cells and the regression of human retinoblastoma cells in rabbit eyes [9]. Minimal retinal damage was observed after intravitreal injection [9].

6.3 Modification of Apoptotic Pathway

A major obstacle in cancer therapy is the resistance of cancer cells to current anticancer treatments: chemotherapy and radiation therapy [93]. Defects in apoptotic programs, which are caused by deregulated expression and function of the components of the apoptotic pathway, contribute to such resistance [94, 95].

Inhibitors of apoptosis proteins (IAPs), which inhibit caspase activity by directly binding to activated caspase-3 and -7, are frequently overexpresssed in malignant tumors [96]. The second mitochondria-derived activator of caspases (Smac) is an important factor that is released from the mitochondria to the cytosol, antagonizes IAPs, and release caspases to promote apoptosis [97, 98]. Based on these mechanisms, one can expect the upregulation of Smac activity in tumor cells to improve resistance to anticancer therapies. Fulda et al. examined this hypothesis using a cell-permeable synthetic peptide composed of Tat-PTD and seven N-terminal amino acids of the Smac protein (AVPIAQK) [10]. The cell-permeable Smac polypeptide was expected to inactivate X-linked IAP (XIAP), disrupt the interaction of XIAP and caspase-9, and consequently induce apoptosis. The peptide enhanced the therapeutic effect of Apo2L/ tumor necrosis factor-related apoptosis-inducing ligand (TRAIL) in an intracranial malignant glioma xenograft model [10]. Moreover, the complete eradication of established tumors was achieved only upon combined treatment with the Smac peptide and Apo2L/TRAIL. In these experiments, no detectable toxicity to normal brain tissue was observed.

Yang et al. examined whether the inhibition of IAPs combined with chemotherapy produced synergistic effects [11]. First of all, they confirmed that the defect in apoptosome activity was dramatically restored by the same seven amino residues of Smac protein through the disruption of XIAP–caspase-9 interaction. On the other hand, SmacN7 peptide did not have any striking effect on the apoptosome activity of normal lung fibroblast cells. They further demonstrated that newly synthesized SmacN7 peptide fused to the cell membrane-permeable polyarginine (SmacN7R8) strongly reversed the resistance to apoptosis, and it displayed a synergistic effect with chemotherapy in vivo (Fig. 4).

Because Survivin, a member of the inhibitor of apoptosis protein (IAP) family, is highly expressed in most tumors, it has been recognized as a promising therapeutic target in cancer [99]. A variety of Survivin antagonists have been reported to rescue the apoptotic pathway and induce apoptosis in

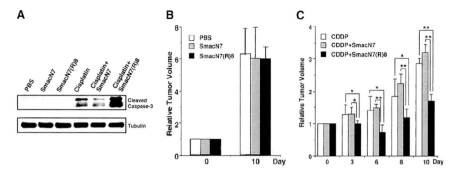

Fig. 4 Effect of SmacN7R8 in combination with chemotherapeutic agent on tumor growth in tumor-bearing mice. Human nonsmall-cell lung carcinoma, NCH-H460, tumor-bearing mice were treated with PBS, SmacN7 (without cell permeability), SmacN7R8 (with cell permeability), Cisplatin, Cisplatin + SmacN7, or Cisplatin + SmacN7R8. (**A**) Western blotting for cleaved caspase-3 in the tumor tissues at 48 h after the treatment. (**B and C**) Tumor volume at indicated days after the treatment. Note: Cell permeable SmacN7R8 sensitized the apoptosis-inducing activity of Cisplatin and potentiated the antitumor activity of Cisplatin. This figure was modified from Ref. [11]; therefore, see Ref. [11] for details

malignant cells; however, the utility of these agents has been limited by the inadequate delivery and permeability into tumor cells. To overcome these problems, Yan et al. generated a recombinant fusion protein composed of Tat-PTD and a dominant-negative mutant of Survivin, T34A mutant [12]. Tat–Surv–T34A induced cell detachment, DNA fragmentation, caspase-3 activation, and mitochondrial release of apoptosis-inducing factor in vitro. Moreover, intraperitoneal injection of the fusion protein into subcutaneous tumor-bearing mice increased aberrant nuclei formation and tumor cell apoptosis, resulting in a 40–50% reduction in growth and mass of the tumor xenografts.

A characteristic of the *Bcl-2* family is the presence of one or more conserved Bcl-2 homology domains (BH1-4) corresponding to four α-helical segments of Bcl-2 [100]. The *Bcl-2* family is categorized into three groups: antiapoptotic proteins (Bcl-2, Bcl-xL, Mcl-1), BH3-only proteins (Bim, Bid, Bad, PUMA), and BH1-3 multidomain proteins (Bax, Bak, Bok). The BH3-only proteins bind to the BH-4 domain of the antiapoptotic proteins, antagonize the function of these proteins, and consequently induce apoptosis of cancer cells. Applying this molecular mechanism, Holinger et al. fused the antennapedia PTD to the BH3 domain and successfully induced the apoptosis of HeLa cells [13]. Similarly, Kashiwagi et al. synthesized a polypeptide composed of Tat-PTD and the BH3 domain of Bim and confirmed that Tat–Bim induced apoptosis of T cell lymphoma (EL4), pancreatic cancer (Panc-2), and melanoma (B16) cells in a dose-dependent fashion [14]. Moreover, local injections of Tat–Bim twice a day for 7 days significantly delayed growth in murine models of pancreatic cancer and melanoma.

6.4 Modification of IGF-I Signaling Pathway

The growth of various kinds of cancer cells depends on insulin-like growth factor-I (IGF-I)-mediated signaling; therefore, inhibiting this pathway has been recognized as a promising strategy. Indeed, direct inhibition of this pathway using a truncated form (dominant-negative form) of the IGF-I receptor (IGF-IR) [101], a specific IGF-IR antibody [102], or a specific IGF-IR antisense oligonucleotide [103] showed a significant therapeutic effect on various experimental tumor xenografts. In addition to such direct inhibition, an indirect method by transducing the functional VHL protein into cancer cells seems to be effective for renal cell carcinoma (RCC). This idea is attributed to the fact that VHL is functionally inactivated in many RCCs [104], and the dysfunction accelerates the growth of RCC cells through the activation of the IGF-I-mediated signaling pathway [15, 105]. Datta et al. fused Tat-PTD to a specific amino acid sequence of the VHL β domain ($VHL_{104-123}$), which binds to the cytoplasmic region of IGF-IR and inhibits IGF-I signaling, and examined the therapeutic effects on RCC [15]. The fusion protein, Tat–FLAG–VHL peptide, inhibited thymidine incorporation into RCC cells by nearly 80% compared with a counterpart protein (Tat–FLAG). Furthermore, the Tat–FLAG–VHL peptide inhibited the tyrosine phosphorylation of MAP kinase, an essential downstream molecule that leads to cell proliferation. Thus, these results suggest that Tat– FLAG–VHL peptide blocks IGF-I-induced proliferation of RCC cells in vitro. Furthermore, i.p. injections of Tat–FLAG–VHL peptide retarded the growth of subcutaneous RCC tumors, and in some cases, reduced the tumor volume, and dramatically inhibited invasiveness into the muscle layer.

6.5 Modification of ErbB2 (HER-2/neu) Expression

The ErbB2 (HER-2/neu) gene is a member of the epidermal growth factor receptor family and is overexpressed in ~30% of breast cancers [106, 107]. Deregulated expression of this gene is associated with lymph node metastasis and a poor prognosis [108, 109]. Therefore, the ErbB2 would serve as an excellent target for the development of novel cancer treatments. One of the critical transcription factors that activate the ErbB2 expression in breast cancer is ESX (ESE-1//ELF3/ERT/Jen) [110]. ESX interacts with DRIP130/CRSP130/Sur-2, a Ras-linked metazoan-specific subunit of human mediator complexes, binds to the ESX-binding site in the ErbB2 promoter, and activates the transcription of the ErbB2 gene [16]. Disruption of ESX–DRIP130 interaction is reported to impair ErbB2 gene expression and reduce the proliferation and viability of ErbB2-expressing breast cancer cells [16]. Asada et al. identified the region essential for ESX–DRIP130 interaction and designed a cell-permeable form of ESX peptide using Tat-PTD [16]. The Tat–ESX peptide reduced the ErbB2 protein level, retarded cell growth, and induced apoptosis in ErbB2-overexpressing breast cancer cells. The important point of their report is that cells with low ErbB2 protein levels were insensitive to the Tat–ESX peptide.

6.6 Application to Dendritic Cell (DC) Vaccines

Dendritic cell (DC)-based vaccines are being developed to treat cancer, and clinical trials are ongoing [111, 112]. A primary goal of the strategy is to elicit responses from cytotoxic lymphocytes (CTL) that can kill tumor cells. In most cases, tumor antigen-derived peptides are loaded into DCs in vitro, and the cells are administered into patients. Expression of the defined tumor antigen in DCs can be achieved by transfecting the cells with cDNA encoding the tumor antigen or by infecting the cells with virus expressing the antigen; however, there are two problems with these methods. First, the transfection of DCs is inefficient, and second, there are practical and theoretical concerns that relate to the use of viral vectors in patients. As an alternative to these genetic modifications, Shibagaki et al. explored PTD-mediated antigen transduction into DCs to elicit CTLs that can lead to tumor rejection in vivo [17]. They demonstrated that a bacterial recombinant model tumor-associated antigen that was fused to Tat-PTD was efficiently transduced into murine lymphocytes and DCs and was processed by proteasomes. The resultant peptides were displayed on the cell surface bound to MHC class I. The transduced DCs were able to elicit CTLs in vivo, and the CTL activity was sufficient to both prevent engraftment with antigen-expressing tumors into mice and lead to a partial regression of the established tumor mass.

6.7 PTD-Mediated Modulation of Deregulated Cell Cycle of Cancer Cells

In nonmalignant cells, the product of the *Rb* gene (pRb) binds to transcription factors belonging to the E2F family and represses their function as transcriptional activators [113]. Cyclin-dependent kinases (Cdks) inactivate pRb, release E2F from the pRb–E2F complex, and consequently upregulate the transcription of late G1 phase-specific genes responsible for S-phase entry. The Cdks are known to be activated through the formation of a complex with cyclins (A–D) and inactivated by p16INK4a, p21, and p27 [114, 115]. This well-organized regulation of the cell cycle is disrupted in malignant cells through genetic alterations, such as inactivation of p16INK4a, amplification of cyclin D1 or Cdk4, or loss or mutation of *Rb gene* [116, 117]. Therefore, reconstitution of the tumor suppressor function of p16INK4, p21, and p27 has been an aim for cancer therapy. As for p16INK4, it has been reported that a 20-amino acid polypeptide in the third ankyrin-like repeat of p16 is sufficient to inhibit cyclin D-Cdk4/6-dependent inactivation of pRb [118]. Based on this knowledge, Guis et al. demonstrated that this p16 polypeptide fused to Tat-PTD (Tat-p16 peptide) was internalized into cultured cells and subsequently induced G1 arrest [119]. As for p21, Ball et al. demonstrated that a 20-amino acid peptide of the C-terminal Cdk-binding domain of p21 conjugated with antennapedia PTD suppressed pRb phosphorylation (inactivation) and consequently induced G_1/S cell cycle arrest (Fig. 5) [120]. As for p27, in order to reconstitute its tumor suppressor function, it was fused to Tat-PTD and applied to human Jurkat

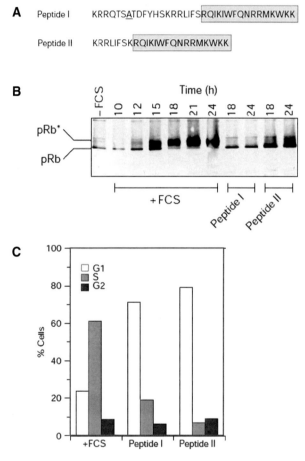

Fig. 5 C-terminal Cdk-binding domain of p21 conjugated with antennapedia PTD suppresses pRb phosphorylation and induces G_1/S cell cycle arrest. (**A**) Peptide sequences of fusion polypeptides composed of C-terminal Cdk-binding domain of p21 (p21$_{141-160}$ [peptide I]; or p21$_{154-160}$ [peptide II]) and antennapedia PTD (*boxed*). (**B**) pRb became hyperphosphorylated between 12 and 15 h after serum was added to starved HaCat cells, but in the presence of peptide I or II remained hypophosphorylated. pRb = hypophosphorylated, pRb* = hyperphosphorylated. (**C**) Cell cycle distribution of HaCat cells after culture in D-MEM medium containing 10% FCS alone or 10% FCS with peptide I or II. Note: Peptide I and II inhibited the phosphorylation of pRb and induced G_1/S cell cycle arrest. This figure was modified from Ref. [120]; therefore, see Ref. [120] for details

T cells in vitro [121]. The Tat-p27 protein dose-dependently induced cell cycle arrest at G1. Snyder et al. demonstrated that the Tat-p27 tumor suppressor protein actually inhibited tumor growth in two mouse models, such as a H1299 subcutaneous solid tumor xenograft model and a more clinical-relevant peritoneal tumor model [122].

6.8 Specific Delivery of PTD-Conjugated Macromolecules to Cancer Cells

Several in vitro studies have reported other possibilities which may enable the delivery of the PTD-conjugated macromolecule specifically to the desired tumor in vivo. First, because tumor cells are reported to have unique glycosaminoglycan on their surface, PTDs, which selectively interact with it, may enables us to selectively target tumor cells [55]. Second, by inserting a tissue- and organelle-specific cleavage recognition site between it and the macromolecule, PTD may be cleaved off, resulting in the accumulation of the PTD-free macromolecules in the desired tissue and organelle [123]. Third, it is also possible to generate a PTD-linked protein drug that specifically acts on tumor cells without affecting normal cells, by applying transformed cell-specific protein activity. Finally, by using a peptide that can be recognized by the tumor-specific membrane proteins, it may be possible to design a variety of proteins that are specifically internalized into desired tissues.

7 Conclusions and Perspectives

Recent advances in molecular and cellular biological techniques have helped to reveal the mechanisms underlying carcinogenesis and tumorigenesis. Based on this knowledge, several ways of discriminating nonmalignant and malignant cells have been proposed, in order to develop PTD-mediated anticancer strategies. Good examples are the exploitation of tumor-specific phenomena, such as dysfunction of p53, suppression of the apoptotic pathway, accelerated IGF-I or ErbB2 (HER-2/neu) signaling pathway, or tumor hypoxia. Each strategy actually showed expected anticancer effects; however, all of them have been achieved only in animal experiments. We are now confronted with the task of applying these strategies to the clinical setting. For that purpose, we cannot ignore the following problems: how to decrease the immunogenicity of PTD-conjugated macromolecules, and how to prepare enough high-quality PTD-conjugated macromolecule. Overcoming these problems should lead to the development of a new generation of anticancer strategies. In addition, the continuation of efforts to explore novel molecular mechanisms responsible for cancer-specific phenomena will pave the way to the development of an innovative PTD-mediated cancer therapy.

References

1. Hanahan D, Weinberg RA. The hallmarks of cancer. *Cell* 2000; **100**: 57–70.
2. Wadia JS, Dowdy SF. Protein transduction technology. *Curr Opin Biotechnol* 2002; **13**: 52–56.
3. Wadia JS, Dowdy SF. Modulation of cellular function by TAT mediated transduction of full length proteins. *Curr Protein Pept Sci* 2003; **4**: 97–104.
4. Harada H, Hiraoka M, Kizaka-Kondoh S. Antitumor effect of TAT-oxygen-dependent degradation-caspase-3 fusion protein specifically stabilized and activated in hypoxic tumor cells. *Cancer Res* 2002; **62**: 2013–2018.
5. Harada H, Kizaka-Kondoh S, Hiraoka M. Optical imaging of tumor hypoxia and evaluation of efficacy of a hypoxia-targeting drug in living animals. *Mol Imaging* 2005; **4**: 182–193.
6. Harada H, Kizaka-Kondoh S, Li G, et al. Significance of HIF-1-active cells in angiogenesis and radioresistance. *Oncogene* 2007; **26**: 7508–7516.
7. Selivanova G, Iotsova V, Okan I, et al. Restoration of the growth suppression function of mutant p53 by a synthetic peptide derived from the p53 C-terminal domain. *Nat Med* 1997; **3**: 632–638.
8. Snyder EL, Meade BR, Saenz CC, Dowdy SF. Treatment of terminal peritoneal carcinomatosis by a transducible p53-activating peptide. *PLoS Biol* 2004; **2**: E36.
9. Harbour JW, Worley L, Ma D, Cohen M. Transducible peptide therapy for uveal melanoma and retinoblastoma. *Arch Ophthalmol* 2002; **120**: 1341–1346.
10. Fulda S, Wick W, Weller M, Debatin KM. Smac agonists sensitize for Apo2L/TRAIL- or anticancer drug-induced apoptosis and induce regression of malignant glioma in vivo. *Nat Med* 2002; **8**: 808–815.
11. Yang L, Mashima T, Sato S, et al. Predominant suppression of apoptosome by inhibitor of apoptosis protein in non-small cell lung cancer H460 cells: therapeutic effect of a novel polyarginine-conjugated Smac peptide. *Cancer Res* 2003; **63**: 831–837.
12. Yan H, Thomas J, Liu T, et al. Induction of melanoma cell apoptosis and inhibition of tumor growth using a cell-permeable Survivin antagonist. *Oncogene* 2006; **25**: 6968–6974.
13. Holinger EP, Chittenden T, Lutz RJ. Bak BH3 peptides antagonize Bcl-xL function and induce apoptosis through cytochrome *c*-independent activation of caspases. *J Biol Chem* 1999; **274**: 13298–13304.
14. Kashiwagi H, McDunn JE, Goedegebuure PS, et al. TAT-Bim induces extensive apoptosis in cancer cells. *Ann Surg Oncol* 2007; **14**: 1763–1771.
15. Datta K, Sundberg C, Karumanchi SA, Mukhopadhyay D. The 104–123 amino acid sequence of the beta-domain of von Hippel-Lindau gene product is sufficient to inhibit renal tumor growth and invasion. *Cancer Res* 2001; **61**: 1768–1775
16. Asada S, Choi Y, Yamada M, et al. External control of Her2 expression and cancer cell growth by targeting a Ras-linked coactivator. *Proc Natl Acad Sci USA* 2002; **99**: 12747–12752.
17. Shibagaki N, Udey MC. Dendritic cells transduced with protein antigens induce cytotoxic lymphocytes and elicit antitumor immunity. *J Immunol* 2002; **168**: 2393–2401.
18. Green M, Loewenstein PM. Autonomous functional domains of chemically synthesized human immunodeficiency virus tat trans-activator protein. *Cell* 1988; **55**: 1179–1188.
19. Frankel AD, Pabo CO. Cellular uptake of the tat protein from human immunodeficiency virus. *Cell* 1988; **55**: 1189–1193.
20. Fawell S, Seery J, Daikh Y, et al. Tat-mediated delivery of heterologous proteins into cells. *Proc Natl Acad Sci USA* 1994; **91**: 664–668.
21. Mann DA, Frankel AD. Endocytosis and targeting of exogenous HIV-1 Tat protein. *Embo J* 1991; **10**: 1733–1739.

22. Ezhevsky SA, Nagahara H, Vocero-Akbani AM, Gius DR, Wei MC, Dowdy SF. Hypophosphorylation of the retinoblastoma protein (pRb) by cyclin D:Cdk4/6 complexes results in active pRb. *Proc Natl Acad Sci USA* 1997; **94**: 10699–10704.

23. Vives E, Brodin P, Lebleu B. A truncated HIV-1 Tat protein basic domain rapidly translocates through the plasma membrane and accumulates in the cell nucleus. *J Biol Chem* 1997; **272**: 16010–16017.

24. Becker-Hapak M, McAllister SS, Dowdy SF. TAT-mediated protein transduction into mammalian cells. *Methods* 2001; **24**: 247–256.

25. Joliot A, Pernelle C, Deagostini-Bazin H, Prochiantz A. Antennapedia homeobox peptide regulates neural morphogenesis. *Proc Natl Acad Sci USA* 1991; **88**: 1864–1868.

26. Joliot AH, Triller A, Volovitch M, Pernelle C, Prochiantz A. alpha-2,8-Polysialic acid is the neuronal surface receptor of antennapedia homeobox peptide. *New Biol* 1991; **3**: 1121–1134.

27. Le Roux I, Joliot AH, Bloch-Gallego E, Prochiantz A, Volovitch M. Neurotrophic activity of the Antennapedia homeodomain depends on its specific DNA-binding properties. *Proc Natl Acad Sci USA* 1993; **90**: 9120–9124.

28. Derossi D, Joliot AH, Chassaing G, Prochiantz A. The third helix of the Antennapedia homeodomain translocates through biological membranes. *J Biol Chem* 1994; **269**: 10444–10450.

29. Elliott G, O'Hare P. Intercellular trafficking and protein delivery by a herpesvirus structural protein. *Cell* 1997; **88**: 223–233.

30. Jarver P, Langel U. The use of cell-penetrating peptides as a tool for gene regulation. *Drug Discov Today* 2004; **9**: 395–402.

31. Astriab-Fisher A, Sergueev DS, Fisher M, Shaw BR, Juliano RL. Antisense inhibition of P-glycoprotein expression using peptide-oligonucleotide conjugates. *Biochem Pharmacol* 2000; **60**: 83–90.

32. Gallazzi F, Wang Y, Jia F, et al. Synthesis of radiometal-labeled and fluorescent cell-permeating peptide-PNA conjugates for targeting the bcl-2 proto-oncogene. *Bioconjug Chem* 2003; **14**: 1083–1095.

33. Ignatovich IA, Dizhe EB, Pavlotskaya AV, et al. Complexes of plasmid DNA with basic domain 47-57 of the HIV-1 Tat protein are transferred to mammalian cells by endocytosis-mediated pathways. *J Biol Chem* 2003; **278**: 42625–42636.

34. Lewin M, Carlesso N, Tung CH, et al. Tat peptide-derivatized magnetic nanoparticles allow in vivo tracking and recovery of progenitor cells. *Nat Biotechnol* 2000; **18**: 410–414.

35. Torchilin VP, Rammohan R, Weissig V, Levchenko TS. TAT peptide on the surface of liposomes affords their efficient intracellular delivery even at low temperature and in the presence of metabolic inhibitors. *Proc Natl Acad Sci USA* 2001; **98**: 8786–8791.

36. Eguchi A, Akuta T, Okuyama H, et al. Protein transduction domain of HIV-1 Tat protein promotes efficient delivery of DNA into mammalian cells. *J Biol Chem* 2001; **276**: 26204–26210.

37. Heng BC, Cao T. Making cell-permeable antibodies (Transbody) through fusion of protein transduction domains (PTD) with single chain variable fragment (scFv) antibodies: potential advantages over antibodies expressed within the intracellular environment (Intrabody). *Med Hypotheses* 2005; **64**: 1105–1108.

38. Troy CM, Stefanis L, Prochiantz A, Greene LA, Shelanski ML. The contrasting roles of ICE family proteases and interleukin-1beta in apoptosis induced by trophic factor withdrawal and by copper/zinc superoxide dismutase down-regulation. *Proc Natl Acad Sci USA* 1996; **93**: 5635–5640.

39. Schwarze SR, Ho A, Vocero-Akbani A, Dowdy SF. In vivo protein transduction: delivery of a biologically active protein into the mouse. *Science* 1999; **285**: 1569–1572.

40. Lindgren M, Hallbrink M, Prochiantz A, Langel U. Cell-penetrating peptides. *Trends Pharmacol Sci* 2000; **21**: 99–103.

41. Zorko M, Langel U. Cell-penetrating peptides: mechanism and kinetics of cargo delivery. *Adv Drug Deliv Rev* 2005; **57**: 529–545.
42. Elmquist A, Lindgren M, Bartfai T, Langel U. VE-cadherin-derived cell-penetrating peptide, pVEC, with carrier functions. *Exp Cell Res* 2001; **269**: 237–244.
43. Rojas M, Donahue JP, Tan Z, Lin YZ. Genetic engineering of proteins with cell membrane permeability. *Nat Biotechnol* 1998; **16**: 370–375.
44. Futaki S, Suzuki T, Ohashi W, et al. Arginine-rich peptides. An abundant source of membrane-permeable peptides having potential as carriers for intracellular protein delivery. *J Biol Chem* 2001; **276**: 5836–5840.
45. Pooga M, Hallbrink M, Zorko M, Langel U. Cell penetration by transportan. *Faseb J* 1998; **12**: 67–77.
46. Morris MC, Vidal P, Chaloin L, Heitz F, Divita G. A new peptide vector for efficient delivery of oligonucleotides into mammalian cells. *Nucleic Acids Res* 1997; **25**: 2730–2736.
47. Derossi D, Calvet S, Trembleau A, Brunissen A, Chassaing G, Prochiantz A. Cell internalization of the third helix of the Antennapedia homeodomain is receptor-independent. *J Biol Chem* 1996; **271**: 18188–18193.
48. Lundberg M, Wikstrom S, Johansson M. Cell surface adherence and endocytosis of protein transduction domains. *Mol Ther* 2003; **8**: 143–150.
49. Richard JP, Melikov K, Vives E, et al. Cell-penetrating peptides. A reevaluation of the mechanism of cellular uptake. *J Biol Chem* 2003; **278**: 585–590.
50. Liu Y, Jones M, Hingtgen CM, et al. Uptake of HIV-1 tat protein mediated by low-density lipoprotein receptor-related protein disrupts the neuronal metabolic balance of the receptor ligands. *Nat Med* 2000; **6**: 1380–1387.
51. Tyagi M, Rusnati M, Presta M, Giacca M. Internalization of HIV-1 tat requires cell surface heparan sulfate proteoglycans. *J Biol Chem* 2001; **276**: 3254–3261.
52. Sandgren S, Cheng F, Belting M. Nuclear targeting of macromolecular polyanions by an HIV-Tat derived peptide. Role for cell-surface proteoglycans. *J Biol Chem* 2002; **277**: 38877–38883.
53. Mai JC, Shen H, Watkins SC, Cheng T, Robbins PD. Efficiency of protein transduction is cell type-dependent and is enhanced by dextran sulfate. *J Biol Chem* 2002; **277**: 30208–30218.
54. Violini S, Sharma V, Prior JL, Dyszlewski M, Piwnica-Worms D. Evidence for a plasma membrane-mediated permeability barrier to Tat basic domain in well-differentiated epithelial cells: lack of correlation with heparan sulfate. *Biochemistry* 2002; **41**: 12652–12661.
55. Console S, Marty C, Garcia-Echeverria C, Schwendener R, Ballmer-Hofer K. Antennapedia and HIV transactivator of transcription (TAT) "protein transduction domains" promote endocytosis of high molecular weight cargo upon binding to cell surface glycosaminoglycans. *J Biol Chem* 2003; **278**: 35109–35114.
56. Anderson RG. The caveolae membrane system. *Annu Rev Biochem* 1998; **67**: 199–225.
57. Fittipaldi A, Ferrari A, Zoppe M, et al. Cell membrane lipid rafts mediate caveolar endocytosis of HIV-1 Tat fusion proteins. *J Biol Chem* 2003; **278**: 34141–34149.
58. Wadia JS, Stan RV, Dowdy SF. Transducible TAT-HA fusogenic peptide enhances escape of TAT-fusion proteins after lipid raft macropinocytosis. *Nat Med* 2004; **10**: 310–315.
59. Kaplan IM, Wadia JS, Dowdy SF. Cationic TAT peptide transduction domain enters cells by macropinocytosis. *J Control Release* 2005; **102**: 247–253.
60. Conner SD, Schmid SL. Regulated portals of entry into the cell. *Nature* 2003; **422**: 37–44.
61. Polyakov V, Sharma V, Dahlheimer JL, Pica CM, Luker GD, Piwnica-Worms D. Novel Tat-peptide chelates for direct transduction of technetium-99m and rhenium into human cells for imaging and radiotherapy. *Bioconjug Chem* 2000; **11**: 762–771.
62. Cai SR, Xu G, Becker-Hapak M, Ma M, Dowdy SF, McLeod HL. The kinetics and tissue distribution of protein transduction in mice. *Eur J Pharm Sci* 2006; **27**: 311–319.

63. Vaupel P, Kallinowski F, Okunieff P. Blood flow, oxygen and nutrient supply, and metabolic microenvironment of human tumors: a review. *Cancer Res* 1989; **49**: 6449–6465.
64. Dang CV, Semenza GL. Oncogenic alterations of metabolism. *Trends Biochem Sci* 1999; **24**: 68–72.
65. Forsythe JA, Jiang BH, Iyer NV, et al. Activation of vascular endothelial growth factor gene transcription by hypoxia-inducible factor 1. *Mol Cell Biol* 1996; **16**: 4604–4613.
66. Semenza GL, Roth PH, Fang HM, Wang GL. Transcriptional regulation of genes encoding glycolytic enzymes by hypoxia-inducible factor 1. *J Biol Chem* 1994; **269**: 23757–23763.
67. Zhong H, De Marzo AM, Laughner E, et al. Overexpression of hypoxia-inducible factor 1alpha in common human cancers and their metastases. *Cancer Res* 1999; **59**: 5830–5835.
68. Brown JM. The hypoxic cell: a target for selective cancer therapy – eighteenth Bruce F. Cain Memorial Award lecture. *Cancer Res* 1999; **59**: 5863–5870.
69. Semenza GL. Targeting HIF-1 for cancer therapy. *Nat Rev Cancer* 2003; **3**: 721–732.
70. Birner P, Schindl M, Obermair A, Plank C, Breitenecker G, Oberhuber G. Overexpression of hypoxia-inducible factor 1alpha is a marker for an unfavorable prognosis in early-stage invasive cervical cancer. *Cancer Res* 2000; **60**: 4693–4696.
71. Birner P, Gatterbauer B, Oberhuber G, et al. Expression of hypoxia-inducible factor-1 alpha in oligodendrogliomas: its impact on prognosis and on neoangiogenesis. *Cancer* 2001; **92**: 165–171.
72. Schindl M, Schoppmann SF, Samonigg H, et al. Overexpression of hypoxia-inducible factor 1alpha is associated with an unfavorable prognosis in lymph node-positive breast cancer. *Clin Cancer Res* 2002; **8**: 1831–1837.
73. Kizaka-Kondoh S, Inoue M, Harada H, Hiraoka M. Tumor hypoxia: a target for selective cancer therapy. *Cancer Sci* 2003; **94**: 1021–1028.
74. Wang GL, Jiang BH, Rue EA, Semenza GL. Hypoxia-inducible factor 1 is a basic-helix-loop-helix-PAS heterodimer regulated by cellular O_2 tension. *Proc Natl Acad Sci USA* 1995; **92**: 5510–5514.
75. Hirota K, Semenza GL. Regulation of hypoxia-inducible factor 1 by prolyl and asparaginyl hydroxylases. *Biochem Biophys Res Commun* 2005; **338**: 610–616.
76. Iliopoulos O, Levy AP, Jiang C, Kaelin Jr WG, Goldberg MA. Negative regulation of hypoxia-inducible genes by the von Hippel-Lindau protein. *Proc Natl Acad Sci USA* 1996; **93**: 10595–10599.
77. Jaakkola P, Mole DR, Tian YM, et al. Targeting of HIF-alpha to the von Hippel-Lindau ubiquitylation complex by O_2-regulated prolyl hydroxylation. *Science* 2001; **292**: 468–472.
78. Harada H, Kizaka-Kondoh S, Hiraoka M. Mechanism of hypoxia-specific cytotoxicity of procaspase-3 fused with a VHL-mediated protein destruction motif of HIF-1alpha containing Pro564. *FEBS Lett* 2006; **580**: 5718–5722.
79. Harada H, Kizaka-Kondoh S, Itasaka S, et al. The combination of hypoxia-response enhancers and an oxygen-dependent proteolytic motif enables real-time imaging of absolute HIF-1 activity in tumor xenografts. *Biochem Biophys Res Commun* 2007; **360**: 791–796.
80. Inoue M, Mukai M, Hamanaka Y, Tatsuta M, Hiraoka M, Kizaka-Kondoh S. Targeting hypoxic cancer cells with a protein prodrug is effective in experimental malignant ascites. *Int J Oncol* 2004; **25**: 713–720.
81. Vousden KH, Lu X. Live or let die: the cell's response to p53. *Nat Rev Cancer* 2002; **2**: 594–604.
82. Momand J, Zambetti GP, Olson DC, George D, Levine AJ. The mdm-2 oncogene product forms a complex with the p53 protein and inhibits p53-mediated transactivation. *Cell* 1992; **69**: 1237–1245.
83. Scheffner M, Werness BA, Huibregtse JM, Levine AJ, Howley PM. The E6 oncoprotein encoded by human papillomavirus types 16 and 18 promotes the degradation of p53. *Cell* 1990; **63**: 1129–1136.

84. Kamijo T, Weber JD, Zambetti G, Zindy F, Roussel MF, Sherr CJ. Functional and physical interactions of the ARF tumor suppressor with p53 and Mdm2. *Proc Natl Acad Sci USA* 1998; **95**: 8292–8297.

85. Vogelstein B, Lane D, Levine AJ. Surfing the p53 network. *Nature* 2000; **408**: 307–310.

86. Sherr CJ, McCormick F. The RB and p53 pathways in cancer. *Cancer Cell* 2002; **2**: 103–112.

87. Roth JA, Nguyen D, Lawrence DD, et al. Retrovirus-mediated wild-type p53 gene transfer to tumors of patients with lung cancer. *Nat Med* 1996; **2**: 985–991.

88. McCormick F. Cancer gene therapy: fringe or cutting edge? *Nat Rev Cancer* 2001; **1**: 130–141.

89. Wu X, Bayle JH, Olson D, Levine AJ. The p53-mdm-2 autoregulatory feedback loop. *Genes Dev* 1993; **7**: 1126–1132.

90. Polsky D, Melzer K, Hazan C, et al. HDM2 protein overexpression and prognosis in primary malignant melanoma. *J Natl Cancer Inst* 2002; **94**: 1803–1806.

91. Mori S, Ito G, Usami N, et al. p53 apoptotic pathway molecules are frequently and simultaneously altered in nonsmall cell lung carcinoma. *Cancer* 2004; **100**: 1673–1682.

92. Berger AJ, Camp RL, Divito KA, Kluger HM, Halaban R, Rimm DL. Automated quantitative analysis of HDM2 expression in malignant melanoma shows association with early-stage disease and improved outcome. *Cancer Res* 2004; **64**: 8767–8772.

93. Lowe SW, Lin AW. Apoptosis in cancer. *Carcinogenesis* 2000; **21**: 485–495.

94. Goyal L. Cell death inhibition: keeping caspases in check. *Cell* 2001; **104**: 805–808.

95. Deveraux QL, Reed JC. IAP family proteins – suppressors of apoptosis. *Genes Dev* 1999; **13**: 239–252.

96. Nachmias B, Ashhab Y, Ben-Yehuda D. The inhibitor of apoptosis protein family (IAPs): an emerging therapeutic target in cancer. *Semin Cancer Biol* 2004; **14**: 231–243.

97. Du C, Fang M, Li Y, Li L, Wang X. Smac, a mitochondrial protein that promotes cytochrome c-dependent caspase activation by eliminating IAP inhibition. *Cell* 2000; **102**: 33–42.

98. Verhagen AM, Ekert PG, Pakusch M, et al. Identification of DIABLO, a mammalian protein that promotes apoptosis by binding to and antagonizing IAP proteins. *Cell* 2000; **102**: 43–53.

99. Altieri DC. Validating survivin as a cancer therapeutic target. *Nat Rev Cancer* 2003; **3**: 46–54.

100. Gross A, McDonnell JM, Korsmeyer SJ. BCL-2 family members and the mitochondria in apoptosis. *Genes Dev* 1999; **13**: 1899–1911.

101. Prager D, Li HL, Asa S, Melmed S. Dominant negative inhibition of tumorigenesis in vivo by human insulin-like growth factor I receptor mutant. *Proc Natl Acad Sci USA* 1994; **91**: 2181–2185.

102. Kalebic T, Tsokos M, Helman LJ. In vivo treatment with antibody against IGF-1 receptor suppresses growth of human rhabdomyosarcoma and down-regulates p34cdc2. *Cancer Res* 1994; **54**: 5531–5534.

103. Lee CT, Wu S, Gabrilovich D, et al. Antitumor effects of an adenovirus expressing antisense insulin-like growth factor I receptor on human lung cancer cell lines. *Cancer Res* 1996; **56**: 3038–3041.

104. Zbar B, Glenn G, Lubensky I, et al. Hereditary papillary renal cell carcinoma: clinical studies in 10 families. *J Urol* 1995; **153**: 907–912.

105. Datta K, Nambudripad R, Pal S, Zhou M, Cohen HT, Mukhopadhyay D. Inhibition of insulin-like growth factor-I-mediated cell signaling by the von Hippel-Lindau gene product in renal cancer. *J Biol Chem* 2000; **275**: 20700–20706.

106. Slamon DJ, Clark GM, Wong SG, Levin WJ, Ullrich A, McGuire WL. Human breast cancer: correlation of relapse and survival with amplification of the HER-2/neu oncogene. *Science* 1987; **235**: 177–182.

107. Slamon DJ, Godolphin W, Jones LA, et al. Studies of the HER-2/neu proto-oncogene in human breast and ovarian cancer. *Science* 1989; **244**: 707–712.
108. Yarden Y, Sliwkowski MX. Untangling the ErbB signalling network. *Nat Rev Mol Cell Biol* 2001; **2**: 127–137.
109. Holbro T, Hynes NE. ErbB receptors: directing key signaling networks throughout life. *Annu Rev Pharmacol Toxicol* 2004; **44**: 195–217.
110. Chang CH, Scott GK, Kuo WL, et al. ESX: a structurally unique Ets overexpressed early during human breast tumorigenesis. *Oncogene* 1997; **14**: 1617–1622.
111. Hsu FJ, Benike C, Fagnoni F, et al. Vaccination of patients with B-cell lymphoma using autologous antigen-pulsed dendritic cells. *Nat Med* 1996; **2**: 52–58.
112. Nestle FO, Alijagic S, Gilliet M, et al. Vaccination of melanoma patients with peptide- or tumor lysate-pulsed dendritic cells. *Nat Med* 1998; **4**: 328–332.
113. Ho A, Dowdy SF. Regulation of G(1) cell-cycle progression by oncogenes and tumor suppressor genes. *Curr Opin Genet Dev* 2002; **12**: 47–52.
114. Sherr CJ, Roberts JM. CDK inhibitors: positive and negative regulators of G1-phase progression. *Genes Dev* 1999; **13**: 1501–1512.
115. Lee MH, Yang HY. Negative regulators of cyclin-dependent kinases and their roles in cancers. *Cell Mol Life Sci* 2001; **58**: 1907–1922.
116. Sherr CJ, McCormick F. The RB and p53 pathways in cancer. *Cancer Cell* 2002; **2**: 103–112.
117. Sherr CJ. The INK4a/ARF network in tumour suppression. *Nat Rev Mol Cell Biol* 2001; **2**: 731–737.
118. Fahraeus R, Paramio JM, Ball KL, Lain S, Lane DP. Inhibition of pRb phosphorylation and cell-cycle progression by a 20-residue peptide derived from p16CDKN2/INK4A. *Curr Biol* 1996; **6**: 84–91.
119. Gius DR, Ezhevsky SA, Becker-Hapak M, Nagahara H, Wei MC, Dowdy SF. Transduced p16INK4a peptides inhibit hypophosphorylation of the retinoblastoma protein and cell cycle progression prior to activation of Cdk2 complexes in late G1. *Cancer Res* 1999; **59**: 2577–2580.
120. Ball KL, Lain S, Fahraeus R, Smythe C, Lane DP. Cell-cycle arrest and inhibition of Cdk4 activity by small peptides based on the carboxy-terminal domain of p21WAF1. *Curr Biol* 1997; **7**: 71–80.
121. Nagahara H, Vocero-Akbani AM, Snyder EL, et al. Transduction of full-length TAT fusion proteins into mammalian cells: TAT-p27Kip1 induces cell migration. *Nat Med* 1998; **4**: 1449–1452.
122. Snyder EL, Meade BR, Dowdy SF. Anti-cancer protein transduction strategies: reconstitution of p27 tumor suppressor function. *J Control Release* 2003; **91**: 45–51.
123. Del Gaizo V, Payne RM. A novel TAT-mitochondrial signal sequence fusion protein is processed, stays in mitochondria, and crosses the placenta. *Mol Ther* 2003; **7**: 720–730.

Pharmaceutical Perspectives of Cancer Therapeutics: Current Therapeutic Uses of Monoclonal Antibodies

Michael D. Axelson and David E. Gerber

1 Introduction

Few cancer therapies have attracted the level of interest given to monoclonal antibodies. These drugs, first approved for cancer treatment in the late 1990s, provide unprecedented target specificity. In so doing, they have begun to fulfill the concept put forth by Paul Ehrlich over 100 years earlier—a "magic bullet" that kills cancer, but does not harm normal tissues [1]. The production of monoclonal antibodies has captured the public's awe and appreciation. The hybridoma technique, which entails the fusion of mouse and human cells into antibody "factories," exemplifies the clinical benefits of biologic research. Perhaps most importantly, monoclonal antibodies offer the promise of effective cancer treatment, without the toxicities associated with conventional chemotherapy.

In a number of instances, monoclonal antibodies have met expectations. The addition of rituximab, an anti-CD20 monoclonal antibody, to standard CHOP chemotherapy increases 2-year overall survival for non-Hodgkin's lymphoma (NHL) from 57% to 70%, without increasing toxicity [2]. Trastuzumab, a monoclonal antibody targeting human epidermal growth factor receptor 2 (HER2), has markedly changed the clinical course of HER2-positive breast cancer. While the 25% of patients with tumors harboring this receptor tyrosine kinase have traditionally had a more aggressive disease and worse clinical outcomes than patients with HER2-negative breast cancers, the availability of trastuzumab has, in essence, reversed this relationship. For patients with early stage HER2-postive breast cancer receiving adjuvant (postoperative) chemotherapy, the addition of trastuzumab to chemotherapy increases disease-free survival 18% and, in a population already experiencing 85% overall survival, increases overall survival an additional 5% [3].

Despite these successes, monoclonal antibodies have not received universal fanfare. While monoclonal antibodies generally do not cause the adverse effects

D.E. Gerber (✉)
Department of Internal Medicine, Division of Hematology & Oncology, University of Texas Southwestern Medical Center, 5323 Harry Hines Boulevard, Dallas, TX 75390, USA
e-mail: david.gerber@utsouthwestern.edu

Y. Lu, R.I. Mahato (eds.), *Pharmaceutical Perspectives of Cancer Therapeutics*, 321
DOI 10.1007/978-1-4419-0131-6_11, © Springer Science+Business Media, LLC 2009

characteristic of conventional chemotherapy—alopecia, nausea and vomiting, and myelosuppression—they are not without toxicities. Class-wide adverse events are related to antibody structure. The presence of mouse proteins in murine, chimeric, and humanized monoclonal antibodies may elicit acute, anaphylactic infusion reactions. Additionally, specific monoclonal antibodies have toxicities related to their individual molecular functions. Antibodies directed against the epidermal growth factor receptor (EGFR) may cause significant dermatologic and gastrointestinal toxicities. Antibodies directed against vascular endothelial growth factor (VEGF) may cause bleeding, clotting, wound healing complications, hypertension, and—through effects on glomerular capillaries—proteinuria. Perhaps the greatest toxicities have occurred with antibodies designed to modify patients' immune responses against cancer and other diseases. Experimental antibodies targeting and neutralizing the molecule cytotoxic T-lymphocyte antigen 4 (CTLA4), which downregulates T cell function, have caused autoimmune colitis that, in some instances, has required colectomy [4]. The monoclonal antibody TGN1412 alters immune responses through binding CD28, a T cell coreceptor. The elicited response is designed to dampen the immune response in autoimmune diseases and augment the immune response in patients with cancer. In a recent phase I clinical trial, 13 healthy volunteers were treated with TGN1412 [5]. Six of these individuals developed a severe cytokine-release syndrome and multiorgan failure.

In an era when the economics of health care have returned to the spotlight, concerns have also been raised about the high costs of monoclonal antibody development and use. One of the earliest hints at the enormous investment and opportunity monoclonal antibodies offer pharmaceutical companies occurred in 2004, when accusations of insider trading, related to the anti-EGFR antibody cetuximab (Erbitux), led to the indictment of ImClone executives and a well-known investor, Martha Stewart. In July 2008, the complex relationship between monoclonal antibody efficacy and cost was highlighted on the front page of *The New York Times* [6]. Largely because of the costs associated with monoclonal antibodies, economic considerations are now being included in oncology practice guidelines and expert recommendations for the first time.

Monoclonal antibodies offer some of the greatest promise and pitfalls in medicine. To provide researchers and clinicians with a greater understanding of this class of therapeutics, this chapter will review the history, production, structure, function, toxicities, and clinical applications of monoclonal antibodies in oncology.

2 History

Paul Ehrlich's concepts of targeting cellular receptors and optimizing the therapeutic index laid the foundation for modern cancer therapy [1]. Ehrlich shared the 1908 Nobel Peace Prize with Ilya Mechnikov, who observed that antibodies alone are not sufficient to kill targeted cells. It is the binding of antibodies, he recognized, that subsequently allows white blood cells to effect cellular destruction. Today, these concepts remain relevant to our understanding of antibody-mediated cytotoxicity. It was not until the establishment of the hybridoma techniques of Georges Kohler and César Milstein [7] in the 1970s, however, that the design of therapeutic monoclonal antibodies became possible. The hybridoma technique involved the fusion of mouse lymphoid cells with immortalized human myeloma cells. The antibodies produced by hybridoma cells were associated with a range of clinical toxicities, including fever, chills, flushing, rash, urticaria, nausea, bronchospasm, dyspnea, hypotension, renal dysfunction, and headache [8, 9], all of which were attributed to antibody interactions with target antigens [10].

In the first monoclonal antibody clinical trial in humans, a patient with lymphoma received Ab 89, which targeted a "human lymphoma antigen." Following infusion, the patient experienced a decrease in the number of viable tumor cells, with no apparent toxicity [11]. Despite such initial reports suggesting few adverse effects, it became clear that with increasing quantities of infused antibody, patients were more likely to have systemic reactions. Ultimately, these reactions were recognized as patient immune responses to these early antibodies, which were composed entirely of murine (mouse) proteins [12, 13]. Human anti-mouse antibodies were recognized early on [14], but only later were they linked to diminished in half-life and efficacy of the therapeutic antibody. As with Ab 89, most early antibody clinical trials focused predominantly on lymphoma. Solid tumors such as melanoma [15] and gastrointestinal malignancies [8] were also studied, although with relatively little success.

Further developments in antibody engineering led to the incorporation of human protein sequences into antibody structures. Chimeric antibodies (approximately 2/3 human protein, 1/3 mouse protein) featured human μ and κ constant regions and murine variable regions [16]. Subsequently designed humanized antibodies (approximately 95% human protein, 5% mouse protein) contained even greater proportions of human proteins. In contrast with the chimeric technique, this process originated with a human antibody framework, to which murine antigen-binding hypervariable domains were added [17]. Chimeric and humanized antibodies provided distinct advantages over their entirely murine predecessors. Decreased murine components led to decreased immunogenicity. Increased human components promoted antibody interaction with patient immune functions— including complement-mediated cytotoxicity (CMC) and antibody-dependent cellular cytotoxicity (ADCC)—thereby enhancing tumor cell kill.

The first two monoclonal antibodies approved by the United States Food and Drug Administration (FDA) for cancer treatment emerged from these techniques. Rituximab, approved in 1997 for the treatment of NHL, is an anti-CD20 chimeric antibody. It contains a human IgG1-κ constant domain and variable regions from the murine monoclonal anti-CD20 antibody IDEC-2B8 [18]. Trastuzumab, approved in 1998 for the treatment of a subset of breast cancer cases, is a humanized antibody directed against HER2. It contains the complementarity-determining region (CDR) of MAb4D5, a murine anti-HER2 antibody, in a human IgG1 backbone [19]. Subsequently approved antibodies for cancer treatment, capitalizing on further advances in bioengineering, have been conjugated to toxins [20] and radioisotopes [21, 22]. Gemtuzumab ozogamicin (Mylotarg) is an anti-CD33 monoclonal antibody conjugated to the calicheamicin toxin that is approved for the treatment of acute myeloid leukemia (AML). Ibritumomab tiuxetan (Zevalin) and Tositumomab (Bexxar) are anti-CD20 antibodies conjugated to the radioisotopes Yttrium-90 and Iodine-131, respectively. In such instances, the antibody's primary function is to target tumor cells and deliver the lethal payload.

3 Antibody Structure and Function

3.1 Antibody Structure

Antibodies are composed of four polypeptide chains, two light chains and two heavy chains, connected by a disulfide bond (see Fig. 1). Together, these make up a protein with a molecular weight of approximately 150,000 Da. Thus, antibodies dwarf other classes of cancer therapies, such as small molecule inhibitors (molecular weight typically 400–500 Da) and conventional cytotoxic chemotherapy drugs (molecular weight typically 100–200 Da). The heavy chain consists of three constant regions and one variable region; the light chain consists of one constant region and one variable region. There are two different light-chain constant regions, kappa (κ) and lambda (λ), which differ in amino acid sequence. κ light chains make up 60% of light chains in endogenous human antibodies and are also the primary light chain in engineered, therapeutic antibodies [23].

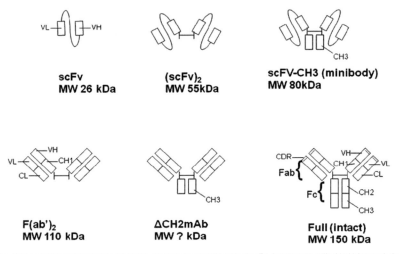

C: constant; CDR: complementarity-determining region; Fab: fragment antigen binding; Fc: fragment crystallizable; H: heavy chain; L: light chain; V: variable

Fig. 1 Antibody structure and fragments

In humans, the genes encoding heavy-chain proteins are located on chromosome 14; light-chain genes are located on chromosomes 2 and 22. Differentiating B cells undergo gene rearrangement of the variable, diversity, and junctional (VDJ) segments, resulting in a wide range of antigen recognition. The variable region is located at the amino terminus of each heavy and light chain. Within the variable region, the complementarity-determining region (CDR) gives an individual antibody its specificity to a single antigen. Heavy-chain constant regions are classified as α, ϵ, γ, δ, and μ, which correspond to immunoglobulin isotypes A (IgA), E (IgE), G (IgG), D (IgD), and M (IgM), respectively. The four isotypes of γ heavy chains correspond to IgG subclasses IgG1, IgG2, IgG3, and IgG4, which differ in ability to mediate host-effector responses (i.e., ADCC and CMC) [24]. They also differ pharmacokinetically; the half-life of IgG3 is only 7 days, in contrast to 21 days for other IgG subclasses [25]. Based on these properties, the development of monoclonal antibodies for cancer therapy has centered on IgG1 and IgG2 immunoglobulins [26].

Presently available therapeutic monoclonal antibodies in oncology are intact IgG molecules. However, antibody fragments are undergoing evaluation in clinical trials. These smaller molecules (molecular weight 26,000–120,000 Da) offer the potential benefits of reduced immunogenicity, improved tumor penetration [27], and more homogeneous tissue distribution [28]. In some cases, monomeric or single-arm antibodies may overcome the tendency of traditional, bivalent antibodies to activate rather than suppress certain cell targets [29]. However, compared with intact monoclonal antibodies, antibody fragments undergo more rapid systemic clearance [30], have lower antigen-binding affinity, and lack effector functions.

To produce antibody fragments, enzymatic degradation with papain yields the Fc (fragment crystallizable) and fragment antigen-binding Fab (fragment antigen binding) regions (Fig. 1). The Fab region recognizes and binds to antigen. The Fc region may be involved in the recruitment of host effector functions by binding Fc receptors (FcR) on host immune cells. Alternatively, the Fc region may be conjugated to radioisotopes or toxins. Following enzymatic degradation, antibodies may be reformulated into single chain variable fragment (scFv), (scFv)$_2$ [31], Fab' or F(ab')$_2$, diabody, or scFv-CH3 (minibody) (see Fig. 1). The scFv and (scFv)$_2$ consist of heavy- and light-chain variable regions connected by a peptide linker or disulfide bond. The Fab' or F(ab')$_2$ is constructed of heavy- and light-chain variable regions, the light-chain constant region, and the CH1 heavy-chain constant region. Diabodies are similar to (scFv)$_2$ but joined end to end rather than side to side. This structure promotes the assembly of a dimeric molecule with two functional antigen-binding sites. Minibodies are similar to (scFv)$_2$ but also contain a CH3 heavy-chain constant domain, which gives them a longer half-life. These fragments may be modified further to impact circulating half-lives, antigen-binding properties, and suitability as a platform for conjugates [27].

3.2 Antibody Production

In the hybridoma technique (see Fig. 2), mice are inoculated with a specific protein, the desired antigenic target, over several months. The mouse is then sacrificed, and splenic lymphocytes are harvested. The murine splenic cells are coincubated and fused with immortalized human myeloma cells *in vitro* [32]. The fused cells grow into colonies that effectively serve as antibody-producing biologic factories. Each colony produces molecularly identical antibodies arising from the same original mouse lymphocyte—hence the term monoclonal. Antibodies are then tested for specificity or desired immune effect.

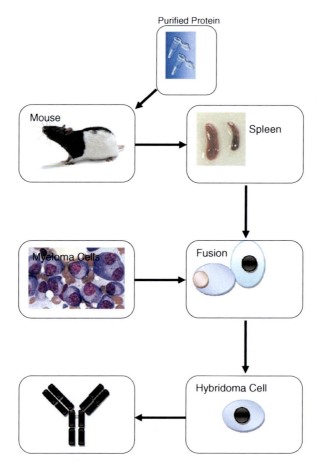

Purified protein consisting of the antigenic target is inoculated in the mice which then develop an immune response. After animal sacrifice, splenic lymphocytes are isolated and co-incubated with immortalized human myeloma cells in vitro. The cells fuse resulting in hybridoma cells and form colonies in cell culture. Selection of the colonies is based on antibody specificity or desired immune effect.

Fig. 2 Monoclonal antibody production: hybridoma

Whereas antibodies produced via the hybridoma technique are composed entirely of murine proteins, it is possible to synthesize antibodies with increasing proportions of human protein via recombinant techniques. Antibody species (i.e., murine, chimeric, humanized, fully human) reflects the proportions of murine and human protein and can be inferred from the suffix of a specific antibody name (see Fig. 3). The production of recombinant antibodies is based on phage display libraries [33]. These antibody libraries come from immunized or nonimmunized donors, synthetic libraries, or a "single pot" library, containing only the antigens against which the immune response is directed. A library of phages (bacterial viruses) contains millions of ligands fused to the gene responsible for the phage coat protein. Expression of the fusion protein and its inclusion into new phage particles take place in bacteria and result in ligand expression on the phage surface while the gene encoding the ligand resides in the phage particle. The phage particles are then passed over a surface that binds and enriches for the desired phage surface ligand. Antibody variable domains encoding binding regions are fused on the surface of phages as minor coat proteins resulting in the expression of a scFv [34]. Further screening of the antibody–phage construct against immobilized antigen allows for selection of higher binding affinities. The antibody gene fragments are then isolated and cloned into an expression vector, usually with a lac-promoter, and the phage protein coat is removed. This phagemid is then expressed in transformed cells allowing for the isolation of single colonies producing a monoclonal antibody [35].

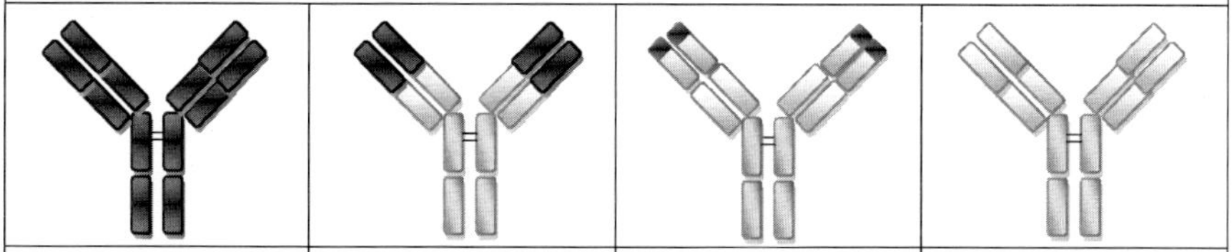

Antibody Species			
Murine	Chimeric	Humanized	Human
100% mouse protein	34% mouse protein	5–10% mouse protein	0% mouse protein
-**mo**mab (mouse)	-**xi**mab (chimera)	-**zu**mab (humanized)	-**mu**mab (human)

Fig. 3 Antibody species

Fully human antibodies may also be developed in mice. This requires inactivation of the murine immunoglobulin gene loci and replacement by human genes encoding the desired heavy and light chains, a process carried out through the use of yeast artificial chromosomes fused into murine embryonic stem cells. The genetically engineered mice are then bred with each other to select for the human genes [36].

3.3 Antibody Function

Monoclonal antibodies exert anticancer effects via three principal mechanisms (see Fig. 4): (1) targeting and inhibition of specific ligands and receptors (Fig. 4a), (2) recruitment of host immune functions (Fig. 4b and c), and (3) transporting a lethal payload (radioisotope, toxin, or drug) to a tumor target (Fig. 4d and e). In some instances, a single antibody may possess multiple antitumor properties.

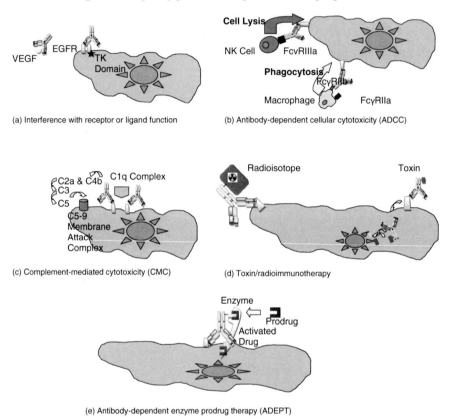

(a) Interference with receptor or ligand function

(b) Antibody-dependent cellular cytotoxicity (ADCC)

(c) Complement-mediated cytotoxicity (CMC)

(d) Toxin/radioimmunotherapy

(e) Antibody-dependent enzyme prodrug therapy (ADEPT)

Fig. 4 Mechanism of killing

3.3.1 Targeting Ligands and Receptors

The discovery and characterization of tumor cell survival and growth signal pathways have improved the understanding of cancer. Capitalizing on this knowledge, monoclonal antibodies targeting specific molecules required for cancer cell survival have been developed. To provide a therapeutic ratio, these molecular targets are ideally unique to, over-expressed in, or mutated in cancer cells as compared to normal tissues. Monoclonal antibody targets may be circulating ligands, such as vascular endothelial growth factor (VEGF), or cell surface receptors, such as members of the HER family. After antibody binding, signal disruption can occur through neutralizing circulating ligand, steric hindrance of ligand binding to receptor, prevention of receptor subunit dimerization, or receptor downregulation. The anti-EGFR antibody cetuximab (Erbitux) binds EFGR, resulting in steric hindrance of receptor dimerization and partial occlusion of the ligand-binding region [37, 38]. The anti-HER2 antibody trastuzumab (Herceptin) prevents receptor homo- and heterodimerization [39].

3.3.2 Recruitment of Host Immune Functions

FcγR and Fc Interactions

In some instances, the mechanism of action for therapeutic antibodies involves not only the binding of antibody to antigen but also the recruitment of immune effects through binding of the Fc region of the antibody to Fc gamma receptors (FcγR) on immune cells. There are six members of the FcγR family, each with distinct binding properties and immune effects. These include FcγRI (CD64), FcγRIIa/b/c (CD32), and FcγRIII a/b (CD16). These receptors are differentially expressed on neutrophils and macrophages (CD64, CD32, and CD16) and natural killer (NK) cells (CD16 only) [40, 41]. The binding of FcγR effects an equilibrium between activation and inhibition of the immune response [41]. FcγRIIb is an inhibitory receptor expressed on macrophages that prevents phagocytosis [42]. FcγRIII is an activating receptor on macrophages and NK cells. The recruitment of immune cells leads to phagocytosis, cytokine release, and tumor cell lysis. Phagocytosis occurs when FcγRIIa on neutrophils or macrophages bind to the Fc regions of antibodies attached to target cells. Macrophages then present antigens from tumor cells that have undergone phagocytosis to activated T cells. The subsequent release of cytokines amplifies immune cell recruitment and increases major histocompatibility complex (MHC) expression. Ultimately, these events result in antibody-dependent cell cytotoxicity (ADCC) and complement-mediated cytotoxicity (CMC).

ADCC

Antibody-dependent cell cytotoxicity (ADCC), occurs when FcγR on effector cells bind to Fc regions of antibodies (Fig. 4b) [43]. The process involves binding of antibody to the target antigen, recognition of the Fc portion by immune effector cells, cross linking of Fc receptors, activation of effector cells, and release of cytotoxic granules containing granzymes, perforin, and granulysin [42]. While many cell types contribute to cytotoxicity, NK cells are considered the principal mediators of ADCC. In preclinical models, depletion of NK cells significantly decreases tumor cell kill in the presence of antibodies [44]. For ADCC, the most relevant Fcγ receptors are FcγRIIb, the inhibitory FcγR, and FcγRIII. Mice deficient in FcγRIIb show increased tumor killing when treated with antibody, while mice deficient in FcγRIII are unable to arrest tumor growth [45].

Polymorphisms in the human FcγRIII, which impact binding of immune cells to Fc, impact antitumor effects [46]. Among lymphoma patients treated with the anti-CD20 monoclonal antibody rituximab, those patients homozygous for the FcγRIIIa 158 V polymorphism have significantly higher response rates than those with the FcγRIIIa 158F polymorphism *in vivo* [47] and *in vitro* [48, 49]. Engineering of IgG antibodies toward increased affinity for FcγRIIIa demonstrates enhanced NK cell activity [50]. The impact of host immune function on tumor cell killing has also been demonstrated by observations that the type, density, and location of immune cell infiltrates in pretreatment colorectal cancer specimens can predict clinical outcomes [51].

CMC

Certain monoclonal antibodies also promote tumor cell killing through complement-mediated cytotoxicity (CMC) (Fig 4c). IgM is the most effective antibody for this mechanism, followed by IgG3 and IgG1 [23]. After binding to antigen, antibody C1q binding sites become available on C_H2 domains, activating the complement cascade, releasing C3a and C5a, and ultimately generating the C5–C9 membrane attack complex [40]. Complement activation has been shown to be an *in vivo* mechanism of action by rituximab in mouse models, even in mice depleted of NK cells or neutrophils [52].

3.3.3 Prior to Delivery of Lethal Payload

Monoclonal antibodies may be conjugated to radioisotopes, toxins, cytokines, enzymes, and drugs (Fig. 4d and e). In these instances, antibodies serve primarily a targeting role, delivering the lethal payload specifically to cancer cells. Despite the promise of these methods, the use of conjugated monoclonal antibodies remains limited. To date, the FDA has approved only three therapeutic conjugated antibodies, two of which incorporate radioisotopes [^{131}I-tositumomab (Bexxar) and ^{90}Y-ibritumomab tiuxetan (Zevalin)] and one that incorporates the calicheamicin toxin [gemtuzumab ozogamicin (Mylotarg)]. ^{90}Y is a pure beta-particle (electron) emitter which has a path length of 5 mm and a half-life of 2.7 days. Because beta particles are not readily visualized, an additional radioisotope is required for imaging. ^{131}I emits both beta particles and gamma rays, thereby providing diagnostic as well as therapeutic radiation. Compared to beta particles, gamma rays have a shorter path length (1 mm) and a longer half-life [53]. Calicheamicin is an antitumor antibiotic that binds the minor groove of DNA and cleaves both DNA strands in a nonspecific fashion [54]. The use of other toxins, such as the ricin A toxin, diphtheria toxin, and *Pseudomonas aeruginosa* exotoxin, has encountered numerous problems in clinical trials. These include local vascular effects, rapid toxin clearance, and toxicity in normal organs expressing the target antigen [55]. Antibody-directed enzyme prodrug therapy (ADEPT) (see Fig 4e) is another antibody modification. First proposed in 1987

[56, 57], ADEPT is a multistep process that begins with the infusion of a monoclonal antibody conjugated to a drug-activating enzyme. After binding of antibody to the target tumor antigen, a prodrug is administered and converted by the enzyme to its active moiety. Ideally, this approach results in a high concentration of active drug at the site of the tumor, with relatively low systemic exposure. Several chemotherapeutic agents (including doxorubicin, methotrexate, 5-fluorouracil, and paclitaxel) and enzymes (including carboxypeptidase G2, aminopeptidase, and β-lactamase) have been studied. To date, this technology remains limited to phase I trials [58].

4 Clinical Uses of Monoclonal Antibodies

4.1 Nontherapeutic Uses of Monoclonal Antibodies

Although the term "monoclonal antibody" is currently most closely associated with therapeutic agents, monoclonal antibodies were used for diagnostic purposes, both *in vivo* and *in vitro*, well before they were used as anticancer drugs. In clinical pathology, the high degree of specificity of monoclonal antibodies often provides confirmation in cases that are not straightforward by microscopic appearance alone. Immunohistochemistry (IHC) is the process of tissue antigen recognition through the binding of antibodies. The antibodies can either be labeled with a dye [e.g., fluorescein isothiocyanate (FITC)] or be counterstained with a second, dye-labeled antibody. The latter of these two processes is more sensitive and is employed more frequently. IHC may contribute to tissue diagnosis. For example, tissue staining with anti-cytokeratin (CK)-7 and anti-thyroid transcription factor (TTF)-1 antibodies may support a diagnosis of non-small cell lung cancer (NSCLC); tissue staining with anti-CK20 antibodies may support a diagnosis of colorectal cancer. IHC may also guide treatment planning. For example, breast cancer tissue staining with anti-estrogen receptor (ER) or anti-progesterone receptor (PR) antibodies may result in the use of the hormone receptor modulator tamoxifen; breast cancer tissue staining with anti-HER2 antibodies may lead to the use of the therapeutic monoclonal antibody trastuzumab or the small molecule tyrosine kinase inhibitor lapatinib. Flow cytometry, a technique first developed in the late 1960s, applies similar principles to particles suspended in a stream of fluid, such as blood and other body fluids. Fluorescence-activated cell sorting (FACS), a specialized form of flow cytometry, provides rapid and objective cell counting and sorting.

Since the early 1990s, murine radioconjugates have been available for diagnostic imaging studies. Satumomab pendetide, an Indium-111 (^{111}In)-labeled antitumor-associated glycoprotein (TAG)-72 IgG1, targets antigens on colorectal and ovarian cancers and is used to image these malignancies [59]. Three other antibodies, two conjugated to Technetium-99m (^{99m}Tc) and one conjugated to ^{111}In are used to image lung, prostate, and colorectal cancers (see Table 1). Despite the promise of

Table 1 FDA approved diagnostic imaging monoclonal antibodies in oncology

Generic name	Trade name	Species	Radionuclide	Structure	Target	Disease	Initial approval date
Satumomab pendetide*	OncoScint	Murine	Indium-111	IgG1	TAG72	Colorectal, ovarian	12.29.1992
Arcitumomab	CEA-Scan	Murine	Technetium-99m	Fab (IgG1)	CEA	Colorectal	6.28.1996
Nofetumomab merpentan	Verluma	Murine	Indium-111	Fab (IgG2)	EGP2	Small cell lung cancer	8.20.1996
Capromab pendetide	ProstaScint	Murine	Indium-111	IgG1	PSMA	Prostate	10.28.1996

*Manufacture and distribution were discontinued in the United States on 2002.

CEA: carcinoembryonic antigen; **EGP**: epithelial glycoprotein 2; **PSMA**: prostate-specific membrane antigen; **TAG**: tumor-associated glycoprotein 72.

these diagnostic antibodies, slow biodistribution and systemic clearance, high liver uptake, and immunogenicity have limited their use. They have been largely replaced by positron emission tomography (PET) scans [60].

4.2 Therapeutic Uses of Antibodies in Other Fields

Although the therapeutic antibodies alemtuzumab, rituximab, and bevacizumab were originally developed as anticancer agents, widely applicable molecular functions have led to their use in other clinical contexts (see Table 2). Because alemtuzumab depletes T lymphocytes, it has been used in hematopoietic stem cell transplant recipients to prevent and treat graft versus host disease [61]. The ability of rituximab to deplete normal B lymphocytes has led to its use in several autoimmune diseases, including immune thrombocytopenic purpura, pemphigus vulgaris, systemic lupus erythematosis, and rheumatoid arthritis (for which it is FDA approved) [62]. Bevacizumab is used topically for the treatment of ocular complications of diabetes and macular degeneration [38]. In addition, monoclonal antibodies are FDA approved for a number of noncancerous conditions. Among others, these include abciximab (ReoPro), a chimeric anti-glycoprotein IIb/IIIa antibody used in the treatment of myocardial infarction and as an adjunct to percutaneous coronary intervention; adalimumab (Humira), a fully human antitumor necrosis alfa (TNFα) antibody approved for the treatment of autoimmune disorders such as ankylosing spondylitis, Crohn's disease, psoriasis, and rheumatoid arthritis; and infliximab (Remicaid), a chimeric anti-TNFα antibody with similar clinical indications as adalimumab.

Table 2 Non-FDA approved uses of cancer-targeted monoclonal antibodies in nonmalignant conditions

Antibody	Diseases
Alemtuzumab	Autoimmune disease – cytopenia
Bevacizumab	Age-related macular degeneration, secondary to choroidal neovascularization
	Diabetic macular edema
	Macular retinal edema, due to retinal vein occlusion
Rituximab	Autoimmune hemolytic anemia
	Evans syndrome, refractory to immunosuppressive therapy
	Graft vs. host disease, chronic, steroid refractory
	Pemphigus vulgaris, severe
	Posttransplant lymphoproliferative disorder
	Systemic lupus erythematosus, refractory to immunosuppressive therapy
	Thrombotic thrombocytopenic purpura, immune or idiopathic

4.3 Therapeutic Uses of Antibodies in Oncology

Currently nine monoclonal antibodies are FDA approved for the treatment of cancer (see Table 3): five for the treatment of hematologic malignancies (see Table 4) and

Table 3 FDA-approved monoclonal antibodies for cancer treatment

Generic name	Trade name	Company	Species	Subclass	Type	Target	Disease	Initial approval date
Rituximab	Rituxan	Genentech	Chimeric	IgG1	Unconjugated	CD20	NHL	11.26.1997
Trastuzumab	Herceptin	Genentech	Humanized	IgG1	Unconjugated	HER2/neu	HER2-positive Breast cancer	9.25.1998
Gemtuzumab ozogamicin	Mylotarg	Wyeth	Humanized	IgG4	Conjugated: Calicheamicin toxin	CD33	AML	5.17.2000
Alemtuzumab	Campath	Bayer	Humanized	IgG1	Unconjugated	CD52	CLL	5.7.2001
^{90}Y Ibritumomab tiuxetan	Zevalin	Biogen Idec	Murine	IgG1	Conjugated: Yttrium-90	CD20	NHL	2.19.2002
^{131}I Tositumomab	Bexxar	GlaxoSmithKline	Murine	IgG2	Conjugated: Iodine-131	CD20	NHL	6.27.2003
Cetuximab	Erbitux	ImClone; Merck; Bristol Myer Squibb	Chimeric	IgG1	Unconjugated	EGFR	CRC; Head and neck	2.12.2004; 3.1.2006
Bevacizumab	Avastin	Genentech	Humanized	IgG1	Unconjugated	VEGF	CRC; NSCLC; Breast cancer	2.26.2004; 10.11.2006; 2.22.2008
Panitumumab	Vectibix	Amgen	Human	IgG2	Unconjugated	EGFR	CRC	9.27.2006

NHL: non-Hodgkin's lymphoma; CLL: chronic lymphocytic leukemia; AML: acute myelogenous leukemia; CRC: colorectal cancer; NSCLC: non-small cell lung cancer; EGFR: epidermal growth factor receptor; VEGF: vascular endothelial growth factor.

Table 4 Selected clinical trials of monoclonal antibodies for the treatment of hematologic malignancies

Antibody	Disease	Trial phase	N	Treatment	Outcomes						References
					RR	p value	PFS	p value	OS	p value	
Alemtuzumab (Campath)	CLL (previously untreated)	3	297	Alemtuzumab Chlorambucil	83% 55%	0.0001	14.6 m 11.7 m	0.0001	NR NR		101
Gemtuzumab ozogamicin (Mylotarg)	AML (relapsed)	2[a]	277	Gemtuzumab ozogamicin	26%[b]		6.2 m[c]		12.6 m[d]		97
90Y-Ibritumomab tiuxetan (Zevalin)	NHL (relapsed/refractory low grade)	3	143	Ibritumomab tiuxetan Rituximab	80% 56%	0.002	11.2m 10.1m	0.173	NR NR		86
	NHL (relapsed low-grade)	2	166	Rituximab	48%		13 m		NR		66
Rituximab (Rituxan)	NHL (previously untreated DLBCL)	3	399	CHOP	63%	0.005	30% 5-y PFS	0.0001	45% 5-yr OS	0.007	2,7
				CHOP + Rituximab	76%		54% 5-y PFS		55% 5-yr OS		
131I-Tositumomab (Bexxar)	NHL (previously untreated low grade)	2	76	Tositumomab	95%		6.1 y		89% 5-yr OS		90

[a]Pooled results of three open-label single-arm phase II studies.
[b]Complete remission (CR).
[c]Relapse-free survival (RFS) among patients achieving CR.
[d]For patients achieving CR. For all patients, median OS was 4.9 months.
AML: acute myeloid leukemia; **CHOP**: cyclophosphamide, hydroxydoxorubicin, vincristine (Oncovin), prednisone; **CLL**: chronic lymphocytic leukemia; **DLBCL**: diffuse large B cell lymphoma; **N**: number of patients; **NHL**: non-Hodgkin's lymphoma; **NR**: not reported; **OS**: overall survival; **PFS**: progression-free survival.

Table 5 Selected clinical trials of monoclonal antibodies for the treatment of solid tumor malignancies

Antibody	Disease	Trial phase	N	Treatment	Outcome						References
					RR	p value	PFS	p value	OS	p value	
Bevacizumab (Avastin)	CRC (metastatic)	3	813	IFL	34.8%	0.004	6.2 m	0.001	15.6 m	0.001	149
				IFL + Bevacizumab	44.8%		10.6 m		20.3 m		
	NSCLC (advanced)	3	878	CP	15%	0.001	4.5 m	0.001	10.3 m	0.003	152
				CP + Bevacizumab	35%		6.2 m		12.3 m		
	Breast cancer (metastatic)	3	722	Paclitaxel	21.2%	0.001	5.9 m	0.001	25.2 m	0.16	150
				Paclitaxel + Bevacizumab	36.9%		11.8 m		26.7 m		
Cetuximab (Erbitux)	Colorectal cancer (metastatic)	3	329	Cetuximab	10.8%	0.007	1.5 m*	0.001	6.9 m	0.48	115
				Cetuximab + Irinotecan	22.9%		4.1 m*		8.6 m		
	HNSCC (locally advanced)	3	424	RT	NR		14.9 m**	0.005	49.0 m	0.03	118
				RT + Cetuximab	NR		24.4 m**		29.3 m		
	HNSCC (advanced)	3	442	Platinum† + 5-FU	20%	0.001	3.3 m	0.001	7.4 m	0.04	120
				Platinum† + 5-FU + Cetuximab	36%		5.6 m		10.1 m		
Panitumumab (Vectibix)	Colorectal cancer (metastatic)	3	463	Best supportive care	0%	0.0001	4.6 m	0.001	20.3 m	0.046	134
				Best supportive care + Panitumumab	10%		7.4 m		25.1 m		
Trastuzumab (Herceptin)	HER2 positive breast cancer (adjuvant)	3	3351	Doxorubicin + Cyclophosphamide → Paclitaxel	–		67.1% 4-yr DFS	0.0001	86.6% 4-yr OS	0.019	3
				Doxorubicin + Cyclophosphamide → Paclitaxel + Trastuzumab	–		85.3% 4-y DFS		91.4% 4-yr OS		
	HER2 + breast cancer (metastatic)	3	469	Anthracycline‡ or Paclitaxel	32%	0.001	4.6 m	0.001	20.3 m	0.046	107
				Anthracycline‡ + Trastuzumab or Paclitaxel + Trastuzumab	50%		7.4 m		25.1 m		

*Time to progression (TTP); **Duration of locoregional control; †Either cisplatin or carboplatin; ‡Either doxorubicin or epirubicin.
CP: carboplatin-paclitaxel; **5-FU**: 5-fluorouracil; **HNSCC**: head and neck squamous cell carcinoma; **IFL**: irinotecan, 5-fluorouracil, leucovorin; **N**: number of patients; **NR**: not reported; **NSCLC**: nonsmall cell lung cancer; **OS**: overall survival; **PFS**: progression-free survival; **RR**: response rate; **RT**: radiotherapy.

four for the treatment of solid tumors (see Table 5). Their structure is distributed as follows: unconjugated (6), radioisotope conjugate (2), and toxin conjugate (1). Their species: murine (2), chimeric (2), humanized (4), and fully human (1). Their subclasses: IgG1 (6), IgG2 (2), and IgG4 (1). Their targets: CD20 (3), CD52 (1), CD33 (1), HER2/neu (1), EGFR (2), and VEGF (1). For the treatment of both hematologic malignancies and solid tumors, antibodies are employed as monotherapy and also in combination with other agents. To date, it appears that the use of monoclonal antibodies as single agents may be more effective against hematologic malignancies, which are generally characterized by fewer molecular aberrations and greater responsiveness to medical therapies than are solid tumors. For solid tumors, monoclonal antibodies may be most effective when combined with conventional chemotherapy, cytotoxic chemotherapy, or radiotherapy.

4.3.1 Hematologic Malignancies

Rituximab

In 1997, rituximab (Rituxan), a chimeric anti-CD20 monoclonal antibody, became the first monoclonal antibody approved by the US FDA for cancer treatment. In addition to being the oldest, rituximab is arguably also the most successful therapeutic antibody in oncology. Because its molecular target is ubiquitous in malignant B cells, rituximab is a component of therapy for most types of B cell non-Hodgkin's lymphoma (NHL). Rituximab also serves as the backbone of the radioimmunoconjugates Yttrium-90 (^{90}Y) Ibritumomab tiuxetan (Zevalin) and Iodine-131 (^{131}I) Tositumomab (Bexxar). Rituximab was developed by combining variable regions of 2B8, a murine anti-CD20 antibody, with a human Fc region [63]. Initially, rituximab was approved for with the treatment of relapsed/refractory follicular NHL (the most common low-grade NHL) based on data collected from several small trials [64]. Eventually rituximab received approval as first-line therapy for the two most common subtypes of NHL: follicular lymphoma and diffuse large B cell lymphoma (DLBCL). Rituximab's place in therapy can be broadly categorized as either initial use in combination with chemotherapy or maintenance monotherapy after achieving remission or significant response.

CD20, the molecular target of rituximab, is an unglycosylated phosphoprotein involved in calcium conductance. It is thought to help regulate B cell proliferation, differentiation, and activation [65]. The expression of CD20 on mature B cells underlies the therapeutic principals of rituximab. First, rituximab is used only in B cell NHL, and not in T cell NHL. Second, because normal B cells express CD20, rituximab has been used in the treatment of autoimmune disorders. Third, because CD20 is not expressed on B cell precursors, normal B cell populations may regenerate after rituximab treatment. The precise mechanism of rituximab's antitumor activity eluded researchers for years. It now appears that rituximab recruits host immune functions, including both ADCC and CMC, to attack targeted CD20-positive cells. Rituximab may also promote apoptosis [66].

As the case for other molecularly targeted therapies, researchers have sought to identify the subset of patients most likely to benefit from rituximab. The molecular markers B cell lymphoma protein 2 (bcl-2) (the first anti-death gene discovered [67]) and bcl-6 appear to provide lymphoma-specific signatures associated with response to rituximab. A retrospective analysis of a large clinical trial comparing CHOP (cyclophosphamide, hydroxydoxorubicin, vincristine, and prednisone) to CHOP plus rituximab (R-CHOP) found that patients with bcl-2-positive lymphomas derived greater response and survival benefits from rituximab than did patients with bcl-2-negative tumors [68]. In this study, bcl-2 positivity was defined as bcl-2 expression in $\geq 50\%$ of tumor cells by IHC. Bcl-6, a marker of germinal center origin and maturity of lymphoma cells, is associated with favorable prognosis in DLBCL [69]. However, the magnitude of benefit from rituximab appears greater in patients with bcl-6-negative lymphomas [70].

Rituximab is now a standard component of first-line treatment for DLBCL, the most common NHL subtype (accounting for over 30% of cases) [71]. The addition of rituximab to standard CHOP chemotherapy significantly increases radiographic response rates, event-free survival, and overall survival, without increasing toxicity [2, 72, 73]. The benefit of rituximab maintenance in DLBCL appears limited to those patients who have not received rituximab as part of their initial therapy [74].

Follicular lymphoma, the most common indolent lymphoma and the second most common NHL overall (approximately 25% of cases) [75] provided the initial clinical experience of rituximab. In phase I studies, one-time doses of 10, 50, 100, 250, and 500 mg/m^2 and weekly doses of 125, 250, and 375 mg/m^2 were evaluated [18, 76]. Common side effects included fever, chills, rash, urticaria, and nausea. In single-agent phase II studies, response rates ranged 46–48% and time to progression (TTP) ranged 10–13 months [64, 76]. Rituximab has also demonstrated benefit when added to combination cytotoxic chemotherapy for advanced follicular lymphoma [77, 78]. In addition, rituximab is used for the treatment of other low-grade CD20-positive lymphomas, such as small lymphocytic lymphoma (SLL) [which is also known as chronic lymphocytic leukemia (CLL)], marginal zone lymphoma, and lymphoplasmacytic lymphoma (also known as Waldenstrom's macroglobulinemia) [63, 79].

Yttrium-90 Ibritumomab Tiuxetan and Iodine-131 Tositumomab

Yttrium-90 (^{90}Y) ibritumomab tiuxetan (Zevalin) and iodine-131 (^{131}I) tositumomab (Bexxar) are collectively known as radioimmunotherapy. Both drugs consist of radioisotopes conjugated to a murine anti-CD20 antibody. They are indicated for the treatment of refractory B cell NHL. NHL is generally considered exquisitely radiosensitive, but the systemic nature of the disease precludes the use of standard external beam radiation therapy in most patients. Radioimmunotherapy capitalizes on the high degree of specificity of monoclonal antibodies to deliver high doses of ionizing radiation to the targeted tumor, while sparing normal tissues. The principles of radioimmunotherapy were first demonstrated by Lym-1, an early murine IgG2a antibody targeting HLA-DR10, a cell surface protein present on over 80% of lymphoma cells. Lym-1 was found to be more effective when conjugated to Iodine-131, with a response rate of 52%, over half of which were complete responses [80].

To limit nonspecific targeting, patients receiving either ibritumomab or tositumomab undergo a multistep treatment process. First, patients receive unlabeled anti-CD20 antibody to clear circulating B lymphocytes and saturate nontumor sites. They then receive a nontherapeutic dose of radiolabeled anti-CD20 antibody and undergo imaging to assess drug biodistribution and localization. Several days later, the therapeutic radiolabeled antibody is administered, dosed by millicurie (mCi) per kilogram body weight. Following treatment, patients are required to take radiation safety precautions (careful disposal of body fluids, including tears and sweat, and condom use) for one week [53].

^{90}Y Ibritumomab tiuxetan and ^{131}I tositumomab are notable for being the only currently approved antibodies for cancer treatment that are composed entirely of murine proteins. Given the adverse effects associated with this species of antibody, and the ability to produce humanized and even fully human antibodies currently, the ongoing use of murine antibodies may not seem intuitive. For radioimmunotherarpy, murine antibodies offer the advantage of rapid clearance from the body. For instance, ibritumomab has an elimination half-life of 30 h, compared to 60 h for rituximab, a chimeric antibody with the same molecular target. Thus, patients remain systemically radioactive for the shortest possible period. While this feature provides a benefit from a radiation therapy standpoint, it does present an immunologic quandary. Because of the high likelihood that a patient will develop anti-mouse antibodies, which could cause life-threatening infusion reactions in the future, ibritumomab and tositumomab are typically administered to a patient only once.

^{90}Y Ibritumomab tiuxetan, also known as IDEC-Y2B8, consists of a murine anti-CD20 IgG1 monoclonal antibody (ibritumomab), a chelator (tiuxetan; isothiocyanobenzyl MX-DTPA), and a radioisotope. During the initial phase, in which dose distribution is assessed, Indium-111 (^{111}I) is used in place of Yttrium-90 because Yttrium-90 is a pure beta emitter and therefore not readily imaged. In contrast, tositumomab is conjugated to the same radioisotope (Iodine-131) for imaging and therapy, as Iodine-131 emits both gamma rays and beta particles. Other differences between Yttrium-90 and Iodine-131 include energy (2.3 MeV for Yttrium-90 vs. 0.61 MeV for Iodine-131) and path length (mean of 5 mm for Yttrium-90 vs. 0.8 mm for Iodine-131) [81]. In a phase I/II trial of ^{90}Y ibritumomab tiuxetan in patients with refractory or relapsed CD20-positive low-grade, intermediate-grade, or mantle cell NHL, the MTD was 0.4 mCi/kg. The response rate was 67%, and 26% of patients achieved a complete response. Among responders, the median time to progression was 13 months [81]. Based on this study and subsequent phase II trials [82, 83], ^{90}Y ibritumomab tiuxetan was approved in February 2002 for relapsed or refractory low-grade NHL [84].

Tositumomab (Bexxar), a murine anti-CD20 IgG2a monoclonal antibody conjugated to Iodine-131, was first used in 1993 for the treatment of NHL refractory to chemotherapy [21]. Tositumomab administration begins with the infusion of unconjugated anti-CD20 antibody and 5 mCi ^{131}I tositumomab on day 1. Whole body gamma counts are obtained over the next 7 days, followed by the infusion of unconjugated anti-CD20 antibody and therapeutic ^{131}I tositumomab to deliver a radiation dose of 75 cGy [85], the MTD determined in phase I studies [21]. Early trials with ^{131}I tositumomab yielded response rates greater than 65% with up to 38% complete response for patients with relapsed or refractory NHL [86, 87]. In patients with previously untreated follicular lymphoma, a single course of ^{131}I tositumomab has yielded a response rate of 95%, a complete response rate of 75%, and 5-year progression-free survival of 59% [88].

Despite early concerns of severe and persistent hematologic toxicity from radioimmunotherapy, ^{131}I tositumomab and ^{90}Y ibritumomab tiuxetan are now being incorporated into combination therapy regimens, some of which include hematopoietic stem cell support. A retrospective analysis demonstrated that patients with NHL who relapse after treatment with ^{90}Y ibritumomab tiuxetan are able to tolerate subsequent courses of chemotherapy without major toxicities [89]. Conversely, radioimmunotherapy appears well tolerated and effective when given following standard chemotherapy. In a phase II trial, patients with advanced stage follicular lymphoma who received ^{131}I tositumomab after six cycles of CHOP [cyclophosphamide, hydroxydoxorubicin, Oncovin (vincristine), prednisone] achieved rates of overall and progression-free survival 23% higher than those seen with CHOP chemotherapy alone [90]. Currently a phase III trial is underway comparing CHOP, rituximab-CHOP, and ^{131}I tositumomab-CHOP in patients with newly diagnosed follicular lymphoma. (ClinicalTrials.gov number, NCT00006721) [90]Y Ibritumomab tiuxetan also appears safe when administered prior to autologous stem cell transplant and does not prolong engraftment time [91].

Despite these promising clinical data, the toxicities, cost, and complexities of administration have limited the use of radioimmunotherapy. The murine antibodies induce an immune response. This may manifest as acute infusion reactions and human anti-murine antibodies (HAMA), which occur in approximately 2% of patients treated with ^{90}Y ibritumomab tiuxetan and 9% of patients treated with ^{131}I tositumomab. Myelosuppression 6–9 weeks after administration is common. Ten percent of patients treated with ^{131}I tositumomab develop hypothyroidism [92]. The most feared complication of radioimmunotherapy is treatment-related myelodysplastic syndrome (MDS) or acute myeloid leukemia (AML). Rates of these late, generally incurable toxicities range 1.5–2.5% for ^{90}Y ibritumomab tiuxetan and 3.5–6.4% for ^{131}I tositumomab [63, 93, 94]. Because ionizing radiation is teratogenic, radioimmunotherapy is contraindicated in all stages of pregnancy.

Gemtuzumab Ozogamicin

Gemtuzumab ozogamicin (Mylotarg) was the first conjugated antibody approved for cancer therapy in the United States. Gemtuzumab ozogamicin, which is approved for the treatment of acute myeloid leukemia (AML), is a humanized IgG4 anti-CD33 monoclonal antibody (hP67.6) conjugated to the toxin calicheamicin [20]. CD33 is an immunoglobulin-like lectin (sugar-binding protein) found on myeloid cells. Its presence is used diagnostically to differentiate AML and acute lymphoblastic leukemia (ALL). After antibody binding, the gemtuzumab–CD33 complex is internalized. Through lysosomal hydrolysis, calicheamicin is released, causing DNA damage. In the three phase II trials that ultimately led to FDA approval, 26% of patients achieved remission, but the remission was typically short lived (median duration 6.4 months) [95]. In early clinical trials, fevers, chills, myelosuppression, and hepatic veno-occlusive disease (VOD) emerged as the primary toxicities of gemtuzumab ozogamicin. VOD, a condition in which the small veins of the liver are obstructed, results in fluid retention, weight gain, hepatomegaly, and hyperbilirubinemia. VOD is a long-recognized complication of hematopoietic stem cell transplant conditioning chemotherapy regimens and appears to occur at significantly higher rates among transplant patients previously treated with gemtuzumab ozogamicin [96]. Accordingly, the use of gemtuzumab ozogamicin is generally limited to AML patients not considered candidates for future transplantation.

Alemtuzumab

Alemtuzumab (Campath) targets CD52, a glycosylphosphatidylinositol-anchored antigen present on mature B and T cells, but not on stem cells. Because CD52 is expressed on a greater lymphoid population than is CD20, alemtuzumab is more immunosuppressive than rituximab. Alemtuzumab was the first humanized antibody produced. In the early 1980s, its murine precursor, CAMPATH-1, was noted to deplete bone marrow B and T cells [97]. In 1988, antigen-binding sites from CAMPATH-1 were incorporated into a human IgG framework, resulting in alemtuzumab [17]. Alemtuzumab was initially approved for relapsed/refractory chronic lymphocytic leukemia (CLL), in which it provides a response rate of approximately 30% and median overall survival of 16 months [98]. Currently, alemtuzumab is also indicated in the first-line setting, based on a phase III trial comparing alemtuzumab to chlorambucil, an alkylating agent that was previously the standard treatment of CLL. In this study, patients randomized to alemtuzumab had a significantly longer time to treatment failure (23.3 vs. 14.7 months; $p = 0.001$), a significantly higher complete response rate (24% vs. 2%; $p < 0.001$), and a significantly lower risk of progression or death (HR 0.58; $p = 0.0001$) [99].

In clinical practice, potential immunosuppression limits the use of alemtuzumab. Up to 50% of patients who would otherwise be candidates for alemtuzumab have infections precluding its use, including *Pneumocystis jiroveci* pneumonia, herpes simplex virus, and cytomegalovirus reactivation [63]. It is recommended that patients undergoing treatment with alemtuzumab receive antimicrobial prophylaxis, including the antibacterial drug trimethoprim-sulfamethoxazole (TMP-SMX), the antiviral drug acyclovir, and the antifungal drug fluconazole [100].

4.3.2 Solid Tumors:

Trastuzumab

Trastuzumab (Herceptin), a humanized monoclonal antibody against the HER2 (human epidermal growth factor receptor 2) antigen, was the first monoclonal antibody approved in the United States for the treatment of a solid organ malignancy. A potent growth regulator of breast cancer cells, HER2 is a transmembrane receptor tyrosine in the same 4-member family as EGFR (HER1). HER2 lacks a ligand-binding domain but activates the intracellular tyrosine kinase domain upon heterodimerizing with other members of the HER family. This event triggers downstream signal transduction via mediators such as the pro-survival Ras-MAPK (mitogen activated protein kinase) pathway and the anti-apoptotic PIK3 (phosphatidylinositol 3-kinase)/AKT/mTor (mammalian target of rapamycin) pathway. The binding of trastuzumab to HER2 is thought to cause cancer cell death by preventing HER2 dimerization and downstream signaling, promoting HER2 internalization and down-regulation, and recruiting ADCC [39, 101, 42].

HER2 is overexpressed in 20–30% of invasive breast cancers [102]. Traditionally, HER2-positive tumors were considered more biologically aggressive than HER2-negative malignancies and were associated with worse clinical outcomes. The availability of trastuzumab for patients with HER2-positive breast cancers has, in essence, inverted this relationship. HER2 status of tumor tissue is determined by IHC and/or fluorescent in situ hybridization (FISH). Breast cancers are considered HER2 positive if IHC staining is 3 + or FISH reveals more than six *HER2* gene copies per nucleus or a FISH ratio (*HER2* gene signals to chromosome 17 signals) of more than 2.2. A negative result is an IHC score of 0 or 1 +, a FISH result of less than four *HER2* gene copies per nucleus, or a FISH ratio of less than 1.8 [103]. If the IHC score is 2 +, this intermediate result is confirmed with FISH.

FDA approval of trastuzumab in 1998 for metastatic breast cancer followed several early phase trials demonstrating single-agent response rates in the 10–20% range [104–106]. In a phase III trial, over 400 patients with untreated, HER2 + breast cancer were randomized to standard chemotherapy with or without trastuzumab. Overall response rate, TTP, duration of response, and OS were all significantly improved in the trastuzumab arm [107]. In these studies, expected adverse events included infusion reactions, fever, and chills. What was not anticipated was the development of cardiac toxicity in a substantial proportion of patients. Cardiomyopathy occurred in 27% of patients treated with anthracycline–cyclophosphamide chemotherapy plus trastuzumab, in 8% of patients treated with anthracycline–cyclophosphamide chemotherapy alone, in 13% of patients treated with paclitaxel chemotherapy plus trastuzumab, and in 1% of patients treated with paclitaxel chemotherapy alone.

Lack of an animal model has hindered the elucidation of a precise mechanism of trastuzumab-associated cardiotoxicity [39]. One hypothesis is that this effect relates to the role of HER2 in cardiac embryonic development [108]. Unlike doxorubicin-associated cardiac dysfunction, trastuzumab-associated cardiotoxicity results in cellular dysfunction, not death, and is generally reversible. Because trastuzumab cardiotoxicity is not dose dependent, serial measurement of left ventricular ejection fraction (LVEF) is recommended throughout the course of therapy. This includes assessments at baseline, every 3 months during therapy, and every 6 months after therapy for up to 5 years [109]. If a patient has an absolute decrease of greater than 15% in LVEF from pretreatment values or an LVEF below the institutional limits of normal and an LVEF absolute decrease of 10% or greater from pretreatment values, trastuzumab therapy should be interrupted. If LVEF returns to normal limits and the LVEF absolute decrease is 15% or less within 4–8 weeks, trastuzumab therapy may be resumed. Permanent discontinuation is recommended when the decline in LVEF persists or if therapy is held on more than three occasions for cardiomyopathy. About 75% of patients with trastuzumab-associated cardiac dysfunction are symptomatic, and about 80% improve with standard medical management of congestive heart failure [107, 110].

In response to the significant rate of cardiac toxicity uncovered in clinical studies for metastatic breast cancer, subsequent trastuzumab trials in the adjuvant (postoperative) setting have been designed to minimize this risk. Specifically, these studies have avoided the concomitant administration of trastuzumab and anthracycline chemotherapy drugs. In the B-31 trial, patients received adjuvant adriamycin– cyclophosphamide chemotherapy, followed by paclitaxel chemotherapy, with or without trastuzumab. In this study, trastuzumab was started only after the completion of adriamycin and continued for up to 1 year. The addition of trastuzumab resulted in a 33% reduction in the risk of death ($p=0.015$). Fewer than 5% of patients experienced serious cardiac events [3]. The Herceptin Adjuvant (HERA) trial enrolled 3,401 patients and compared 1 or 2 years of adjuvant (postoperative) trastuzumab with observation alone after neoadjuvant (preoperative) or adjuvant (postoperative) chemotherapy. The unadjusted HR for risk of death with trastuzumab compared to observation was 0.66 (95% CI, 0.47–0.91; $p=0.0115$) [111]. The optimal duration of trastuzumab in the adjuvant setting remains unknown. In the Finland Herceptin (FinHer) Study, the subset of 232 HER2+ patients were randomized to receive adjuvant chemotherapy with or without nine weekly doses of trastuzumab. The addition of this relatively short course of trastuzumab significantly improved 3-year recurrence-free survival (89% vs. 78%; hazard ratio for recurrence or death, 0.42; 95% CI, 0.21–0.83; $p=0.01$) [112].

Cetuximab

Cetuximab (Erbitux), previously known as C225, is a chimeric IgG1 monoclonal antibody that binds to EGFR. EGFR, which is expressed in multiple cancer types (among them colorectal, lung, head and neck, and pancreatic), has been studied as a potential target for cancer therapy since the early 1980s [113]. EGFR contributes to cellular proliferation, migration, angiogenesis, and inhibition of apoptosis. Overall, the effects of cetuximab resemble those of EGFR small molecule tyrosine kinase inhibitors [e.g., erlotinib (Tarceva)]. Cetuximab binding blocks EGFR tyrosine kinase activation, thereby abrogating downstream signaling via intracellular mediators. Specifically, antibody binding causes a conformational change that sterically hinders EGFR dimerization [38]. In contrast to EGFR small molecule tyrosine kinase inhibitors, however, cetuximab appears to provide further antitumor effect by recruiting host immune functions (CMC and ADCC). Cetuximab also leads to long-term EGFR downregulation by promoting EGFR internalization and degradation [114]. The main clinical toxicities of cetuximab are rash, diarrhea, hypomagnesemia, and infusion reactions.

Cetuximab was first approved, in combination with cytotoxic chemotherapy, for the treatment of recurrent or refractory metastatic colorectal cancer. In a phase III clinical trial of patients with metastatic colorectal progressing on irinotecan-based chemotherapy, the addition of cetuximab provided a median time to progression of 4.1 months [115]. In the Erbitux plus Irinotecan for Metastatic Colorectal Cancer (EPIC) study, patients with metastatic colorectal cancer progressing on oxaliplatin-containing regimens were randomized to irinotecan with or without cetuximab. Patients in the cetuximab arm achieved statistically significantly longer progression-free survival (4.0 vs. 2.6 months) (HR, 0.692; 95% CI, 0.617–0.776; $p<0.0001$), higher radiographic response rate (16.4% vs. 4.2%; $p<0.0001$), and better scores in a quality-of-life analysis ($p=0.047$). However, the median overall survival was comparable between treatments: 10.7 months with cetuximab-irinotecan and 10.0 months with irinotecan alone (hazard ratio [HR], 0.975; 95% CI, 0.854–1.114; $p=0.71$). The investigators attributed this finding to the high rate (47%) of subsequent cetuximab use among patients randomized to irinotecan alone [116]. More recently, cetuximab has been added to first-line chemotherapy regimens. In the Cetuximab Combined with Irinotecan in First-Line Therapy for Metastatic Colorectal Cancer (CRYSTAL) trial, 1,217 patients were randomized to FOLFIRI (folinic acid, 5-fluorouracil, irinotecan) with or without cetuximab. The addition of cetuximab provided a statistically significant but clinically modest increase in median progression-free survival: 8.9 vs. 8.0 months ($p=0.036$) [117].

Cetuximab is also FDA approved for the treatment of locally advanced and metastatic head and neck squamous cell carcinoma (HNSCC). In a phase III trial, patients with locally advanced HNSCC were randomized to radiation therapy with or without cetuximab. The addition of cetuximab provided a clinically meaningful improvement in median overall survival (49 vs. 29 months; HR, 0.74 (95% CI, 0.57–0.97) [118]. An unexpected toxicity observed in clinical studies of cetuximab plus radiation for HNSCC was cardiopulmonary arrest, which resulted in an FDA-mandated black box warning. It is not clear if this is related to hypomagnesemia or other electrolyte disturbances. Because cisplatin-based concomitant chemoradiation is generally considered the standard treatment of locoregionally advanced HNSCC, many clinicians reserve radiation plus cetuximab for those patients who would not tolerate cisplatin-based concomitant chemoradiation. It has been proposed that the apparent synergy between cetuximab and radiation therapy is due to interference with the function of EGFR in the repair of double stranded DNA breaks caused by ionizing radiation [119]. In the recurrent/metastatic setting, cetuximab has been combined with chemotherapy for the treatment of recurrent HNSCC. The addition of cetuximab to cisplatin and 5-FU chemotherapy increased median OS from 7.4 months to 10.1 months (HR, 0.80; 95% CI, 0.64–0.99; $p = 0.04$) [120].

Compared to the clinically meaningful benefit of trastuzumab in the treatment of breast cancer, the impact of cetuximab, particularly in the treatment of colorectal cancer, may appear rather modest. One potential explanation for these differences is the ability to predict treatment response and to identify those patients most likely to benefit from therapy. For trastuzumab, this has been achieved through the early recognition that its clinical effect was limited to the 25% of breast cancer cases that overexpress HER2/neu. For cetuximab, identifying the optimal patient population remains elusive. Many clinical trials employing cetuximab for the treatment of colorectal cancer have limited enrollment to those patients whose tumors express EGFR [115–117]. Indeed, the formal FDA approval is for colorectal tumors with positive EGFR staining by IHC. However, it has been demonstrated that the effect of cetuximab may be independent of the degree of tumor EGFR expression [121]. This lack of correlation has been attributed to differences in EGFR expression between primary and metastatic tumor lesions, heterogeneous EGFR expression within an individual tumor, changes in EGFR expression over time, unreliable and inconsistent IHC scoring, and the contribution of host effector functions (e.g., ADCC) to the antitumor effects of cetuximab [121–124]. As observed in clinical trials of EGFR small molecule tyrosine kinase inhibitors [e.g., erlotinib (Tarceva)] [125], cetuximab-treated patients who develop an acneiform rash appear to have significantly improved outcomes compared to patients who do not develop this effect [126, 127]. In lung and colorectal cancer patients, EGFR gene copy number assessed by FISH may predict response to cetuximab [128, 129]. More recently, attention has turned to the mutation status of K-ras, a proto-oncogenic mediator in the EGFR signal transduction pathway. When K-ras is mutated, as occurs in approximately 25% of lung cancer cases [130] and over 30% of colorectal cancer cases [131], downstream pro-survival pathways are constitutively activated despite EGFR inhibition. As a result, cetuximab appears to provide no benefit to these patients. In one series of patients with refractory colorectal cancer treated with cetuximab, objective response rates were 40% for patients with wild-type K-ras, vs. 0% for patients with mutated K-ras. Median overall survival was 43 and 27 months, respectively [131]. In addition, expression levels of the EGFR ligands epiregulin and amphiregulin appear to correlate with response to cetuximab. Patients with colorectal tumors featuring high levels of epiregulin and amphiregulin are more likely to have disease control with cetuximab [132].

Panitumumab

Panitumumab (Vectibix) is the first fully human (i.e., no murine protein components) monoclonal antibody approved by the FDA for use in cancer therapy. Formerly called ABX-EGF, panitumumab is an IgG2 antibody directed against EGFR. Panitumumab was initially developed using XenoMouse transgenic technology, whereby mouse immunoglobulin genes are replaced by DNA sequences encoding human antibodies. Based on observations from earlier clinical trials with cetuximab, the frequency and severity of rash was considered a pharmacodynamic endpoint in panitumumab dose-finding studies [133]. As expected, the fully human protein structure of panitumumab is associated with fewer hypersensitivity reactions and a longer half-life than are comparable antibodies featuring murine components. In panitumumab clinical trials, 4% of patients experienced hypersensitivity reactions (1% serious). In contrast, with the chimeric anti-EGFR antibody cetuximab, hypersensitivity reactions have been reported in 19% of patients (3% serious) [122]. Consequently, premedication with an antihistamine (e.g., diphenhydramine) is required for cetuximab, but not for panitumumab. With a half-life 50% longer than that of cetuximab, panitumumab is dosed every 2 weeks as compared to weekly dosing for cetuximab. FDA approval of panitumumab for colorectal cancer followed a phase III clinical trial in which 463 patients with EGFR-positive chemotherapy-refractory metastatic colorectal cancer were randomized to panitumumab plus best supportive care vs. best supportive care alone. Patients receiving panitumumab had significantly higher objective response rates (10% vs. 0%; $p<0.0001$) and longer progression-free survival (HR, 0.54; 95% CI, 0.44–0.66; $p<0.0001$). Median progression-free survival was only days longer in the panitumumab arm (8 weeks vs. 7.3 weeks); however, *mean* progression-free survival was 13.8 weeks for panitumumab and 8.5 weeks for supportive care alone [134]. Whether panitumumab's IgG2 structure—which is generally considered to lack the immune function recruitment properties of IgG1—is clinically relevant remains unknown.

Bevacizumab

Bevacizumab (Avastin) is a humanized IgG1 monoclonal antibody that targets vascular endothelial growth factor (VEGF). VEGF is the principal mediator of angiogenesis, the growth of new blood vessels from preexisting vasculature. Angiogenesis is an essential component of tumor development and progression, as tumor cells cannot survive more than 2–3 mm from their blood supply [135]. The binding of VEGF to the extracellular domain of VEGF receptors (VEGFR) on vascular endothelial cells activates an intracellular tyrosine kinase. The activated tyrosine kinase generates downstream signals resulting in vascular proliferation [136]. Bevacizumab appears not only to disrupt angiogenesis but also to normalize preexisting tumor blood vessels. That is, it decreases tumor vessel tortuosity and tumor interstitial pressure, effects that may promote the delivery of other anticancer therapies [137, 138]. With approval for three of the most common malignancies—breast, lung, and colorectal cancer—bevacizumab has become one of the most widely used monoclonal antibodies in oncology.

Because bevacizumab affects normal as well as malignant angiogenesis, it is associated with several toxicities. Patients receiving bevacizumab may experience bleeding, clotting (primarily arterial [139]), hypertension, and—through effects on glomerular capillaries—proteinuria [140]. Wound healing complications and reports of gastrointestinal perforation have led to recommendations that major surgical procedures not be performed within 8 weeks of bevacizumab administration [141]. Bevacizumab is contraindicated in patients with squamous cell histology nonsmall cell lung cancer because in phase II clinical trials, these patients experienced unacceptably high levels of life-threatening hemoptysis [142]. The safety of bevacizumab in patients with primary or metastatic brain tumors remains unclear. In a phase II trial of irinotecan chemotherapy plus bevacizumab for recurrent glioblastoma multiforme, 1 of 35 patients developed intracranial hemorrhage, which occurred during the tenth cycle of therapy [143]. While the presence of brain metastases was an exclusion criteria in bevacizumab phase III clinical trials for lung, breast, and colorectal cancers, more recent experience suggests that rates of CNS bleeding are not increased in patients with previously treated (i.e., surgery and/or radiation) brain metastases [144–146].

Currently, bevacizumab is FDA approved in combination with chemotherapy for advanced colorectal, breast, and lung cancers. For colorectal cancer, it is administered at a dose of 10 mg/kg every 2 weeks with FOLFOX (5-FU, leucovorin, oxaliplatin) or FOLFIRI (5-FU, leucovorin, irinotecan) regimens [147–149]. For breast cancer, it is given at a dose of 10 mg/kg every 3 weeks with paclitaxel chemotherapy. FDA approval in February 2008 of this combination followed a randomized phase III clinical trial in which the addition of bevacizumab significantly improved median progression-free survival (11.8 months vs. 5.9 months) but not overall survival [150]. The approval was granted despite the fact that an FDA Oncologic Drugs Advisory Committee voted narrowly (5 to 4) against recommending approval in December 2007 [151]. For nonsmall cell lung cancer (nonsquamous histology), bevacizumab administration is 15 mg/kg every 3 weeks with carboplatin-paclitaxel chemotherapy. In a phase III trial of this regimen, despite the exclusion of patients at high risk for bleeding (preexisting hemoptysis, brain metastases, anticoagulation, and squamous cell histology), there were 15 treatment-related deaths, 5 from pulmonary hemorrhage [152]. Given the high cost of bevacizumab, preliminary results of a

European study in which patients with advanced NSCLC were randomized to cisplatin-gemcitabine chemotherapy alone, cisplatin-gemcitabine plus bevacizumab 7.5 mg/kg, or cisplatin-gemcitabine plus bevacizumab 15 mg/kg were greeted with interest, as both doses of bevacizumab were associated with prolonged progression-free survival [153].

Because the development and proliferation of most tumors are thought to depend on angiogenesis, bevacizumab has also been studied in several other clinical settings. For the treatment of renal cell carcinoma, single-agent bevacizumab 10 mg/kg significantly prolonged time to progression compared to placebo [154]. In a subsequent phase III renal cell carcinoma study, patients randomized to interferon alfa-2a plus bevacizumab had a median progression-free survival of 10.2 months, compared to 5.4 months for patients randomized to interferon alfa-2a alone [155]. For the treatment of recurrent glioblastoma multiforme, which is traditionally associated with a median survival of 3–6 months, irinotecan chemotherapy plus bevacizumab resulted in 46% 6-month progression-free survival and 77% 6-month overall survival rates [156]. Other malignancies under study include ovarian cancer, (ClinicalTrials.gov, NCT00262847) hepatocellular cancer, gastric cancer [140], pancreatic cancer [157], and non-Hodgkin's lymphoma (ClinicalTrials.gov, NCT00486759).

The individual tailoring of anti-angiogenic therapies is particularly challenging. The VEGF pathway involves both tumor and patient biology. VEGF may be secreted by tumor cells or by host stromal cells. VEGFR may be present on tumor cells or on host endothelial cells. Consequently, the factors that predict response to bevacizumab remain largely unclear. Tumor and serum levels of VEGF do not seem to correlate with response [157, 158], nor do tumor levels of VEGFR. In a recent retrospective analysis of tissue specimens from the phase III trial of paclitaxel plus bevacizumab for metastatic breast cancer, the VEGF-2578 AA and VEGF-1154 A polymorphisms were associated with outcomes [159]. Expression of CD31 (a marker of vascular endothelial cells) and platelet-derived growth factor receptor (PDGFR)-β have also been linked to response to bevacizumab in breast cancer studies [160]. Preclinical models suggest that both tumor and nontumor cell types may be involved in inherent and acquired resistance to antiangiogenic therapy. For instance, inherent anti-VEGF refractoriness is associated with infiltration of tumor tissue by $CD11b^+Gr1^+$ myeloid cells, and recruitment of these myeloid cells appears to confer refractoriness. Furthermore, combining anti-VEGF treatment with an antibody-targeting myeloid cells inhibited the growth of refractory tumors more effectively than anti-VEGF therapy alone [161]. Other proposed mechanisms of resistance to bevacizumab include the upregulation of alternate pro-angiogenic pathways and increased pericyte coverage of tumor vasculature [162]. Given the cost and toxicities of anti-angiogenic therapies such as bevacizumab, further defining these molecular characteristics and applying them to patient selection is likely to be a research priority in the future.

4.4 Characterizing "Targeted Therapy": Comparing Monoclonal Antibodies and Small Molecule Kinase Inhibitors

In oncology, the ubiquitous term "targeted therapy" generally refers to monoclonal antibodies and small molecule inhibitors. While drugs in each class often share molecular targets and have similar clinical indications, monoclonal antibodies and small molecule kinase inhibitors (which are alternatively referred to as small molecule tyrosine kinase inhibitors, tyrosine kinase inhibitors, small molecule inhibitors, or small molecules) have several key differences that impact their clinical use (see Table 6). As previously discussed, monoclonal antibodies generally have a single molecular target. In many instances, small molecule inhibitors have multiple molecular targets. While this property may lead to greater antitumor effects, it also increases toxicities. As a result, small molecule inhibitors are often used as monotherapy [e.g., sorafanib (Nexavar) for hepatocellular carcinoma and renal cell carcinoma, bortezomib (Velcade) in multiple myeloma, erlotinib (Tarceva) in nonsmall cell lung cancer, and imatinib (Gleevec) in chronic myelogenous leukemia and gastrointestinal stromal tumors], whereas monoclonal antibodies are often administered in combination with other treatment modalities, such as cytotoxic chemotherapy or radiation therapy. Because monoclonal antibodies are proteins, they would be denatured

Table 6 Classes of targeted cancer therapy

Property	Small molecule TKIs	Monoclonal antibodies
Size	~500 Da	~150,000 Da
Administration	Oral*	Intravenous
Dosing	Daily or twice daily[†]	Every 7–21 days
Half-life	Hours	Days
Specificity	+++	+++++
Targets	Intracellular (kinases)	Extracellular (cell surface receptors, soluble ligands)
Mechanisms of action	Inhibition of growth signals	Direct inhibitory effects, ADCC, CMC, receptor internalization
Drug interactions	Multiple (via CYP450)	None
Immunogenicity	None	Infusion reactions, HAMA, HACA
Cost	$$$	$$$$$

*Two of the ten FDA-approved small molecule TKIs (bortezomib, temsirolimus) are administered intravenously.

[†]Bortezomib is given either weekly or every 3 days with periodic rest periods; temsirolimus is given weekly.

HAMA: human anti-murine antibodies; **HACA**: human anti-chimeric antibodies; **ADCC**: antibody-dependent cellular cytotoxicity; **CMC**: complement-mediated cytoxicity; **CYP450**: cytochrome P450; **TKI**: tyrosine kinase inhibitor.

in the gastrointestinal tract and are thus administered intravenously. In contrast, the majority of small molecule inhibitors are administered orally. The metabolism of small molecule inhibitors via cytochrome P450 enzymes leads to multiple potential interactions with drugs such as azole antifungals, macrolide antibacterials, certain anticonvulsants, and warfarin.

In cases of shared molecular targets, functional differences between monoclonal antibodies and small molecule inhibitors may underlie apparent differences in clinical outcomes [163]. For instance, the anti-EGFR antibody cetuximab and the small molecule EGFR inhibitor erlotinib both result in attenuation of EGFR tyrosine kinase-mediated pro-survival and anti-apoptotic signal transduction. Cetuximab attaches to the extracellular domain of EGFR and prevents ligand binding, receptor dimerization, and activation of the intracellular tyrosine kinase. Erlotinib crosses the cell membrane and directly interferes with tyrosine kinase function. However, cetuximab also engages host immune functions and leads to long-term EGFR downregulation by promoting the internalization and degradation of the EGFR complex. Neither effect occurs with erlotinib.

5 Toxicities and Limitations of Monoclonal Antibodies

5.1 Infusion Reactions

Most toxicities associated with monoclonal antibodies reflect the molecular targets and mechanism of the individual antibody. Indeed, monoclonal antibodies and small molecule kinase inhibitors targeting similar pathways often have similar toxicity profiles. For instance, both the anti-VEGF antibody bevacizumab and the VEGF receptor (VEGFR) tyrosine kinase inhibitors sorafenib (Nexavar) and sunitinib (Sutent) are associated with bleeding, clotting, and hypertension. Acneiform rash and diarrhea occur with the anti-EGFR antibodies cetuximab and panitumumab, as well as with the EGFR tyrosine kinase inhibitors erlotinib and gefitinib (Iressa).

In contrast, infusion reactions, which are due to the nature of antibody production and structure, represent a class effect of monoclonal antibodies. To address these potentially fatal events, clinical researchers have examined such factors as duration of infusion [164]; the role of premedication with antihistamines, acetaminophen, and/or corticosteroids; and the molecular etiology of antibody infusion reactions. Infusion reactions may be broadly characterized as cytokine-dependent or hypersensitivity reactions [165]. Cytokine-dependent reactions arise from the interaction of a monoclonal antibody with molecular targets on tumor cells, blood cells, or effector cells, resulting in the release of inflammatory cytokines such as TNF α and interleukin (IL)-6 [166]. In a hypersensitivity reaction, the structure of a monoclonal antibody is recognized as an antigen by the patient's immune system. IgE is produced and sensitizes tissue mast cells and circulating basophils, resulting in the release of histamines, leukotrienes, and prostaglandins. The clinical features of these molecularly distinct syndromes overlap considerably and include bronchospasm, dyspnea, tachycardia, hypotension, urticaria, angioedema, and fever [167]. Because infusion reactions represent cytokine-dependent as well as hypersensitivity processes, the incidence of these adverse events is not always predicted by antibody species. For instance, the humanized (5% mouse, 95% human) antibody trastuzumab causes infusion reactions in up to 40% of patients during the initial treatment [168]. In contrast, infusion reactions have been reported in only 12% of patients treated with the chimeric (1/3 mouse, 2/3 human) antibody cetuximab [169]. However, severe infusion reactions—which are most commonly due to hypersensitivity—occur in fewer than 1% of patients receiving trastuzumab, but in 3% of patients treated with cetuximab. Rituximab, a clinically potent chimeric antibody, is associated with the highest rate of infusion reactions (almost 80% overall and approximately 10% serious). In general, most infusion reactions occur with the initial antibody dose, with decreased frequency for subsequent administrations. Indeed, one retrospective series suggests that antihistamine premedication might be discontinued after two uneventful administrations of cetuximab [170].

Recently, it has been observed that patients in the southeastern United States (treated at selected centers in Tennessee and North Carolina) have a markedly higher incidence of cetuximab-associated severe infusion reactions (22%) than has been seen nationally (3%) [171]. These regional differences appear due to a higher incidence of preexisting serum IgE antibodies directed against galactose-α-1, 3-galactose, a moiety present on the Fab region of the cetuximab heavy chain [172].

5.2 Drug Delivery

With a molecular weight of approximately 150,000 Da, monoclonal antibodies are essentially 1,000 times larger than conventional cytotoxic chemotherapy drugs (MW typically 100–200 Da) and 500 times larger than small molecule kinase inhibitors. Consequently, issues of drug delivery have arisen, particularly related to the central nervous system (CNS). This observation has been most pronounced with the use of trastuzumab in patients with breast cancer. In some series, up to 25–50% of patients develop "sanctuary" brain metastases, a finding that has been attributed to trastuzumab's enhanced control of systemic disease but apparent failure to cross the blood–brain barrier [173]. Because primary and metastatic brain tumors together affect approximately 200,000 people per year in the United States, the delivery of antibody-based therapeutics to the CNS compartment has received considerable attention. The observed efficacy of the anti-VEGF antibody bevacizumab for the treatment of high-grade gliomas may reflect the distribution of its molecular target; circulating VEGF is present on the systemic side of the blood–brain barrier. Direct intra-tumoral injection and convection-enhanced delivery, which provides a positive pressure gradient via a motor-driven pump, have been employed for the administration of ^{131}I-TNT (tumor necrosis treatment)-1/B (Cotara). This monoclonal antibody binds to the histone H1–DNA complex, a universally expressed intracellular antigen that becomes available for targeting in the necrotic core of tumors due to increased cell membrane permeability [174].

The development of smaller antibody-based therapeutics may improve drug delivery (see Fig. 1). For example, a ~3 kDa antibody fragment (about 1/50 the size of an intact monoclonal antibody) comprising two CDRs (V_HCDR1 and V_LCDR3) and a framework region (V_HFR2) targeted against the Epstein–Barr virus (EBV) envelope antigen gp350/220 was shown to have similar antigen recognition as its parent molecule but superior capacity to penetrate tumors in murine EBV-induced tumors [175]. Other antibody fragments under study include ^{131}I Mel-14 F(ab')$_2$, which targets glycoproteins present in melanoma and glioma cells [176], and ranibizumab-F(ab)$_2$, which targets VEGF for the treatment of ocular diseases [177]. Minibodies are genetically engineered constructs, 80 kDa in size, that maintain antigen binding but have improved tumor uptake compared to their parent antibodies. The T84.66 (cT84.66) minibody is an antibody construct (VL-linker-VH-CH3) that binds carcinoembryonic antigen (CEA) and has been conjugated to Iodine-123. In a pilot trial of 10 patients with colon cancer, cT84.66 targeted the tumor [178]. Further studies are underway to examine the pharmacokinetics and biodistribution of this therapeutic agent.

6 Areas of Current and Future Development

6.1 Antibody Engineering

The utilization of monoclonal antibodies as a therapeutic platform continues to evolve. The progression from murine to entirely human antibodies represents only one aspect of this process. Refined bioengineering is leading to improvements in techniques of toxin, radioisotope, and drug conjugation. As previously described, the use of antibody fragments may overcome issues related not only to the large size of intact monoclonal antibodies but also to their immunogenicity. However, it will take years to implement these developments into clinical practice. In the near future, the greatest clinical advances in antibody therapy are likely to come not from improved antibody design and production, but rather from an improved understanding of the diseases these drugs target. Specifically, the identification and elucidation of the processes that underlie the development and progression of cancer will result in new molecular targets for antibody therapy.

6.2 Targets

In the evaluation of potential targets for antibody-based therapy, a number of properties are considered. Ideally, these targets have selective cell-surface expression present of malignant cell but not on normal cells, have high cell-surface density, and be anchored to the cell surface membrane (rather than secreted). By promoting the binding of antibodies to malignant but not normal cells, these characteristics optimize the therapeutic margin. A recent review of molecular therapeutics examined over 1,000 candidate drugs that entered clinical study between 1990 and 2006 [26]. During this period, the 10 most frequently targeted molecules were epithelial cell adhesion molecule (EpCAM), EFGR, mucin-1 (MUC1/CanAg), CD20, CEA, HER2, CD22, CD33, Lewis Y antigen, and prostate-specific membrane antigen (PSMA). Four of these molecules (EGFR, CD20, HER2, and CD33) are targeted by seven of the monoclonal antibodies currently approved for cancer therapy.

Table 7 lists monoclonal antibodies currently in late-phase clinical development. These drugs target a number of molecules, including CD20, CD22, EGFR, EpCAM, insulin-like growth factor-1 receptor (IGF-1R), and cytotoxic T lymphocyte antigen-4 (CTLA-4). Targeting CTLA-4, a molecule involved in

Table 7 Selected monoclonal Ab oncology phase III trials

Condition	Drug	Target	Start date	NCT
Colon cancer	Edrecolomab	17-1A	5.1997	NCT00002968
			7.1997	NCT00309517
Ovarian cancer; peritoneal cavity	^{90}Y monoclonal antibody HMFG1	HMFG-1	12.1998	NCT00004115
SCLC	BEC2 and BCG	Anti-idiotypic	9.1999	NCT00006352
AML	Lintuzumab	CD33	3.2000	NCT00006045
Lymphoma	Epratuzumab	CD22	9.2001	NCT00022685
Neuroblastoma	Ch14.18 with chemotherapy	GD2	10.2001	NCT00026312
RCC	^{124}I-cG250	G250	8.2004	NCT00087022
			3.2208	NCT00606632
Melanoma, metastases	MDX-010	CTLA4	9.2004	NCT00094653
Mycosis Fungoides	Zanolimumab	CD4	7.2005	NCT00127881
Kidney cancer	cG250 (Rencarex)	MN	9.2005	NCT00209183
Melanoma	Tremelimumab (CP-675,206)	CTLA4	3.2006	NCT00257205
NSCLC	CP-751, 871	IGF-1R	3.2008	NCT00596830
FL	Ofatumumab-HuMax-CD20	CD20	3.2006	NCT00394836
CLL			6.2006	NCT00349349
Prostate cancer	Denosumab	RANKL	4.2006	NCT00321620
HNSCC	Zalutumumab	EGFR	10.2006	NCT00382031

AML: acute myelogenous leukemia; **BCG**: *Bacillus Calmette-Guérin*; **CLL**: chronic lymphocytic leukemia; **CTLA4**: Cytotoxic T-Lymphocyte Antigen 4; **EGFR**: epidermal growth factor recptor; **FL**: follicular lymphoma; **GD2**: disialoganglioside; **HMFG-1**: human milk fat globulin 1; **HNSCC**: head and neck squamous cell cancer; **IGF1-R**: insulin like growth factor receptor 1; **MN**: a cell surface antigen found on 90% of renal cell carcinomas; **NSCLC**: non-small cell lung cancer; **RANKL**: Receptor activator of nuclear factor kappa B ligand; **RCC**: Renal Cell Carcinoma; **SCLC**: small cell lung cancer.

suppression of T cell function, appears to promote immune rejection of tumors. The anti-CTLA-4 monoclonal antibodies ipilumumab and tremilimumab are currently under study for the treatment of melanoma, a malignancy generally considered resistant to cytotoxic chemotherapy and potentially sensitive to immune-based approaches [179, 180]. Anti-IGF-1R antibodies have demonstrated encouraging activity in a variety of malignancies, including breast, liver, colorectal, and prostate cancer, as well as sarcomas. In a study of carboplatin-paclitaxel chemotherapy plus the anti-IGF-1R antibody CP-751,871 for the treatment of metastatic NSCLC, 72% of patients with squamous cell tumors achieved an objective response [181]. These early results are particularly encouraging because recent therapeutic advances for NSCLC have not been highly applicable to squamous cell histology, which is relatively insensitive to EGFR inhibition and is contraindicated with anti-VEGF therapy because of bleeding complications. IGF-1R serves as an example of a target that may be more appropriate for monoclonal antibodies than for small molecule tyrosine kinase inhibitors. Exquisite target specificity is likely to be clinically important, as IGF-1R has extensive sequence homology to the insulin receptor, which would promote significant hyperglycemia if inhibited [182].

6.3 Economics

Economic considerations may impact the future development and use of monoclonal antibodies. As increasing attention turns to the cost of health care, the price tag of these treatments is likely to come under scrutiny. For instance, 5-fluorouracil and leucovorin, the standard treatment of metastatic colorectal cancer until the mid-1990s, has an adjusted 2004 cost of $63 for 8 weeks of treatment. State-of-the-art combination chemotherapy regimens for this disease, featuring monoclonal antibodies such as bevacizumab and cetuximab, cost over $30,000 for 8 weeks of treatment [183]. These treatments have doubled the median survival of patients with metastatic colorectal cancer, a clinically meaningful benefit that, to date, has made it difficult to consider limiting the use of these drugs. In a survey study of medical oncologists, respondents generally believed that treatments up to $300,000 per quality-adjusted life-year were reasonable, and 78% stated that cost should not impact access to "effective" care. However, 71% felt that rising drug costs would lead to treatment rationing in the near future [184]. While patent expiration typically results in the availability of less-expensive generic medications, this process may be less straightforward for monoclonal antibodies. The molecular techniques used to develop monoclonal antibodies often include a number of patents. Furthermore, the FDA has yet to set out clear guidelines for the development of follow-along biologic agents or bio-similar agents [185]. It will be several years before this transition is tested. Rituximab and trastuzumab, approved in the late 1990s, are not expected to come off patent protection until 2015.

References

1. Strebhardt K, Ullrich A. Paul Ehrlich's magic bullet concept: 100 years of progress. *Nature Reviews Cancer* 2008; **8**: 473–480.
2. Coiffier B et al. CHOP Chemotherapy plus rituximab compared with CHOP alone in elderly patients with diffuse large-B-cell lymphoma. *The New England Journal of Medicine* 2002; **346**: 235–242.
3. Romond EH et al. Trastuzumab plus adjuvant chemotherapy for operable HER2-positive breast cancer. *The New England Journal of Medicine* 2005; **353**: 1673–1684.
4. Antonia S et al. Natural history of diarrhea associated with the anti-CTLA4 monoclonal antibody CP-675,206. *Journal of Clinical Oncology (Meeting Abstracts)* 2007; **25**: 3038.
5. Sheridan C. TeGenero fiasco prompts regulatory rethink. *Nature Biotechnology* 2006; **24**: 475–476.
6. Kolata G, Adrew P. Costly cancer drug offers hope, but also a dilemma. *New York Times* 6 July 2008: A1.
7. Köhler G, Milstein C. Continuous cultures of fused cells secreting antibody of predefined specificity. *Nature* 1975; **256**: 495–497.
8. Oldham RK. Monoclonal antibodies in cancer therapy. *Journal of Clinical Oncology* 1983; **1**: 582–590.
9. Oldham RK, Dillman RO. Monoclonal antibodies in cancer therapy: 25 years of progress. *Journal of Clinical Oncology* 2008; **26**: 1774–1777.
10. Dillman RO. Toxicities and side effects associated with intravenous infusions of murine monoclonal antibodies. *Journal of Biological Response Modifiers* 1986; **5**: 73–84.
11. Nadler LM et al. Serotherapy of a patient with a monoclonal antibody directed against a human lymphoma-associated antigen. *Cancer Research* 1980; **40**: 3147–3154.
12. Dillman RO et al. Murine monoclonal antibody therapy in two patients with chronic lymphocytic leukemia. *Blood* 1982; **59**: 1036–1045.
13. Ritz J, Schlossman SF. Utilization of monoclonal antibodies in the treatment of leukemia and lymphoma. *Blood* 1982; **59**: 1–11.
14. Miller RA, Maloney DG, McKillop J, Levy R. In vivo effects of murine hybridoma monoclonal antibody in a patient with T-cell leukemia. *Blood* 1981; **58**: 78–86.
15. Houghton AN et al. Mouse monoclonal IgG3 antibody detecting GD3 ganglioside: a phase I trial in patients with malignant melanoma. *Proceedings of the National Academy of Sciences of the United States of America* 1985; **82**: 1242–1246.
16. Boulianne GL, Hozumi N, Shulman MJ. Production of functional chimaeric mouse/human antibody. *Nature* 1984; **312**: 643–646.
17. Riechmann L, Clark M, Waldmann H, Winter G. Reshaping human antibodies for therapy. *Nature* 1988; **332**: 323–327.
18. Maloney DG et al. Phase I clinical trial using escalating single-dose infusion of chimeric anti-CD20 monoclonal antibody (IDEC-C2B8) in patients with recurrent B-cell lymphoma. *Blood* 1994; **84**: 2457–2466.
19. Carter P et al. Humanization of an anti-p185HER2 antibody for human cancer therapy. *Proceedings of the National Academy of Sciences of the United States of America* 1992; **89**: 4285–4289.
20. Sievers EL et al. Selective ablation of acute myeloid leukemia using antibody-targeted chemotherapy: a phase I study of an anti-CD33 calicheamicin immunoconjugate. *Blood* 1999; **93**: 3678–3684.
21. Kaminski MS et al. Radioimmunotherapy of B-cell lymphoma with [131I]anti-B1 (anti-CD20) antibody. *The New England Journal of Medicine* 1993; **329**: 459–465.
22. Knox SJ et al. Yttrium-90-labeled anti-CD20 monoclonal antibody therapy of recurrent B-cell lymphoma. *Clinical Cancer Research* 1996; **2**: 457–470.
23. Strome SE, Sausville EA, Mann D. A mechanistic perspective of monoclonal antibodies in cancer therapy beyond target-related effects. *Oncologist* 2007; **12**: 1084–1095.

24. Nimmerjahn F, Ravetch JV. Divergent immunoglobulin G subclass activity through selective Fc receptor binding. *Science* 2005; **310**: 1510–1512.
25. Morell A, Terry W, Waldmann T. Metabolic properties of IgG subclasses in man. *Journal of Clinical Investigation* 1970; **49**: 673–680.
26. Reichert JM, Valge-Archer VE. Development trends for monoclonal antibody cancer therapeutics. *Nature Reviews Drug Discovery* 2007; **6**: 349–356.
27. Loo L, Robinson MK, Adams GP. Antibody engineering principles and applications. *Cancer Journal* 2008; **14**: 149–153.
28. Colcher D et al. Pharmacokinetics and biodistribution of genetically-engineered antibodies. *QJ Nuclear Medicine* 1998; **42**: 225–241.
29. Martens T et al. A novel one-armed anti-c-met antibody inhibits glioblastoma growth in vivo. *Clinical Cancer Research* 2006; **12**: 6144–6152.
30. Wochner RD, Strober W, Waldmann TA. The role of the kidney in the catabolism of bence jones proteins and immunoglobulin fragments. *Journal of Experimental Medicine* 1967; **126**: 207–221.
31. Sharkey RM, Goldenberg DM. Targeted therapy of cancer: new prospects for antibodies and immunoconjugates. *CA Cancer Journal for Clinicians* 2006; **56**: 226–243.
32. Mechetner E. *Development and Characterization of Mouse Hybridomas* Monocolonal Antibodies. Ed. Maher Albitar. SpringerLink: New York, 2007, pp. 1–13.
33. Hoogenboom HR et al. Antibody phage display technology and its applications. *Immunotechnology* 1998; **4**: 1–20.
34. McCafferty J, Griffiths AD, Winter G, Chiswell DJ. Phage antibodies: filamentous phage displaying antibody variable domains. *Nature* 1990; **348**: 552–554.
35. Donzeau M, Knappik A. *Recombinant Monoclonal Antibodies* Monocolonal Antibodies. Ed. Maher Albitar. SpringerLink: New York, 2007, pp. 15–31.
36. Yang X-D et al. Development of ABX-EGF, a fully human anti-EGF receptor monoclonal antibody, for cancer therapy. *Critical Reviews in Oncology/Hematology* 2001; **38**: 17–23.
37. Masui H, Moroyama T, Mendelsohn J. Mechanism of antitumor activity in mice for anti-epidermal growth factor receptor monoclonal antibodies with different isotypes. *Cancer Research* 1986; **46**: 5592–5598.
38. McKillop D et al. Metabolism and enantioselective pharmacokinetics of Casodex in man. *Xenobiotica* 1993; **23**: 1241–1253.
39. Hudis CA. Trastuzumab – mechanism of action and use in clinical practice. *The New England Journal of Medicine* 2007; **357**: 39–51.
40. Adams GP, Weiner LM. Monoclonal antibody therapy of cancer. *Nature Biotechnology* 2005; **23**: 1147–1157.
41. Desjarlais JR, Lazar GA, Zhukovsky EA, Chu SY. Optimizing engagement of the immune system by anti-tumor antibodies: an engineer's perspective. *Drug Discovery Today* 2007; **12**: 898–910.
42. Iannello A, Ahmad A. Role of antibody-dependent cell-mediated cytotoxicity in the efficacy of therapeutic anti-cancer monoclonal antibodies. *Cancer and Metastasis Reviews* 2005; **24**: 487–499.
43. Steplewski Z, Lubeck MD, Koprowski H. Human macrophages armed with murine immunoglobulin G2a antibodies to tumors destroy human cancer cells. *Science* 1983; **221**: 865–867.
44. van Ojik HH et al. CpG-A and B Oligodeoxynucleotides enhance the efficacy of antibody therapy by activating different effector cell populations. *Cancer Research* 2003; **63**: 5595–5600.
45. Clynes RA, Towers TL, Presta LG, Ravetch JV. Inhibitory Fc receptors modulate in vivo cytoxicity against tumor targets. *Nature Medicine* 2000; **6**: 443–446.
46. Shields RL et al. High resolution mapping of the binding site on human IgG1 for FcγRI, FcγRII, FcγRIII, and FcRn and Design of IgG1 variants with improved binding to the FcγR. *Journal of Biologic Chemistry* 2001; **276**: 6591–6604.

47. Cartron G et al. Therapeutic activity of humanized anti-CD20 monoclonal antibody and polymorphism in IgG Fc receptor FcγRIIIa gene. *Blood* 2002; **99**: 754–758.
48. Weng W-K, Levy R. Two immunoglobulin G fragment C receptor polymorphisms independently predict response to rituximab in patients with follicular lymphoma. *Journal of Clinical Oncology* 2003; **21**: 3940–3947.
49. Treon SP et al. Polymorphisms in FcγRIIIA (CD16) receptor expression are associated with clinical response to rituximab in Waldenstrom's macroglobulinemia. *Journal of Clinical Oncology* 2005; **23**: 474–481.
50. Bowles JA et al. Anti-CD20 monoclonal antibody with enhanced affinity for CD16 activates NK cells at lower concentrations and more effectively than rituximab. *Blood* 2006; **108**: 2648–2654.
51. Galon J et al. Type, density, and location of immune cells within human colorectal tumors predict clinical outcome. *Science* 2006; **313**: 1960–1964.
52. Di Gaetano N et al. Complement activation determines the therapeutic activity of rituximab in vivo. *Journal of Immunology* 2003; **171**: 1581–1587.
53. Cheson BD. Radioimmunotherapy of non-Hodgkin lymphomas. *Blood* 2003; **101**: 391–398.
54. Walker S et al. Cleavage behavior of calicheamicin gamma 1 and calicheamicin T. *Proceedings of the National Academy of Sciences of the United States of America* 1992; **89**: 4608–4612.
55. Ricart AD, Tolcher AW. Technology Insight: cytotoxic drug immunoconjugates for cancer therapy. *Nature Clinical Practice Oncology* 2007; **4**: 245–255.
56. Bagshawe K. Antibody directed enzymes revive anti-cancer prodrugs concept. *British Journal of Cancer* 1987; **56**: 531–532.
57. Senter PD et al. Anti-tumor effects of antibody-alkaline phosphatase conjugates in combination with etoposide phosphate. *Proceedings of the National Academy of Sciences of the United States of America* 1988; **85**: 4842–4846.
58. Kratz F, Müller Ivonne A, Ryppa C, Warnecke A. Prodrug strategies in anticancer chemotherapy. *ChemMedChem* 2008; **3**: 20–53.
59. Maguire RT, Pascucci VL, Maroli AN, Gulfo JV. Immunoscintigraphy in patients with colorectal, ovarian, and prostate cancer. Results with site-specific immunoconjugates. *Cancer* 1993; **72**: 3453–3462.
60. Frangioni JV. New technologies for human cancer imaging. *Journal of Clinical Oncology* 2008; **26**: 4012–4021.
61. Gómez-Almaguer D et al. Alemtuzumab for the treatment of steroid-refractory acute graft-versus-host disease. *Biology of Blood and Marrow Transplantation* 2008; **14**: 10–15.
62. Browning JL. B cells move to centre stage: novel opportunities for autoimmune disease treatment. *Nature Reviews Drug Discovery* 2006; **5**: 564–576.
63. Cheson BD, Leonard JP. Monoclonal antibody therapy for B-cell non-Hodgkin's lymphoma. *The New England Journal of Medicine* 2008; **359**: 613–626.
64. McLaughlin P et al. Rituximab chimeric anti-CD20 monoclonal antibody therapy for relapsed indolent lymphoma: half of patients respond to a four-dose treatment program. *Journal of Clinical Oncology* 1998; **16**: 2825–2833.
65. Cragg M, Walshe C, Ivanov A, Glennie M. The biology of CD20 and its potential as a target for mAb therapy. *Current Directions in Autoimmunity* 2005; **8**: 140–174.
66. Stolz C et al. Targeting Bcl-2 family proteins modulates the sensitivity of B-cell lymphoma to Rituximab-induced apoptosis. *Blood* 2008; **112**: 3312–3321.
67. Reed JC. Bcl-2-family proteins and hematologic malignancies: history and future prospects. *Blood* 2008; **111**: 3322–3330.
68. Mounier N et al. Rituximab plus CHOP (R-CHOP) overcomes bcl-2–associated resistance to chemotherapy in elderly patients with diffuse large B-cell lymphoma (DLBCL). *Blood* 2003; **101**: 4279–4284.
69. Lossos IS et al. Expression of a single gene, BCL-6, strongly predicts survival in patients with diffuse large B-cell lymphoma. *Blood* 2001; **98**: 945–951.

70. Winter JN et al. Prognostic significance of Bcl-6 protein expression in DLBCL treated with CHOP or R-CHOP: a prospective correlative study. *Blood* 2006; **107**: 4207–4213.
71. Harris NL et al. A revised European-American classification of lymphoid neoplasms: a proposal from the International Lymphoma Study Group. *Blood* 1994; **84**: 1361–1392.
72. Pfreundschuh M et al. CHOP-like chemotherapy plus rituximab versus CHOP-like chemotherapy alone in young patients with good-prognosis diffuse large-B-cell lymphoma: a randomised controlled trial by the MabThera International Trial (MInT) Group. *The Lancet Oncology* 2006; **7**: 379–391.
73. Feugier P et al. Long-term results of the R-CHOP study in the treatment of elderly patients with diffuse large B-cell lymphoma: a study by the Groupe d'Etude des Lymphomes de l'Adulte. *Journal of Clinical Oncology* 2005; **23**: 4117–4126.
74. Habermann TM et al. Rituximab-CHOP versus CHOP alone or with maintenance rituximab in older patients with diffuse large B-cell lymphoma. *Journal of Clinical Oncology* 2006; **24**: 3121–3127.
75. Armitage JO, Weisenburger DD. New approach to classifying non-Hodgkin's lymphomas: clinical features of the major histologic subtypes. Non-Hodgkin's Lymphoma Classification Project. *Journal of Clinical Oncology* 1998; **16**: 2780–2795.
76. Maloney DG et al. IDEC-C2B8: results of a phase I multiple-dose trial in patients with relapsed non-Hodgkin's lymphoma. *Journal of Clinical Oncology* 1997; **15**: 3266–3274.
77. Hiddemann W et al. Frontline therapy with rituximab added to the combination of cyclophosphamide, doxorubicin, vincristine, and prednisone (CHOP) significantly improves the outcome for patients with advanced-stage follicular lymphoma compared with therapy with CHOP alone: results of a prospective randomized study of the German Low-Grade Lymphoma Study Group. *Blood* 2005; **106**: 3725–3732.
78. van Oers MHJ et al. Rituximab maintenance improves clinical outcome of relapsed/resistant follicular non-Hodgkin lymphoma in patients both with and without rituximab during induction: results of a prospective randomized phase 3 intergroup trial. *Blood* 2006; **108**: 3295–3301.
79. Keating MJ et al. Early results of a chemoimmunotherapy regimen of fludarabine, cyclophosphamide, and rituximab as initial therapy for chronic lymphocytic leukemia. *Journal of Clinical Oncology* 2005; **23**: 4079–4088.
80. DeNardo GL et al. Maximum-tolerated dose, toxicity, and efficacy of (131)I-Lym-1 antibody for fractionated radioimmunotherapy of non-Hodgkin's lymphoma. *Journal of Clinical Oncology* 1998; **16**: 3246–3256.
81. Witzig TE et al. Phase I/II trial of IDEC-Y2B8 radioimmunotherapy for treatment of relapsed or refractory CD20+ B-cell non-Hodgkin's lymphoma. *Journal of Clinical Oncology* 1999; **17**: 3793–3803.
82. Gordon LI et al. Durable responses after ibritumomab tiuxetan radioimmunotherapy for CD20+ B-cell lymphoma: long-term follow-up of a phase 1/2 study. *Blood* 2004; **103**: 4429–4431.
83. Witzig TE et al. Treatment with ibritumomab tiuxetan radioimmunotherapy in patients with rituximab-refractory follicular non-Hodgkin's lymphoma. *Journal of Clinical Oncology* 2002; **20**: 3262–3269.
84. Witzig TE et al. Randomized controlled trial of yttrium-90-labeled ibritumomab tiuxetan radioimmunotherapy versus rituximab immunotherapy for patients with relapsed or refractory low-grade, follicular, or transformed B-cell non-Hodgkin's lymphoma. *Journal of Clinical Oncology* 2002; **20**: 2453–2463.
85. Vose JM et al. Multicenter phase II study of iodine-131 tositumomab for chemotherapy-relapsed/refractory low-grade and transformed low-grade B-cell non-Hodgkin's lymphomas. *Journal of Clinical Oncology* 2000; **18**: 1316–1323.
86. Horning SJ et al. Efficacy and safety of tositumomab and iodine-131 tositumomab (Bexxar) in B-cell lymphoma, progressive after rituximab. *Journal of Clinical Oncology* 2005; **23**: 712–719.

87. Kaminski MS et al. Pivotal study of iodine I 131 tositumomab for chemotherapy-refractory low-grade or transformed low-grade B-cell non-Hodgkin's lymphomas. *Journal of Clinical Oncology* 2001; **19**: 3918–3928.
88. Kaminski MS et al. 131I-tositumomab therapy as initial treatment for follicular lymphoma. *The New England Journal of Medicine* 2005; **352**: 441–449.
89. Ansell SM et al. Subsequent chemotherapy regimens are well tolerated after radio-immunotherapy with yttrium-90 ibritumomab tiuxetan for non-Hodgkin's lymphoma. *Journal of Clinical Oncology* 2002; **20**: 3885–3890.
90. Press OW et al. Phase II trial of CHOP chemotherapy followed by tositumomab/iodine I-131 tositumomab for previously untreated follicular non-Hodgkin's lymphoma: five-year follow-up of southwest oncology group protocol S9911. *Journal of Clinical Oncology* 2006; **24**: 4143–4149.
91. Nademanee A et al. A phase 1/2 trial of high-dose yttrium-90-ibritumomab tiuxetan in combination with high-dose etoposide and cyclophosphamide followed by autologous stem cell transplantation in patients with poor-risk or relapsed non-Hodgkin lymphoma. *Blood* 2005; **106**: 2896–2902.
92. Kaminski MS et al. Radioimmunotherapy with iodine 131I tositumomab for relapsed or refractory B-cell non-Hodgkin lymphoma: updated results and long-term follow-up of the University of Michigan experience. *Blood* 2000; **96**: 1259–1266.
93. Czuczman MS et al. Treatment-related myelodysplastic syndrome and acute myelogenous leukemia in patients treated with ibritumomab tiuxetan radioimmunotherapy. *Journal of Clinical Oncology* 2007; **25**: 4285–4292.
94. Bennett JM et al. Assessment of treatment-related myelodysplastic syndromes and acute myeloid leukemia in patients with non-Hodgkin lymphoma treated with tositumomab and iodine I131 tositumomab. *Blood* 2005; **105**: 4576–4582.
95. Larson RA, Sievers EL, Michael R. Loken Jacques JM, van Dongen Irwin D, Bernstein Frederick R. Appelbaum Mylotarg Study Group. Final report of the efficacy and safety of gemtuzumab ozogamicin (Mylotarg) in patients with CD33-positive acute myeloid leukemia in first recurrence. *Cancer* 2005; **104**: 1442–1452.
96. Wadleigh M et al. Prior gemtuzumab ozogamicin exposure significantly increases the risk of veno-occlusive disease in patients who undergo myeloablative allogeneic stem cell transplantation. *Blood* 2003; **102**: 1578–1582.
97. Hale G et al. Removal of T cells from bone marrow for transplantation: a monoclonal antilymphocyte antibody that fixes human complement. *Blood* 1983; **62**: 873–882.
98. Keating MJ et al. Therapeutic role of alemtuzumab (Campath-1H) in patients who have failed fludarabine: results of a large international study. *Blood* 2002; **99**: 3554–3561.
99. Hillmen P et al. Alemtuzumab compared with chlorambucil as first-line therapy for chronic lymphocytic leukemia. *Journal of Clinical Oncology* 2007; **25**: 5616–5623.
100. Thursky KA et al. Spectrum of infection, risk and recommendations for prophylaxis and screening among patients with lymphoproliferative disorders treated with alemtuzumab. *British Journal of Haematology* 2006; **132**: 3–12.
101. Carson WE et al. Interleukin-2 enhances the natural killer cell response to Herceptin-coated Her2/*neu*-positive breast cancer cells. *European Journal of Immunology* 2001; **31**: 3016–3025.
102. Slamon DJ et al. Human breast cancer: correlation of relapse and survival with amplification of the HER-2/neu oncogene. *Science* 1987; **235**: 177–182.
103. Wolff AC et al. American Society of Clinical Oncology/College of American Pathologists guideline recommendations for human epidermal growth factor receptor 2 testing in breast cancer. *Journal of Clinical Oncology* 2007; **25**: 118–145.
104. Vogel CL et al. Efficacy and safety of trastuzumab as a single agent in first-line treatment of HER2-overexpressing metastatic breast cancer. *Journal of Clinical Oncology* 2002; **20**: 719–726.

105. Cobleigh MA et al. Multinational study of the efficacy and safety of humanized anti-HER2 monoclonal antibody in women who have HER2-overexpressing metastatic breast cancer that has progressed after chemotherapy for metastatic disease. *Journal of Clinical Oncology* 1999; **17**: 2639–2648.

106. Baselga J et al. Phase II study of weekly intravenous recombinant humanized anti-p185HER2 monoclonal antibody in patients with HER2/neu-overexpressing metastatic breast cancer. *Journal of Clinical Oncology* 1996; **14**: 737–744.

107. Slamon DJ et al. Use of chemotherapy plus a monoclonal antibody against HER2 for metastatic breast cancer that overexpresses HER2. *The New England Journal of Medicine* 2001; **344**: 783–792.

108. Lee K-F et al. Requirement for neuregulin receptor erbB2 in neural and cardiac development. *Nature* 1995; **378**: 394–398.

109. Ewer SM, Ewer MS. Cardiotoxicity profile of trastuzumab. *Drug Safety* 2008; **31**: 459–467.

110. Seidman A et al. Cardiac dysfunction in the trastuzumab clinical trials experience. *Journal of Clinical Oncology* 2002; **20**: 1215–1221.

111. Smith I et al. 2-year follow-up of trastuzumab after adjuvant chemotherapy in HER2-positive breast cancer: a randomised controlled trial. *The Lancet* 2007; **369**: 29–36.

112. Joensuu H et al. Adjuvant docetaxel or vinorelbine with or without trastuzumab for breast cancer. *The New England Journal of Medicine* 2006; **354**: 809–820.

113. Kawamoto T et al. Growth stimulation of A431 cells by epidermal growth factor: identification of high-affinity receptors for epidermal growth factor by an anti-receptor monoclonal antibody. *Proceedings of the National Academy of Sciences of the United States of America* 1983; **80**: 1337–1341.

114. Thomas SM, Grandis JR. Pharmacokinetic and pharmacodynamic properties of EGFR inhibitors under clinical investigation. *Cancer Treatment Reviews* 2004; **30**: 255–268.

115. Cunningham D et al. Cetuximab monotherapy and cetuximab plus irinotecan in irinotecan-refractory metastatic colorectal cancer. *The New England Journal of Medicine* 2004; **351**: 337–345.

116. Sobrero AF et al. EPIC: Phase III trial of cetuximab plus irinotecan after fluoropyrimidine and oxaliplatin failure in patients with metastatic colorectal cancer. *Journal of Clinical Oncology* 2008; **26**: 2311–2319.

117. Van Cutsem E et al. Randomized phase III study of irinotecan and 5-FU/FA with or without cetuximab in the first-line treatment of patients with metastatic colorectal cancer (mCRC): The CRYSTAL trial. *Journal of Clinical Oncology (Meeting Abstracts)* 2007; **25**: 4000.

118. Bonner J et al. Radiotherapy plus cetuximab for squamous-cell carcinoma of the head and neck. *The New England Journal of Medicine* 2006; **354**: 567–578.

119. Katchen B, Buxbaum S. Disposition of a new, nonsteroid, antiandrogen, alpha,alpha,alpha-trifluoro-2-methyl-4'-nitro-m-propionotoluidide (Flutamide), in men following a single oral 200 mg dose. *Journal of Clinical Endocrinology & Metabolism* 1975; **41**: 373–379.

120. Vermorken JB et al. Platinum-based chemotherapy plus cetuximab in head and neck cancer. *The New England Journal of Medicine* 2008; **359**: 1116–1127.

121. Chung KY et al. Cetuximab shows activity in colorectal cancer patients with tumors that do not express the epidermal growth factor receptor by immunohistochemistry. *Journal of Clinical Oncology* 2005; **23**: 1803–1810.

122. Messersmith WA, Hidalgo M. Panitumumab, a monoclonal anti epidermal growth factor receptor antibody in colorectal cancer: another one or the one? *Clinical Cancer Research* 2007; **13**: 4664–4666.

123. Saltz L. Epidermal growth factor receptor-negative colorectal cancer: is there truly such an entity? *Clinical Colorectal Cancer* 2005; **5(Suppl.2)**: S98–S100.

124. Scartozzi M et al. Epidermal Growth Factor Receptor (EGFR) status in primary colorectal tumors does not correlate with EGFR expression in related metastatic sites:

implications for treatment with EGFR-targeted monoclonal antibodies. *Journal of Clinical Oncology* 2004; **22**: 4772–4778.

125. Wacker B et al. Correlation between development of rash and efficacy in patients treated with the epidermal growth factor receptor tyrosine kinase inhibitor erlotinib in two large phase III studies. *Clinical Cancer Research* 2007; **13**: 3913–3921.

126. Jonker D et al. Cetuximab for the treatment of colorectal cancer. *The New England Journal of Medicine* 2007; **357**: 2040–2048.

127. Saltz L et al. Bevacizumab (Bev) in combination with XELOX or FOLFOX4: Updated efficacy results from XELOX-1/ NO16966, a randomized phase III trial in first-line metastatic colorectal cancer. *Journal of Clinical Oncology (Meeting Abstracts)* 2007; **25**: 4028.

128. Hirsch FR et al. Increased EGFR gene copy number detected by fluorescent in situ hybridization predicts outcome in non-small-cell lung cancer patients treated with cetuximab and chemotherapy. *Journal of Clinical Oncology* 2008; **26**: 3351–3357.

129. Personeni N et al. Clinical usefulness of EGFR gene copy number as a predictive marker in colorectal cancer patients treated with cetuximab: a fluorescent in situ hybridization study. *Clinical Cancer Research* 2008; **14**: 5869–5876.

130. Massarelli E et al. KRAS mutation is an important predictor of resistance to therapy with epidermal growth factor receptor tyrosine kinase inhibitors in non-small-cell lung cancer. *Clinical Cancer Research* 2007; **13**: 2890–2896.

131. De Roock W et al. KRAS wild-type state predicts survival and is associated to early radiological response in metastatic colorectal cancer treated with cetuximab. *Annals of Oncology* 2008; **19**: 508–515.

132. Khambata-Ford S et al. Expression of epiregulin and amphiregulin and K-ras mutation status predict disease control in metastatic colorectal cancer patients treated with cetuximab. *Journal of Clinical Oncology* 2007; **25**: 3230–3237.

133. Rowinsky EK et al. Safety, pharmacokinetics, and activity of ABX-EGF, a fully human anti-epidermal growth factor receptor monoclonal antibody in patients with metastatic renal cell cancer. *Journal of Clinical Oncology* 2004; **22**: 3003–3015.

134. Van Cutsem E et al. Open-label phase III trial of panitumumab plus best supportive care compared with best supportive care alone in patients with chemotherapy-refractory metastatic colorectal cancer. *Journal of Clinical Oncology* 2007; **25**: 1658–1664.

135. Cardones A, Banez L. VEGF inhibitors in cancer therapy. *Current Pharmaceutical Design* 2006; **12**: 387–394.

136. Ellis LM, Hicklin DJ. VEGF-targeted therapy: mechanisms of anti-tumour activity. *Nature Reviews Cancer* 2008; **8**: 579–591.

137. Willett CG et al. Direct evidence that the VEGF-specific antibody bevacizumab has antivascular effects in human rectal cancer. *Nature Medicine* 2004; **10**: 145–147.

138. Jain RK. Normalization of tumor vasculature: an emerging concept in antiangiogenic therapy. *Science* 2005; **307**: 58–62.

139. Scappaticci FA et al. Arterial thromboembolic events in patients with metastatic carcinoma treated with chemotherapy and bevacizumab. *Journal of the National Cancer Institute* 2007; **99**: 1232–1239.

140. Reinacher-Schick A, Pohl M, Schmiegel W. Drug insight: antiangiogenic therapies for gastrointestinal cancers-focus on monoclonal antibodies. *Nature Clinical Practice Gastroenterology and Hepatology* 2008; **5**: 250–267.

141. Hurwitz H, Shermini S. Bevacizumab in the treatment of metastatic colorectal cancer: safety profile and management of adverse events. *Seminars in Oncology* 2006; **33**: s26–s34.

142. Johnson DH et al. Randomized phase II trial comparing bevacizumab plus carboplatin and paclitaxel with carboplatin and paclitaxel alone in previously untreated locally advanced or metastatic non-small-cell lung cancer. *Journal of Clinical Oncology* 2004; **22**: 2184–2191.

143. Vredenburgh JJ et al. Bevacizumab plus irinotecan in recurrent glioblastoma multiforme. *Journal of Clinical Oncology* 2007; **25**: 4722–4729.

144. Akerley WL et al. Acceptable safety of bevacizumab therapy in patients with brain metastases due to non-small cell lung cancer. *Journal of Clinical Oncology (Meeting Abstracts)* 2008; **26**: 8043.
145. Dansin E et al. Safety of bevacizumab-based therapy as first-line treatment of patients with advanced or recurrent non-squamous non-small cell lung cancer (NSCLC): MO19390 (SAiL). *Journal of Clinical Oncology (Meeting Abstracts)* 2008; **26**: 8085.
146. Lynch TJ et al. Preliminary treatment patterns and safety outcomes for non-small cell lung cancer (NSCLC) from ARIES, a bevacizumab treatment observational cohort study (OCS). *Journal of Clinical Oncology (Meeting Abstracts)* 2008; **26**: 8077.
147. Fuchs CS et al. Randomized, controlled trial of irinotecan plus infusional, bolus, or oral fluoropyrimidines in first-line treatment of metastatic colorectal cancer: results from the BICC-C study. *Journal of Clinical Oncology* 2007; **25**: 4779–4786.
148. Giantonio BJ et al. Bevacizumab in combination with oxaliplatin, fluorouracil, and leucovorin (FOLFOX4) for previously treated metastatic colorectal cancer: results from the eastern cooperative oncology group study E3200. *Journal of Clinical Oncology* 2007; **25**: 1539–1544.
149. Hurwitz H et al. Bevacizumab plus irinotecan, fluorouracil, and leucovorin for metastatic colorectal cancer. *The New England Journal of Medicine* 2004; **350**: 2335–2342.
150. Miller K et al. Paclitaxel plus bevacizumab versus paclitaxel alone for metastatic breast cancer. *The New England Journal of Medicine* 2007; **357**: 2666–2676.
151. Spalding B. Thumbs up for Avastin. *Nature Biotechnology* 2008; **26**: 365–365.
152. Sandler A et al. Paclitaxel-carboplatin alone or with bevacizumab for non-small-cell lung cancer. *The New England Journal of Medicine* 2006; **355**: 2542–2550.
153. Manegold C et al. Randomised, double-blind multicentre phase III study of bevacizumab in combination with cisplatin and gemcitabine in chemotherapy-naive patients with advanced or recurrent non-squamous non-small cell lung cancer (NSCLC): BO17704. *Journal of Clinical Oncology (Meeting Abstracts)* 2007; **25**: LBA7514.
154. Yang J et al. A randomized trial of bevacizumab, an anti-vascular endothelial growth factor antibody, for metastatic renal cancer. *The New England Journal of Medicine* 2003; **349**: 427–434.
155. Escudier B et al. Bevacizumab plus interferon alfa-2a for treatment of metastatic renal cell carcinoma: a randomised, double-blind phase III trial. *The Lancet* 2007; **370**: 2103–2111.
156. Vredenburgh JJ et al. Phase II Trial of bevacizumab and irinotecan in recurrent malignant glioma. *Clinical Cancer Research* 2007; **13**: 1253–1259.
157. Kindler HL et al. A double-blind, placebo-controlled, randomized phase III trial of gemcitabine (G) plus bevacizumab (B) vs. gemcitabine plus placebo (P) in patients (pts) with advanced pancreatic cancer (PC): A preliminary analysis of Cancer and Leukemia Group B (CALGB). *Journal of Clinical Oncology (Meeting Abstracts)* 2007; **25**: 4508.
158. Longo R, Gasparini G. Challenges for patient selection with VEGF inhibitors. *Cancer Chemotherapy and Pharmacology* 2007; **60**: 151–170.
159. Schneider BP et al. Association of vascular endothelial growth factor and vascular endothelial growth factor receptor-2 genetic polymorphisms with outcome in a trial of paclitaxel compared with paclitaxel plus bevacizumab in advanced breast cancer: ECOG 2100. *Journal of Clinical Oncology* 2008; **26**: 4672–4678.
160. Yang SX et al. Gene expression profile and angiogenic markers correlate with response to neoadjuvant bevacizumab followed by bevacizumab plus chemotherapy in breast cancer. *Clinical Cancer Research* 2008; **14**: 5893–5899.
161. Shojaei F et al. Tumor refractoriness to anti-VEGF treatment is mediated by $CD11b^+Gr1^+$ myeloid cells. *Nature Biotechnology* 2007; **25**: 911–920.
162. Bergers G, Hanahan D. Modes of resistance to anti-angiogenic therapy. *Nature Reviews Cancer* 2008; **8**: 592–603.
163. Bunn PA, Jr., Thatcher N. Conclusion. *Oncologist* 2008; **13**: 37–46.
164. Sehn LH et al. Rapid infusion rituximab in combination with corticosteroid-containing chemotherapy or as maintenance therapy is well tolerated and can safely be delivered in the community setting. *Blood* 2007; **109**: 4171–4173.

165. Chung CH. Managing premedications and the risk for reactions to infusional mono-clonal antibody therapy. *Oncologist* 2008; **13**: 725–732.

166. Winkler U et al. Cytokine-release syndrome in patients with B-cell chronic lymphocytic leukemia and high lymphocyte counts after treatment with an anti-CD20 monoclonal antibody (Rituximab, IDEC-C2B8). *Blood* 1999; **94**: 2217–2224.

167. Breslin S. Cytokine-release syndrome: overview and nursing implications. *Clinical Journal of Oncology Nursing* 2007; **11**: 37–42.

168. Herceptin (trastuzumab) Package Insert. South San Franciso, CA: Genentech, Inc., Nov 2006.

169. Erbitux (cetuximab) Package Insert. New York: ImClone Systems Inc and Princeton, NJ: Bristol-Myers Squibb Company, Oct 2007.

170. Timoney J et al. Cetuximab use without chronic antihistamine premedication. *Journal of Clinical Oncology (Meeting Abstracts)* 2006; **24**: 13521.

171. O'Neil BH et al. High incidence of cetuximab-related infusion reactions in tennessee and North Carolina and the association with atopic history. *Journal of Clinical Oncology* 2007; **25**: 3644–3648.

172. Chung C et al. Cetuximab-induced anaphylaxis and IgE specific for galactose-{alpha}-1,3-galactose. *The New England Journal of Medicine* 2008; **358**: 1109–1117.

173. Cheng X, Hung M-C. Breast cancer brain metastases. *Cancer and Metastasis Reviews* 2007; **26**: 635–643.

174. Patel S et al. Safety and feasibility of convection-enhanced delivery of Cotara for the treatment of malignant glioma: initial experience in 51 patients. *Neurosurgery* 2005; **56**: 1243–1253.

175. Qiu X-Q et al. Small antibody mimetics comprising two complementarity-determining regions and a framework region for tumor targeting. *Nature Biotechnology* 2007; **25**: 921–929.

176. Cope DA et al. Enhanced delivery of a monoclonal antibody F(ab')$_2$ fragment to subcutaneous human glioma xenografts using local hyperthermia. *Cancer Research* 1990; **50**: 1803–1809.

177. Pieramici DJ, Rabena MD. Anti-VEGF therapy: comparison of current and future agents. *Eye* 2008; **22**: 1330–1336.

178. Wong JYC et al. Pilot trial evaluating an ^{123}I-labeled 80-kilodalton engineered anticarcinoembryonic antigen antibody fragment (cT84.66 Minibody) in patients with colorectal cancer. *Clinical Cancer Research* 2004; **10**: 5014–5021.

179. Ribas A et al. Phase III, open-label, randomized, comparative study of tremelimumab (CP-675,206) and chemotherapy (temozolomide [TMZ] or dacarbazine [DTIC]) in patients with advanced melanoma. *Journal of Clinical Oncology (Meeting Abstracts)* 2008; **26**: LBA9011.

180. Weber JS et al. Safety and efficacy of ipilimumab with or without prophylactic budesonide in treatment-naïve and previously treated patients with advanced melanoma. *Journal of Clinical Oncology (Meeting Abstracts)* 2008; **26**: 9010.

181. Karp DD et al. High activity of the anti-IGF-IR antibody CP-751,871 in combination with paclitaxel and carboplatin in squamous NSCLC. *Journal of Clinical Oncology (Meeting Abstracts)* 2008; **26**: 8015.

182. Rodon J, DeSantos V, Ferry RJ Jr., Kurzrock R. Early drug development of inhibitors of the insulin-like growth factor-I receptor pathway: Lessons from the first clinical trials. *Molecular Cancer Therapeutics* 2008; **7**: 2575–2588.

183. Schrag D. The price tag on progress – chemotherapy for colorectal cancer. *The New England Journal of Medicine* 2004; **352**: 317–319.

184. Nadler ES, Eckert B, Neumann PJ. Do oncologists believe new cancer drugs offer good value? *Journal of Clinical Oncology (Meeting Abstracts)* 2005; **23**: 6011.

185. Grabowski H. Follow-on biologics: data exclusivity and the balance between innovation and competition. *Nature Reviews Drug Discovery* 2008; **7**: 479–488.

Cancer Vaccines

Zsuzsanna Tabi

1 Introduction

The role of the immune system in preventing the development of tumours was first suggested by Paul Ehrlich in the early 1900s. Half a century later, Lewis Thomas and McFarlaine Burnet introduced the concept of immunosurveillance, meaning that immune cells while continuously patrolling the body recognise special antigens present only on transformed cells and eliminate these cells. They suggested that the type of cell responsible for tumour immunosurveillance is the T cell [1]. Direct experimental evidence confirming this hypothesis came from immunodeficient mouse strains, where the lack of certain components of the cellular immune response, such as interferon (IFN)-γ, perforin, and tumour necrosis factor-related apoptosis-inducing ligand (TRAIL), lead to significantly more aggressive growth of experimental tumours [2]. More importantly, late onset of spontaneously occurring adenocarcinoma has been observed in IFN-γ and perforin-deficient mice [3]. Indirect evidence in humans is the survival benefit of cancer patients with tumours infiltrated with activated CD8 + T cells, observed in numerous cancers such as ovarian, prostate, colorectal, and mesothelioma [4–8].

The components of the immunosurveillance are the innate immune system, consisting of monocytes, macrophages, dendritic cells (DC), natural killer (NK) and NKT cells, and the adaptive immune system, represented by DC, B-cells, and T cells (Fig. 1).

The first cancer vaccine was used by W.B. Coley in the 1890s who, based on his observation that in some cancer patients advanced tumours disappeared following acute streptococcal infection, used a mixture of several bacterial strains and injected straight into tumours. The treatment had varying success to cure established solid tumours. The reason why this treatment may have worked in some patients did not become clear until the 1980s when bacterial

Z. Tabi (✉)
Department of Oncology, School of Medicine, Cardiff University, Velindre Hospital, Whitchurch, Cardiff, CF14 2TL, UK
e-mail: zsuzsanna.tabi@velindre-tr.wales.nhs.uk

Y. Lu, R.I. Mahato (eds.), *Pharmaceutical Perspectives of Cancer Therapeutics*, DOI 10.1007/978-1-4419-0131-6_12, © Springer Science+Business Media, LLC 2009

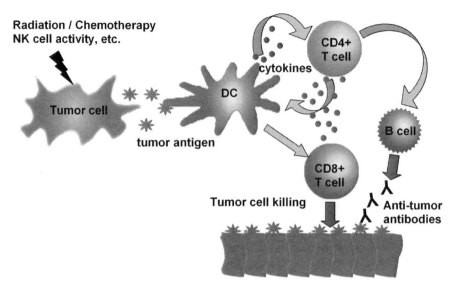

Fig. 1 Tumour immunosurveillance and the role of the main immune cell types. The immune response against cancer may be initiated by cells of the innate immune system, by external damage to the tumour cells and via other mechanisms. Tumour antigens, taken up by dendritic cells (DC), are carried into secondary lymphoid organs where T cell priming occurs. CD4+ T cells provide help for B cell and CD8+ T cell responses. CD8+ tumour-antigen-specific T cells become activated and migrate to the periphery where they recognise and destroy malignant cells

products, described as pathogen-associated molecular patterns (PAMP), were discovered to have immunostimulatory effects on DC, which represent a link between the innate and the adaptive immune system. DC stimulated with bacterial products may be able to break anergy and tolerance of tumour-specific T cells, as discussed later. Coley's treatment has a modern day counterpart: superficial bladder cancer is successfully treated with bacillus Calmette-Guerin (BCG) sprayed into the bladder. The ensuing immune response eliminates stage 1 cancer in an adjuvant setting in >80% of patients.

When tumour cells encounter immune attack, due to their high mutation rate, some cells may develop resistance to the immunological pressure. The tumour developing from these cells is called "edited" as it is the result of an active anti-tumour response [9]. Edited tumours are less immunogenic than those not yet attacked by immune cells. Clinically manifesting tumours have escaped immune recognition, thus cancer vaccines need to target weakly immunogenic tumours which likely possess multiple mechanisms to evade the immune system. So it may not be surprising that the first generation of cancer vaccines showed a disappointing lack of clinical efficacy, although enhanced tumour-specific immune responses can be detected in vaccine recipients. The possible reasons for the lack of success are that (a) single antigenic entities are unlikely to work as the tumour develops immune escape mutants, (b) bulky solid tumours are unlikely to be eliminated by activated immune cells due to immunosuppressive mechanisms of the tumour, and (c) patients with inoperable, multi-resistant, advanced disease are unlikely to respond to cancer vaccines. However, the lessons may show the way towards improved cancer vaccines. Treatment of less advanced patients, targeting several tumour antigens and multiple epitopes, combining vaccines with treatments which block tumour evasion and deliver adjuvant effects is more likely to succeed than the single agents used up to now.

In this chapter, the main approaches in present cancer vaccine development for the treatment of solid tumours, current research directions, and critical challenges are discussed and some ongoing phase III trials are listed.

2 Cell-Based Vaccines

2.1 Adoptive T Cell Transfer (ACT)

Large numbers of activated CD8+ T cells infiltrating the tumour have a positive prognostic value in colon, prostate, ovarian, and other cancers [4–8], indicating a key effect of CD8+ T cells in tumour-immunity. T cell-based vaccines can be made by ex vivo expanding or manipulating tumour-specific T cells and injecting them back into the patient. The transferred T cells need to fulfil complex requirements, in order to act as potent tumour killers. They need to break the immune evasive mechanisms of tumours, infiltrate tumour tissues and eliminate tumour cells with a high degree of specificity followed by long-lasting protection.

2.1.1 T Cell Differentiation Status

The first requirement for ACT is obtaining sufficient numbers of tumour-antigen-specific T cells with the right level of differentiation and activation status. Although several expansion protocols can achieve high cell numbers for transfer ($\sim 10^5$ cells isolated from the tumour, expanded up to 10^{11} in vitro), these T cells are not necessarily effective in vivo [10]. The reason for this is the nature of the expansion which in the past often consisted of prolonged in vitro cultures, resulting in large numbers of highly differentiated effector T cells. Recently, it has been demonstrated that a relatively short in vitro culture period of T cells results in cells more effective in adoptive immunotherapy [11]. These T cells contain heterogeneous T cell populations. Effector or effector memory T cells can attack tumour cells immediately upon cell transfer but they are short-lived cells, while central memory T cells require antigen-specific stimulation before proliferation and effector function but tend to adapt better to the environment and persist longer [12]. The longer persistence of transferred T cells with early memory phenotype than that of more differentiated T cells correlates with the length of their telomeres at the time of transfer and also with improved clinical responses [13]. Large numbers of T cells can be obtained for transfer from patients vaccinated with relevant antigens, although these T cells may have already undergone expansion and differentiation in vivo [14]. Other approaches to generate potent T cells for transfer may include the use of common γ-chain cytokines such as interleukin (IL)-15 and IL-7 during in vitro T cell expansion [15], rather than IL-2, which drives terminal T cell differentiation. Interestingly, maturation of naïve CD8 + T cells into effector cells is inhibited by IL-21 but the resulting T cells are more effective in mediating tumour regression upon adoptive transfer than IL-2 expanded T cells [16].

2.1.2 T Cell Subtype

Traditionally, CD8 + T cells are regarded as the key T cell subset-mediating tumour rejection via direct cytotoxicity of tumour-antigen expressing, major histocompatibility complex (MHC) Class I positive targets. The role of CD4 + T cells is less well understood, but it is generally accepted that CD4 + Treg cells can suppress CD8 + T cell function in a tumour-antigen-specific manner, while Th1 cells provide help via IL-2 and IFNγ-production to CD8 + T cells. CD4 + T cells may also prevent tumour-angiogenesis and tumour-progression via simultaneous tumour necrosis factor receptor 1 (TNFR1) and IFN-γ signalling [17]. Interestingly, in experimental models of tumour rejection, CD4 + T cells were shown to suppress the growth of MHC Class II negative tumours [18] via an indirect mechanism. While the presence of IL-17 by transfecting tumour cells with IL-17 induces more potent anti-tumour CTL responses [19], a recent study demonstrated that Th17 (T helper-17)-polarised CD4 + T cells can directly eliminate tumour cells [20]. In a mouse model of melanoma, adoptive transfer of TRP-1-specific in vitro polarised Th0, Th1 or Th17 T cells into mice with established tumours resulted in complete cure and long-term survival, unexpectedly, not when Th1 but when Th17 cells were transferred [20]. In the model, Th17 cells had a survival advantage following transfer and their anti-tumour action was nearly entirely IFN-γ mediated. However, the ratio of IFN-γ and IL-17 produced by T cells in tumour tissues may be crucial, as TGF-β-induced IL-17-production by CD8 + T cells may promote tumour growth [21]. While the presence of CD4 + T cells is reportedly beneficial in adoptively transferred T cell-mediated tumour regression [11], the exact role of Th17 cells in the treatment of human cancer is awaiting confirmation.

2.1.3 Improving ACT by Lymphodepletion and IL-2 Treatment of Recipients

Significant progress with ACT of cancer was achieved by the transfer of ex vivo expanded, tumour-antigen-specific T cells, isolated from tumour-infiltrating lymphocytes (TIL), into patients who have received lymphodepleting chemotherapy and high-dose IL-2-treatment. The 50% objective response rate in heavily pretreated metastatic melanoma patients [11, 22] makes ACT in cancer the most promising immunological approach to date. Treatment with cyclophosphamide before cell transfer increases the rate of regression of established tumours in patients with metastatic melanoma, resistant to standard therapies. Cyclophosphamide (60 mg/kg for 2 days), followed by fludarabine (25 mg/m^2) for 5 days before T cell transfer in a cohort of 35 patients, resulted in objective clinical responses in 18 patients, including complete remission in 3 [11, 22]. The effect of lymphodepletion with these drugs may depend on the removal of CD4 + CD25 + Foxp3 + regulatory T cells (Treg cells, will be discussed later), as both cyclophosphamide and fludarabine have anti-Treg effects. Another possible explanation for the beneficial effect of lymphodepletion is that depleting host T cells in a non-selective manner before the transfer of tumour-specific T cells removes a significant pool of cells which would be competing for cytokines necessary for T cell growth and effector function (cytokine sink). A third possibility is that lymphodepletion not only spares professional antigen-presenting cells of myeloid origin (myeloid dendritic cells) but increases their activation and maturation status while simultaneously inducing tumour-cell apoptosis. These events may lead to the generation of broader anti-tumour T cell responses via cross-presentation of tumour antigens derived from dying cancer cells. DC cytokine production may amplify the in vivo effector function of transferred T cells. Ongoing preclinical investigations are going a step further by increasing the intensity of lymphodepletion to a level which causes myeloablation and requires hematopoietic stem cell (HSC) transplantation. The expansion of transferred T cells is supported by the haematopoietic stem cells in mice in a non-specific manner [23]. Further improvement has been achieved by giving full-body irradiation to melanoma patients with 2 or 12 Gy treated with cyclophosphamide and fludarabine chemotherapy as described above [12] (Fig. 2). The results, both by the RECIST criteria or by analysing 3-year survival rates, indicate that increasing lymphodepletion improves the anti-tumour effect of adoptively transferred T cells.

The administration of high dose IL-2 to lymphopenic patients receiving adoptive T cell transfer is beneficial for the in vivo expansion and effector function of transferred T cells. High-dose IL-2 alone (720,000 U/kg every 8 h for 2–3 days) can cause tumour regression in some patients with advanced melanoma. However, IL-2 is also able to promote the rapid in vivo expansion of CD4 + CD25 + Treg cells. Furthermore, toxicity (vascular leakage and hypotension) is also a limiting factor in many patients. Thus, IL-2 is probably not the best cytokine to use in this context, and other cytokines which also signal via the common γ-chain receptor, especially IL-15, may better be able to support the persistence and activity of transferred T cells without supporting Treg cells [24, 25]. Alternatively, simultaneous blocking or elimination of Treg cells [26] during IL-2 administration may improve the efficiency of transferred T cells.

Fig. 2 Cancer immunotherapy by the adoptive transfer of T cells. (a) Tumour tissue, containing tumour infiltrating lymphocytes (TIL) is removed from melanoma. Special tissue culture conditions favour T cell growth in vitro. (b) T cells are selected for tumour-reactivity and (c) tumour-reactive T cells are grown into large numbers. (d) The selected T cells are injected back into the patient who has been lymphodepleted by chemotherapy (CT) and radiation therapy (RT)

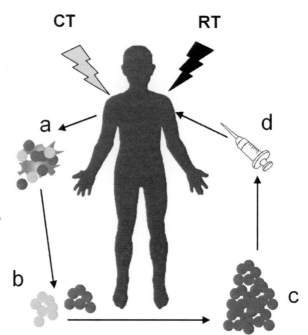

2.1.4 Modification of Transferred T Cells or the Host Environment

Therapy with ACT is especially promising in metastatic melanoma, while in other cancers the success is more modest [12] – the reason for this is not clear, but may depend on the quality of T cells present among tumour infiltrating lymphocytes (TIL) used for expansion. The input T cells should ideally have broad specificity and high avidity for tumour antigens. As this is not always the case even in melanoma, there is a great interest in creating such T cells by genetic modification. T cells after in vitro expansion should be able to infiltrate the tumour, exert effector function and persist in the host. Genes encoding TCRs isolated from cells with high avidity for known tumour antigens can be cloned into vectors, and these constructs can redirect the specificity of T cells to target cancer cells [27–29]. The first such clinical trial, in which melanoma patients were treated with autologous T cells transduced with a high-affinity TCR recognising MART-1 antigen, provided encouraging results [27]. This approach also makes it possible to achieve a relatively early differentiation stage from hematopoietic stem cells for the transferred T cells, which helps their persistence in the host following transfer [30]. Alternatively, reverting effector T cells to a less differentiated state by modulating transcription factors [31] is another idea presently in experimental phase. Retrovirally mediated TCR gene transfer may result in prolonged survival of transferred T cells, but the anti-tumour activity maybe lost due to specific loss of gene expression, as reported recently [32]. Genetic modification can also be used to generate T cells capable of tumour cell recognition in an MHC-unrestricted manner. This approach is based on introducing a chimeric antigen receptor (CAR) into T cells. CARs contain an extracellular domain that recognises a tumour-associated antigen and a fusion partner representing an intracellular signalling domain. The intracellular domain usually consists of the ζ-chain of the TCR complex and triggers T cell proliferation and effector function [33]. CAR modified, prostate-specific membrane antigen (PSMA)-targeted human T cells efficiently killed prostate cancer xenotransplants in mice [34]. Tumour eradication was directly proportional to the in vivo effector-to-tumour cell ratio. T cells needed to survive for at least 1 week to induce durable remissions. This approach holds promise as it overrides MHC restriction. However, further optimisation is necessary in order to allow co-stimulatory signalling and long-term survival of T cells.

Tumour-homing of adoptively transferred cells can be improved by making the tumour environment less immunosuppressive for these cells. Aberrant activation of signal transducer and activator of transcription (STAT)3 is responsible for immunosuppression in many cancers. Intraperitoneal injection of a STAT3 inhibitor into mice with intracranial glioma resulted in elevated IL-15 levels, improved T cell persistence leading to improved survival [35], indicating yet another new approach for making ACT work more efficiently.

Autologous T cell transfer in combination with lymphodepleting chemotherapy and non-specific adjuvant treatment does not represent an easy off-the-shelf treatment, but so far it has provided dramatic evidence for the power of immunotherapy even in advanced patients with bulky, metastatic tumours, resistant to conventional treatments. Further optimisation of this system, which shows so much promise, will reveal if ACT is a viable approach in the treatment of not only melanoma but also other types of cancers.

2.2 Dendritic Cell Vaccines

Dendritic cells (DC) are professional antigen-presenting cells (APC) which, unlike other APC, can migrate into lymph nodes and prime naïve T cells. DC are uniquely adept at antigen cross-presentation. The cross-presentation pathway in DC allows CD8 + T cell stimulation with antigen exogenous to DC, such as tumour-associated antigen derived from necrotic or apoptotic tumour cells. DC control immunity and tolerance via interactions with both the innate and the adaptive immune systems. They have three activation levels, such as immature (iDC), intermediate, and mature DC (mDC). These three stages can be described clearly by distinct phenotype and function. Immature DC typically reside in the tissues where they encounter pathogens and take up antigen. Antigen uptake in the presence of microbial products, called pathogen-associated molecular patterns (PAMP), or molecules released by stressed or dying cells (heat shock proteins, HMGB-1, S100 proteins, etc.), called damage-associated molecular patterns (DAMP), trigger DC maturation. During maturation, intermediate DC upregulate MHC Class II and co-stimulatory molecules and chemokine receptor CCR7, the latter guiding them to lymph nodes. The main function of DC in the lymph nodes is antigen presentation to T cells. CD40-CD40L engagement, due to DC–T cell interaction in the lymph node, triggers transient IL-12 production which is the main cytokine necessary for enabling mature DC to prime naïve T cells and generate Th1-type responses. DC function can be fundamentally altered by tumours: tumour cells display neither PAMPs nor DAMPs while they produce granulocyte–monocyte colony-stimulating factor (GM-CSF), transforming growth factor (TGF)-β and IL-10 which negatively influence DC maturation, migration, cytokine production, and T cell stimulatory capacity. These tumour-conditioned DC may even stimulate the proliferation and activation of T regulatory cells [36]. The aim of DC-based cancer vaccines is to generate a large number of DC ex vivo, load them with tumour antigen and mature them for the generation of efficient anti-tumour T cell immunity upon injection into patients. What seems a straightforward idea becomes extremely complex when searching for optimum efficiency, especially as our present understanding of the workings of the immune system in cancer is still incomplete. The method of DC generation, the nature of the antigen, the way of loading the antigen, the optimum level of DC maturation, and the manner of delivery are all questions which might be easily answered in preclinical models but require constant trial modifications in groups of patients with advanced disease. The main approaches and the present standing of DC vaccines are summarised here.

2.2.1 Ex Vivo Generation of Autologous DC

Large numbers of DC can be generated from peripheral blood cells or bone marrow cells by different methods. The most frequently used approach utilises GM-CSF and IL-4 for the generation of immature DC, which takes ∼5 days, and can be carried out in a closed culture system [37]. Other methods may differentiate CD34+ hematopoietic progenitors with IL-3, IL-6, and stem cell factor (SCF), or with GM-CSF, tumour necrosis factor (TNF)-α and Flt-3 ligand [38], IFN-β and IL-3 [39], or with IFNα or TNFα alone [40, 41]. Alternatively, DC can be directly isolated from the blood, requiring no further in vitro differentiation. The numbers of DC obtainable this way may be low, and if derived from cancer patients, often carry functional abnormalities [42–44]. DC are very diverse and all the above methods generate DC with slightly different phenotypic and functional features. Monocyte-derived DC are most popular, probably because of the homogeneity and relatively stable phenotype of the cells.

Immature DC, generated by any of these methods and loaded with antigens ex vivo, as discussed below, have to be matured, as only this would enable them to migrate to lymph nodes and present antigen to T cells. Early trials indicated that immature DC are unable to stimulate T cell responses and may even generate tumour-specific regulatory T cells [45]. However, the strength and complexity of the ex vivo provided maturation signal should be finely balanced, as the antigen-loaded DC, injected back into the patients, should be able to migrate to the lymph node but their full maturation should only occur within the lymph node, otherwise T cell priming will not take place. Maturation ex vivo is usually induced with Toll-like receptor (TLR) agonists, such as PAMPs, alone or in combination, or with a mixture of cytokines, such as tumour necrosis factor (TNF)-α, IL-6, IL-1, prostaglandin-E, IFN-γ, and CD40-ligand (CD40L) [46]. Some of these agents are capable of inducing full maturation, including the induction of IL-12 production, which is believed to be undesirable before DC reach their destination in vivo.

A recently published "fast-DC" protocol, stimulating monocytes for only 2 days ex vivo in the presence of IFN-γ and lipopolysaccharide (LPS), reported tumour-peptide-specific responses (to Her/2b) and decreased tumour volumes in vaccinated breast cancer patients [47], the mechanism being dependent on a delayed IL-12 burst. Alternatively, maturation can be induced in vivo following administration of the antigen-loaded DC with systemically applied antibodies cross-linking stimulatory molecules on DC, such as anti-CD40 antibody [48].

2.2.2 Antigen Loading In Vitro

When antigen is loaded onto DC ex vivo, the choice of the optimal antigen is based on the following criteria: (1) expressed on the majority of tumour cells in most or all patients with the same type of tumour, (2) not expressed on healthy cells, (3) necessary for the maintenance of tumour growth, i.e. antigen escape mutants should not be viable, (4) able to induce robust CD4+ and CD8+ T cell responses against the tumour, and (5) immunogenic in several major MHC haplotypes. Alternatively, when tumour-cell lysates are loaded onto DC, the nature of antigen is not defined. The most frequently used approaches to load DC with tumour-cell antigens are listed below.

Exogenous Antigens

Tumour Cell Lysate: This method was used extensively in preclinical models and in clinical trials with some original success in selected melanoma patients [49], followed by mixed results in subsequent clinical trials. Recently it has been demonstrated that freeze-thawing does not mimic well in vivo tumour cell death, and cross-presentation of tumour material may not be efficient [50]. There are also some problems with the design of this approach: some tumours are not easily accessible, thus tumour material cannot be obtained. As the antigen repertoire is unknown, it is difficult to design efficient monitoring. Potential improvements include the introduction of treatments which would make tumour cell death more immunogenic. Originally, necrotic cell death was thought to be immunogenic while apoptotic was not. These categories are now being replaced by more sophisticated markers of immunogenicity, such as calreticulin surface expression and release of high mobility group box-1 (HMGB1); a signal of tissue damage. The impact of applying inducers of immunogenic tumour cell death, such as anthracyclins, gamma irradiation or UVC-induced apoptosis [51, 52], to tumour cells before preparing the lysates has yet to be assessed in DC vaccines.

Peptides, Proteins and Recombinant Proteins: Using whole tumour antigens has several advantages, the main one being that they are able to generate immune responses against unknown epitopes in any HLA type. However, as they have a rather limited availability at clinical grade, an easier approach is the use of overlapping peptides, spanning the entire length of proteins, synthesised at the required good manufacturing practice (GMP) grade. With the expanding library of new tumour antigens representing potential new or tested T cell epitopes, loading DC with known amounts of synthetic peptides became the most popular area of DC vaccine studies. The variation in the approaches include the use of poly- vs. single epitopes; a mixture of Class I- and Class II-restricted peptides vs. Class I-restricted peptides alone, and long peptides vs. short peptides. Objective clinical responses in up to 25% of patients were achieved in phase I/II clinical trials in melanoma, prostate, and bladder cancer patients with metastatic disease. The treatment resulted in long-term survivors (3/10) in a cohort of melanoma patients [53]. Patients who survived longer were those who mounted melanoma peptide-specific immunity to at least two melanoma peptides. The conclusion from early trials and preclinical experiments is that DC loaded with long peptides representing poly-epitopes, and including both Class I- and Class II-restricted epitopes are more efficient in generating T cell responses and objective clinical responses.

A significant improvement on exogenously loaded antigens is represented by recombinant proteins which deliver DC stimulatory compounds together with the antigen. The best example is the vaccine Sipuleucel-T (APC8015), where DC are loaded ex vivo with a recombinant fusion protein, consisting of prostatic acid phosphatase (PAP) linked to GM-CSF. This vaccine is undergoing a phase III randomised placebo-controlled trial (discussed later).

Endogenous Antigens

The use of tumour-antigen-encoding cDNA or mRNA seems attractive as this approach provides unselected endogenous expression of tumour antigens in DC. As cDNA transfection of DC is very inefficient, this method is better suited for infection of DC with viral vectors expressing defined antigens. Loading tumour-derived mRNA has also been attempted, and optimisation of the method is ongoing [54, 55]. One of the advantages of the autologous tumour-derived mRNA approach is that it delivers antigen with the relevant mutations to DCs. Endogenous antigen presentation favours CD8+ T cell stimulation, which may result in the lack of stimulating CD4+ T helper responses, thus limiting the usefulness of the method. Another method to target DC is the docking of glycosylated tumour antigens alone or coupled to antibodies specific for C-type lectin receptors DEC-205 [56] or DC-SIGN [57].

2.2.3 Delivery of DC Vaccines

Depending on the site of injection of antigen-loaded DC, their homing pattern, and their ability to generate anti-tumour T cell responses varies. In prostate cancer, patients were injected with DC-enriched peripheral blood mononuclear cells (PBMC), which were cultured for 2 days ex vivo, with recombinant mouse PAP intradermally (i.d.), intravenously (i.v.), or intralymphatically (i.l.) into lymphatic vessels in the feet. CD4+ T cell proliferative responses were primed by all three treatments; however, i.d. and i.l. vaccination routes were superior to the i.v. route in generating CTL responses [58]. These observations were confirmed by other studies, making i.d. the most common route of DC vaccine administration. Direct administration into draining lymph nodes is also promising but requires more technical skill.

2.3 Tumour Cell: DC Hybrids

The fusion of irradiated tumour cells with DC generates immune responses which could eliminate established tumours in mice [59]. Functionally active fusions have also been generated using human cells. The fused cells express a broad array of tumour-associated antigens, including yet unidentified ones, and also deliver DC-mediated co-stimulatory signals. However, unless the tumour cells are autologous to the patient being vaccinated, there is a possibility of invoking a predominant response against allogeneic MHC molecules rather than tumour antigens. Fusion of DCs with breast carcinoma cells upregulates the expression of co-stimulatory molecules, maturation markers such as CCR7 and IL-12 [60]. Interestingly, the fused DC stimulate mixed T cell responses by activating both effector and regulatory T cells, where the effector responses are relatively weak. In this model, the presence of IL-12, IL-18, and a TLR 9 agonist skews the response towards effector T cell development. It should also be considered that although irradiated fused tumour cells are unable to divide, they can still produce immunosuppressive substances, such as TGF-β, which may impair DC function. In a preclinical model, specific targeting of TGF-β in the tumour environment by transfecting the tumour cells before their fusion with DC with an adenoviral vector encoding TGF-β-R interrupted TGF-β signalling and enhanced the efficacy of the fusion vaccine [61]. These results confirm the need for a multi-level approach when developing cancer vaccines.

3 Antigen Vaccines

3.1 Peptide- and Protein-Based Vaccines, Adjuvants

Unlike cell-based vaccines, synthetic peptides are easy to obtain in large quantities at clinical grade. Peptide vaccines, injected with incomplete Freund's adjuvant (IFA), can induce efficient T cell responses in mice to prevent progression and metastasis of established tumours. The immunogenicity of peptide epitopes can be increased by amino acid modifications, which increase the binding affinity of the peptide to MHC molecules and generate more robust T cell responses cross-reacting with the wild-type sequence. These peptides with higher biological potency than wild-type sequences are called heteroclitic peptides. Successful modification of a MART-1 peptide [62], to generate cross-reactive T cells has been demonstrated in a small cohort of melanoma patients. Inclusion of Class II-restricted peptides, especially in the form of physical linking of Class I- and Class II-restricted epitopes from the same tumour antigen, further improves the antigenicity of peptide vaccines, probably by the simultaneous stimulation of CD4 + and CD8 + T cell responses. This has been demonstrated against NY-ESO-1 sequences in melanoma [63] and Her/2-sequences in breast and ovarian cancer [64]. Natural processing of long peptides may prevent the generation of cryptic epitopes, i.e. sequences which are not generated by natural processing of antigens. T cells specific against cryptic epitopes cannot recognise and kill tumour cells [65].

The limitation of peptide vaccines is due to strict MHC-restriction rules. For stimulation of T cells regardless of MHC Class I and Class II haplotypes, overlapping peptides, representing T cell epitope clusters, can be used [66]. Peptide vaccines need to be taken up and processed in vivo by DC. Peptides injected alone are unable to trigger DC maturation, and immature DC-presenting antigen may generate T cell tolerance or regulatory T cells. Adjuvants, given simultaneously with the peptide vaccines, are needed to mature DC in vivo and also to induce cross-presentation of the antigen. In turn, these DC secure the generation of antigen-specific, long-lived effector T cells able to migrate to the tumour site. The combination of TLR agonists and CD40L applied together indeed had a synergistic effect to induce more potent CD8 + T cell responses in a CD4-independent manner [67]; but, the combination applied with a tumour vaccine did not lead to tumour eradication because T cells accumulated primarily in the draining lymph nodes and did not migrate to the tumour [66]. Covalent linking of a TLR agonist to a multiepitope peptide may result in the appropriate T cell stimulation, including tumour infiltration in vivo. Promising data have been obtained in experimental models, including covalent linking of a Her/2 CTL epitope and an influenza CD4 + T cell epitope followed by the conjugation of the peptides to the surface of liposomes via a Pam3CSS anchor, a synthetic lipopeptide with TLR2 agonist activity. Injection of mice with this construct has protected them against Her/2 + tumour challenge. More importantly, in a therapeutic setting, treatment of established tumours with the liposomal vaccine resulted not only in delayed tumour growth but also in the complete rejection of tumours in 60% of animals [68].

Although recombinant proteins are more difficult to generate at a clinical grade, there are some promising early phase clinical trials. One example is vaccinating with recombinant NY-ESO-1, a cancer-testis antigen, of patients with cancers known to express NY-ESO-1. Recombinant NY-ESO-1 antigen co-injected with Montanide ISA-51 and the TLR-9-agonist CpG7909 in a water–oil emulsion subcutaneously in 18 patients generated specific IgG antibodies in all patients. The immune complexes aided the cross-presentation of antigen resulting in the stimulation of CD8+ T cell responses [69]. This approach can be further improved, such as with increased numbers of vaccinations, using multiple TLR agonists.

3.2 Recombinant Viral Vector Vaccines

Recombinant cancer vaccines consist of tumour antigens encoded by viral vectors. This approach allows antigen to be delivered at a high concentration both endogenously and for cross-presentation, while DC maturation signals are also provided. Good viral vectors can accommodate one or more genes encoding tumour antigens and also co-stimulatory molecules. Several viruses can be considered as vectors for tumour antigens, such as vaccinia, fowlpox, canarypox, and adenovirus. Immunological memory against some of these viruses can be limiting because of the presence of pre-existing antibodies with the ability to neutralise the recombinant virus particles before they reach their destinations. Vaccinia is becoming an increasingly useful vector, as global immunisation with vaccinia ended in the 1980s. Phase I and II clinical trials demonstrated excellent safety and the generation of humoral and cellular immune responses, as summarised by Harrop [70].

One of the directions to improve clinical benefit is to include genes for co-stimulatory molecules, such as B7.1, ICAM-1, and LFA-3 (TRICOM) [71] together with that for tumour antigen. Furthermore, a prime-boost regime of vaccine delivery using two different recombinant viruses can also improve immunological results, as indicated by preclinical experiments. The reason behind this twofold: one is, that the antibody generated against the first vector may limit the efficacy of the same vector in a repeated application. The second is that a relatively larger number of T cells are activated by the viral part of the vaccine than by the tumour antigen in the "prime" vaccination. Use of a different vector ensures that only tumour-antigen-specific T cells are reactivated by the "boost" treatment. Although several early phase cancer vaccine trials have used this protocol, the clinical benefits are variable [72–78]. There is an obvious need to further improve the efficiency of viral vaccines which may be done via carefully designed combination with existing treatments and the inclusion of immune response modifiers.

4 Immune Response Modifiers

Non-specific immune stimulation of cancer patients has been tried for many years. Typically, the adjuvant is injected at the site of the tumour followed by a massive activation of macrophages and release of inflammatory cytokines.

These may break immunological tolerance and initiate an avalanche of immunological events which lead to the attack of the tumour cell by the immune system.

4.1 Adjuvants

BCG: Superficial bladder cancer can be effectively treated with Bacillus Calmette-Guerin (BCG) intravesical immunotherapy, by reducing tumour recurrence, disease progression, and mortality. The treatment induces inflammation of the bladder with infiltration of a broad range of cells such as macrophages, T lymphocytes, B lymphocytes, and NK cells. Inflammatory cytokines, such as IL-1, IL-2 and IL-6, IFNγ, and TNFα, can be measured in the urine for many hours after treatment. The adjuvant effect is likely to be mediated by TLR signalling, especially via TLR2 and TLR4.

Montanides: Montanides are a group of oil/surfactant based adjuvants in which different surfactants are combined with a non-metabolisable mineral oil, a metabolisable oil, or a mixture of the two. They are prepared for use as an emulsion with aqueous antigen solution. The surfactant for e.g. Montanide ISA 50 (ISA = Incomplete Seppic Adjuvant) is mannide oleate, a major component of the surfactant in Freund's adjuvants. The various Montanide ISA group of adjuvants are used as water-in-oil emulsions, oil-in-water emulsions, or water-in-oil-in-water emulsions.

CpG-ODN: Synthetic oligodeoxynucelotides (ODN) containing CpG motifs stimulate cells via TLR9. The stimulatory effect is due to mimicking bacterial DNA which is rich in unmethylated CpG sequences, while in mammalian DNA these sequences are rare and methylated. In man, TLR9 is expressed on plasmacytoid DC and B cells, while in mice it is also expressed on myeloid DC and monocytes. CpG-ODN activate both innate and adaptive immune responses, stimulate Th1-type immune responses, mature DC, and induce CTL responses. They promote IFN-α and TNF-α production. In melanoma patients, enhanced CD8 + T cell responses were observed in vaccine + CpG-ODN recipients, but the outcome was not affected. Interestingly, CpG-ODN can protect immune cells from the damaging effects of chemo- and radiotherapy.

Iscomatrix: Immunostimulatory complex of a purified saponin fraction, cholesterol and phospholipid, which under defined conditions form cage-like structures typically 40 nm in diameter. The principal advantage of this combination is the reduction of toxicity of saponin component. Iscomatrix particulate vaccines are likely to be phagocytosed by macophages and induce cytokines such as IL-12 and IFN-γ. They have a significant potential in cancer vaccine development [79].

MPL (monophosphoryl lipid A): Although the effectiveness of LPS as an immunomodulator has long been known, the pharmacologic use of purified LPS (or lipid A) as an adjuvant is precluded by its toxicity. LPS is highly pyrogenic and promotes systemic inflammatory response syndrome. MPL comprises the lipid A portion of LPS from which the (R)-3-hydroxytetradeca-noyl group and the 1-phosphate have been removed by successive acid and base hydrolysis in an effort to uncouple the immunomodulatory effects of lipid A from its toxicity. LPS and MPL induce similar cytokine profiles, but MPL is at least 100-fold less toxic. Several vaccines containing MPL have been approved, including an HPV vaccine in Australia and a hepatitis B vaccine in Europe.

4.2 Cytokines

Cytokines behave as messengers in the immune system. They are secreted by immune cells and can act in an autocrine or a paracrine fashion, functioning either locally or at a distance to modulate immune responses. In cancer therapy, cytokines are often used to enhance immunity.

IL-2 is primarily a T cell growth factor, but its receptor is also expressed on B cells and NK cells. IL-2, when administered in high doses, increases the number of T cells, B cells, and NK cells in the blood, the activity of NK cells, and the serum levels of TNFα, IL-1β, and IFN-γ. Furthermore, IL-2 has been shown to preferentially expand Treg cells which can suppress effector T cells, preventing them from killing tumour cells. IL-2 is approved for the treatment of metastatic kidney cancer and metastatic melanoma. High-dose IL-2 treatment requires close monitoring because of toxic side effects such as capillary leak syndrome and subsequent severe hypotension. There are attempts to modify the IL-2 molecule, such as by amino acid replacements, in order to preserve its biological activity without the toxicity.

IFN-α has an antiproliferative and anti-angiogenic effect on tumour cells, upregulates tumour antigens, increases the lytic capacity of NK cells and the expression of MHC Class I molecules on various cell types. It is a powerful activator of a wide range of immune cells. IFNα is approved for the treatment of metastatic melanoma and AIDS-related Kaposi's sarcoma. High-dose IFN-α applied to resected Stage 3 and 2B melanoma patients results in disease-free and overall survival benefits, including some long-term survivors. Its side effects include depression, lack of energy, and dehydration.

IFN-γ is known to increase the expression of MHC Class I and II, adhesion molecules, and molecules associated with antigen processing, as well as activate macrophages, NK cells, T cells, and DC. Although its systemic application seemed promising in metastatic carcinoma, its significant toxicity has limited its widespread use. Current approaches, such as gene transfection or liposomal application, achieve stable and high local concentrations in the tumour environment without inducing side effects.

GM-CSF stimulates the maturation of granulocyte precursors and the development of monocytes and dendritic cells. It is approved in stem cell and bone marrow transplant patients to reconstitute granulocytes and myeloid cells. Its main application in cancer treatment is not necessarily the induction of anti-tumour immune responses but the shortening of the period of time a patient is neutropenic after chemotherapy. However, its effect as an immunotherapeutic agent needs to be evaluated.

4.3 Antibodies and Ligands with Immunological Targets

Ontak or denileukin diftitox: A recombinant IL-2 – diphteria-toxin (DT) fusion protein. It binds to cells expressing high-affinity IL-2R (CD25). The fusion protein is internalised via receptor-mediated endocytosis and proteolytically cleaved within the endosome, liberating the enzymatically active portion of the DT, the A fragment. DT fragment A is released into the cytosol-inhibiting protein synthesis and leading to cell death. In vivo treatment with Ontak depletes Treg cells significantly, resulting in enhanced Th1-type immune responses and substantial development of antigen-specific CD8 T cells upon vaccination.

Antagonistic CTLA-4 antibody: CTLA-4 (cytotoxic T-lymphocyte activating factor-4) is a CD28-family protein and a powerful negative regulator of T cell responses. B7-1 and B7-2 molecules, present on DC, serve as ligands for both CD28 co-stimulatory molecules and CTLA-4 inhibitory molecules on T cells. In association with T cell receptor binding of peptide antigen presented on MHC molecules, signal by CD28 binding provides a co-stimulatory signal for T cells, whereas CTLA-4 triggers inhibition of T cell function (Fig. 3). CTLA-4 block-ade by antibodies attenuates the negative signal and thus promotes T cell proliferation and effector function. In mice, antibodies to CTLA-4 can promote tumour rejection and tumour immunity. Anti-tumour activity has been observed in metastatic melanoma [80] and other malignancies after treatment with anti-CTLA-4 antibodies, as well as the potential for autoimmune-related toxicities.

Recombinant CD40L: CD40L is expressed on activated T cells. CD40 is a cell surface molecule expressed on B cells, monocytes, and DC, a member of the TNFR superfamily. CD40 signalling is a strong inducer of DC maturation, stimulating both innate and adaptive immune responses. CD40–CD40L inter-action, representing "T cell help", enables DC to undergo full maturation and stimulate primary anti-tumour T cell responses. Apart from this indirect effect, ~70% of solid tumours also express CD40, and a direct trigger of tumour cell apoptosis by a poorly understood mechanism has also been implied. CD40L administered to patients as a soluble protein or as trimers is undergoing phase I trials [81]. CD40-directed agonistic antibodies have also been evaluated in preclinical models (Fig. 3). The combination of anti-CD40 agonist antibody with chemotherapy cures established implanted tumours and protects from re-challenge with the same tumour.

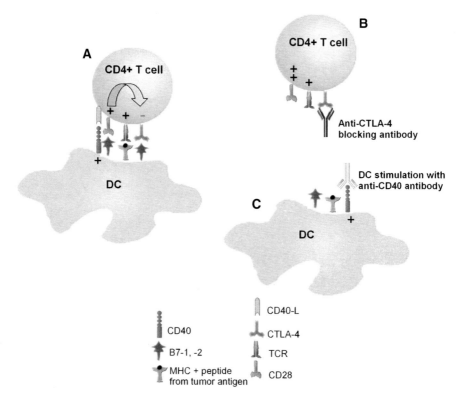

Fig. 3 Boosting DC–T cell interaction by monoclonal antibodies. (A) CD4 + T cells require MHC + peptide and TCR interaction (signal 1) and co-stimulation via B7-1, -2, and CD28 interaction (signal 2). CD40L and CD40 interaction delivers a maturation signal for DC and enables them to stimulate CD8 + T cells. CD4 + T cell activity is downregulated by B7-1,-2 and CTLA-4 interaction. (B) T cell stimulation can be improved by switching off CTLA-4 using an antagonising anti-CTLA-4 antibody. This enhances positive co-stimulation via CD28 signalling. (C) DC maturation can be boosted in vivo by injecting synthetic CD40L or agonising anti-CD40 antibody as shown. These DC are able to prime naive CD8 + T cells even in the absence of T cell help

5 Combination of Cancer Vaccines with Chemo- and Radiotherapy

Cancer vaccine trials are often conducted in advanced patients resistant to conventional treatments such as chemo- or radiotherapy. Although early treatment with immune therapy is not likely to happen soon, well-designed combinations of established treatments with immune therapy would be an important step towards achieving the full potential of cancer vaccines.

5.1 Combined Chemo-immunotherapy

Chemotherapy (CT), using cytotoxic agents, destroys dividing cells in a nonspecific manner, resulting in a mainly apoptotic elimination of all rapidly dividing cells. The long-held belief that CT is detrimental for not only the tumour but also the cells of the immune system is not supported by the latest results studying the activation and functional status of T cells in peripheral blood mononuclear cells (PBMC) and tumour-draining lymph nodes during CT [82, 83]. CT can crucially influence the survival and behaviour of immune cells at multiple levels: (1) Tumour cells killed by CT provide a wide range of tumour-associated antigens (TAA) for the immune system. (2) Depending on the type of CT, TAA uptake can happen in an immunogenic or a non-immunogenic way. (3) CT can remove immune inhibitory cells or effects produced by tumour cells. (4) CT generates lymphopenia, which creates "space" for tumour-specific T cells to expand and removes competition for important inflammatory cytokines. A more detailed analysis of these immunologically beneficial effects of CT, waiting to be exploited in combined immunological approaches, is discussed below.

Antigen release following CT-induced tumour cell death: Whatever the type of tumour cell death following CT, it is certain that a huge amount of TAA is released from the affected cells. In mice, antigen-presenting cells carrying TAA accumulate in draining lymph nodes following CT. High concentration of exogenous antigen can be cross-presented by DC to CD8+ T cells, so TAA released following CT is expected to favour this type of antigen presentation. The nature of TAA is also interesting, as important, but yet unknown, tumour antigens including tumour-rejection antigens may be released and thus this mix of TAA represents the most complete and relevant array of antigens for immune recognition in an autologous manner.

The type of tumour cell death: CT of bulky solid tumours results mainly in apoptotic cell death but non-apoptotic mechanisms, such as necrosis, autophagy, and mitotic catastrophe also occur, as reviewed by Okada [84]. Apoptotic cells are normally not immunogenic when taken up by macrophages or DC. However, regardless the mode of CT-induced cell death, when it happens on a massive scale and in a highly synchronised manner, the anti-inflammatory default mechanism to clear these cells may easily be overwhelmed. Accumulation of monocytes, B cells, DC, and macrophages occurs at the site of tumour cell death, and beside the huge amount and range of TAA taken up by these cells, it is expected that heat shock proteins and HMGB1 (from cells that die by apoptosis) are also released. These molecules represent damage-associated molecular patterns (DAMP) which serve as adjuvants to initiate DC maturation. Based simply on this quantitative argument, it would be expected that TAA-specific T cell responses are generated in the draining lymph nodes following CT. An improved definition of immunogenic cell death may enable us to exploit better the wave of CT-induced tumour cell death for immune therapies. The question of immunogenic vs. non-immunogenic cell death focused for a long time simply on the difference between apoptotic vs. necrotic cell death, without definitive conclusions. It seems now that the key to immunogenic cell death is the translocation of certain, normally intracellular, molecules on the cell surface during apoptosis. Calreticulin has been indicated as such a molecule, and its cell surface expression can be induced by anthracyclins, γ-irradiation, and UVC light [51, 52]. Anthracyclins inhibit DNA and RNA synthesis by intercalating between base pairs of the DNA/RNA strand, thus preventing the replication of cancer cells. They are used to treat a wide range of cancers, including breast, uterine, ovarian, and lung cancers, so it is feasible to consider them for the design of combination chemo-immunotherapy.

Removal of tumour-associated immunosuppressive effects by CT: As most tumours produce TGFβ, IL-10, IL-6, and growth factors, it can be expected that simply by decreasing the tumour burden, the level of these inhibitory factors will fall. Standard, platinum-based chemotherapy of ovarian cancer patients decreases the level of Ca125 systemically. Ca125 itself has suppressive effects on NK and maybe on other cell types. Indeed, CT in these patients was associated with improved T cell responses [83]. A similar effect may be responsible for the immune stimulation observed in pancreatic cancer patients treated with gemcitabine. In these patients, there was no decrease in the proportion of Treg cells, but the numbers of T cells producing IFN-γ and expressing CD69 increased [85]. Gemcitabine also stimulated TNF-α and IL-2 production in a small group of lung cancer patients, reviewed by Nowak et al. [86].

CT-induced lymphopenia: Earlier in this chapter we discussed the beneficial effects of lymphodepleting chemotherapies for generating a more favourable environment for adoptive T cell transfer. All chemotherapy, not only lymphodepleting drugs, is associated with a certain level of lymphopenia as a side effect which, in the treatment of solid tumours, is usually not symptomatic. The altered immune cell composition in the tumour tissue, draining lymph nodes, or even in the blood during treatment with different agents, has not been studied in a systematic manner. Cyclophosphamide and fludarabine have confirmed anti-Treg cell properties in the circulation [87–89], but little is known about the effect of these and other drugs on other inhibitory cell subsets such as myeloid suppressor cells or tolerogenic DC. It is important to determine if routine chemotherapy regimes are adequate to eliminate inhibitory cell types or if a specific combination of drugs should be used to achieve this in chemo-immunotherapy approaches.

Chemo-immunotherapy in the clinic: Combination of standard chemotherapy with therapeutic vaccines or non-specific immune therapy is being tested presently in cancer patients. They are in early phases with small numbers of patients, so it is not yet possible to draw conclusions about efficacy.

5.2 Combined Radio-immunotherapy

Radiation therapy (RT) is a successful therapeutic approach in cancer treatment. Besides its cytotoxic effects on tumour cells, RT also has immunomodulatory effects. The ability of peripheral blood T cells to proliferate to PPD (purified protein derivative of *Mycobacterium tuberculosis*) was impaired in breast cancer patients 45 days after finishing RT [90], and impaired mitogen-induced proliferation was also observed in cervical cancer patients on the last day of receiving 25 fractions of pelvic RT [91]. T cell receptor cross-linking by CD3–CD28 antibody coated beads also revealed proliferative impairment of T cells in prostate cancer patients (Fig. 4). On the other hand, sublethal irradiation of the tumour in vitro or in vivo is considered immunostimulatory as it upregulates MHC Class I, ICAM-1 and Fas molecules, adhesion molecules (ICAM-1, PECAM-1, and VCAM-1), and heat shock proteins; stimulates IFN-γ secretion; facilitates the migration of CD8 T cells to the irradiated tissue; and makes tumour cells more susceptible to T cell-mediated killing [92–94]. The mechanism behind the inhibition of distant tumours after local RT, called abscopal effect, is little understood, but accumulating evidence points towards immunological effector function. RT is known to cause immunogenic tumour cell death, releasing not only tumour antigens but also DAMPs, such as HMGB1, which signal tissue injury and contribute to the cross-presentation of tumour-associated antigens [95]. Standard therapies have been shown to initiate immune responses in prostate cancer patients, demonstrated by antibody

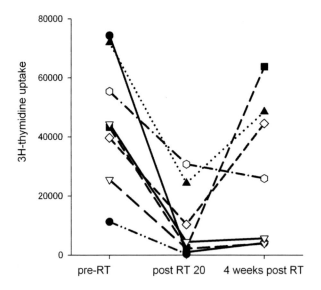

Fig. 4 Radiation therapy impairs T cell proliferative capacity in prostate cancer patients. PBMC were isolated from peripheral blood of patients undergoing a total of 20 fractions of localised pelvic and lymph node radiation therapy for the treatment of locally advanced prostate cancer. Samples were collected before the first fraction of RT, after 20 fractions, and 4 weeks after the patients received the last cycle of RT. PBMC were stimulated in vitro with CD3–CD28 T cell expander beads (Dynal) at 2×10^5 cells per well for 3 days. ^{3}H-thimidine was added to the cells for the last 12 h of culture, and isotope uptake was measured by a Wallace Betaplate counter. The results are expressed as mean ^{3}H-thymidine uptake from triplicate cultures. Each line represents T cell proliferation data from an individual patient. After 20 fractions of RT, T cells from each patient displayed impaired proliferative ability

production against tumour-associated antigens after androgen deprivation therapy, followed by further enhancement of these antibody titres by RT [96]. Thus it seems that localised RT exerts a complex effect both on the tumour and on the bystander cells, including lymphocytes, which may critically influence cellular immune responses.

Results of preclinical models and clinical trials indicate that certain combinations of immunotherapy and radiotherapy can achieve synergistic effects with potential clinical benefit. Synthetic CpG oligonucleotides (TLR9 agonists) dramatically enhance the effect of single-dose or fractionated radiotherapy in a mouse model [97]. The combination not only increased tumour response but also generated memory responses protecting from re-challenge. Localised irradiation of a subcutaneous, carcioembryonic antigen (CEA)-expressing tumour, in combination with the CEA-encoding TRICOM vaccine induced significant CD8 + T cell influx into the tumour with subsequent arrest of tumour growth [92]. In the first clinical trial combining external beam RT with a vaccine, prostate cancer patients received a poxviral vaccine, encoding prostate-specific antigen (PSA), three times monthly before RT [98]. This treatment resulted not only in increased levels of PSA-specific T cell responses but also caused epitope spreading, indicating the presence of active anti-tumour immune responses. The trial also indicated that local radiotherapy does not have a negative effect on vaccine-induced PSA-specific T cell responses, which might be explained by preferential resistance of memory cells to RT [99].

6 Ongoing Phase III Cancer Immunotherapy Trials

6.1 Cancer Vaccines

6.1.1 Sipuleucel-T (APC8015)

Sipuleucel is made by Dendreon Corp. (Seattle, WA). It is a vaccine for patients with hormone-resistant metastatic prostate cancer. Peripheral blood collected from patients by leukapheresis is enriched for CD54 + cells (monocytes and DC) and loaded ex vivo with a fusion protein consisting of PAP and GM-CSF. The antigen is targeted to GMCSF-R + antigen-presenting cells via the fusion partner, GM-CSF [100]. Promising early phase trials indicated beneficial effects by reduced PSA levels and prolonged time to progression (TTP) in patients with anti-PAP immune responses [101]. The first phase III clinical trial shows a significant positive effect on overall survival (OS) but not on TTP which was the primary endpoint of the trial. In order to obtain FDA approval, the trial has been extended to study Sipuleucel's effect in 500 patients. The survival data from this study are expected by 2010.

6.1.2 Stimuvax

Stimuvax[®] (L-BLP25) is a vaccine developed in Europe by Merck KGaA and in the United States by its affiliate, EMD Serono Inc. Stimuvax is a liposome vaccine, targeting non-small cell lung cancer (NSCLC) patients with unresectable stage IIIB tumour. The major component of Stimuvax is the synthetic human MUC-1 protein, consisting of a 20-amino acid tandem repeat sequence on its extracellular domain. MUC-1 is expressed on normal epithelial as well as on tumour cells, but on tumours it is abnormally glycosylated. The vaccine also contains an adjuvant (MPL; monophosphoryl lipid A) and both are enclosed in a liposomal vehicle.

Randomised phase II trials indicated improved survival in patients at 3 years in the Stimuvax arm (49%) compared to best supportive care alone (27%). In the subgroup of patients with stage IIIB disease, a 17.3 month difference in median survival compared to patients receiving best supportive care alone (30.6 months vs. 13.3 months respectively) was observed [102]. Side effects were mild to moderate, such as flu-like symptoms, gastro-intestinal and mild injection site reactions. Based on these phase II results, Stimuvax has entered its phase III development, and the START (Stimulating Targeted Antigenic Responses to NSCLC) trial is a multi-centre, randomised, double-blind, placebo-controlled study that will evaluate patients with documented unresectable stage IIIA or IIIB NSCLC who have had a response or stable disease after at least two cycles of platinum-based chemo-radiotherapy. The study will involve more than 1,300 patients in approximately 30 countries. Treatment administered will consist of a single i.v. dose of 300 mg/m^2 cyclophosphamide followed by 8-weekly subcutaneous immunisations with Stimuvax. Maintenance immunisations will then be given at 6-week intervals. One of the potential benefits of Stimuvax is that the MUC-1 protein is not specific for lung; it is also expressed on breast, colon, and prostate tumours. An early phase trial has already been reported in prostate cancer [103].

6.1.3 TroVax

TroVax[®] is Oxford BioMedica's therapeutic cancer vaccine, consisting of the 5T4 antigen [104] encoded by a modified vaccinia Ankara (MVA) virus. Early phase clinical trials reported potent CD4+ T cell and antibody responses in colorectal and prostate cancer patients [105, 106]. Time to progression was significantly longer in patients who developed 5T4-specific cellular responses compared with those who did not (5.6 vs. 2.3 months, respectively). However, there were no objective clinical responses.

TRIST (by Sanofi-Aventis) is a phase III clinical trial of TroVax in renal cell carcinoma, taking place across approximately 120 centres in the USA and Western and Eastern Europe. Trovax is administered in combinations with IL-2, IFN-α, and sunitinib (a tyrosine kinase inhibitor) to combat advanced or metastatic renal cell carcinoma to 700 patients, with the primary endpoint being the rate of overall survival. It is hoped that TroVax will prove to be effective against a wide range of cancers. Phase III trials are also planned in colorectal and breast cancer.

6.1.4 Prostvac (TM)

For the potential treatment of prostate cancer, Bavarian Nordic is developing PROSTVAC-VF-TRICOM, a prime-boost vaccine regimen that consists of a priming injection with a recombinant attenuated vaccinia virus expressing PSA and triad of co-stimulatory molecules (TRICOM: ICAM-1, B7.1, and LFA-3) and a booster injection with a fowlpox virus expressing the same combination. In clinical trials to date, Prostvac(TM) has been investigated in 464 patients over 10 years. The results from the latest phase II prospective randomised placebo-controlled study of 125 patients with advanced prostate cancer after 4 years of follow-up show that patients receiving Prostvac(TM) had a statistically significantly longer median overall survival by 8.5 months ($p = 0.015$) compared to the control group [71, 107]. In addition, it also had a favourable safety and tolerability profile. Based on these promising results, Bavarian Nordic together with the National Cancer Institute expects to initiate phase III studies for Prostvac(TM) for the approval of this therapy.

6.1.5 GVAX

GVAX has been developed by Cell Genesys, Inc. for the treatment of symptomatic hormone-refractory advanced prostate cancer. The vaccine consists of two allogeneic tumour cell lines transfected with an adenoviral vector encoding GM-CSF.

Early phase studies with different doses of the vaccine achieved median survival of 34.9 months after treatment with the high dose of immunotherapy and 24.0 months with the low dose. Radiation therapy alone resulted in a median survival of 26.2 months. The median time to bone scan progression in the radiation therapy group was 5.0 months with the high dose and 2.8 months with the low dose. In the rising-PSA group receiving the low dose, the median time to bone scan progression was 5.9 months and median survival was 37.5 months. No dose-limiting or autoimmune toxicities were seen; the most common adverse events were injection site reaction and fatigue.

Ongoing phase III trials (VITAL-1 and VITAL-2) were comparing GVAX + Taxotere with Taxotere + Prednisone in randomised, blinded. The primary endpoint was improved overall survival. Both trials have recently been halted. In September 2008 VITAL-2, which has enrolled 408 patients, has been halted because of the high proportion of deaths in patients receiving the vaccine (67 patients) compared with those in the control arm (47 patients). In October 2008 VITAL-1, which has recruited 626 patients has also been terminated on the advise of the study's Independent Data Monitoring Committee which indicated that the trial had less than a 30% chance of meeting its predefined primary endpoint of an improvement in survival.

6.1.6 Lucanix

NovaRx Corp. launched a study of therapeutic vaccine Lucanix™ (belagenpumatucel-L) in non-small cell lung cancer (NSCLC) patients. Belagenpumatucel-L is a TGF-β2 antisense gene-modified allogeneic tumour cell vaccine that demonstrates enhancement of tumour-antigen recognition as a result of TGF-β2 inhibition. In a phase II trial, 75 patients (stages II–IV) received a total of 550 vaccinations as monthly i.d. injections of Lucanix. No significant adverse events were observed. A dose-related survival difference was demonstrated in patients who received more or at least 2.5×10^7 cells/injection. In late-stage (IIIB and IV, $n = 61$) patients, a 15% partial response rate was achieved. The estimated probabilities of surviving 1 and 2 years were 68% and 52%, respectively, for the higher dose groups combined and 39% and 20%, respectively, for the low-dose group. Immune function was explored in the 61 advanced-stage (IIIB and IV) patients. Increased cytokine production (IFN-γ, IL-6, IL-4) at week 12, compared with patients with progressive disease, was observed among clinical responders. Furthermore, positive T cell responses to belagenpumatucel-L showed a correlation trend with clinical responsiveness in patients achieving stable disease or better [108]. Phase II results showed that 50% of patients with stable disease who received Lucanix after one front-line regimen of chemotherapy lived for more than 44 months vs. fewer than for 10–12 months for those receiving standard care. Patients receiving Lucanix after zero to five prior chemo-treatments had a 1-year survival of 61% and a 2-year survival of 41%, a striking improvement for late-stage patients, who typically have a 1-year survival rate of less than 30%.

The phase III trial is designated as STOP for its expected endpoints – survival, tumour-free survival, overall survival, and progression-free survival, where overall survival is the primary endpoint. It is expected to enroll up to 700 patients with advanced-stage disease who have been treated with at least one prior platinum-based chemotherapy regimen. Patients will be randomised to receive Lucanix or placebo, administered i.d., once monthly for 18 months and then once at 21 months and at 24 months.

6.1.7 Telovac (GV1001)

Pharmexa's Telovax is a telomerase peptide vaccine for the treatment of locally advanced or metastatic pancreatic cancer. Telomerase is a common tumour antigen overexpressed in most tumour types and, importantly, recent studies suggest that tumour stem cells are also telomerase positive [109]. As telomerase is important in the maintenance of telomeres and replicative immortality, it is expected that tumours cannot develop resistance to telomerase-based therapies.

Early phase trials targeting the catalytic component of telomerase, TERT (telomerase reverse transcriptase) with peptides, mRNA, plasmid, or viral DNA established that TERT-specific CD8+ and CD4+ T cell responses can be generated. Anti-tumour effects were demonstrated against a wide range of tumours [110]. Pharmexa has shown in phase II trials that patients receiving GV1001 had a median lifetime of 8.6 months vs. 5 months for those on standard chemotherapy.

Telovac is 16-mer peptide which can be presented by multiple MHC Class II and also processed into Class I epitopes. Patients receive the vaccine in two combinations with gemcitabine and capecitabine chemotherapy, either together with chemotherapy for 8 weeks or starting 1 week after chemotherapy (in week 9). GM-CSF is coinjected with the vaccine. The primary endpoint is survival at 12 months. The aim is to enroll 1,100 patients.

6.2 Biological Therapies

6.2.1 Oncophage

In April 2008, Oncophage® (vitespen; formerly HSPPC-96) was approved in Russia for the treatment of kidney cancer patients at intermediate risk for disease recurrence. The company, Antigenics, expects to submit to the European Regulatory Agency before the end of 2008.

Oncophage is a vaccine made from individual patients' tumour. Patients have surgery to remove part or all of the cancerous tissue, which is used to isolate heat shock protein gp96 and its associated peptides. The complexes are extracted and purified from each sample, then sterilely filtered and placed into vials.

More than 750 cancer patients in more than a dozen clinical trials around the world have received Oncophage. Many of these patients had advanced disease, including kidney cancer, melanoma, and colon cancer, and had not responded to traditional cancer treatments.

Oncophage has also been evaluated in two international phase III trials in kidney cancer and metastatic melanoma, as well as studies in several other cancers, such as non-small cell lung cancer, lymphoma, colorectal cancer, pancreatic cancer, and gastric cancer. Data from Antigenics' phase III trial of Oncophage in kidney cancer showed a 45% improvement in recurrence-free survival associated with Oncophage in a well-defined subgroup of earlier stage (better-prognosis) patients, although a significant improvement was not observed in the overall patient population [111].

In a phase III study of Oncophage in metastatic melanoma, overall median survival was 29% longer in patients who received at least 10 injections of Oncophage compared with physician's choice regimen. Patients in the M1a and M1b substages receiving a larger number of immunisations survived longer than those receiving fewer treatments. The results suggest that patients with less-advanced disease who are able to receive 10 or more treatments are a promising candidate population [112].

6.2.2 Ipilimumab

Ipilimumab, a fully humanised monoclonal antibody targeting CTLA-4 on CD4 + T cells, is undergoing phase III trials in advanced melanoma patients. The trials are conducted by Medarex and Bristol Myers Squibb. One placebo-controlled monotherapy trial targets patients with fully resected stage III melanoma, another trial is comparing the effect of chemotherapy (Dacarbazine) and Ipilimumab with chemotherapy alone, while the third one is combining a gp100 peptide vaccine with Ipilimumab in HLA-A2$^+$ melanoma patients.

Pfizer's phase III anti-CTLA-4 antibody (Tremelimumab) trial has recently been halted as no beneficial effect over chemotherapy alone has been observed. The safety profile of the antibody is also a problem, as it may cause rash, diarrhoea, hepatitis, bowel inflammation, loss of pituitary hormone function, and hypothyroidism.

7 Summary

The website http://ClinicalTrials.gov contains the most complete and regularly updated list of ongoing cancer vaccine clinical trials. At the time of writing this chapter, cancer vaccines are represented by 782 entries in the database (including hematologic malignancies), 292 of which are open trials. This indicates a continued interest in cancer vaccines, possibly encouraged by some of the obvious successes, such as ACT, which clearly demonstrate the enormous power of the immune system to combat cancer.

The design of cancer vaccines, which utilise the patients' own immune system ultimately to recognise and destroy cancer cells without serious side effects, is progressing with every single trial. Earlier attempts with single agents failed, as vaccine-induced immune responses did not translate into clinical responses, but ongoing and future trials are built on the lessons learned. Interesting features of immune therapies, which showed clinical benefit, are that tumour responses are often delayed, and the treatment may only stabilise the disease rather than leading to tumour regression. These features should be considered when designing primary endpoints. One area which has received relatively little attention in past clinical trials is how to neutralise the complex immunosuppressive networks in cancer. This problem is addressed now by several ongoing trials. There is also a growing interest in combination therapies, where immunotherapy is applied as an adjuvant to traditional treatments. Also, combination of different immunotherapies, or co-application with biological response modifiers, opens new avenues for investigation. There is hope of achieving not only additive but synergistic effects with well-designed new treatments.

The ultimate aim of cancer immunologists, to make cancer vaccines part of standard of care in oncology, is firmly on the way to becoming a reality.

Abbreviations

ACT: adoptive T cell transfer
APC: antigen-presenting cell
BCG: Bacillus Calmette-Guerin
CAR: chimeric antigen receptor
CD40L: CD40-ligand
CT: chemotherapy
CTL: cytotoxic T lymphocyte
CTLA-4: cytotoxic T lymphocyte antigen-4
DAMP: damage associated molecular patterns
DC: dendritic cell
DT: diphteria toxin
GM-CSF: granulocyte–monocyte colony stimulating factor
GMP: good manufacturing procedures
HMGB-1: high mobility group box 1
HSC: hematopoietic stem cell
i.d.: intradermal
i.l.: intralymphatic
i.v.: intravenous
IFA: incomplete Freud's adjuvant
IFN: interferon
IL: interleukin
LPS: lipopolysaccharide
MPL: monophosphoryl lipid
MVA: modified vaccinia Ankara
NK: natural killer
NKT: natural killer T
NSCLC: non-small cell lung cancer
PAMP: pathogen-associated molecular pattern
PAP: prostate-associated antigen
PBMC: peripheral blood mononuclear cells
PPD: purified protein derivative
PSA: prostate-specific antigen
PSMA: prostate-specific membrane antigen
RT: radiation therapy
SCF: stem cell factor
TAA: tumour-associated antigen
TERT: telomerase reverse transcriptase
TGF: transforming growth factor

Th: T helper
TIL: tumour infiltrating lymphocytes
TLR: toll-like receptor
TNF: tumour necrosis factor
TRAIL: TNF-related apoptosis inducing ligand
Treg: T regulatory
TTP: time to progression

Acknowledgment The author thanks Mr B. Keszei for his assistance with the illustrations.

References

1. Burnet FM. Immunological aspects of malignant disease. *Lancet* 1967; **1**: 1171–1174.
2. Street SE, Cretney E, Smyth MJ. Perforin and interferon-gamma activities independently control tumor initiation, growth, and metastasis. *Blood* 2001; **97**: 192–197.
3. Street SE, Trapani JA, MacGregor D, Smyth MJ. Suppression of lymphoma and epithelial malignancies effected by interferon gamma. *J Exp Med* 2002; **196**: 129–134.
4. Sato E et al. Intraepithelial CD8+ tumor-infiltrating lymphocytes and a high CD8+/regulatory T cell ratio are associated with favorable prognosis in ovarian cancer. *Proc Natl Acad Sci USA* 2005; **102**: 18538–18543.
5. Kärjä V et al. Tumour-infiltrating lymphocytes: A prognostic factor of PSA-free survival in patients with local prostate carcinoma treated by radical prostatectomy. *Anticancer Res* 2005; **25**: 4435–4438.
6. Galon J et al. Type, density, and location of immune cells within human colorectal tumors predict clinical outcome. *Science* 2006; **313**: 1960–1964.
7. Anraku M et al. Impact of tumor-infiltrating T cells on survival in patients with malignant pleural mesothelioma. *J Thorac Cardiovasc Surg* 2008; **135**: 823–829.
8. Leffers N et al. Prognostic significance of tumor-infiltrating T-lymphocytes in primary and metastatic lesions of advanced stage ovarian cancer. *Cancer Immunol Immunother* 2008; doi: 10.1007/s0026200805835.
9. Dunn GP et al. Cancer immunoediting: from immunosurveillance to tumor escape. *Nat Immunol* 2002; **3**: 991–998.
10. Gattinoni L et al. Acquisition of full effector function in vitro paradoxically impairs the in vivo antitumor efficacy of adoptively transferred CD8+ T cells. *J Clin Invest* 2005; **115**: 1616–1626.
11. Dudley ME et al. Adoptive cell transfer therapy following non-myeloablative but lymphodepleting chemotherapy for the treatment of patients with refractory metastatic melanoma. *J Clin Oncol* 2005; **23**: 2346–2357.
12. Rosenberg SA et al. Adoptive cell transfer: a clinical path to effective cancer immunotherapy. *Nat Rev Cancer* 2008; **8**: 299–308.
13. Zhou J et al. Telomere length of transferred lymphocytes correlates with in vivo persistence and tumor regression in melanoma patients receiving cell transfer therapy. *J Immunol* 2005; **175**: 7046–7052.
14. Powell DJ et al. Adoptive transfer of vaccine-induced peripheral blood mononuclear cells to patients with metastatic melanoma following lymphodepletion. *J Immunol* 2006; **177**: 6527–6539.
15. Liu S, Riley J, Rosenberg S, Parkhurst M. Comparison of common gamma-chain cytokines, interleukin-2, interleukin-7, and interleukin-15 for the in vitro generation of human tumor-reactive T lymphocytes for adoptive cell transfer therapy. *J Immunother* 2006; **29**: 284–293.

16. Hinrichs CS et al. IL-2 and IL-21 confer opposing differentiation programs to CD8 + T cells for adoptive immunotherapy. *Blood* 2008; **111**: 5326–5333.
17. Müller-Hermelink N et al. TNFR1 signaling and IFN-gamma signaling determine whether T cells induce tumor dormancy or promote multistage carcinogenesis. *Cancer Cell* 2008; **13**: 507–518.
18. Perez-Diez A et al. CD4 cells can be more efficient at tumor rejection than CD8 cells. *Blood* 2007; **109**: 5346–5354.
19. Benchetrit F et al. Interleukin-17 inhibits tumor cell growth by means of a T-cell-dependent mechanism. *Blood* 2002; **99**: 2114–2121.
20. Muranski P et al. Tumor-specific Th17-polarized cells eradicate large established melanoma. *Blood* 2008; **112**: 362–373.
21. Nam JS et al. Transforming growth factor beta subverts the immune system into directly promoting tumor growth through interleukin-17. *Cancer Res* 2008; **68**: 3915–3923.
22. Dudley ME et al. Cancer regression and autoimmunity in patients after clonal repopulation with antitumor lymphocytes. *Science* 2002; **298**: 850–854.
23. Wrzesinski C et al. Hematopoietic stem cells promote the expansion and function of adoptively transferred antitumor CD8 T cells. *J Clin Invest* 2007; **117**: 492–501.
24. Perera LP et al. Development of smallpox vaccine candidates with integrated interleukin-15 that demonstrate superior immunogenicity, efficacy, and safety in mice. *J Virol* 2007; **81**: 8774–8783.
25. Sato N, Patel HJ, Waldmann TA, Tagaya Y. The IL-15/IL-15Ralpha on cell surfaces enables sustained IL-15 activity and contributes to the long survival of CD8 memory T cells. *Proc Natl Acad Sci USA* 2007; **104**: 588–593.
26. Colombo MP, Piconese S. Regulatory-T-cell inhibition versus depletion: the right choice in cancer immunotherapy. *Nat Rev Cancer* 2007; **7**: 880–887.
27. Morgan RA et al. Cancer regression in patients after transfer of genetically engineered lymphocytes. *Science* 2006; **314**: 126–129.
28. Cohen CJ et al. Enhanced antitumor activity of T cells engineered to express T-cell receptors with a second disulfide bond. *Cancer Res* 2007; **67**: 3898–3903.
29. Morgenroth A et al. Targeting of tumor cells expressing the prostate stem cell antigen (PSCA) using genetically engineered T-cells. *Prostate* 2007; **67**: 1121–1131.
30. Zhao Y et al. Extrathymic generation of tumor-specific T cells from genetically engineered human hematopoietic stem cells via Notch signaling. *Cancer Res* 2007; **67**: 2425–2429.
31. Gattinoni L, Powell DJ, Rosenberg SA, Restifo NP. Adoptive immunotherapy for cancer: building on success. *Nat Rev Immunol* 2006; **6**: 383–393.
32. Rubinstein MP et al. Loss of T cell-mediated antitumor immunity after construct-specific downregulation of retrovirally encoded T-cell receptor expression in vivo. *Cancer Gene Ther* 2009; **16**: 171–183.
33. Sadelain M, Rivière I, Brentjens R. Targeting tumours with genetically enhanced T lymphocytes. *Nat Rev Cancer* 2003; **3**: 35–45.
34. Gade TP et al. Targeted elimination of prostate cancer by genetically directed human T lymphocytes. *Cancer Res* 2005; **65**: 9080–9088.
35. Fujita M et al. Inhibition of STAT3 promotes the efficacy of adoptive transfer therapy using type-1 CTLs by modulation of the immunological microenvironment in a murine intracranial glioma. *J Immunol* 2008; **180**: 2089–2098.
36. Ghiringhelli F et al. Tumor cells convert immature myeloid dendritic cells into TGF-{beta}-secreting cells inducing CD4 + CD25 + regulatory T cell proliferation. *J Exp Med* 2005; **202**: 919–929.
37. Dohnal AM et al. Comparative evaluation of techniques for the manufacturing of dendritic cell-based cancer vaccines. *J Cell Mol Med* 2008: E-pub.
38. Curti A et al. Dendritic cell differentiation from hematopoietic CD34 + progenitor cells. *J Biol Regul Homeost Agents* 2001; **15**: 49–52.

39. Trakatelli M et al. A new dendritic cell vaccine generated with interleukin-3 and interferon-beta induces CD8+ T cell responses against NA17-A2 tumor peptide in melanoma patients. *Cancer Immunol Immunother* 2006; **55**: 469–474.
40. Banchereau J, Pascual V, Palucka AK. Autoimmunity through cytokine-induced dendritic cell activation. *Immunity* 2004; **20**: 539–550.
41. Iwamoto S et al. TNF-alpha drives human CD14+ monocytes to differentiate into CD70+ dendritic cells evoking Th1 and Th17 responses. *J Immunol* 2007; **179**: 1449–1457.
42. Bharadwaj U et al. Elevated interleukin-6 and G-CSF in human pancreatic cancer cell conditioned medium suppress dendritic cell differentiation and activation. *Cancer Res* 2007; **67**: 5479–5488.
43. Ratta M et al. Dendritic cells are functionally defective in multiple myeloma: the role of interleukin-6. *Blood* 2002; **100**: 230–237.
44. Pinzon-Charry A et al. Numerical and functional defects of blood dendritic cells in early- and late-stage breast cancer. *Br J Cancer* 2007; **97**: 1251–1259.
45. Jonuleit H et al. A comparison of two types of dendritic cell as adjuvants for the induction of melanoma-specific T-cell responses in humans following intranodal injection. *Int J Cancer* 2001; **93**: 243–251.
46. Nicolette CA et al. Dendritic cells for active immunotherapy: optimizing design and manufacture in order to develop commercially and clinically viable products. *Vaccine* 2007; **25**: S2 B47–60.
47. Czerniecki BJ et al. Targeting HER-2/neu in early breast cancer development using dendritic cells with staged interleukin-12 burst secretion. *Cancer Res* 2007; **67**: 1842–1852.
48. Tong AW, Stone MJ. Prospects for CD40-directed experimental therapy of human cancer. *Cancer Gene Ther* 2003; **10**: 1–13.
49. Nestle FO et al. Vaccination of melanoma patients with peptide- or tumor lysate-pulsed dendritic cells. *Nat Med* 1998; **4**: 328–332.
50. Hatfield P et al. Optimization of dendritic cell loading with tumor cell lysates for cancer immunotherapy. *J Immunother* 2008; **31**: 620–632.
51. Obeid M et al. Calreticulin exposure dictates the immunogenicity of cancer cell death. *Nat Med* 2007; **13**: 54–61.
52. Obeid M et al. Calreticulin exposure is required for the immunogenicity of gamma-irradiation and UVC light-induced apoptosis. *Cell Death Differ* 2007; 14: 1848–1850.
53. Fay JW et al. Long-term outcomes in patients with metastatic melanoma vaccinated with melanoma peptide-pulsed CD34(+) progenitor-derived dendritic cells. *Cancer Immunol Immunother* 2006; **55**: 1209–1218.
54. Miura S et al. Appropriate timing of CD40 ligation for RNA-Pulsed DCs to induce antitumor immunity. *Scand J Immunol* 2008; **67**: 385–391.
55. Michiels A et al. Delivery of tumor-antigen-encoding mRNA into dendritic cells for vaccination. *Methods Mol Biol* 2008; **423**: 155–163.
56. Bonifaz L et al. Efficient targeting of protein antigen to the dendritic cell receptor DEC-205 in the steady state leads to antigen presentation on major histocompatibility complex class I products and peripheral CD8+ T cell tolerance. *J Exp Med* 2002; **196**: 1627–1638.
57. Tacken PJ et al. Effective induction of naive and recall T-cell responses by targeting antigen to human dendritic cells via a humanized anti-DC-SIGN antibody. *Blood* 2005; **106**: 1278–1285.
58. Fong L et al. Dendritic cells injected via different routes induce immunity in cancer patients. *J Immunol* 2001; **166**: 4254–4259.
59. Gong J, Chen D, Kashiwaba M, Kufe D. Induction of antitumor activity by immunization with fusions of dendritic and carcinoma cells. *Nat Med* 1997; **3**: 558–561.
60. Vasir B et al. Fusions of dendritic cells with breast carcinoma stimulate the expansion of regulatory T cells while concomitant exposure to IL-12, CpG oligodeoxynucleotides, and

anti-CD3/CD28 promotes the expansion of activated tumor reactive cells. *J Immunol* 2008; **181**: 808–821.

61. Zhang M, Berndt BE, Chen JJ, Kao JY. Expression of a soluble TGF-beta receptor by tumor cells enhances dendritic cell/tumor fusion vaccine efficacy. *J Immunol* 2008; **181**: 3690–3697.

62. Lienard D et al. Ex vivo detectable activation of Melan-A-specific T cells correlating with inflammatory skin reactions in melanoma patients vaccinated with peptides in IFA. *Cancer Immun* 2004; **4**: 4.

63. Zeng G et al. Generation of NY-ESO-1-specific CD4+ and CD8+ T cells by a single peptide with dual MHC class I and class II specificities: a new strategy for vaccine design. *Cancer Res* 2002; **62**: 3630–3635.

64. Knutson K, Schiffman K, Disis M. Immunization with a HER-2/neu helper peptide vaccine generates HER-2/neu CD8 T-cell immunity in cancer patients. *J Clin Invest* 2001; **107**: 477–484.

65. Gnjatic S et al. CD8(+) T cell responses against a dominant cryptic HLA-A2 epitope after NY-ESO-1 peptide immunization of cancer patients. *Proc Natl Acad Sci USA* 2002; **99**: 11813–11818.

66. van der Burg SH et al. Improved peptide vaccine strategies, creating synthetic artificial infections to maximize immune efficacy. *Adv Drug Deliv Rev* 2006; **58**: 916–930.

67. Ahonen CL et al. Combined TLR and CD40 triggering induces potent CD8+ T cell expansion with variable dependence on type I IFN. *J Exp Med* 2004; **199**: 775–784.

68. Roth A et al. Induction of effective and antigen-specific antitumour immunity by a liposomal ErbB2/HER2 peptide-based vaccination construct. *Br J Cancer* 2005; **92**: 1421–1429.

69. Valmori D et al. Vaccination with NY-ESO-1 protein and CpG in Montanide induces integrated antibody/Th1 responses and CD8 T cells through cross-priming. *Proc Natl Acad Sci USA* 2007; **104**: 8947–8952.

70. Harrop R, John J, Carroll MW. Recombinant viral vectors: cancer vaccines. *Adv Drug Deliv Rev* 2006; **58**: 931–947.

71. Arlen PM et al. Preclinical and clinical studies of recombinant poxvirus vaccines for carcinoma therapy. *Crit Rev Immunol* 2007; **27**: 451–462.

72. Lindsey KR et al. Evaluation of prime/boost regimens using recombinant poxvirus/tyrosinase vaccines for the treatment of patients with metastatic melanoma. *Clin Cancer Res* 2006; **12**: 2526–2537.

73. Kaufman HL et al. Poxvirus-based vaccine therapy for patients with advanced pancreatic cancer. *J Transl Med* 2007; **5**: 60.

74. Adamina M et al. Heterologous prime-boost immunotherapy of melanoma patients with Influenza virosomes, and recombinant Vaccinia virus encoding 5 melanoma epitopes and 3 co-stimulatory molecules. A multi-centre phase I/II open labeled clinical trial. *Contemp Clin Trials* 2008; **29**: 165–181.

75. Hallermalm K et al. Pre-clinical evaluation of a CEA DNA prime/protein boost vaccination strategy against colorectal cancer. *Scand J Immunol* 2007; **66**: 43–51.

76. Doehn C et al. Drug evaluation: Therion's rV-PSA-TRICOM + rF-PSA-TRICOM prime-boost prostate cancer vaccine. *Curr Opin Mol Ther* 2007; **9**: 183–189.

77. Jäger E et al. Recombinant vaccinia/fowlpox NY-ESO-1 vaccines induce both humoral and cellular NY-ESO-1-specific immune responses in cancer patients. *Proc Natl Acad Sci USA* 2006; **103**: 14453–14458.

78. Fiander AN et al. Prime-boost vaccination strategy in women with high-grade, noncervical anogenital intraepithelial neoplasia: clinical results from a multicenter phase II trial. *Int J Gynecol Cancer* 2006; **16**: 1075–1081.

79. Skene CD, Sutton P. Saponin-adjuvanted particulate vaccines for clinical use. *Methods* 2006; **40**: 53–59.

80. Downey SG et al. Prognostic factors related to clinical response in patients with meta-static melanoma treated by CTL-associated antigen-4 blockade. *Clin Cancer Res* 2007; **13**: 6681–6688.
81. Loskog A, Tötterman TH. CD40L - a multipotent molecule for tumor therapy. *Endocr Metab Immune Disord Drug Targets* 2007; **7**: 23–28.
82. Fattorossi A et al. Neoadjuvant therapy changes the lymphocyte composition of tumor-draining lymph nodes in cervical carcinoma. *Cancer* 2004; **100**: 1418–1428.
83. Coleman S et al. Recovery of CD8+ T-cell function during systemic chemotherapy in advanced ovarian cancer. *Cancer Res* 2005; **65**: 7000–7006.
84. Okada H, Mak TW. Pathways of apoptotic and non-apoptotic death in tumour cells. *Nat Rev Cancer* 2004; **4**: 592–603.
85. Bang S et al. Differences in immune cells engaged in cell-mediated immunity after chemotherapy for far advanced pancreatic cancer. *Pancreas* 2006; **32**: 29–36.
86. Nowak AK, Lake RA, Robinson BW. Combined chemoimmunotherapy of solid tumours: improving vaccines? *Adv Drug Deliv Rev* 2006; **58**: 975–990.
87. Beyer M et al. Reduced frequencies and suppressive function of CD4+CD25hi regula-tory T cells in patients with chronic lymphocytic leukemia after therapy with fludar-abine. *Blood* 2005; **106**: 2018–2025.
88. Audia S et al. Increase of CD4+ CD25+ regulatory T cells in the peripheral blood of patients with metastatic carcinoma: a Phase I clinical trial using cyclophosphamide and immunotherapy to eliminate CD4+ CD25+ T lymphocytes. *Clin Exp Immunol* 2007; **150**: 523–530.
89. Brode S, Raine T, Zaccone P, Cooke A. Cyclophosphamide-induced type-1 diabetes in the NOD mouse is associated with a reduction of CD4+CD25+Foxp3+ regulatory T cells. *J Immunol* 2006; **177**: 6603–6612.
90. Mozaffari F et al. NK-cell and T-cell functions in patients with breast cancer: effects of surgery and adjuvant chemo- and radiotherapy. *Br J Cancer* 2007; **97**: 105–111.
91. Santin AD et al. Effects of concurrent cisplatinum administration during radiotherapy vs. radiotherapy alone on the immune function of patients with cancer of the uterine cervix. *Int J Radiat Oncol Biol Phys* 2000; **48**: 997–1006.
92. Chakraborty M et al. External beam radiation of tumors alters phenotype of tumor cells to render them susceptible to vaccine-mediated T-cell killing. *Cancer Res* 2004; **64**: 4328–4337.
93. Garnett CT et al. Sublethal irradiation of human tumor cells modulates phenotype resulting in enhanced killing by cytotoxic T lymphocytes. *Cancer Res* 2004; **64**: 7985–7994.
94. Reits EA et al. Radiation modulates the peptide repertoire, enhances MHC class I expression, and induces successful antitumor immunotherapy. *J Exp Med* 2006; **203**: 1259–1271.
95. Apetoh L et al. The interaction between HMGB1 and TLR4 dictates the outcome of anticancer chemotherapy and radiotherapy. *Immunol Rev* 2007; **220**: 47–59.
96. Nesslinger NJ et al. Standard Treatments Induce Antigen-Specific Immune Responses in Prostate Cancer. *Clin Cancer Res* 2007; **13**: 1493–1502.
97. Mason KA et al. Targeting toll-like receptor 9 with CpG oligodeoxynucleotides enhances tumor response to fractionated radiotherapy. *Clin Cancer Res* 2005; **11**: 361–369.
98. Gulley JL et al. Combining a recombinant cancer vaccine with standard definitive radiotherapy in patients with localized prostate cancer. *Clin Cancer Res* 2005; **11**: 3353–3362.
99. Tabi Z et al. *Memory T Cell Resistance to Functional Impairment and Apoptosis During Radiation Therapy in Cancer.* Unpublished.
100. Small EJ et al. Immunotherapy of hormone-refractory prostate cancer with antigen-loaded dendritic cells. *J Clin Oncol* 2000; **18**: 3894–3903.

101. Burch PA et al. Immunotherapy (APC8015, Provenge) targeting prostatic acid phosphatase can induce durable remission of metastatic androgen-independent prostate cancer: a Phase 2 trial. *Prostate* 2004; **60**: 197–204.

102. Sangha R, Butts C. L-BLP25: a peptide vaccine strategy in non small cell lung cancer. *Clin Cancer Res* 2007; **13**: s4652–4654.

103. North SA, Graham K, Bodnar D, Venner P. A pilot study of the liposomal MUC1 vaccine BLP25 in prostate specific antigen failures after radical prostatectomy. *J Urol* 2006; **176**: 91–95.

104. Southall PJ et al. Immunohistological distribution of 5T4 antigen in normal and malignant tissues. *Br J Cancer* 1990; **61**: 89–95.

105. Harrop R et al. Vaccination of colorectal cancer patients with modified vaccinia Ankara delivering the tumor antigen 5T4 (TroVax) induces immune responses which correlate with disease control: a phase I/II trial. *Clin Cancer Res* 2006; **12**: 3416–3424.

106. Amato RJ et al. Vaccination of prostate cancer patients with modified vaccinia ankara delivering the tumor antigen 5T4 (TroVax): a phase 2 trial. *J Immunother* 2008; **31**: 577–585.

107. Madan RA et al. Analysis of overall survival in patients with nonmetastatic castration-resistant prostate cancer treated with vaccine, nilutamide, and combination therapy. *Clin Cancer Res* 2008; **14**: 4526–4531.

108. Nemunaitis J et al. Phase II study of belagenpumatucel-L, a transforming growth factor beta-2 antisense gene-modified allogeneic tumor cell vaccine in non-small-cell lung cancer. *J Clin Oncol* 2006; **24**: 4721–4730.

109. Phatak P et al. Telomere uncapping by the G-quadruplex ligand RHPS4 inhibits clonogenic tumour cell growth in vitro and in vivo consistent with a cancer stem cell targeting mechanism. *Br J Cancer* 2007; **96**: 1223–1233.

110. Cortez-Gonzalez X, Zanetti M. Telomerase immunity from bench to bedside: round one. *J Transl Med* 2007; **5**: 12.

111. Wood C et al. An adjuvant autologous therapeutic vaccine (HSPPC-96; vitespen) versus observation alone for patients at high risk of recurrence after nephrectomy for renal cell carcinoma: a multicentre, open-label, randomised phase III trial. *Lancet* 2008; **372**: 145–154.

112. Testori A et al. Phase III comparison of vitespen, an autologous tumor-derived heat shock protein gp96 peptide complex vaccine, with physician's choice of treatment for stage IV melanoma: the C-100-21 Study Group. *J Clin Oncol* 2008; **26**: 955–962.

RNA Interference for Cancer Therapy

Kun Cheng and Bin Qin

1 Introduction

Evolved as a defense mechanism against RNA virus, RNA interference (RNAi) is the phenomenon in which small interfering RNA (siRNA) of 21–23 nucleotides in length silences the target gene by binding to its complementary mRNA and triggering the degradation of target mRNA [1]. It was first found in *Caenorhabditis elegans* that introduction of foreign small double-stranded RNA (dsRNA) can lead to potent degradation of the complementary mRNA [2]. This finding generated huge interest in the application of siRNA for the biomedical research community. Potent knockdown of the target gene with high sequence specificity makes RNAi a powerful tool to uncover gene functions, understand the effects of selective gene silencing, and explore potential therapeutics for complex diseases [3]. The discovery of RNAi is one of the most dramatic findings over the past decade in the field of molecular biology [4]. As illustrated by the histogram in Fig. 1, the number of publications related to "RNAi" increased dramatically from 5 in 1998 to over 2000 in 2007.

Over the past two decades, the idea of developing novel therapeutics targeting disease at the molecular level using gene modulation approach has attracted great attention [5]. The advances in molecular and cell biology, especially the completion of human genome project in 2003, have led to elucidation of the molecular pathological mechanisms underlying malignant transformation of various cancers. As a result, it brings new opportunities for novel therapeutic approaches, such as gene modulation. Gene targeted therapeutics is an effective strategy for a broad range of cancers because (i) different tumor types share a relatively small number of deficient pathways; (ii) drugs targeting a particular gene may be effective in treating tumor with a mutation of the target gene as well as any upstream genes of the target and (iii) many strategies are available to develop gene therapeutics once a target disease gene is identified [2].

K. Cheng (✉)
Department of Pharmaceutical Sciences, University of Missouri-Kansas City,
Kansas City, MO 64110, USA
e-mail: chengkun@umkc.edu

Y. Lu, R.I. Mahato (eds.), *Pharmaceutical Perspectives of Cancer Therapeutics*,
DOI 10.1007/978-1-4419-0131-6_13, © Springer Science+Business Media, LLC 2009

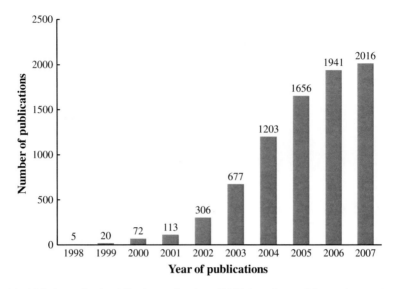

Fig. 1 PubMed search of publications related to "RNA interference" for each year since its discovery in 1998

Thus far, 66.5% of gene therapy clinical trials aimed at the treatment of cancer [6]. Among all gene modulation approaches, RNAi is the most revolutionized and promising method for treating cancer. The RNAi technology has moved remarkably toward therapeutic application and there are already 12 ongoing clinical trials using siRNA (www.clinicaltrial.gov). Furthermore, RNAi holds great promises in cancer research because the inactivation of oncogenes could block or reverse the tumorigenesis, whereas silencing of tumor suppressor genes contributes to the better understanding of tumorigenesis [7]. On the other hand, many large pharmaceutical companies showed great interest and have begun to invest in developing RNAi-based drugs for various diseases. This will further drive the transformation of RNAi toward therapeutic products [6].

In this chapter, we will highlight the RNAi mechanism, utility of RNAi in screening oncogenes, and cancer-associated genes involved in different cellular pathways. We will also discuss the challenges in developing siRNA therapeutics, as well as the targeted delivery of siRNA.

2 RNA Interference Mechanism and Limitations for In Vivo Application

2.1 Mechanism of RNAi

The silencing process of siRNA is an ATP-dependent and post-transcriptional event occurred in the cytoplasm. The RNA-induced silencing complex (RISC) model is shown in Fig. 2. RNAi can be trigged by vector-based short hairpin RNA (shRNA), long dsRNA, or synthetic siRNA. In the RNAi process, the long dsRNA and shRNA are cleaved by the endogenous enzyme, dicer, into fragments of 21–23 nucleotide in length with a two-nucleotide 3'-overhang. The short siRNA is then unwound by an ATP-dependent helicase and the antisense strand is incorporated into a multiprotein, RISC, which is the key step in RNAi. Subsequently, the incorporated antisense strand guides the RISC to its homologous mRNA for endonucleolytic cleavage of the mRNA [8, 9]. It is noteworthy that only one of the strands from siRNA is incorporated into the RISC, whereas many scientists previously believed that the whole duplex was incorporated. The stability at the 5' end of the two strands determines which strand enters RISC, and the strand with the less-stable 5' end is more likely to be incorporated. To be functional against target mRNA, the antisense strand must be the one incorporated into the RISC [10].

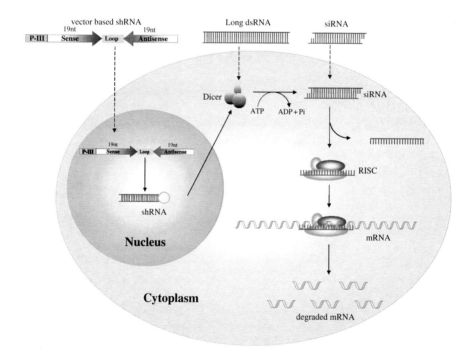

Fig. 2 Mechanism of RNA interference. RNAi can be trigged by vector-based short hairpin RNA (shRNA), long dsRNA, or siRNA. Long dsRNA and shRNA are cleaved by Dicer into fragments of 21–23 nucleotide siRNAs. The siRNA is then unwound by an ATP-dependent helicase and the antisense strand is incorporated into a multiprotein, RISC, which is the key step in RNAi. Subsequently, the incorporated antisense strand guides the RISC to its homologous targeted mRNA for the endonucleolytic cleavage

2.2 siRNA Design

The design of siRNA sequences for a target gene is the first critical step in its therapeutic applications. Bearing in mind the complexities of the RNAi mechanism, designing siRNA has to be conducted very cautiously to achieve potent silencing effect while minimize off-target effects [5, 11]. So far, there are no universally accepted rules or softwares to design siRNAs, instead, numerous online siRNA design tools are available through academic institutions and commercial siRNA suppliers (Table 1). Each software uses different rational design algorithms and the optimal sequence needs to be determined experimentally by comparing silencing effect of several candidates [5, 9].

Table 1 Online siRNA design tools

Name of program	Provider	URL
RNAi OligoRetriever	Cold Spring Harbor Laboratories	http://katahdin.cshl.org:9331/RNAi/html/rnai.html
RNAxs	University of Vienna	http://rna.tbi.univie.ac.at/cgi-bin/RNAxs
DEQOR	Scionics Computer Innovation	http://cluster-1.mpi-cbg.de/Deqor/deqor.html
siRNA Selection Program	Whitehead Institute	http://jura.wi.mit.edu/bioc/siRNAext
siRNA Selector	The Wistar Institute	http://bioinfo.wistar.upenn.edu/siRNA/siRNA.htm
sIR: siRNA Information Resource	University of Texas Southwestern Medical Center	http://biotools.swmed.edu/siRNA/
siRNA Target Finder	Ambion, Inc.	http://www.ambion.com/techlib/misc/siRNA_finder.html
siDESIGN® Center	Dharmacon Research, Inc.	http://www.dharmacon.com/DesignCenter/DesignCenterPage.aspx
BLOCK-iT™ RNAi Designer	Invitrogen, Inc.	https://rnaidesigner.invitrogen.com/rnaiexpress/
BIOPREDsi	Qiagen Sciences Inc.	http://www.biopredsi.org/start.html
siRNA Target Finder	Gen script corporation	https://www.genscript.com/ssl-bin/app/rnai

Nevertheless, many studies have been done to summarize the designing criteria, such as sequence length, G/C content and localization of target sequence within the mRNA [12–17]. Based on the molecular mechanism of RISC assembly, Ui-Tei et al. proposed four practical guidelines: (i) A/U at the 5′ end of the antisense strand; (ii) G/C at the 5′ end of the sense strand; (iii) at least five A/U residues in the 5′ terminal of the antisense strand; and (iv) the absence of GC stretch of >9 nt in length [13]. To identify siRNA-specific features related to its activity, Khvorova et al. performed a systematic analysis of 180 siRNAs targeting every other positions of two different mRNAs and summarized three important criteria for siRNA design: moderate or low G/C content (30–52%), low internal stability at the 5′ antisense-end, and lack of internal repeats. In addition, three sense strand base preferences were revealed: (i) presence of an A at position 3 and 19 in the sense strand; (ii) presence of a U in position 10 of the sense strand; (iii) absence of a G or C at position 19, and a G at position 13 of the sense strand [12]. Considering the fact that high internal stability prevents efficient unwinding, low internal stability of the sense 3′ end and the overall low internal stability of the duplex (low G/C content) are preferable for high activity because it can promotes strand selection and entry into the RISC. However, very low stability should be avoided since it may decrease the affinity of siRNA to its complementary mRNA and subsequently affect its cleavage at the binding site [12].

In summary, all currently used selection criteria can be divided into "related" (group 1) or "unrelated" (group 2) parameters based on the stability of siRNA termini [18]. As per the rules for group 1, the ability of siRNA antisense strand to enter into RISC is critical for the mRNA cleavage. siRNA strands with less stable 5′ end enters RISC faster than other strands that explains why the 5′ end of the antisense strand needs to be A/U rich and 3′ end G/C rich. The unrelated (group 2) rules include (i) presence of a specific nucleotide at a certain position; (ii) the stability of secondary structure of the target mRNA; (iii) the stability of the siRNA antisense strand; and (iv) the percentage of a particular nucleotide in the siRNA [18].

In addition to the properties of siRNA, structure and accessibility of the target site should also be considered as a criterion in designing potent siRNA. For the first time, Tafer et al. described a comprehensive analysis of the effect of target mRNA structure on RNAi and developed a new siRNA design tool, RNAxs, which combines known siRNA selection criteria with target mRNA accessibility. RNAxs was calibrated with two data sets of 573 siRNAs for 38 genes and then tested on an independent set of 360 siRNAs targeting additional four genes. Compared to previously reported criteria which only considered the siRNA duplex sequence, RNAxs significantly improved the prediction of effective siRNAs after incorporating the selection criteria for target site accessibility [19].

2.3 siRNA Versus shRNA

Generally, there are two strategies to introduce siRNA into mammalian cells: (i) chemical synthesis strategy in which the synthetic siRNA is directly introduced into target cells or (ii) DNA-based (plasmid or viral vector) strategy in which the siRNA is produced via intracellular processing of the expressed RNA hairpin transcript (Fig. 2). There are advantages and disadvantages associated with each strategy.

The most common strategy is to directly introduce chemically synthesized double-stranded siRNA of 21–23 nucleotides into mammalian cells. There are several advantages of using synthetic siRNA: (i) easy to synthesize and use; (ii) high transfection efficiency into the cells with potent and specific gene silencing effect; (iii) the amount and purity of siRNA can be controlled easily; (iv) quick initiation of gene silencing effect; and (v) various modifications can be introduced to enhance siRNA's stability and targeting specificity [9]. However, the silencing effect of synthesized siRNA is transient because there is no siRNA replication in mammalian cells [20]. Consequently, repeated treatment of siRNA is needed and the subsequently high cost limits its application in animal and clinical studies [21].

Considering the limitations of synthetic siRNA, the DNA-based shRNA strategy has been developed as it provides a stable expression of siRNA in the treated cells and the cost is much lower. Typically, synthetic siRNA mediates silencing effects for 2–3 days post-transfection, while the shRNA expression vector produces siRNAs continuously in cells and silence the expression of target gene for weeks or even months [22]. Another advantage of shRNA is that the multiple siRNA expression cassettes can be constructed within one vector so that it can knockdown several different sites of a target gene or several different genes simultaneously.

In the DNA-based expression vector, shRNA is expressed in cells under the control of an RNA polymerase II or polymerase III promoter. Polymerase II promoter can induce tissue-specific RNA expression but also induces the interferon response in many mammalian cells [9]. Thus, the application of polymerase II promoter is limited and polymerase III promoter is commonly used in shRNA applications. Polymerase III promoters have a relatively simple structure, a well-defined transcription initiation and a termination signal consisting of five thymidines. More importantly, the transcript is cleaved after the second uridine of the termination site, which yields a transcript resembling the end of synthetic siRNA [22]. To date, there are two RNA polymerase III promoters, the human H1 promoter (H1) and the human U6 small nuclear promoter (U6), available to drive the shRNA expression. It is however notable that H1 and U6 promoters may give different silencing efficiency. Makinen et al. have demonstrated the difference between U6 and H1 promoters in a lentiviral vector-mediated RNAi using green fluorescent protein (GFP) as a target gene. The U6 promoter was found to be more efficient than H1 in silencing GFP in vitro. It persistently silenced 80% of the GFP gene for several months. In addition, U6 promoter also showed higher in vivo silencing effect in mouse brain for at least 9 months [23]. This result is in agreement with another study using AAV as a vector to express shRNA under U6 or H1 promoter [24]. The U6 promoter-derived caspase 8 siRNA successfully silenced the caspase expression, while the H1 promoter-driven shRNA failed to show the silencing effect. Although the exact reason was not clear, it was conceivable that the U6 promoter's high expression may contribute to this difference [24].

To study the function of genes involved in cell growth or survival, a tightly regulated siRNA expression is required. Recently, several tetracycline-responsive variants of U6 and H1 promoters have been developed as inducible promoter systems to drive conditional shRNA expression [25, 26]. Generally, a tetracycline operator (tetO) sequence, which has a high-binding affinity for tetracycline repressor (tetR), is inserted near the TATA box of the promoter. Once the tetR binds to the tetO sequence, the tetR will prevent RNA polymerase III from binding to the promoter to initiate the transcription. Subsequently, adding analogs with higher affinity for tetR will cause the tetR to dissociate from tetO and the transcription is restored [25]. Therefore the inducible shRNA expression system is not only a useful tool for basic research on gene function but also a potential approach for therapeutic applications [25].

Although DNA-based shRNA expression vector has been widely used in gene function study as well as therapeutic application, most vectors only contain one single siRNA expression cassette [27]. To maximize the efficiency and versatility, shRNA expression vector containing multiple tandem expression cassettes have been developed. Up to six tandem cassettes can be successfully constructed into one single shRNA expression vector and produces different shRNA simultaneously [27]. Accordingly, these vectors can silence multiple genes or maximize the silencing effect by targeting different regions of the same gene [27, 28]. The multiple shRNA expression vector is best suited for cancer treatment where multiple pathways are needed to be targeted simultaneously.

Chen et al. has constructed a multiple shRNA expression vector targeting the mRNA of vascular endothelial growth factor (VEGF), human telomerase reverse transcriptase (hTERT) and antiapoptotic factor Bcl-XI. The multiple expression vector was injected intratumorally into the tumor formed by human laryngeal squamous carcinoma (Hep-2) cells implanted in nude mice. Significant reduction in VEGF, Htert, and Bcl-XI mRNAs and protein levels were observed and tumor growth of treated group was obviously smaller than that of the control group with blank vector. This result demonstrated the potential application of multiple gene silencing using shRNA vector in cancer therapy [29].

2.4 Virus-Based shRNA Expression Vector

The shRNA expression vector can be plasmid-based or viral-based. Although plasmid-based shRNA expression vectors have been successfully developed in many applications, they usually have low transfection efficiency, especially in primary cells and non-dividing cells [9]. To overcome problems associated with the plasmid vector, viral vectors including adenoviral, adeno-associated viral (AAV), retroviral and lentiviral vectors, have been developed. Although lentiviral vector can express integrated siRNA efficiently in a wide variety of actively dividing, non-dividing and primary cells, its infrequent insertional mutagenesis limited its therapeutic application [30]. As a relatively safe and efficient vector for a wide variety of cell types, adenoviral vector is a popular vector for therapeutic delivery of shRNA [31]. Jung et al. generated adenoviral vector encoding shRNA against pituitary tumor transforming 1 (PTTG1) and treated hepatoma cells. The PTTG1 expression was specifically silenced, leading to activation of p53 and induction of cell apoptosis. Intratumoral delivery of the adenoviral vector significantly inhibits the tumor growth in nude mice [31].

In addition, AAV is another promising vector for shRNA therapies because of its unique features: (i) lack of immune and inflammatory responses; (ii) ability to infect dividing and non-dividing cells over a broad host range; (iii) long-term shRNA expression after integration into host chromosome [24]. Tomar et al. created a series of modified AAV vectors expressing shRNAs targeting p53 or caspase 8 under the control of H1 or U6 promoter. An enhanced green fluorescent protein (EGFP) was also cloned in the vector as a report gene to monitor the infection efficiency. Results demonstrated that the AAV-based vector was efficient in infecting and expressing shRNA in mammalian cells [24].

2.5 Limitations of siRNA Therapeutic Application

Initially, the application of RNAi was emerged as a powerful tool for gene knockdown experiments to understand gene functions. However, the impressive in vitro results of RNAi soon spurred researcher's interest to develop RNAi therapeutics. In 2002, Mc Caffrey et al. reported the first proof-of-concept study of in vivo gene silencing by synthetic siRNA and shRNA [32]. siRNA and luciferase plasmid were co-injected into mice and luciferase expression was monitored using quantitative whole body imaging. Specific inhibition of luciferase expression by an average of 81% in mice was detected in 11 independent experiments [32]. Later, Song et al. reported the first in vivo therapeutic application of siRNA targeting the gene *Fas* (encoding the Fas receptor) to protect mice from liver failure and fibrosis [33]. The synthetic siRNA was injected into mice by hydrodynamic tail vein injection and 88% of hepatocytes took up the siRNA after 24 h. Both mRNA and protein expressions of *Fas* gene were reduced and the effects persisted for 10 days. Furthermore, the siRNA treatment protected mice from fulminant hepatitis and hepatic fibrosis in two different animal models [33].

Notwithstanding these exciting studies for potential therapeutic application, several important considerations should be emphasized [5, 34]. Both studies administrated siRNA into mice using hydrodynamic injection in which a large volume (1 ml/20 g body weight) was rapidly injected into the tail vein within a short period of several seconds. Apparently, it is not applicable for human beings because about 3.5 liters of solution is needed to be injected into a 70 kg patient within a few minutes [5].

The major bottleneck in the development of siRNA therapeutics is the efficient delivery of siRNA to target cells. The difficulty is mainly due to the pharmacokinetic profiles of siRNA. To reach the target site, systemically administered siRNAs need to overcome several biological barriers: moving from the bloodstream into tissues, passing through the extracellular space, crossing the cell membrane, and then entering the cytoplasm to silence the target mRNA. In the plasma, single-stranded RNA is degraded by nucleases within seconds, whereas double-stranded RNA molecules have a longer half-life of approximate 6 minutes in rats. However, it is still far below the stability requirements for systemic administration [35]. The cellular uptake of naked siRNA is also very limited because of its negative charge and large molecular weight. Subsequently, to bypass these problems associated with siRNA, local administration of siRNA becomes the favorable approach and most of the current siRNA clinical trials are based on the local delivery of naked siRNA (Table 2) [5]. Nevertheless, systemic delivery is the desired route for most siRNA therapies.

Tremendous efforts have been made to overcome these challenges, cationic liposome and positively charged polymers are currently being used as the most common method to complex with negatively charged siRNA for systemic delivery [30, 36]. Other in vivo delivery approaches include conjugation with cholesterol, aptamer, peptide; complexation with antibody–protamine fusion protein; or encapsulation in cyclodextrin nanoparticles [35, 37–39].

To improve the in vivo stability of siRNA, various chemical modifications have been developed in relevant subunits, such as sugar, base, and phosphate moieties. One of the simplest modifications is the introduction of phosphorothioate (PS) linkage, which can enhance the resistance of siRNA to nucleases and subsequently increase the in vivo half-life. However, extensive phosphorothioate linkages are not desirable because it extensively bind to serum protein and can be toxic in vivo [40]. In addition, PS modification has shown reduced siRNA activity compared to unmodified siRNA [41]. Alternatively, modification of the 2'-OH group in the ribose is another common method to increase the stability against nucleases while not affect the silencing effect. Typically, 2'-O-methyl (2'-OMe) and 2'-O-fluoro (2'-F) modifications are among the most prominent methods. On account of the unfavorable pharmacokinetic properties, 2'-F modified siRNAs are less potent than unmodified siRNAs in the animal [42]. In contrast, incorporation of 2'-OMe modified nucleotides in siRNA is well tolerated and siRNA with every other 2'-OMe modification is resistant to nuclease and enhanced activity has been observed [43].

Contrary to antisense oligonucleotides, chemical modifications for siRNA should be designed cautiously so that they do not affect the silencing effect of siRNA. Once inside the cells, siRNA duplex will be unwound and the antisense strand will be incorporated into the RISC, followed by binding to its homologous target mRNA for endonucleolytic cleavage. Taking these facts into consideration, any modification of the antisense strand (especially the 5' end) should be avoided and most of reported modifications are located in the sense strand [11, 44].

Table 2 Current clinical trails of siRNA

Company	Target disease	Status	Route	Delivery method
Sirna Therapeutics, Inc.	Age-related macular degeneration	Phase I clinical trail completed in October 2007	Intravitreal	Naked siRNA
Allergan, Inc.	Choroid neovascularization and age-related macular degeneration	Phase II	Intravitreal	Naked siRNA
Hadassah Medical Organization	Chronic myeloid leukemia			SV40 Vectors
Opko Health, Inc.	Wet age-related macular degeneration	Phase III	Intravitreal	Naked siRNA
Opko Health, Inc.	Diabetic macular edema	Phase II clinical trial completed in March 2007	Intravitreal	Naked siRNA
Alnylam Pharmaceuticals	Respiratory syncytial virus infections	Phase II clinical trial completed in November 2007	Administrated by nebulization	Naked siRNA
TransDerm, Inc.	Pachyonychia congenita	Phase Ib clinical trial began in January 2008	Injected into callus on the bottom of foot	Naked siRNA
Acuity Pharmaceuticals	Wet age-related macular degeneration	Phase II	Intravitreal	Naked siRNA
Calando Pharmaceuticals	Cancer	Received approval for phase I clinical trial in March 2008	Intravenous	Nanoparticles entrapped siRNA
Quark Pharmaceuticals	Wet age-related macular degeneration	Phase I/IIa	Intravitreal	Naked siRNA
Quark Pharmaceuticals Nucleonics, Inc.	Acute renal failure Chronic hepatitis B virus (HBV) infection	Phase I Received approval for phase I clinical trial in May 2007	Intravenous	Naked siRNA Plasmid-based shRNA

Information resource: www.clinicaltrial.gov and Internet.

There are usually two potential side effects associated with siRNA, off-target effect and induction of interferon (IFN). siRNA was assumed to be highly specific for target mRNA and even a single base mismatch was believed to protect mRNA from degradation [45]. However, recent studies have shown that mRNA having less than 100% complementarity with the siRNA can also be silenced [46–50]. This phenomenon is called off-target effect and it may cause undesired effects as well as toxicity. Sometimes, siRNA can silence non-target genes containing only 11–15 contiguous nucleotides of identity to the siRNA [46]. Fedorov et al. evaluated 176 randomly selected siRNAs to determine the relationship between cell survival and off-target effects. Twenty-nine percent of the tested siRNAs induced sequence-independent changes in cell viability, indicating the off-target derived phenotypes are much more extensive than originally anticipated [49]. The $5'$ end of siRNA antisense strand was found as the primary determinant for regulation of the off-target effects [50]. Subsequently, chemical modification, especially the $2'$-O-methyl substitution in the antisense strand, was found to be able to substantially eliminate the off-target effects [51]. In addition, computer algorithms have been developed to address the off-target problem [52]. Nevertheless, the off-target effects emphasize the need to spend more effort in the design and validation of siRNAs before conducting experiments.

Soon after the discovery of RNAi, the application of RNAi to mammalian cells was not successful due to the fact that dsRNA >30bp in mammalian cells can trigger the nonspecific interferon responses, which limits its therapeutic application [53]. This immune response is believed to be caused by the activation of the dsRNA-dependent protein kinase R (PKR), $2',5'$-oligoadenylate synthetase or Toll-like receptors (TLR) [54]. In 2001, for the first time, Elbashir et al. succeeded in silencing a target gene in human cells without inducing IFN response using a 21-nt siRNA [55]. The sequence of siRNA maybe too short to be recognized by the dsRNA-dependent sensors. However, even unmodified siRNA sometimes induces innate immune responses which represent a significant barrier to the therapeutic application of siRNA [56]. Till now, chemical modifications have been the best strategy to abrogate the immunostimulatory activity of siRNA. By selective incorporation of small number (<20% of all nucleotides) of $2'$-O-methyl uridine or guanosine into one strand of the siRNA, the immune stimulation can be completely abrogated without disrupting its silencing activity [54, 57].

3 Screening for Therapeutic Targets in Malignancy

The great potential of RNAi in cancer therapy has been recognized since its discovery in 1998. The first step toward the treatment of cancer using RNAi is the understanding of the tumorigenic process and identifying genes which are responsible for tumor cell's initiation and progression. Currently, majority of new anti-cancer therapeutics under development are directed against existing targets, while only a few drugs are developed against novel targets. It is mainly because that identifying new targets for cancer therapy is a difficult, time-consuming, and expensive process. Consequently, many key genes or proteins related to cancer have not been selected as targets for drug development [58]. Traditionally, homologous recombination was the only method to determine the function of the interested genes, such as oncogenes or tumor suppressor genes. However, the production of knockout animal using recombinant technology is very time consuming and complicated. Alternatively, potent and specific gene silencing ability make RNAi-based screening a novel tool to identify genes which are responsible for certain aspects in cancer biology [7]. siRNA/shRNA has been successfully performed to determine the function of a specific gene in cancer biology without generating knockout animals. Generally, two methods can be used to uncover the biomarkers related with tumorigenesis: (i) use siRNA directly to establish knockdown cell lines or (ii) use RNAi library to screen the important genes involved in tumorigenesis.

3.1 Gene KnockDown Cells

Gene knockdown cells is an easy and fast way to study the function of interested gene in vitro using cell lines. Ganesan et al. used siRNA to knock down the expression of BRCA1 (breast cancer 1, early onset) in female somatic cells and observed the destabilization of the silenced state of inactivative X chromosome (Xi). These observations suggested that the loss of BRCA1 in female cells may lead to Xi perturbation as well as destabilization of its silenced state [59]. To explore the oncogenic potential of leucyl-tRNA synthetase 1 (LARS1) in lung cancer, Shin et al. knocked down LARS1 in lung cancer cells using siRNA and then examined the tumor behavior. Knockdown cells showed reduced ability to form colonies in soft agar and slow migration through transwell membrane. Consequently, LARS1 was identified as a potential biomarker for the migration and growth of lung cancer cells [60]. Compared to the transit knockdown effect of synthetic siRNA, retroviral vector-based shRNA provides a specific and stable inhibition of target gene in tumor cells. Brummelkamp et al. developed a retroviral vector to stably silence the expression of oncogenic K-RAS (V12) allele in human tumor cells. Knockdown of this gene resulted in a loss of the anchorage-independent growth and tumorigenicity, indicating the K-RAS gene as a potential therapeutic target for treating lung cancer [61].

Since this gene knockdown method can only screen one gene at one time, it is granted another name, "gene by gene" method. Obviously, this method is too tedious and expensive for multiple gene screening [62]. Alternatively, RNAi library provides a powerful tool to identify cancer-related genes in a large-scale pattern. Generally, the cells are transfected with RNAi library followed by biological screens. Cells reacting significantly are analyzed for the corresponding siRNA, and subsequently the gene responsible for the reaction can be identified [7]. Two strategies, transfected cell array and RNAi barcode screens, have been developed for screening of cancer-related genes in mammalian cells.

3.2 Transfected Cell Array

Transfected cell array (TCA) is a one-by-one arrayed approach using reverse transfection to interrogate phenotypes in a well-based format (Fig. 3). Two types of RNAi libraries, siRNA and plasmid-based shRNA libraries, can be used for this screening. While siRNA provides a fast and transit gene silencing effect, plasmid-based shRNA library provides a stable silencing effect from several days to several weeks so that it is possible to examine phenotypes that develop over a longer time span [63]. For screening, siRNA or shRNA targeting different genes are dissolved in gelatin solution and then plated at high density on a solid support array using a robotic arrayer or dispensing printer. Subsequently, the array is placed in tissue culture dish and covered with sufficient number of cells to achieve confluence at the end of the assay. Up to 6000 distinct siRNA or shRNA can be spotted in the same array and each spot can be covered by 30–500 cells. As cells reach the attached siRNA/shRNA, the siRNA/shRNA will be incorporated and a potential knockdown phenotype becomes detectable. The incorporation efficiency can be monitored by fluorescein-conjugated siRNA or shRNA encoding a reporter gene, green fluorescence protein (GFP) [5, 7, 62].

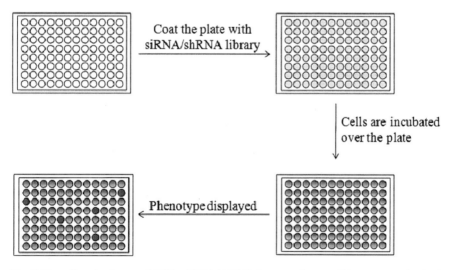

Fig. 3 Transfected cell array (TCA). siRNA/shRNA is arrayed on a solid support and mixed with cationic lipid to enhance the transfection efficiency. Then the cells are plated and grown on the solid support. As these cells uptake the siRNA/shRNA, phenotypes corresponding to specific silencing become detectable and the corresponding gene will be identified

High resolution imaging system with image analysis software is necessary to analyze the array. Gene silencing effect can be detected by fluorescein-labeled antibodies for a specific protein. Induction of apoptosis can be detected by reagents like Annexin V and the cell morphology can be observed directly under microscope [7]. This technique provides broad applications for high-throughput, low-cost, and large-scale loss-of-function studies in mammalian cells [62].

There are three advantages of TCA: (i) each well is only transfected with one siRNA/shRNA and thus the screening sensitivity is high; (ii) it provides high-throughput screening of cells within their micro-environment, which is important for gene function study; and (iii) fewer cells per gene are required than standard microwell plate-based methods, which is particularly important for primary cells since the number of isolated cells are often very limited [5, 64]. However, the major challenge of this approach is to produce and array large number of siRNA/shRNA, as well as the requirement of upfront investment in the infrastructure such as the liquid handling robots [64].

3.3 RNAi Barcode Screens

Another commonly used RNAi screening method uses pooled shRNA library and it is also known as RNAi barcode screens. shRNA libraries are mainly used in this pooled base assays and it is a promising approach to identify novel targets for cancer therapy.

The screening protocol is illustrated in Fig. 4. shRNA library is constructed and then packaged into retroviruses, which are used to infect target cells. Appropriate amounts of viruses are added to cells so that each cell, on average, contains a single integrated virus and each individual shRNA infects ~1000 cells. The shRNA expression cassette consists of two unique components, the shRNA sequence and a unique DNA sequence which is called barcode [62]. The barcode is designed to rapidly identify individual shRNA vector associated with a specific phenotype [65]. After infection, cells or clones which display a specific phenotype, such as resistance to a small molecular inhibitor, are isolated and shRNA sequences are identified using PCR and sequencing [58, 64]. By comparing barcode from cells treated in different conditions, researchers can assess the effects of a given individual shRNA on the cell's response to a specific treatment, subsequently the function of the related gene will be determined [63]. For example, to search for components of the p53 tumor-suppressor pathway Berns et al. constructed a large set of retroviral vectors encoding 23742 distinct shRNAs targeting 7914 different human genes. One known and five new modulators of the p53-dependent proliferation arrest were identified using colony formation assays. Inhibition of each of these five genes resulted in resistance to three different p53-depedent proliferation arrests, indicating them as the possible tumor suppressor genes [65]. All these studies highlighted the power of large-scale RNAi screen in identifying cancer-related genes in

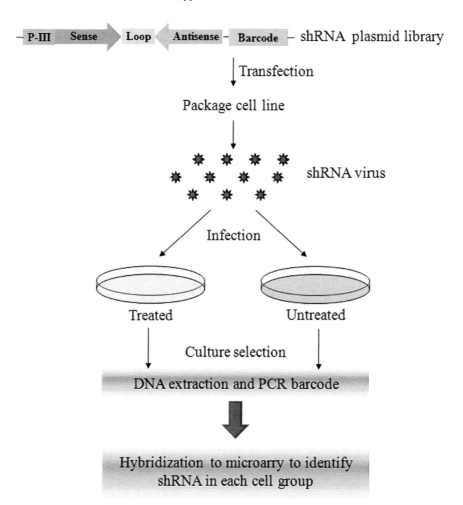

Fig. 4 siRNA barcode screen. First, plasmids encoding shRNA and barcode sequences are packaged into retroviruses which are used to infect cells at a concentration of 1 virus per cell. Cells are divided and treated with different culture conditions. DNA is then extracted from selected cells and the barcode is recovered by PCR. The abundance of each barcode can be determined by hybridization to a DNA microarray containing the complement of these sequences. Finally, the shRNA in each cell group will be identified

mammalian cells. However, the major limitation of this screening method is the difficulty in isolation of small number of cells exhibiting specific phenotype from a large cell population. Therefore, growth selection is commonly used to induce colony formation [64].

Bearing in mind the fact that the high-quality RNAi libraries have only become available recently and most groups are in the process of carrying out their exploratory studies, the large-scale RNAi library screen is still in its early stage [66].

4 siRNA Gene Targets Involved in Carcinogenesis

Cancer is fundamentally the unlimited and continuous growth of cells caused by the loss of normal cell behavior including proliferation, differentiation, and apoptosis [67]. It is essentially a genetic disease affected by three types of gene alterations: oncogene activation, tumor-suppressor gene suppression, and stability gene dysfunction [2]. Unlike other genetic diseases, wherein only one mutated gene can cause disease, cancer is usually caused by multiple gene alternations. Vogelstein et al. have summarized various cancer genes and related pathways in a comprehensive review [2]. Table 3 listed the genes which have been investigated for RNAi therapy of several common cancers including breast, prostate, and lung cancer.

4.1 Genes Involved in Tumorgenesis

Oncogene normally encodes positive signals for cell growth and division, whereas tumor-suppressor gene prevents cells to develop to cancer by inhibiting cell proliferation. Stability genes are responsible for keeping genetic alterations, which happens in normal cells, to a minimum level by different repairing mechanisms. Thus, when they are inactivated, mutations in normal genes will occur at a high rate resulting in high chance of tumorigenesis [2]. For the treatment of cancer, the oncogene level should be reduced while the tumor-suppressor gene and stability gene levels should be restored. Subsequently, oncogenes are the primary targets of RNAi-based cancer therapy. On the contrary, the application of RNAi in tumor-suppressor gene and stability gene is mainly focused on the identification or elucidation of the correlated mechanisms.

4.2 Genes Involved in Tumor–Host Interactions

Another important targets of RNAi therapy are genes involved in the tumor–host interactions. As neoplastic cells grow and spread within the host environment, there are several steps required, such as the new blood vessel formation (angiogenesis) to obtain sufficient oxygen and nutrients, breaking down of the extracellular matrix (ECM) to invade surrounding tissues and metastasize, and the improved motility of tumor cells and immune evasion [3, 68]. Particularly, the role of angiogenesis in tumor growth has been well recognized since Folkman hypothesized that the inhibition of angiogenesis could be an effective approach for treating cancer [69]. Tumor angiogenesis is controlled by the balance of numerous activators and inhibitors. Activators include VEGF, the transcription factor for hypoxia-inducible factor-1 (HIF-1α), and fibroblast growth factor (FGF). Among them, VEGF has been proved the key contributor to tumor angiogenesis and growth [70]. Although blocking VEGF or VEGF

Table 3 Genes investigated in the RNAi therapy for breast cancer, lung cancer, and prostate cancer

Cancer type	Target gene	Results	Model	References
Breast cancer	Brother of the regulator of imprinted sites (BORIS)	Induce apoptosis	MDA-MB-231 cell line and non-malignant epithelial cell lines	125
	Adenine nucleotide translocator 2(ANT2)	Induces apoptosis/inhibits tumor growth	MDA-MB-231 cell line/in vitro and in vivo	126
	Wilms tumor 1(WT1)	Inhibits tumor growth	MCF-7 cell line	127
	Wnt-1	Induces apoptosis	MCF-7 cell line	128
	Plasminogen activator inhibitor type I (PAI-1)		MDA-MB-231 cell line	129
	Cytoprotective factors	Enhance radiosensitivity	MCF-7 cell line	130
	Heparanase	Reduce invasion and adhesion in vitro; less vascularization and metastatic	MDA-MB-435 cell line and xenograft model	131
	Vascular endothelial growth factor (VEGF) gene	Induces apoptosis; inhibits tumor growth	MCF-7 cell line	132
	Integrin alpha(v)beta(3)	Increases radiosensitivity; induces apoptosis	MDA-MB-435 cell line	133
	Survivin	Induces apoptosis; suppresses cell proliferation	MCF-7 cell line	134
	Cyclin D1	Inhibits proliferation	MCF-7 cell line	135
	Urokinase plasminogen Activator (uPA) and uPA receptor	Decrease angiogenic potential	MDA-MB-231 cell line; ZR-75-1 cell line	136
	X-linked inhibitor of apoptosis (XIAP)	Suppresses tumor growth; induces apoptosis	MCF-7 cell line; xenograft model	137
	Human UDP-glucose dehydrogenase		ZR-75-1 cell line	138
	HER2/neu gene	Induces apoptosis; inhibits proliferation	SK-BR-3 cell line; BT-474 cell line; MCF-7 cell line; MDA-MB-468 cell line	139
	Epidermal growth factor (EGF) receptor	Inhibits tumor growth	MDA-MB-231 cell line; xenograft model	140
	Hdm2 oncogene	Inhibits tumor growth	MCF-7 xenografts	141

Table 3 (continued)

Cancer type	Target gene	Results	Model	References
Lung cancer	Cytochrome P450 1A1 (CYP1A1) and telomerase (hTERT)	Rapid cell death	A549 cell line	142
	Mutant K-ras gene	Induces apoptosis; inhibits tumor growth	H441 cells line	143
	MDM2 (murine double minute 2)	Enhances radiosensitivity	A549 cell line	144
	Type I insulin-like growth factor receptor (IGF-IR)	Induces apoptosis; inhibits tumor growth	A549 cell line; xenograft model	145
	Pituitary transforming gene (PTTG)	Inhibits tumor growth	H1299 cell line; xenograft model	146
	EGFR	Enhances chemosensitivity to gefitinib	Lung adenocarcinoma cell lines	147
	Akt	Enhances chemosensitivity to cisplatin	Non-small cell lung cancer (NSCLC) cells	148
	Heme oxygenase-1 (HO-1)	Enhances chemosensitivity to cisplatin	A549 cell line	149
	Class III beta-tubulin (betaIII-tubulin)	Enhances chemosensitivity to cisplatin	NCI-H460 cell line; Calu-6 cell line	150
	Fibroblast growth factor receptor 1 oncogene partner	Inhibits tumor growth	Lung cancer cells	151
	Cyclin A1	Induces apoptosis	H157 and H596 cell lines	152
	NBS1	Enhances radiosensitivity	H1299/wtp53 cell line; H1299/mp53 cell line	153
	Ganglioside GD3 synthase gene	Inhibits tumor growth; induces apoptosis	human lung cancer cells	154

Table 3 (continued)

Cancer type	Target gene	Results	Model	References
Prostate cancer	Androgen Receptor; androgen-regulated (PAR) gene	Inhibits tumor growth	Mice bearing exponentially growing castration-resistant tumors; LNCaP cell line; PC3 cell line	155
	Decoy receptor 2 (DcR2; TRAIL-R4)	Reduces tumorigenic potential	DU145 cell lines; LNCaP cell lines	156
	Midkine (MK)	Inhibits tumor growth	PC3 cell line; xenograft model	157
	Fatty acid synthase (FAS)	Inhibits tumor cell growth; induces apoptosis	Prostate tumor cells	158
	Signal transducer and activator of transcription (STAT)-3	Inhibits tumor cell growth; induces apoptosis	PC3 cell line; LNCaP cell line; xenograft model	159
	Signal transducer and activator of transcription (STAT)-6	Induce apoptosis; inhibit cell migration	DU145 cell line	160
	Polo-like kinase (Plk) 1	Induces apoptosis	LNCaP cell line; DU145 cell line; PC3 cell line	161
	MAT-8 gene	Inhibits tumor cell growth	LNCaP cell line; PC3 cell line	162
	Vinexinbeta	Enhances chemotherapy sensitization to paclitaxel	PC-3 cell line	163
	Metallothionein (MT)	Inhibits tumor cell growth; induces cell death	LNCaP cell line; PC-3 cell line	164
	Acid ceramidase (AC)	Inhibits tumor growth; enhances chemotherapy sensitization	DU145 cell line; xenograft model	165
	Urokinase plasminogen activator (uPA) promoter	Dramatic reduction of tumor cell invasion and angiogenesis in vitro; inhibits tumor growth	PC3 cell line; DU145 cell line; metastasis model	166
	Akt kinase	Enhances chemotherapy sensitization to paclitaxel	DU-145 cell line	167
	Heat-shock protein 27 (Hsp27)	Enhances chemotherapy sensitization	LNCaP cell line; PC-3 cell line	168

receptor inhibits essential pathways involved in tumor progression and metastasis, anti-VEGF siRNA showed more effective anti-angiogenesis effect than siRNA targeting VEGF receptor [70].

5 Nonviral Delivery Systems for siRNA

The crucial challenge of in vivo application of RNAi therapy is developing efficient delivery system to transport the siRNA into the tissue and finally into the cytoplasm or shRNA into the nucleus of target cells [4]. Several studies have demonstrated efficient delivery of siRNA in vivo as well as its therapeutic effect in animal model. Recently in 2008, FDA approved the first clinical study using targeted cyclodextrin-containing nanoparticle for the systemic delivery of an anti-cancer siRNA, RONDEL^{TM}, developed by Calando Pharmaceutical Inc.

Although there are several reports of local delivery of naked siRNA into eye, lung, or other tissues without employing any carriers [71], it is not the preferred administration route for most RNAi cancer therapies. The large molecular weight and negative charges are two major obstacles which hinder the systemic delivery of naked siRNA. A series of carriers, including cationic lipids, peptides, synthetic or biodegradable polymers have been developed to enhance the cross-membrane capability of siRNA. Although plasmid DNA (pDNA) and siRNA have similar composition and identical negative charges/nucleotide ratio, they condense into different structures with cationic lipid/polymer, due to their difference in the molecular weight and molecular topography. siRNA alone cannot be efficiently condensed into particles of nanometric dimensions while all pDNA can be condensed into nanoparticles of 60–100 nm when it is complexed with catiomic lipid [72]. Unlike pDNA, the electrostatic interaction between siRNA and cationic lipid is relatively uncontrolled and the encapsulation of siRNA is therefore incomplete [72]. Since plasmid-based shRNA shares the same properties with pDNA in classic gene therapy, the same delivery strategies developed before for pDNA can also be used for shRNA. In this chapter we will focus on the nonviral delivery systems for synthetic siRNA, which has a very different structure and properties from the previously investigated pDNA.

5.1 Components of the Delivery System for siRNA

Generally, an efficient siRNA delivery system should contain the following components: a cationic group, an endosomal disrupting group, and a tumor-specific ligand. To neutralize the negatively charged siRNA, cationic lipid or polymer is commonly used in all siRNA delivery systems [73]. The complexation can induce endocytosis by charge-mediated interaction with negative charges on the cell membrane surface. After entering the cytoplasm, the anti-cancer efficacy of siRNA will not display unless it is released from the endosome and silence the target mRNA. For this reason, fusogenic agents that can disrupt the endosome are generally required for the delivery system. Nonspecific delivery of therapeutics to normal cells and subsequent side effects is the major hurdle for all cancer therapies. Many unique receptors or antigens overexpressed on the surface of cancer cells provide good targets to design tumor-targeted delivery systems. Coupling tumor-specific ligands to the carrier surface can trigger specific cells internalization of siRNA via ligand–receptor binding interaction.

Figure 5 is the schematic diagram for a typical siRNA delivery system. In this system, siRNA are entrapped inside or condensed with the cationic materials (lipids, polymer, or peptides). Tumor-specific ligands (antibody, antibody fragments, peptides) are conjugated directly on the surface of the system or linked through flexible hydrophilic polymers, like PEG. For some polymer carriers, such as PEI and PAMAM dendrimers, endosomal release can be achieved without addition of the endosome disrupting agent due to their own special "proton-sponge" mechanism endorsed by their instinct secondary and tertiary amine structures [74]. However, for other polymers, such as PLL, the endosomal release agent is necessary in order to deliver siRNA efficiently into cytoplasm.

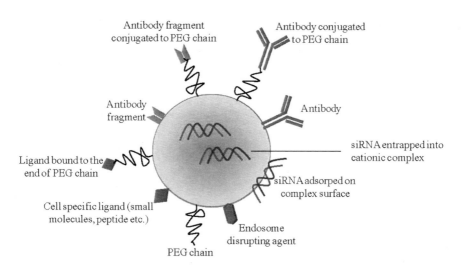

Fig. 5 Schematic diagram of the siRNA delivery system. A cationic group is universal in all siRNA delivery systems to condense siRNA into nanosized complex. To release the siRNA from the endosome after endocytosis, an endosomal disrupting agent is also essential. PEG modification is also important to improve the pharmacokinetic profile of the complex, as well as to avoid the nonspecific uptake by RES. To achieve the targeted delivery to tumor cells, various ligands including antibody, antibody fragments, peptides, small molecules should be modified to the complex directly or via PEG as a linker

5.2 Cationic Lipids and Polymers

5.2.1 Cationic Lipid

Since the first introduction in 1987 for pDNA transfection, numerous cationic lipids have been developed for in vitro and in vivo delivery of nucleic acids, including siRNA recently [75]. Cationic lipid is currently the most common carrier to deliver siRNA into mammalian cells because it is technically simple, easy to formulate, and can be conjugated for specific applications [76]. Many commercial cationic liposomes (such as lipofectamine, oligofectamine, and RNAifect) are available for the in vitro transfection of siRNA. Generally, the cationic liposome is formulated by the mixture of cationic lipid, neutral helper lipid, and cholesterol at different ratios. Cationic lipid is a positively charged amphiphile system composed of a cationic head group and a lipid hydrophobic moiety. The cationic headgroup is a very important factor for the transfection efficiency. Mével M. et al. have synthesized a series of cationic lipids containing different headgroups including arginine methyl ester, lysine methyl ester, homo-arginine methyl ester, ethylenediamine, guanidinium, diaminopropane, and imidazolium. The transfection efficiency of these lipids, alone or with the colipid DOPE (L-alpha-Dioleoyl phosphatidylethanolamine), were evaluated in HEK293-T7 cells. The cationic lipid with imidazolium headgroup/DOPE lipoplex was proved to be the most efficient transfection reagent with low toxicity [77].

Based on the differences of their structure characteristics, cationic lipids can be classified into three groups: (i) monovalent aliphatic lipids which have a single amine function in the head group, e.g., N-[1-(2,3-dioleyloxy)propyl]-N,N,N-trimethylammonium chloride (DOTMA) and N-[1-(2,3-dioleoyloxy)propyl]-N,N,N-trimethylammonium chloride (DOTAP); (ii) multivalent aliphatic lipids containing more than one amine function in the head group, e.g., dioctadecyla-midoglycylspermine (DOGS); and (iii) cationic cholesterol derivatives, e.g., 3beta-[N-(N′,N′-dimethylaminoethane)-carbamoyl] cholesterol (DC-Chol) [76].

5.2.2 Poly(ethyleneimine)

Poly(ethyleneimine) (PEI) is a series of synthetic polymers in branched or linear form with different molecular weights, ranging from 1 kDa to more than 1000 kDa [78]. It is well known as an efficient cationic polymer to introduce nucleic acids into mammalian cells. Its high cationic charge density can condense and compact pDNA into nanosized complex. In addition, the buffering capacity of PEI allows the nucleic acid to escape from the endosome through the "proton-sponge" effect [79]. The transfection efficiency of PEI is affected by the properties including molecular weight, degree of branching, branched or linear, and functionalized group modification. Generally, low molecular weight with branched architecture shows higher transfection efficiency and less cytotoxicity [78]. A novel low-molecular weight PEI, F25-LMW PEI, was obtained by fractionation of a commercially available 25-kDa PEI using size exclusion chromatography. Compared to the 25-kDa PEI, F25-LMW PEI showed higher transfection efficiency of siRNA with low toxicity in various cell lines and in the presence of serum, suggesting its potential in in vivo application [80, 81].

In addition, numerous modifications have been carried out in PEI to enhance the transfection efficiency and decrease the cytotoxicity. PEI was modified with different degrees of PEG substitution and the in vitro transfection efficiency was evaluated for siRNA and pDNA. The transfection efficiency of siRNA/PEG-PEI complex was much less dependent on the PEGylation of PEI or on the N/P (PEI nitrogen/nucleic acid phosphate) ratio, which was critical for pDNA delivery [82]. PEGylation of PEI can improve the stability of siRNA complex against RNase digestion and heparin displacement. Both chain length and graft density of PEG strongly affect the stability and silencing efficiency of siRNA [83]. PEI was also modified by ketalization of the branches and ketalized PEI efficiently compacted siRNA into polyplexes with 80–200 nm in diameter. In vitro study demonstrated that the ketalization not only enhanced the transfection efficiency of siRNA but also reduced the cytotoxicity [84]. In order to achieve targeted delivery of siRNA to tumor cells, tumor-specific ligands, such as RGD and folate, have been conjugated to PEI using PEG as a linker [85, 86].

5.2.3 Chitosan

Chitosan is a natural, biodegradable linear amino polysaccharide composed of N-acetyl-D-glucosamine and d-glucosamine subunits. Due to its low toxicity, low immunogenicity, and excellent biocompatibility, chitosan has been widely utilized as a delivery carrier for protein, peptide, pDNA, and siRNA. The physico-chemical properties of chitosan/DNA complex depend on the type, molecular weight, and deacetylation degree of the chitosan [76]. It can compact DNA into small particles (200–500 nm) due to its cationic polyelectrolyte nature. To explore the application of chitosan in siRNA delivery, Katas et al. prepared chitosan/siRNA complex using two ionic cross-linking methods: simple complexation and ionic gelation using sodium tripolyphosphate (TPP) [87]. Both methods formed nanosized particles less than 500 nm and the silencing effect was evaluated in CHO K1 and HEK293 cells. The association of siRNA with chitosan is a key factor for its silencing effect. Due to the high-binding capacity and loading efficiency, entrapping siRNA in the chitosan–TPP complex using ionic gelation method showed better effect than the simple chitosan/siRNA complexation [87]. Besides the preparation method, molecular weight and deacetylation degree of chitosan also affect the silencing effect of siRNA [88]. Low-molecular weight (~10 kDa) chitosan showed little knockdown effect of target gene, while the highest silencing effect was achieved by the chitosan with high molecular weight (114 and 170 kDa) and high degree of deacetylation (84%), which formed a stable complex of ~200 nm [88].

de Martimprey et al. have developed a novel chitosan coated nanoparticle for the delivery of siRNA against Ret/PTC1 junction oncogene. The coated chitosan provides a strong electrostatic interaction with siRNA, while the core is composed of a biodegradable polymer, poly(isobutylcyanoacrylate). Complex formation with the nanoparticles protected the Ret/PTC1 siRNA from in vivo degradation and the siRNA complex significantly inhibited the tumor growth after intratumoral administration [89]. Another novel chitosan-based siRNA nanoparticle was developed by Howard et al. [90]. Nanoparticles sized from 40 to 600 nm were rapidly uptaken into NIH 3T3 cells within 1 h, followed by accumulation over 24 h. The siRNA nanoparticles knocked down endogenous enhanced green fluorescent protein (EGFP) gene expression in H1299 human lung carcinoma cells and murine peritoneal macrophages. In addition, effective in vivo silencing was demonstrated in bronchiole epithelial cells of transgenic mice after nasal administration of the siRNA/chitosan nanoparticles [90].

5.2.4 Dendrimer

Dendrimer is a highly branched polymer with three-dimensional structures synthesized using divergent or convergent method. The architecture of dendrimer generally consists of three regions: the core; the interior branches composed of tertiary amine groups which play a critical role in the endosomal releasing of dendrimer; and the periphery which includes many terminal function groups [91]. It has been extensively studied for the delivery of nucleic acid because the molecular weight, molecular size, and shape can be precisely controlled [78]. The primary amine groups of dendrimer condense and compact DNA into nanosized particles, while the internal tertiary amino groups act as proton-sponge in the endosome.

Polyamidoamine (PAMAM) is the most commonly used and commercially available dendrimer and its potential application as an siRNA carrier has been explored. The PAMAM/siRNA complex is affected by the siRNA molecular weight, dendrimer generation, and charge ratio between PAMAM and siRNA. High generation, large charge ratio, and large siRNA tend to form stable, uniform complex in nanosize. The effect of PAMAM on siRNA delivery is somewhat contradictory since unmodified PAMAM did not show any promising effect in siRNA delivery, but modified PAMAM did enhance siRNA delivery [92, 93]. Juliano et al. conjugated the Tat peptide, a cell-penetrating peptide, to PAMAM G5 dendrimer and formed complexes with antisense oligonucleotide and siRNA separately. The bioactivity was evaluated in NIH 3T3 MDR cells. The PAMAM complex only showed moderate effect for the delivery of antisense oligonucleotide, but not the siRNA [94]. In another approach, PAMAM dendrimer(G3) was conjugated with α-cyclodextrin and then utilized as an siRNA carrier. The complexes can significantly silence the target mRNA in NIH3T3 cells in the presence of serum. Intercellular distribution studies showed that the carrier allowed siRNA to distribute in the cytoplasm [92]. Furthermore, an internally quaternized and surface-acetylated

PAMAM (QPAMAM-NHAc) was developed for the delivery of siRNA. Surface modification of the amino groups to amide significantly decrease PAMAM's toxicity. Enhanced cellular uptake and homogeneous cytoplasm distribution of siRNA after complexation with QPAMAM-NHAc was observed by confocal microscopy [93].

5.3 Cell-Penetrating Peptide

Cell-penetrating peptide (CPP) is a short sequence of amino acids (less than 20 amino acid) that are capable of carrying active molecule to cross the plasma membrane and enter the cytoplasm of mammalian cells. Based on its composition, the CPP is divided into two categories: the amphiphathic helical peptides, such as transportan and model amphipathic peptide (MAP); and the arginine rich peptides, such as Tat (48-60) [95]. CPP has been widely used to deliver numerous biological or non-biological cargos including protein, nucleic acid, antibody, imaging agent, and liposomes into cells [95].

Recently, CPPs have been utilized to improve the delivery of siRNA into mammalian cells both in vitro and in vivo. Two different CPPs, penetratin and transportan, have been conjugated to the 5′ end of siRNA via disulfide bond. The CPP–siRNA conjugates efficiently reduced the expression of reporter gene in cells [96]. In another study, siRNA targeting p38MAPK (mitogen-activated protein kinase) was conjugated to two CPPs, Tat (48-60) and penetratin, respectively. As shown in Fig. 6, both the Tat (48-46) and penetratin–siRNA

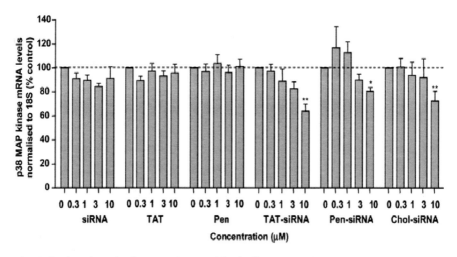

Fig. 6 Conjugation of cell-penetrating peptides facilitates siRNA-mediated p38 MAP kinase silencing without transfection reagents. L929 cells were incubated for 24 h with siRNA in the absence of Lipofectamine-2000. p38 MAP kinase mRNA levels were determined using RT-PCR and normalized to 18s (**$P<0.01$; *$P<0.05$). (Adopted from *Bioconjugate Chemistry* 2007; 18:1450–1459)

conjugates knocked down about 40% of the p38MAPK gene expression at high concentration of 10 μM in in vitro transfection, whereas unconjugated siRNA did not show silencing effect at the concentration of 0.3–10 μM. However, the silencing effect of the CPP conjugated siRNA was not observed in mice by i.t. instillation [38].

In addition to Tat (48-60) and penetratin, another short amphipathic peptide, MPG, was applied to deliver siRNA into cultured cells [97]. Contrary to Tat (48-60) and penetratin, MPG was utilized to form stable complexes with siRNA rather than covalently conjugated to siRNA. MPG peptide can form nanoparticles with siRNA rapidly through electrostatic interactions and peptide–peptide interaction [97]. It has been successfully applied in an in vivo delivery of Oct-3/4 siRNA into mouse blastocytes. It forms stable nanoparticles with siRNA and protects siRNA from degradation [98].

5.4 Cyclodextrin

Cyclodextrin has been extensively used to increase the solubility of hydrophobic drug in pharmaceutical industry for many years. In the mid-1990s, some groups began to design cyclodextrin-containing cationic polymer for gene delivery due to its low toxicity and little immune responses. Numerous cationic cyclodextrin polymers have been synthesized through grafting cyclodextrin to other cationic polymers including chitosan, PEI, and dendrimer [99]. Recently, cyclodextrin polycation systems were also utilized for siRNA delivery. In 2008, a targeted nanoparticle consisting of PEG and cationic cyclodextrin was approved by FDA for a phase I clinical trial of a systemic siRNA therapy.

Davis et al. have developed a cyclodextrin-containing cationic carrier to condense siRNA to colloidal particles of 50 nm in diameter (Fig. 7). The carrier protects siRNA from degradation and the surface modified PEG stabilizes the siRNA complex in biological fluids. In addition, some PEG molecules were linked to a tumor-specific ligand, transferrin, to achieve the in vivo tumor-targeted delivery. Systemic administration of EWS-FL11 siRNA using the novel carrier significantly inhibited tumor growth in a murine model of metastatic Ewing's sarcoma [100]. Furthermore, they evaluated safety of the same system in cynomolgus monkeys after multiple, systemic administration of siRNA. The system is well tolerated at doses of 3 and 9 mg siRNA/kg and no system-specific antibody response was detected after multiple injections. Only mild immune response was observed at a very high dose, 27 mg siRNA/kg [101]. These results provided strong evidence for the safety and efficacy of the cyclodextrin-containing carrier for siRNA delivery.

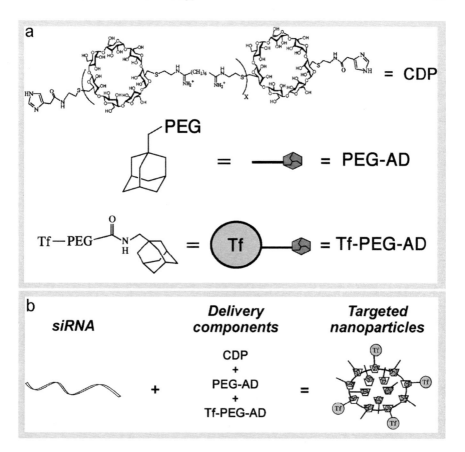

Fig. 7 Schematic diagram of the cyclodextrin-containing delivery system. (**a**) Components of the delivery system. The CDP condenses siRNA and protects it from degradation. The AD-PEG stabilizes the complexes in systemic circulation via inclusion compound formation. The AD-PEG-transferrin (Tf-PEG-AD) conjugate confers a targeting ligand to the complex. (**b**) Assembly of the targeted delivery systems. CDP, AD-PEG, and Tf-PEG-AD are combined and added to siRNA to generate stable complex. (Adopted from *Cancer Research* 2005; 65: 8984–8992)

5.5 Atelocollagen

Atelocollagen is a highly purified, pepsin treated type I collagen with low immunogenicity and positive charge. It has been widely used in wound-healing, vessel prosthesis, and as bone cartilage substitute and hemostatic agent [102]. Atelocollagen can form complex with siRNA as nanosized particles with a diameter of 100–300 nm. The complex provides nuclease resistance, efficient cellular uptake, prolonged release, and increased in vivo half-life for siRNA [103]. Since atelocollagen is a liquid at 4°C and becomes gel at 37°C, it can be used as a site-specific in vivo delivery system for nucleic acid including siRNA [104]. In an in vivo study with site-specific administration, VEGF siRNA with atelocollagen efficiently suppressed tumor growth and tumor angiogenesis in a prostate cancer xenograft model [104]. Similar silencing effect was also observed in an orthotopic xenograft model of human testicular cancer using site-specific in vivo administration of siRNA/atelocollagen complex [103]. Moreover, atelocollagen can be used for systemic siRNA delivery. After i.v. injection, siRNA/atelocollagen complex was delivered to tumors within 24 h and stayed intact for 3 days. Accordingly, the delivered siRNA showed significant reduction of target gene expression in bone-metastatic prostate tumor cells [105].

6 Ligand-Targeted Delivery of siRNA to Tumor Cells

To develop an efficient siRNA cancer therapy, targeted delivery of siRNA to tumor cells is the primary requisite to overcome nonspecific side effects, as well as increase the therapeutic effect. Most cancer cells express unique or over-expressed receptors/antigens on their cell surface which can bind various ligands including antibodies, antibody fragments, small molecules, peptides, and aptamers. A number of tumor-specific ligands have been modified to the siRNA delivery system to enhance the specific cellular uptake in tumor cells. The most commonly used ligands are described below.

6.1 Antibodies

Antibody is a fundamental substance in immune response and it is composed of a pair of heavy chains and a pair of light chains. The variable regions of antibody can recognize and bind to specific epitope of antigen in a high affinity [106]. In the past decades, monoclonal antibody-mediated targeted delivery has spurred great attention in cancer therapy and the intact monoclonal antibody has been used for the targeted delivery of various therapeutics including nucleic acids [107]. However, the large size of intact antibody molecule (Mw 159 kDa) limits its application to some extent. Alternatively, antibody fragments were successfully exploited as ligands for targeted drug delivery to tumor cells because they have a small molecular weight and remain the same binding specificity as the parent antibody with low immunogenicity [106, 108]. The most frequently used antibody fragments are $F(ab')_2$, Fab' and single-chain Fv fragment (scFv), all of which lack the Fc domain and the complement-activating region. Both Fab' and scFv have only one binding region, while $F(ab')_2$, which consisted of two Fab' linked by a disulphide bond, is bivalent and thus have higher binding affinity than Fab' and scFv [108]. Compared to intact antibody, antibody fragments have several advantages: (i) antibody fragments avoid the possibility of binding with non-target cells caused by the interaction of Fc domain with Fc receptor in normal cells; (ii) the size of antibody fragments are much smaller than that of entire antibody, thus the tissue penetration will be improved; (iii) the cost and manufacture time of antibody fragments are lower than that of the whole antibody because antibody fragments can be easily produced in bacteria in a large scale [106].

In 2005, Song et al. evaluated the first in vivo study of an antibody-mediated siRNA delivery system [39]. A Fab antibody fragment (F105) against HIV-1 envelope was fused to protamine and the fusion protein (F-105P) was able to deliver siRNA only into cells expressing HIV-1 envelope. Systemic administration of F-105P/siRNA complex into mice delivered siRNA into HIV-1 expressing tumors, but not the HIV-1 negative tumors and other normal cells. Administration of F105-P with siRNAs targeting oncogenes including c-my, MDM2, and VEGF inhibited the growth of HIV-1 expressing tumor cells. Furthermore, the authors fused Her-2 scFv with protamine and it could deliver siRNA specifically to the Her-2 expressing tumor cells in a breast cancer xenograft model in vivo [39].

Instead of designing antibody fusion protein, immunoliposome prepared with antibody-conjugated cationic lipid is another approach for siRNA delivery. After complexing with immunoliposome, siRNA can be specifically delivered into tumor cells [109, 110]. Antibody or antibody fragment can be conjugated to the surface of cationic liposome or to the terminus of polyethylene glycol (PEG), which is grafted on the surface of liposome. For example, scFV can be covalently coupled to liposome via a reaction between cysteine at the 3'-end of the protein and a maleimide group on the liposome. The modification does not affect the immunological activity and targeting ability of the scFv [111].

Pirollo et al. developed a nanoimmunoliposome modified with anti-TfR scFV to deliver siRNA to tumor cells. A fluorescein-labeled siRNA was delivered via systemic injection and it was specifically distributed into primary and metastatic tumor cells [110]. Later, the authors developed a similar nanoimmunoliposome for an anti-Her-2 siRNA. To enhance the endosomal release, a pH-sensitive histidine–lysine peptide was included in the complex. The in vitro results showed that the complexes can sensitize human cancer cells to chemotherapeutics. Furthermore, systemic delivery of the siRNA significantly inhibit tumor growth in a pancreatic cancer model [109].

6.2 Transferrin

Transferrin is a very common ligand used to target tumor cells. It is an 80 kDa monomeric glycoprotein which can form complex with ferric ion and facilitate the cellular uptake of iron through binding with transferrin receptor (TfR). Through a circle of endocytosis and exocytosis of transferrin meditated by TfR, the iron was delivered into the cells [112]. TfR is a transmembrane glycoprotein consisting of two subunits linked by a disulfide bond and each of the monomer binds one transferrin molecule. The X-ray crystal structure studies revealed that the TfR is composed of three parts: an NH_2-terminal cytoplasmic region containing internalization motif Tyr-Thr-Arg-Phe, a transmembrane region, and a large extracellular domain which contains binding site for transferrin [113]. TfR is widely expressed in human body, including red blood cells, thyroid cells, hepatocytes, intestinal cells, brain, and the blood–brain barrier. However, there are overexpression of TfR on the surface of tumor cells since high level of iron is essential for the tumor growth [113]. Therefore, transferrin is widely used as a targeting ligand in the targeted delivery of antitumor agents including nucleic acids and proteins to tumor cells with high TfR expression. Generally, the transferrin is directly conjugated to anti-cancer drug or to the surface of delivery vehicles, such as liposome, nanoparticle, and complex [100, 113–115]. In an in vitro study, cationic liposomes associated with transferrin were complexed with siRNA at different lipid/siRNA ratios. Transferrin modified liposome efficiently delivered siRNA into cells via endocytosis [115].

Bartllet et al. designed a transferrin modified nanoparticle to deliver siRNA targeting ribonucleotide reductase subunit M2 (RRM2) to tumors. After intravenous administration of the transferrin modified nanoparticles at a dose of 2.5 mg siRNA/kg for three consecutive days, significant inhibition of tumor growth was observed in the A/J mice bearing Neuro2A tumors, whereas the unmodified nanoparticles formulation showed much less effect [116]. Furthermore, they employed positron emission tomography (PET)/computer tomography (CT) to study the whole-body biodistribution profiles and localization of siRNA in the tumor site. Simultaneously, they measure the gene knockdown effect of siRNA using bioluminescent imaging (BLI) in the mice bearing luciferase-expressing Neuro2A tumors. Transferrin modified nanoparticles reduced tumor luciferase activity by 50% compared to unmodified nanoparticles. However, both nanoparticles showed similar pharmacokinetic profiles and tumor localization. Compartmental modeling suggested that the major advantage of the targeted nanoparticles was the increased cellular uptake in tumor cells rather than the overall localization at tumor site [114].

A similar TfR-meditated delivery system was applied to deliver siRNA-targeting EWS-FLI1 gene in a murine model of metastatic Ewing's sarcoma. Systemic treatments of TfR-targeted siRNA formulation significantly inhibited the engraftment of TC71-LUC cells, while elimination of the anti-cancer effects was observed when removing transferrin from the delivery system [100].

6.3 Folic Acid

Folate receptor has been intensively studied as a target for tumor-specific drug delivery because it has a limited distribution in normal tissues, but a significant overexpression on a series of malignant tumors including carcinoma of ovary, breast, kidney, brain, endometrium, colon, and hematopoietic cells of myelogenous origin [117]. Folate receptor is represented by a family of glycopolypeptides including four isoforms: FR-α, β, γ, and δ. Both FR-α and FR-β are membrane-associated proteins which are attached to the plasma membrane by glycosyl phosphatidylinositol (GPI) anchor [118]. Folic acid, a necessary vitamin for the body, has a high affinity for folate receptor ($K_d = 10^{-10}$ M), even after bioconjugation with therapeutic drugs. For this reason, folic acid has been exploited as a ligand for tumor targeting via conjugation to numerous chemotherapeutic agents, liposomes, and imaging agents [119].

Zhang et al. conjugated folic acid to the 5′-end of a 17 nt oligodeoxynucleotide (ODN). Subsequently, siRNAs targeting αV integrin gene were tethered to the folic acid–ODN conjugate through base pair interaction between a 15 nt "hook-like structure" of the ODN and a "complimentary hook" sequence at the 3′-end extension of the siNRA's sense strand. After treating with folate–ODN/siRNA complex, about 80% inhibition of the αV integrin mRNA was observed in HUVEC cells. It is concluded that the delivery process was folate receptor mediated since the siRNA/ODN complex without folate conjugation failed to show any silencing effect [117].

6.4 Arginine-Glycine-Aspartic Acid (RGD) Peptide

RGD peptide is a popular tool for the targeted delivery of therapeutic agents to $\alpha_v\beta_3$ integrin, which is a type of cell surface receptor distributing in tumor neovasculature, melanoma, and glioblastoma. Each year, a number of RGD peptides have been developed based on the module of "arginine-glycine-aspartic acid" sequence. It was found that all the RGD–peptide ligands are cyclic and have at least one ring structure [120]. RGD peptides were widely exploited in the targeted drug delivery, imaging agent and nucleic acids via conjugating multiple RGD peptides with carrier systems like liposomes or nanoparticles. Self-assembling nanoparticles constructed by RGD–PEG–PEI has been prepared to deliver siRNA targeting vascular endothelial growth factor receptor-2 (VEGF R2) to angiogenic vasculature in neuroblastoma N2A tumor-bearing mice [121]. After systemic administration, the siRNA nanoparticles was selectively uptaken by tumor cells and inhibited tumor angiogenesis and growth [121].

6.5 Aptamer

Aptamer is a globular-shaped oligonucleotide that is identified by the systematic evolution of ligands by exponential enrichment (SELEX) process. It has the similar composition as natural nucleic acid, but the nucleotides of aptamer have 2′-modified sugars to enhance the nuclease resistance [122]. Since its discovery in 1990, aptamer has become a valuable research tool. Aptamers can specifically bind to target protein with high affinity, therefore it can be utilized in the targeted delivery of siRNA [37, 123]. For example, prostate-specific membrane antigen (PSMA) is a type II protein synthesized by prostatic epithelium and it is overexpressed in the most advanced androgen-resistant prostate cancer cells. PSMA is believed to be an ideal target for the targeted drug delivery systems to prostate cancer [124]. McNamara et al. have developed a PSMA aptamer–siRNA chimeras to deliver functional siRNA into prostate cancer cells. The aptamer portion of the chimeras guided siRNA to prostate tumor cells and then the siRNA silenced the target gene. Significant inhibition of tumor growth was observed in a mouse xenograft model bearing PSMA-positive prostate cancer cells, LNCaP, after treatment with the aptamer–siRNA chimeras (Fig. 8b).

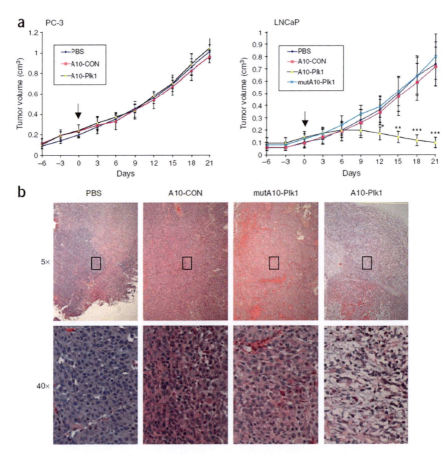

Fig. 8 Antitumor activity of aptamer–siRNA chimera in a mouse xenograft model of prostate cancer. (**a**) Chimeric siRNA and PBS were administered intratumorally in mice bearing either PSMA-negative prostate cancer cells, PC-3 (*left panel*) or PSMA-positive cells, LNCaP (*right panel*). Tumors were measured every 3 days and analyzed using a one-way ANOVA (***$P<0.0001$; **$P<0.001$; *$P<0.01$, $n=$ 6–8). (**b**) Histology of LNCaP tumors treated with chimeric RNAs. Formalin-fixed tumors were embedded in paraffin and stained with hematoxylin and eosin. (Adopted from *Nature Biotechnology* 2006; 24: 1005–1015)

However, the antitumor effect was not observed in mouse xenograft model bearing PSMA-negative prostate cancer cells (Fig. 8a), PC-3, indicating that the antitumor effect of the siRNA chimeras was mediated by the recognition of aptamer to PSMA [123]. In a similar study, PSMA aptamer was conjugated to siRNA via a streptavidin linker. The aptamer–siRNA conjugates can be uptaken by cells and mediate specific silencing effect without the help of cationic lipids [37].

7 Perspectives

As one of the most exciting discoveries in the last decade, RNAi has exhibited the greatest potential for treating cancer, one of the most devastating diseases. siRNA can be used for large-scale screening to identify cancer-related genes, or it can be used directly as a therapeutics to silence specific genes which are involved in the tumor growth and differentiation. Since its discovery in 1998, RNAi technology has moved remarkably toward therapeutic application and there are already 12 ongoing RNAi clinical trials .

Compared to 66.5% of gene therapy clinical trials aiming at the treatment of cancer, only 2 of the 12 siRNA clinical trials are designed for cancer therapy, indicating the siRNA cancer therapy is still in its infancy. Same as the therapeutic application of pDNA, the major bottleneck for a successful siRNA therapy is the efficient delivery. Scientists have gained extensive experiences in the delivery of pDNA and these experiences can be utilized for the delivery of plasmid-based shRNA. However, the same experience cannot be transferred to siRNA directly since siRNA is very different from pDNA in terms of the molecular weight, molecular topography, and in vivo stability. In addition, compared to pDNA, siRNA is more difficult to be condensed into nanosized complex. Nevertheless, many nonviral vectors have been developed for siRNA delivery and one of them was recently approved for phase I clinical trial.

Generally, in order to develop an effective siRNA drug for cancer therapy, there are three primary requirements: (i) targeted delivery of siRNA to the tumor site in the body, (ii) passage of the siRNA through cell membrane, and (iii) targeting at a specific gene which is crucial in the tumorgenesis. For the targeted delivery, numerous ligands have been employed on the surface of the siRNA delivery system. The most promising ligands are antibody fragments, aptamers, and peptide which can bind to specific antigen on the tumor cell surface. In addition, PEG surface modification is necessary to overcome the pharmacokinetic problems associated with cationic complexes, such as the nonspecific protein binding and uptake by the reticuloendothelial system (RES). Furthermore, all siRNA delivery system should contain a cationic group to condense siRNA into nanosized particles, as well as to enhance the cellular uptake. Specificity of siRNA is another important issue in its therapeutic application since many siRNAs can induce off-target effects and nonspecific immunoresponses. Careful designing and backbone modification have been proved to be the best approaches to address these limitations.

In summary, we should look forward to successful clinical reports of siRNA cancer therapies and results from ongoing clinical trials will help us in further understanding and developing siRNA-based therapeutics against cancer in the near future.

References

1. Cheng K, Mahato RI. Gene modulation for treating liver fibrosis. *Crit Rev Ther Drug Carrier Syst* 2007; **24**: 93–146.
2. Vogelstein B, Kinzler KW. Cancer genes and the pathways they control. *Nat Med* 2004; **10**: 789–799.
3. Masiero M, Nardo G, Indraccolo S, Favaro E. RNA interference: implications for cancer treatment. *Mol Aspects Med* 2007; **28**: 143–166.
4. Takeshita F, Ochiya T. Therapeutic potential of RNA interference against cancer. *Cancer Sci* 2006; **97**: 689–696.
5. Cejka D, Losert D, Wacheck V. Short interfering RNA (siRNA): tool or therapeutic? *Clin Sci (Lond)* 2006; **110**: 47–58.
6. Edelstein ML, Abedi MR, Wixon J. Gene therapy clinical trials worldwide to 2007 – an update. *J Gene Med* 2007; **9**: 833–842.
7. Fuchs U, Borkhardt A. The application of siRNA technology to cancer biology discovery. *Adv Cancer Res* 2007; **96**: 75–102.
8. Nykanen A, Haley B, Zamore PD. ATP requirements and small interfering RNA structure in the RNA interference pathway. *Cell* 2001; **107**: 309–321.
9. Dykxhoorn DM, Novina CD, Sharp PA. Killing the messenger: short RNAs that silence gene expression. *Nat Rev Mol Cell Biol* 2003; **4**: 457–467.
10. Schwarz DS, Hutvagner G, Du T, Xu Z, Aronin N, Zamore PD. Asymmetry in the assembly of the RNAi enzyme complex. *Cell* 2003; **115**: 199–208.
11. Mahato RI, Cheng K, Guntaka RV. Modulation of gene expression by antisense and antigene oligodeoxynucleotides and small interfering RNA. *Expert Opin Drug Deliv* 2005; **2**: 3–28.
12. Reynolds A, Leake D, Boese Q, Scaringe S, Marshall WS, Khvorova A. Rational siRNA design for RNA interference. *Nat Biotechnol* 2004; **22**: 326–330.
13. Ui-Tei K, Naito Y, Takahashi F, Haraguchi T, Ohki-Hamazaki H, Juni A, et al. Guidelines for the selection of highly effective siRNA sequences for mammalian and chick RNA interference. *Nucleic Acids Res* 2004; **32**: 936–948.
14. Milhavet O, Gary DS, Mattson MP. RNA interference in biology and medicine. *Pharmacol Rev* 2003; **55**: 629–648.
15. Naito Y, Yamada T, Ui-Tei K, Morishita S, Saigo K. siDirect: highly effective, target-specific siRNA design software for mammalian RNA interference. *Nucleic Acids Res* 2004; **32**: W124–W129.
16. Amarzguioui M, Lundberg P, Cantin E, Hagstrom J, Behlke MA, Rossi JJ. Rational design and in vitro and in vivo delivery of Dicer substrate siRNA. *Nat Protoc* 2006; **1**: 508–517.
17. Sanguino A, Lopez-Berestein G, Sood AK. Strategies for in vivo siRNA delivery in cancer. *Mini Rev Med Chem* 2008; **8**: 248–255.
18. Matveeva O, Nechipurenko Y, Rossi L, Moore B, Saetrom P, Ogurtsov AY, et al. Comparison of approaches for rational siRNA design leading to a new efficient and transparent method. *Nucleic Acids Res* 2007; **35**: e63.

19. Tafer H, Ameres SL, Obernosterer G, Gebeshuber CA, Schroeder R, Martinez J, et al. The impact of target site accessibility on the design of effective siRNAs. *Nat Biotechnol* 2008; **26**: 578–583.
20. Zeng Y, Cullen BR. RNA interference in human cells is restricted to the cytoplasm. *RNA* 2002; **8**: 855–860.
21. Aagaard L, Rossi JJ. RNAi therapeutics: principles, prospects and challenges. *Adv Drug Deliv Rev* 2007; **59**: 75–86.
22. Brummelkamp TR, Bernards R, Agami R. A system for stable expression of short interfering RNAs in mammalian cells. *Science* 2002; **296**: 550–553.
23. Makinen PI, Koponen JK, Karkkainen AM, Malm TM, Pulkkinen KH, Koistinaho J, et al. Stable RNA interference: comparison of U6 and H1 promoters in endothelial cells and in mouse brain. *J Gene Med* 2006; **8**: 433–441.
24. Tomar RS, Matta H, Chaudhary PM. Use of adeno-associated viral vector for delivery of small interfering RNA. *Oncogene* 2003; **22**: 5712–5715.
25. Henriksen JR, Lokke C, Hammero M, Geerts D, Versteeg R, Flaegstad T, et al. Comparison of RNAi efficiency mediated by tetracycline-responsive H1 and U6 promoter variants in mammalian cell lines. *Nucleic Acids Res* 2007; **35**: e67.
26. Lin X, Yang J, Chen J, Gunasekera A, Fesik SW, Shen Y. Development of a tightly regulated U6 promoter for shRNA expression. *FEBS Lett* 2004; **577**: 376–380.
27. Wang S, Shi Z, Liu W, Jules J, Feng X. Development and validation of vectors containing multiple siRNA expression cassettes for maximizing the efficiency of gene silencing. *BMC Biotechnol* 2006; **6**: 50.
28. Jazag A, Kanai F, Ijichi H, Tateishi K, Ikenoue T, Tanaka Y, et al. Single small-interfering RNA expression vector for silencing multiple transforming growth factor-beta pathway components. *Nucleic Acids Res* 2005; **33**: e131.
29. Chen SM, Wang Y, Xiao BK, Tao ZZ. Effect of blocking VEGF, hTERT and Bcl-xl by multiple shRNA expression vectors on the human laryngeal squamous carcinoma xenograft in nude mice. *Cancer Biol Ther* 2007; **7**.
30. De Paula D, Bentley MV, Mahato RI. Hydrophobization and bioconjugation for enhanced siRNA delivery and targeting. *RNA* 2007; **13**: 431–456.
31. Cho-Rok J, Yoo J, Jang YJ, Kim S, Chu IS, Yeom YI, et al. Adenovirus-mediated transfer of siRNA against PTTG1 inhibits liver cancer cell growth in vitro and in vivo. *Hepatology* 2006; **43**: 1042–1052.
32. McCaffrey AP, Meuse L, Pham TT, Conklin DS, Hannon GJ, Kay MA. RNA interference in adult mice. *Nature* 2002; **418**: 38–39.
33. Song E, Lee SK, Wang J, Ince N, Ouyang N, Min J, et al. RNA interference targeting Fas protects mice from fulminant hepatitis. *Nat Med* 2003; **9**: 347–351.
34. Shackel NA, Rockey DC. Intrahepatic gene silencing by RNA interference. *Gastroenterology* 2004; **126**: 356–358; discussion 358–359.
35. Soutschek J, Akinc A, Bramlage B, Charisse K, Constien R, Donoghue M, et al. Therapeutic silencing of an endogenous gene by systemic administration of modified siRNAs. *Nature* 2004; **432**: 173–178.
36. Meyer M, Wagner E. Recent developments in the application of plasmid DNA-based vectors and small interfering RNA therapeutics for cancer. *Hum Gene Ther* 2006; **17**: 1062–1076.
37. Chu TC, Twu KY, Ellington AD, Levy M. Aptamer mediated siRNA delivery. *Nucleic Acids Res* 2006; **34**: e73.
38. Moschos SA, Jones SW, Perry MM, Williams AE, Erjefalt JS, Turner JJ, et al. Lung delivery studies using siRNA conjugated to TAT(48–60) and penetratin reveal peptide induced reduction in gene expression and induction of innate immunity. *Bioconjug Chem* 2007; **18**: 1450–1459.
39. Song E, Zhu P, Lee SK, Chowdhury D, Kussman S, Dykxhoorn DM, et al. Antibody mediated in vivo delivery of small interfering RNAs via cell-surface receptors. *Nat Biotechnol* 2005; **23**: 709–717.

40. Nawrot B, Sipa K. Chemical and structural diversity of siRNA molecules. *Curr Top Med Chem* 2006; **6**: 913–925.

41. Chiu YL, Rana TM. siRNA function in RNAi: a chemical modification analysis. *RNA* 2003; **9**: 1034–1048.

42. Manoharan M. RNA interference and chemically modified small interfering RNAs. *Curr Opin Chem Biol* 2004; **8**: 570–579.

43. Czauderna F, Fechtner M, Dames S, Aygun H, Klippel A, Pronk GJ, et al. Structural variations and stabilising modifications of synthetic siRNAs in mammalian cells. *Nucleic Acids Res* 2003; **31**: 2705–2716.

44. Chiu YL, Ali A, Chu CY, Cao H, Rana TM. Visualizing a correlation between siRNA localization, cellular uptake, and RNAi in living cells. *Chem Biol* 2004; **11**: 1165–1175.

45. Elbashir SM, Martinez J, Patkaniowska A, Lendeckel W, Tuschl T. Functional anatomy of siRNAs for mediating efficient RNAi in Drosophila melanogaster embryo lysate. *Embo J* 2001; **20**: 6877–6888.

46. Jackson AL, Bartz SR, Schelter J, Kobayashi SV, Burchard J, Mao M, et al. Expression profiling reveals off-target gene regulation by RNAi. *Nat Biotechnol* 2003; **21**: 635–637.

47. Scacheri PC, Rozenblatt-Rosen O, Caplen NJ, Wolfsberg TG, Umayam L, Lee JC, et al. Short interfering RNAs can induce unexpected and divergent changes in the levels of untargeted proteins in mammalian cells. *Proc Natl Acad Sci USA* 2004; **101**: 1892–1897.

48. Birmingham A, Anderson EM, Reynolds A, Ilsley-Tyree D, Leake D, Fedorov Y, et al. 3′ UTR seed matches, but not overall identity, are associated with RNAi off-targets. *Nat Methods* 2006; **3**: 199–204.

49. Fedorov Y, Anderson EM, Birmingham A, Reynolds A, Karpilow J, Robinson K, et al. Off-target effects by siRNA can induce toxic phenotype. *RNA* 2006; **12**: 1188–1196.

50. Jackson AL, Burchard J, Schelter J, Chau BN, Cleary M, Lim L, et al. Widespread siRNA "off-target" transcript silencing mediated by seed region sequence complementarity. *RNA* 2006; **12**: 1179–1187.

51. Jackson AL, Burchard J, Leake D, Reynolds A, Schelter J, Guo J, et al. Position-specific chemical modification of siRNAs reduces "off-target" transcript silencing. *RNA* 2006; **12**: 1197–1205.

52. Naito Y, Yamada T, Matsumiya T, Ui-Tei K, Saigo K, Morishita S. dsCheck: highly sensitive off-target search software for double-stranded RNA-mediated RNA interference. *Nucleic Acids Res* 2005; **33**: W589–W591.

53. Stark GR, Kerr IM, Williams BR, Silverman RH, Schreiber RD. How cells respond to interferons. *Annu Rev Biochem* 1998; **67**: 227–264.

54. Kim JY, Choung S, Lee EJ, Kim YJ, Choi YC. Immune activation by siRNA/liposome complexes in mice is sequence- independent: lack of a role for Toll-like receptor 3 signaling. *Mol Cells* 2007; **24**: 247–254.

55. Elbashir SM, Harborth J, Lendeckel W, Yalcin A, Weber K, Tuschl T. Duplexes of 21-nucleotide RNAs mediate RNA interference in cultured mammalian cells. *Nature* 2001; **411**: 494–498.

56. Sledz CA, Holko M, de Veer MJ, Silverman RH, Williams BR. Activation of the interferon system by short-interfering RNAs. *Nat Cell Biol* 2003; **5**: 834–839.

57. Judge AD, Bola G, Lee AC, MacLachlan I. Design of noninflammatory synthetic siRNA mediating potent gene silencing in vivo. *Mol Ther* 2006; **13**: 494–505.

58. Iorns E, Lord CJ, Turner N, Ashworth A. Utilizing RNA interference to enhance cancer drug discovery. *Nat Rev Drug Discov* 2007; **6**: 556–568.

59. Ganesan S, Silver DP, Greenberg RA, Avni D, Drapkin R, Miron A, et al. BRCA1 supports XIST RNA concentration on the inactive X chromosome. *Cell* 2002; **111**: 393–405.

60. Shin SH, Kim HS, Jung SH, Xu HD, Jeong YB, Chung YJ. Implication of leucyl-tRNA synthetase 1 (LARS1) over-expression in growth and migration of lung cancer cells detected by siRNA targeted knock-down analysis. *Exp Mol Med* 2008; **40**: 229–236.

61. Brummelkamp TR, Bernards R, Agami R. Stable suppression of tumorigenicity by virus-mediated RNA interference. *Cancer Cell* 2002; **2**: 243–247.
62. Silva JM, Mizuno H, Brady A, Lucito R, Hannon GJ. RNA interference microarrays: high-throughput loss-of-function genetics in mammalian cells. *Proc Natl Acad Sci USA* 2004; **101**: 6548–6552.
63. Silva J, Chang K, Hannon GJ, Rivas FV. RNA-interference-based functional genomics in mammalian cells: reverse genetics coming of age. *Oncogene* 2004; **23**: 8401–8409.
64. Micklem DR, Lorens JB. RNAi screening for therapeutic targets in human malignancies. *Curr Pharm Biotechnol* 2007; **8**: 337–343.
65. Berns K, Hijmans EM, Mullenders J, Brummelkamp TR, Velds A, Heimerikx M, et al. A large-scale RNAi screen in human cells identifies new components of the p53 pathway. *Nature* 2004; **428**: 431–437.
66. Sachse C, Echeverri CJ. Oncology studies using siRNA libraries: the dawn of RNAi-based genomics. *Oncogene* 2004; **23**: 8384–8391.
67. Hunt KK, Vorburger SA, Swisher SG. *Gene Therapy for Cancer*. Humana Press: Totowa, 2007.
68. Pai SI, Lin YY, Macaes B, Meneshian A, Hung CF, Wu TC. Prospects of RNA inter-ference therapy for cancer. *Gene Ther* 2006; **13**: 464–477.
69. Folkman J. Tumor angiogenesis: therapeutic implications. *N Engl J Med* 1971; **285**: 1182–1186.
70. Hadj-Slimane R, Lepelletier Y, Lopez N, Garbay C, Raynaud F. Short interfering RNA (siRNA), a novel therapeutic tool acting on angiogenesis. *Biochimie* 2007; **89**: 1234–1244.
71. de Fougerolles A, Vornlocher HP, Maraganore J, Lieberman J. Interfering with disease: a progress report on siRNA-based therapeutics. *Nat Rev Drug Discov* 2007; **6**: 443–453.
72. Spagnou S, Miller AD, Keller M. Lipidic carriers of siRNA: differences in the formulation, cellular uptake, and delivery with plasmid DNA. *Biochemistry* 2004; **43**: 13348–13356.
73. Heidel JD. Linear cyclodextrin-containing polymers and their use as delivery agents. *Expert Opin Drug Deliv* 2006; **3**: 641–646.
74. Boussif O, Lezoualc'h F, Zanta MA, Mergny MD, Scherman D, Demeneix B, et al. A versatile vector for gene and oligonucleotide transfer into cells in culture and in vivo: polyethylenimine. *Proc Natl Acad Sci USA* 1995; **92**: 7297–7301.
75. Felgner PL, Gadek TR, Holm M, Roman R, Chan HW, Wenz M, et al. Lipofection: a highly efficient, lipid-mediated DNA-transfection procedure. *Proc Natl Acad Sci USA* 1987; **84**: 7413–7417.
76. Morille M, Passirani C, Vonarbourg A, Clavreul A, Benoit JP. Progress in developing cationic vectors for non-viral systemic gene therapy against cancer. *Biomaterials* 2008; **29**: 3477–3496.
77. Mevel M, Breuzard G, Yaouanc JJ, Clement JC, Lehn P, Pichon C, et al. Synthesis and Transfection Activity of New Cationic Phosphoramidate Lipids: High Efficiency of an Imidazolium Derivative. *Chembiochem* 2008; **9**: 1462–1471.
78. Akhtar S, Benter IF. Nonviral delivery of synthetic siRNAs in vivo. *J Clin Invest* 2007; **117**: 3623–3632.
79. Zhang S, Zhao B, Jiang H, Wang B, Ma B. Cationic lipids and polymers mediated vectors for delivery of siRNA. *J Control Release* 2007; **123**: 1–10.
80. Hobel S, Prinz R, Malek A, Urban-Klein B, Sitterberg J, Bakowsky U, et al. Polyethy-lenimine PEI F25-LMW allows the long-term storage of frozen complexes as fully active reagents in siRNA-mediated gene targeting and DNA delivery. *Eur J Pharm Biopharm* 2008; **70**: 29–41.
81. Werth S, Urban-Klein B, Dai L, Hobel S, Grzelinski M, Bakowsky U, et al. A low molecular weight fraction of polyethylenimine (PEI) displays increased transfection efficiency of DNA and siRNA in fresh or lyophilized complexes. *J Control Release* 2006; **112**: 257–270.

82. Malek A, Czubayko F, Aigner A. PEG grafting of polyethylenimine (PEI) exerts different effects on DNA transfection and siRNA-induced gene targeting efficacy. *J Drug Target* 2008; **16**: 124–139.
83. Mao S, Neu M, Germershaus O, Merkel O, Sitterberg J, Bakowsky U, et al. Influence of polyethylene glycol chain length on the physicochemical and biological properties of poly(ethylene imine)-graft-poly(ethylene glycol) block copolymer/SiRNA polyplexes. *Bioconjug Chem* 2006; **17**: 1209–1218.
84. Shim MS, Kwon YJ. Controlled delivery of plasmid DNA and siRNA to intracellular targets using ketalized polyethylenimine. *Biomacromolecules* 2008; **9**: 444–455.
85. de Wolf HK, Snel CJ, Verbaan FJ, Schiffelers RM, Hennink WE, Storm G. Effect of cationic carriers on the pharmacokinetics and tumor localization of nucleic acids after intravenous administration. *Int J Pharm* 2007; **331**: 167–175.
86. Kim SH, Mok H, Jeong JH, Kim SW, Park TG. Comparative evaluation of target-specific GFP gene silencing efficiencies for antisense ODN, synthetic siRNA, and siRNA plasmid complexed with PEI-PEG-FOL conjugate. *Bioconjug Chem* 2006; **17**: 241–244.
87. Katas H, Alpar HO. Development and characterisation of chitosan nanoparticles for siRNA delivery. *J Control Release* 2006; **115**: 216–225.
88. Liu X, Howard KA, Dong M, Andersen MO, Rahbek UL, Johnsen MG, et al. The influence of polymeric properties on chitosan/siRNA nanoparticle formulation and gene silencing. *Biomaterials* 2007; **28**: 1280–1288.
89. de Martimprey H, Bertrand JR, Fusco A, Santoro M, Couvreur P, Vauthier C, et al. siRNA nanoformulation against the ret/PTC1 junction oncogene is efficient in an in vivo model of papillary thyroid carcinoma. *Nucleic Acids Res* 2008; **36**: e2.
90. Howard KA, Rahbek UL, Liu X, Damgaard CK, Glud SZ, Andersen MO, et al. RNA interference in vitro and in vivo using a novel chitosan/siRNA nanoparticle system. *Mol Ther* 2006; **14**: 476–484.
91. Dufes C, Uchegbu IF, Schatzlein AG. Dendrimers in gene delivery. *Adv Drug Deliv Rev* 2005; **57**: 2177–2202.
92. Tsutsumi T, Hirayama F, Uekama K, Arima H. Evaluation of polyamidoamine dendrimer/alpha-cyclodextrin conjugate (generation 3, G3) as a novel carrier for small interfering RNA (siRNA). *J Control Release* 2007; **119**: 349–359.
93. Patil ML, Zhang M, Betigeri S, Taratula O, He H, Minko T. Surface-Modified and Internally Cationic Polyamidoamine Dendrimers for Efficient siRNA Delivery. *Bioconjug Chem* 2008; **19**: 1396–1403.
94. Kang H, DeLong R, Fisher MH, Juliano RL. Tat-conjugated PAMAM dendrimers as delivery agents for antisense and siRNA oligonucleotides. *Pharm Res* 2005; **22**: 2099–2106.
95. Gupta B, Levchenko TS, Torchilin VP. Intracellular delivery of large molecules and small particles by cell-penetrating proteins and peptides. *Adv Drug Deliv Rev* 2005; **57**: 637–651.
96. Muratovska A, Eccles MR. Conjugate for efficient delivery of short interfering RNA (siRNA) into mammalian cells. *FEBS Lett* 2004; **558**: 63–68.
97. Crombez L, Charnet A, Morris MC, Aldrian-Herrada G, Heitz F, Divita G. A non-covalent peptide-based strategy for siRNA delivery. *Biochem Soc Trans* 2007; **35**: 44–46.
98. Zeineddine D, Papadimou E, Chebli K, Gineste M, Liu J, Grey C, et al. Oct-3/4 dose dependently regulates specification of embryonic stem cells toward a cardiac lineage and early heart development. *Dev Cell* 2006; **11**: 535–546.
99. Davis ME, Pun SH, Bellocq NC, Reineke TM, Popielarski SR, Mishra S, et al. Self-assembling nucleic acid delivery vehicles via linear, water-soluble, cyclodextrin-containing polymers. *Curr Med Chem* 2004; **11**: 179–197.
100. Hu-Lieskovan S, Heidel JD, Bartlett DW, Davis ME, Triche TJ. Sequence-specific knockdown of EWS-FLI1 by targeted, nonviral delivery of small interfering RNA inhibits tumor growth in a murine model of metastatic Ewing's sarcoma. *Cancer Res* 2005; **65**: 8984–8992.

101. Heidel JD, Yu Z, Liu JY, Rele SM, Liang Y, Zeidan RK, et al. Administration in non-human primates of escalating intravenous doses of targeted nanoparticles containing ribonucleotide reductase subunit M2 siRNA. *Proc Natl Acad Sci USA* 2007; **104**: 5715–5721.

102. Ochiya T, Nagahara S, Sano A, Itoh H, Terada M. Biomaterials for gene delivery: atelocollagen-mediated controlled release of molecular medicines. *Curr Gene Ther* 2001; **1**: 31–52.

103. Minakuchi Y, Takeshita F, Kosaka N, Sasaki H, Yamamoto Y, Kouno M, et al. Atelocollagen-mediated synthetic small interfering RNA delivery for effective gene silencing in vitro and in vivo. *Nucleic Acids Res* 2004; **32**: e109.

104. Takei Y, Kadomatsu K, Yuzawa Y, Matsuo S, Muramatsu T. A small interfering RNA targeting vascular endothelial growth factor as cancer therapeutics. *Cancer Res* 2004; **64**: 3365–3370.

105. Takeshita F, Minakuchi Y, Nagahara S, Honma K, Sasaki H, Hirai K, et al. Efficient delivery of small interfering RNA to bone-metastatic tumors by using atelocollagen in vivo. *Proc Natl Acad Sci USA* 2005; **102**: 12177–12182.

106. Ikeda Y, Taira K. Ligand-targeted delivery of therapeutic siRNA. *Pharm Res* 2006; **23**: 1631–1640.

107. Zhang Y, Zhang YF, Bryant J, Charles A, Boado RJ, Pardridge WM. Intravenous RNA interference gene therapy targeting the human epidermal growth factor receptor prolongs survival in intracranial brain cancer. *Clin Cancer Res* 2004; **10**: 3667–3677.

108. Allen TM. Ligand-targeted therapeutics in anticancer therapy. *Nat Rev Cancer* 2002; **2**: 750–763.

109. Pirollo KF, Rait A, Zhou Q, Hwang SH, Dagata JA, Zon G, et al. Materializing the potential of small interfering RNA via a tumor-targeting nanodelivery system. *Cancer Res* 2007; **67**: 2938–2943.

110. Pirollo KF, Zon G, Rait A, Zhou Q, Yu W, Hogrefe R, et al. Tumor-targeting nanoimmunoliposome complex for short interfering RNA delivery. *Hum Gene Ther* 2006; **17**: 117–124.

111. Xu L, Huang CC, Huang W, Tang WH, Rait A, Yin YZ, et al. Systemic tumor-targeted gene delivery by anti-transferrin receptor scFv-immunoliposomes. *Mol Cancer Ther* 2002; **1**: 337–346.

112. Agarwal A, Saraf S, Asthana A, Gupta U, Gajbhiye V, Jain NK. Ligand based dendritic systems for tumor targeting. *Int J Pharm* 2008; **350**: 3–13.

113. Li H, Qian ZM. Transferrin/transferrin receptor-mediated drug delivery. *Med Res Rev* 2002; **22**: 225–250.

114. Bartlett DW, Su H, Hildebrandt IJ, Weber WA, Davis ME. Impact of tumor-specific targeting on the biodistribution and efficacy of siRNA nanoparticles measured by multimodality in vivo imaging. *Proc Natl Acad Sci USA* 2007; **104**: 15549–15554.

115. Cardoso AL, Simoes S, de Almeida LP, Pelisek J, Culmsee C, Wagner E, et al. siRNA delivery by a transferrin-associated lipid-based vector: a non-viral strategy to mediate gene silencing. *J Gene Med* 2007; **9**: 170–183.

116. Bartlett DW, Davis ME. Impact of tumor-specific targeting and dosing schedule on tumor growth inhibition after intravenous administration of siRNA-containing nanoparticles. *Biotechnol Bioeng* 2008; **99**: 975–985.

117. Zhang K, Wang Q, Xie Y, Mor G, Sega E, Low PS, et al. Receptor-mediated delivery of siRNAs by tethered nucleic acid base-paired interactions. *RNA* 2008; **14**: 577–583.

118. Salazar MD, Ratnam M. The folate receptor: what does it promise in tissue-targeted therapeutics? *Cancer Metastasis Rev* 2007; **26**: 141–152.

119. Low PS, Henne WA, Doorneweerd DD. Discovery and development of folic-acid-based receptor targeting for imaging and therapy of cancer and inflammatory diseases. *Acc Chem Res* 2008; **41**: 120–129.

120. Temming K, Schiffelers RM, Molema G, Kok RJ. RGD-based strategies for selective delivery of therapeutics and imaging agents to the tumour vasculature. *Drug Resist Updat* 2005; **8**: 381–402.

121. Schiffelers RM, Ansari A, Xu J, Zhou Q, Tang Q, Storm G, et al. Cancer siRNA therapy by tumor selective delivery with ligand-targeted sterically stabilized nanoparticle. *Nucleic Acids Res* 2004; **32**: e149.

122. Hicke BJ, Stephens AW. Escort aptamers: a delivery service for diagnosis and therapy. *J Clin Invest* 2000; **106**: 923–928.

123. McNamara JO, 2nd, Andrechek ER, Wang Y, Viles KD, Rempel RE, Gilboa E, et al. Cell type-specific delivery of siRNAs with aptamer-siRNA chimeras. *Nat Biotechnol* 2006; **24**: 1005–1015.

124. Silver DA, Pellicer I, Fair WR, Heston WD, Cordon-Cardo C. Prostate-specific membrane antigen expression in normal and malignant human tissues. *Clin Cancer Res* 1997; **3**: 81–85.

125. Dougherty CJ, Ichim TE, Liu L, Reznik G, Min WP, Ghochikyan A, et al. Selective apoptosis of breast cancer cells by siRNA targeting of BORIS. *Biochem Biophys Res Commun* 2008; **370**: 109–112.

126. Jang JY, Choi Y, Jeon YK, Kim CW. Suppression of adenine nucleotide translocase-2 by vector-based siRNA in human breast cancer cells induces apoptosis and inhibits tumor growth in vitro and in vivo. *Breast Cancer Res* 2008; **10**: R11.

127. Navakanit R, Graidist P, Leeanansaksiri W, Dechsukum C. Growth inhibition of breast cancer cell line MCF-7 by siRNA silencing of Wilms tumor 1 gene. *J Med Assoc Thai* 2007; **90**: 2416–2421.

128. Wieczorek M, Paczkowska A, Guzenda P, Majorek M, Bednarek AK, Lamparska-Przybysz M. Silencing of Wnt-1 by siRNA induces apoptosis of MCF-7 human breast cancer cells. *Cancer Biol Ther* 2007; **7**.

129. Meryet-Figuieres M, Resina S, Lavigne C, Barlovatz-Meimon G, Lebleu B, Thierry AR. Inhibition of PAI-1 expression in breast cancer carcinoma cells by siRNA at nanomolar range. *Biochimie* 2007; **89**: 1228–1233.

130. Sutton D, Kim S, Shuai X, Leskov K, Marques JT, Williams BR, et al. Efficient suppression of secretory clusterin levels by polymer-siRNA nanocomplexes enhances ionizing radiation lethality in human MCF-7 breast cancer cells in vitro. *Int J Nanomed* 2006; **1**: 155–162.

131. Zhang ZH, Chen Y, Zhao HJ, Xie CY, Ding J, Hou YT. Silencing of heparanase by siRNA inhibits tumor metastasis and angiogenesis of human breast cancer in vitro and in vivo. *Cancer Biol Ther* 2007; **6**: 587–595.

132. Zhang X, Xu WH, Ge YL, Hou L, Li Q. Effect of siRNA transfection targeting VEGF gene on proliferation and apoptosis of human breast cancer cells. *Xi Bao Yu Fen Zi Mian Yi Xue Za Zhi* 2007; **23**: 14–17.

133. Cao Q, Cai W, Li T, Yang Y, Chen K, Xing L, et al. Combination of integrin siRNA and irradiation for breast cancer therapy. *Biochem Biophys Res Commun* 2006; **351**: 726–732.

134. Guan HT, Xue XH, Wang XJ, Li A, Qin ZY. Effects of siRNA targeted to survivin in suppressing proliferation and inducing apoptosis in breast cancer MCF-7 cells. *Zhonghua Zhong Liu Za Zhi* 2006; **28**: 326–330.

135. Jiang L, Chen RS, Li JC. siRNA-cyclin D1 inhibit cell proliferation in breast cancer MCF-7 cell line. *Fen Zi Xi Bao Sheng Wu Xue Bao* 2006; **39**: 118–122.

136. Subramanian R, Gondi CS, Lakka SS, Jutla A, Rao JS. siRNA-mediated simultaneous downregulation of uPA and its receptor inhibits angiogenesis and invasiveness triggering apoptosis in breast cancer cells. *Int J Oncol* 2006; **28**: 831–839.

137. Zhang Y, Wang Y, Gao W, Zhang R, Han X, Jia M, et al. Transfer of siRNA against XIAP induces apoptosis and reduces tumor cells growth potential in human breast cancer in vitro and in vivo. *Breast Cancer Res Treat* 2006; **96**: 267–277.

138. Huh JW, Choi MM, Yang SJ, Yoon SY, Choi SY, Cho SW. Inhibition of human UDP-glucose dehydrogenase expression using siRNA expression vector in breast cancer cells. *Biotechnol Lett* 2005; **27**: 1229–1232.

139. Faltus T, Yuan J, Zimmer B, Kramer A, Loibl S, Kaufmann M, et al. Silencing of the HER2/neu gene by siRNA inhibits proliferation and induces apoptosis in HER2/neu-overexpressing breast cancer cells. *Neoplasia* 2004; **6**: 786–795.

140. Wu WD, Fang CH, Yang ZX, Bao JJ. Effects of RNA interference on epidermal growth factor receptor expression in breast cancer cells: a study in tumor-bearing nude mice. *Nan Fang Yi Ke Da Xue Xue Bao* 2008; **28**: 60–64.

141. Liu TG, Yin JQ, Shang BY, Min Z, He HW, Jiang JM, et al. Silencing of hdm2 oncogene by siRNA inhibits p53-dependent human breast cancer. *Cancer Gene Ther* 2004; **11**: 748–756.

142. Mohammed K, Shervington A. Can CYP1A1 siRNA be an effective treatment for lung cancer? *Cell Mol Biol Lett* 2008; **13**: 240–249.

143. Zhang Z, Jiang G, Yang F, Wang J. Knockdown of mutant K-ras expression by adenovirus-mediated siRNA inhibits the in vitro and in vivo growth of lung cancer cells. *Cancer Biol Ther* 2006; **5**: 1481–1486.

144. Guo W, Ahmed KM, Hui Y, Guo G, Li JJ. siRNA-mediated MDM2 inhibition sensitizes human lung cancer A549 cells to radiation. *Int J Oncol* 2007; **30**: 1447–1452.

145. Dong AQ, Kong MJ, Ma ZY, Qian JF, Xu XH. Down-regulation of IGF-IR using small, interfering, hairpin RNA (siRNA) inhibits growth of human lung cancer cell line A549 in vitro and in nude mice. *Cell Biol Int* 2007; **31**: 500–507.

146. Kakar SS, Malik MT. Suppression of lung cancer with siRNA targeting PTTG. *Int J Oncol* 2006; **29**: 387–395.

147. Yamanaka S, Gu Z, Sato M, Fujisaki R, Inomata K, Sakurada A, et al. siRNA targeting against EGFR, a promising candidate for a novel therapeutic application to lung adenocarcinoma. *Pathobiology* 2008; **75**: 2–8.

148. Lee MW, Kim DS, Min NY, Kim HT. Akt1 inhibition by RNA interference sensitizes human non-small cell lung cancer cells to cisplatin. *Int J Cancer* 2008; **122**: 2380–2384.

149. Kim HR, Kim S, Kim EJ, Park JH, Yang SH, Jeong ET, et al. Suppression of Nrf2-driven heme oxygenase-1 enhances the chemosensitivity of lung cancer A549 cells toward cisplatin. *Lung Cancer* 2008; **60**: 47–56.

150. Gan PP, Pasquier E, Kavallaris M. Class III beta-tubulin mediates sensitivity to chemotherapeutic drugs in non small cell lung cancer. *Cancer Res* 2007; **67**: 9356–9363.

151. Mano Y, Takahashi K, Ishikawa N, Takano A, Yasui W, Inai K, et al. Fibroblast growth factor receptor 1 oncogene partner as a novel prognostic biomarker and therapeutic target for lung cancer. *Cancer Sci* 2007; **98**: 1902–1913.

152. Cho NH, Choi YP, Moon DS, Kim H, Kang S, Ding O, et al. Induction of cell apoptosis in non-small cell lung cancer cells by cyclin A1 small interfering RNA. *Cancer Sci* 2006; **97**: 1082–1092.

153. Ohnishi K, Scuric Z, Schiestl RH, Okamoto N, Takahashi A, Ohnishi T. siRNA targeting NBS1 or XIAP increases radiation sensitivity of human cancer cells independent of TP53 status. *Radiat Res* 2006; **166**: 454–462.

154. Ko K, Furukawa K, Takahashi T, Urano T, Sanai Y, Nagino M, et al. Fundamental study of small interfering RNAs for ganglioside GD3 synthase gene as a therapeutic target of lung cancers. *Oncogene* 2006; **25**: 6924–6935.

155. Xu XF, Zhang ZY, Ge JP, Cheng W, Zhou SW, Zhang X *et al.* RNA interference-mediated silencing of the PAR gene inhibits the growth of PC3 cells via the induction of G2/M cell cycle arrest and apoptosis. *J Gene Med* 2007; **9**: 1065–1070.

156. Sanlioglu AD, Karacay B, Koksal IT, Griffith TS, Sanlioglu S. DcR2 (TRAIL-R4) siRNA and adenovirus delivery of TRAIL (Ad5hTRAIL) break down in vitro tumorigenic potential of prostate carcinoma cells. *Cancer Gene Ther* 2007; **14**: 976–984.

157. Takei Y, Kadomatsu K, Goto T, Muramatsu T. Combinational antitumor effect of siRNA against midkine and paclitaxel on growth of human prostate cancer xenografts. *Cancer* 2006; **107**: 864–873.

158. Bandyopadhyay S, Pai SK, Watabe M, Gross SC, Hirota S, Hosobe S, et al. FAS expression inversely correlates with PTEN level in prostate cancer and a PI 3-kinase inhibitor synergizes with FAS siRNA to induce apoptosis. *Oncogene* 2005; **24**: 5389–5395.

159. Zhang L, Gao L, Zhao L, Guo B, Ji K, Tian Y, et al. Intratumoral delivery and suppression of prostate tumor growth by attenuated Salmonella enterica serovar typhimurium carrying plasmid-based small interfering RNAs. *Cancer Res* 2007; **67**: 5859–5864.

160. Das S, Roth CP, Wasson LM, Vishwanatha JK. Signal transducer and activator of transcription-6 (STAT6) is a constitutively expressed survival factor in human prostate cancer. *Prostate* 2007; **67**: 1550–1564.

161. Reagan-Shaw S, Ahmad N. Silencing of polo-like kinase (Plk) 1 via siRNA causes induction of apoptosis and impairment of mitosis machinery in human prostate cancer cells: implications for the treatment of prostate cancer. *FASEB J* 2005; **19**: 611–613.

162. Grzmil M, Voigt S, Thelen P, Hemmerlein B, Helmke K, Burfeind P. Up-regulated expression of the MAT-8 gene in prostate cancer and its siRNA-mediated inhibition of expression induces a decrease in proliferation of human prostate carcinoma cells. *Int J Oncol* 2004; **24**: 97–105.

163. Mizutani K, Nagata K, Ito H, Ehara H, Nozawa Y, Deguchi T. Possible roles of vinexinbeta in growth and paclitaxel sensitivity in human prostate cancer PC-3 cells. *Cancer Biol Ther* 2007; **6**: 1800–1804.

164. Yamasaki M, Nomura T, Sato F, Mimata H. Metallothionein is up-regulated under hypoxia and promotes the survival of human prostate cancer cells. *Oncol Rep* 2007; **18**: 1145–1153.

165. Saad AF, Meacham WD, Bai A, Anelli V, Elojeimy S, Mahdy AE, et al. The functional effects of acid ceramidase overexpression in prostate cancer progression and resistance to chemotherapy. *Cancer Biol Ther* 2007; **6**: 1455–1460.

166. Pulukuri SM, Rao JS. Small interfering RNA directed reversal of urokinase plasminogen activator demethylation inhibits prostate tumor growth and metastasis. *Cancer Res* 2007; **67**: 6637–6646.

167. Priulla M, Calastretti A, Bruno P, Azzariti A, Paradiso A, Canti G, et al. Preferential chemosensitization of PTEN-mutated prostate cells by silencing the Akt kinase. *Prostate* 2007; **67**: 782–789.

168. Rocchi P, Jugpal P, So A, Sinneman S, Ettinger S, Fazli L, et al. Small interference RNA targeting heat-shock protein 27 inhibits the growth of prostatic cell lines and induces apoptosis via caspase-3 activation in vitro. *BJU Int* 2006; **98**: 1082–1089.

MicroRNAs as Therapeutic Targets for Cancer

Guofeng Cheng, Michael Danquah, and Ram I. Mahato

1 Introduction

MicroRNAs (miRNAs) are a recently discovered family of endogenous, non-coding RNA molecules approximately 22 nt in length [1]. They modulate gene expression post-transcriptionally by binding to the complementary sequence in the coding or 3′ untranslated region of target messenger RNAs (mRNAs) [1]. miRNAs are transcribed from genomic DNA by RNA polymerase II but not further translated into protein (non-coding RNA). Eventually, they are processed from primary transcripts known as pri-miRNAs to short stem-loop structures called pre-miRNA and finally to become functionally mature miRNA. Mature miRNA molecules are partially complimentary to target mRNA where they either repress translation or direct destructive cleavage [2]. The first miRNA was described in 1993 by Lee and colleagues, who found miRNA-*lin-4* is essential for the normal temporal control of diverse post-embryonic development in *Caenorhabditis elegans* by negatively regulating the level of LIN-14 protein via antisense RNA–RNA interaction [3]. miRNAs have a large-scale effect as a new layer of gene regulation mechanism. It has been estimated that the vertebrate genome encodes up to 1000 unique miRNAs, which can regulate expression of at least 30% of genes [4, 5].

Cancer is an intricate genetic disease attributed to the breakdown of gene regulatory networks governing the balance between oncogenes and tumor-suppressor genes. That cancer results from a deregulation of this highly regulated network suggests the use of gene modulation as a therapeutic approach for treating cancer. To date, several approaches such as antisense oligonucleotides (ODN), aptamers, ribozymes, and small interfering RNAs (siRNAs) have been explored as tools for modulating the production of aberrant proteins. Recent evidence indicates that miRNAs play an important role in cancer pathogenesis by functioning as novel oncogenes or tumor-suppressor genes and altered

R.I. Mahato (✉)
Department of Pharmaceutical Sciences, University of Tennessee Health Science
Center, Memphis, TN, 38103, USA
e-mail: rmahato@utmem.edu

Y. Lu, R.I. Mahato (eds.), *Pharmaceutical Perspectives of Cancer Therapeutics*,   441
DOI 10.1007/978-1-4419-0131-6_14, © Springer Science+Business Media, LLC 2009

expressions of specific miRNA genes have been identified as signatures for certain cancer types [6– 8]. Since miRNAs are powerful regulators of gene expression and can regulate more than one target, they have the potential to serve as a new class of therapeutic targets for treating cancer by artificially manipulating their expression levels.

This chapter highlights the role of miRNAs in the initiation and progression of human cancer, their utility as diagnostics and prognostics and focuses on the potential of miRNAs as therapeutic targets for cancer treatment. We also describe the current strategies for modulating miRNAs to exploit them as therapeutics.

2 Gene Regulation

2.1 Type of Nucleic Acids Used for Gene Modulation

One of the major developments in modern biomedical research resulting from the fields of molecular biology and genetics is gene modulation-based gene therapy. During the past 30 years, several approaches of gene regulation have been developed to artificially alter the expression of a given gene (Fig. 1). These include antisense oligodeoxynucleotides (ODN), triplex-

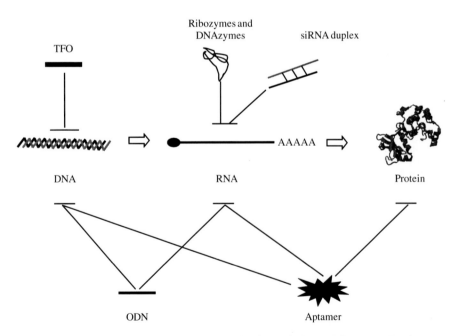

Fig. 1 Schematic representation of gene modulation by TFO, ODN, Ribozymes, DNAzymes, siRNA duplex, and aptamer

forming oligonucleotides (TFOs), aptamers, ribozymes and DNAzymes, and small interfering RNA (siRNA). Among them, aptamers can regulate endogenous gene expression at both genomic and transcription levels [9]. TFOs and ODNs can exert their functions through binding the promoter region or open reading frame of target regions [10]. Ribozymes and DNAzymes can catalytically cleave the target gene [9]. All current approaches for gene regulation have been applied to selectively turn off specific genes in diseased tissue. This blockage of active target molecules by gene regulation has a potential to be developed into efficacious gene therapies for human diseases. Recently, RNA interference (RNAi), which is small interfering RNA (siRNA)-mediated specific gene silencing has become an important tool for analyzing gene function at the transcription level [11] and also provides a potentially therapeutic tool for treating genetic or acquired disease [12].

2.2 RNA Interference

RNAi was first described in *C. elegans* in 1998 by Andrew Fire and Craig C. Mello, who demonstrated substantially more effective gene silencing using dsRNA than either strand individually [11]. As per RNAi, introduction of dsRNA into organism results into the 21- or 22-nt dsRNA fragments that bear 2- or 3-nt 3' overhangs upon cleavage by Dicer. These 21-nt dsRNAs, which are referred to as siRNAs, are then selectively incorporated into a RNA-induced silencing complex (RISC). Then a RISC undergoes an ATP-dependent activation step that involves unwinding of the double-stranded siRNA component to give a single-stranded guide RNA that targets RISC to homologous mRNAs. After mRNA binding, a RISC cleaves the target mRNA at the center of the region that is complementary to the guide RNA. dsRNAs can be produced by first chemical synthesis and the following in vitro annealing or are transcribed by plasmid or viral vectors encoding short hairpin RNA (shRNA). Due to its high specificity and efficiency, extensive efforts have led to the development of this technique as a potentially therapeutic strategy through gene regulation at the transcription level.

2.3 miRNA Versus siRNA

Both siRNA and miRNA are small RNAs of 18–25 nt in length that exert their functions by incorporating into related RISCs (Fig. 2). However, unlike siRNA, miRNAs are a class of endogenous molecules that are transcribed by RNA polymerase II from genomic DNA. In the nucleus, miRNA are usually transcribed by RNA polymerase II into pri-miRNAs which are large precursor RNAs. These transcripts are then processed by an RNase III enzyme

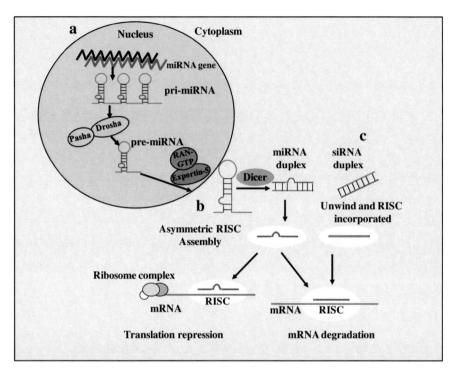

Fig. 2 The biogenesis and function of miRNAs and siRNA pathway. (**a**) The primary miRNA (pri-miRNA) is transcribed from genome by RNA polymerase II, then is processed into precursor miRNA (pre-miRNA) by the Drosha/Pasha microprocessor complex and exported to cytoplasm by exportin-5. (**b**) pre-miRNA becomes a bioactive miRNA duplex upon removing the loop by Dicer. The miRNA duplex is unwinded into single-stranded mature miRNA, which is subsequently incorporated into related RISC. Asymmetric RISC including mature miRNA inhibits the translation of the target gene or cleaves mRNA of target gene. (**c**) Upon arrival in the cytoplasm, siRNA duplex is unwinded and the guide siRNA strand is incorporated into related RISC. The RISC specifically degrades the mRNA of target gene

Drosha and its double-stranded binding domain protein Pasha into ~70 nt long stem-loop structures known as pre-miRNAs [13– 15]. The pre-miRNAs are then exported out of the nucleus by the GTP-driven exportin 5 transporter and further processed by the RNase III Dicer-TRBP microprocessor complex in the cytoplasm [16– 18]. This results in the release of a double-stranded RNA duplex composed of the mature miRNA bound to its complementary strand. The mature miRNA strand is separated from its complement due to differences in thermodynamic stability at the 5′ end and loaded into the RNA-induced silencing complex (RISC) where it has the capacity to regulate target genes; the unused strand is degraded [19]. The bound mRNAs either remain untranslated resulting in a decrease in the proteins they encode or are degraded by the RISC resulting in a decreased number of transcripts. miRNAs are involved in numerous cellular processes including development, differentiation, proliferation, apoptosis, and the stress response [20]. As to siRNA-mediated RNAi, it is an evolutionary mechanism for protecting the genome against invasion by mobile genetic elements such as transposons and viruses. siRNAs directly trigger a sequence-specific post-transcriptional degradation of homologous genes by binding to its complementary mRNA, which is not limited to 3′ UTR. The siRNA sequence is required to strictly complement with target mRNA. It is recently noted that siRNA-mediated gene silencing could induce unwanted off-target effect and immune response.

3 Identification of miRNA Targets

As mentioned above, miRNAs function by binding to complementary sites on target mRNAs to induce cleavage or repression of productive translation. As such, identification of miRNA targets is a key step for analyzing miRNA function in organisms. Up to now, some miRNA targets have been identified and their functions assigned. For example, the *lin-4* and *let-7* miRNAs control developmental timing in *C. elegans* [21, 22]; *lsy-6* miRNA regulates left–right asymmetry in the nervous system [23]; *bantam* miRNA controls tissue growth [24]; *bantam* and *miR-14* control apoptosis [24]; *miR-181* is involved in hematopoietic differentiation [25]; *miR-375* regulates insulin secretion [26]; and *miR-373* and *miR-520c* stimulate cancer cell migration and invasion [27].

Computational prediction of miRNA targets provides an alternative approach to assigning biological functions of miRNAs. Several softwares with different governing algorithms have been developed and applied for prediction of a large number of targets genes for miRNA as listed in Table 1. In the following section, we introduce some of the softwares used for the prediction of miRNA targets. TargetScan is an algorithm developed by Lewis et al. for predicting miRNA targets in vertebrates [28]. Using this software, genes involved in transcriptional regulation were enriched even though the functions of the predicted target genes encompassed a broad range of activities. TargetScans criterion for target detection involves the existence of perfect complementarity to the "seed-region" of miRNA and the degree of complementarity of surrounding regions. Later, the authors improved the TargetScan algorithm and developed it into TargetScanS [5]. This updated software successfully predicated all of the known miRNA–target interaction and has been used in the prediction of over 5300 human genes as potential targets of miRNAs. The miRanda software was initially designed to predict miRNA target genes in *Drosophila melanogaster* [29] and utilizes dynamic programming to rapidly identify sites with a high-degree of miRNA complementarity. This software was also applied for prediction of human miRNA in targets [29, 30]. About 2000 putative human miRNA target genes were identified, suggesting that 10% or more of human genes are regulated by miRNAs. The RNAhybrid program presented by Rehmsmeier et al., which is

Table 1 List of some softwares used for predicting miRNA target

Name	Website	Applied proposes
TargetScan	http://www.targetscan.org/	Worm/fly/mammalian
miRanda	http://www.microrna.org/microrna/ getGeneForm.do	Human/fly/zebrafish
PicTar	http://pictar.bio.nyu.edu/	Vertebrates/fly/ nematode
RNAhybrid	http://bibiserv.techfak.uni-bielefeld.de/rnahybrid/	Worm
MicroTar	http://tiger.dbs.nus.edu.sg/microtar/	Worm/fly/mouse
ViTa	http://vita.mbc.nctu.edu.tw/	Virus
miRU	http://bioinfo3.noble.org/miRU.htm	Plants
RNAhybrid	http://bibiserv.techfak.uni-bielefeld.de/rnahybrid/	C. elegans
STarMir	http://sfold.wadsworth.org/starmir.pl	Worm/mammalian

the identification target miRNA based on energetically optimal binding sites for a small RNA within a large RNA sequences [31], can predict known and new miRNA targets. Because cross-species comparisons provide powerful criteria for identifying miRNA target genes, Kerk et al. developed Pic Tar algorithm to compare a group of orthologous 3′UTR from multiple species and retain the 3′UTRs with seeding match for miRNAs [32]. Then those candidate targets were further filtered according to their thermodynamic stability. They utilized this method to predict vertebrate miRNA targets and suggested that about 200 transcripts are regulated by a single miRNA. Yousef et al. also presented a machine learning approach for predicting miRNA target site based on the naïve Bayer (NB) classifiers [33]. They used the classifier as a filter for the output of the miRanda tool and demonstrated that the filtering step decreases the false-positive prediction by miRanda significantly. Calculation of mRNA secondary structures and favorable hybridization between miRNA and target mRNA can also be used to predict miRNA target such as RNAhybrid [31] and STarMir [34]. The microRNA.org site (http://www.microrna.org) is a resource for miRNA target predictions and miRNA expression that is widely used by the research community [35]. Other annotated miRNA databases such as miRBase [36], miRGen [37], Argonaute [38], miRNAMap [39], and smiRNAdb [40] could also provide some valuable information for predicting miRNA target.

Experimental validation of predicated miRNA targets is crucial for understanding miRNA functions as well as the biological significance of results from computational prediction. This is necessary since computational methods are not warranted due to the associated risk of false-positive prediction. Although experimental validation of miRNA target genes is challenging compared to computational validation, more and more miRNA target genes from various species have been identified using a combination of computational and biological approaches. Experimental validation is performed against two types of predicted miRNA targets that have different regulatory mechanisms: translational repression of target mRNAs and cleavage of target mRNAs. Methods such as reporter gene [41– 43], gene mutation [44– 46], rapid amplification of 5′ complementary DNA end (5′ RACE) [47], and proteomics [48] have been applied for experimental validation of computationally predicated miRNA targets that are translationally regulated. In addition, microarray analysis, which provides a powerful and high-throughput method for observing cleaved target mRNAs, was also used to identify a large number of human miRNA targets that appear to be cleaved by miRNAs [49]. Recently, German et al. directly sequenced miRNA–mRNA pairs and identified miRNA targets from the mRNA cleaved site, which provided a novel method for predicting miRNA target [50]. However, there is no clear agreement as to which experimental procedures should be followed to demonstrate a predicated miRNA target is a target of specific miRNA. It is therefore necessary to experimentally confirm predicated targets by using a combination of techniques.

4 Roles of miRNAs in Cancer

4.1 miRNA Profile in Cancer

Several studies have shown that miRNAs are involved in cancers since they regulate the expression of genes responsible for cell growth and apoptosis [6, 7]. Calin and coworkers were the first to provide evidence regarding the involvement of miRNAs in cancers based on a study characterizing the frequently deleted and downregulated chromosome 13q14 in human chronic lymphocytic leukemia (CLL) [51]. They observed that this chromosome which is deleted in a majority of B-cell chronic lymphocytic leukemia contained two miRNAs: miR-15 and miR-16. Subsequently, numerous studies have been undertaken to identify the differentially expressed miRNAs between cancer and normal tissues to further understand their biological functions in tumor development. Because miRNA array technology allows hundreds of miRNAs to be studied simultaneously and enables the observation of altered profiles, investigation of miRNA profiles between cancer and normal tissues were initially carried out by miRNA array to identify miRNAs functions. To date, several microarray-based approaches have been used for miRNA profiling analysis. These include miChip which is a microarray platform for identifying miRNA expression profiles based on locked nucleic acid (LNA) oligonucleotide capture probes [52], an oligonucleotide microarray [53], and a novel bead-based flow cytometric technique designed by Lu et al. Using this novel technique, Lu and colleagues analyzed the expression of 217 miRNAs in 332 tissue samples, including many different types of tumors [54].

The miRNA expression profile seems to be tissue specific: different types of tumors have distinctive patterns of miRNA expression, and the miRNA profiles also reflect the developmental origin of tissues [54] as indicated in Table 2. In the following section, we highlight some representative miRNA

Table 2 Loss of some miRNA expression profiles in cancer

Tumors/Cells	miRNA profiles	Identified methods	Comments	References
B-cell chronic lymphocytic leukemia (B-CLL)	MiR-123,miR-220,and miR-192 down MiR-190,miR-183-prec.miR-33,miR-19a,miR-140,miR-123,miR-10b,miR-15b-prec.miR-92-1,miR-188,miR-154,miR-227,miR-101,miR-141-prec.miR-153-prec.miR-196-2,miR-134,miR-141,miR-132,and miR-181b-prec up	Microarray, confirmed by northern blot and real-time RT-PCR	miRNA profiles are associated with biological behavior and prognosis in B-CLL	146
Glioblastoma	MiR-128,miR-181a,miR-181b,and miR-181c down MiR-221 up	Microarray, confirmed by northern blot	The alternation of miRNAs is associated with glioblastoma	147
Breast cancer	miR-125b, miR-145, miR-21, and miR-155down	Microarray, confirmed by northern blot	miRNAs expression correlates with specific breast cancer biopathologic features	115
Hepatocellular carcinoma	MiR-92,miR-20,miR-18, miR-99a, and miR-18 prec up	Microarray, confirmed by northern blot	miRNAs are potentially involved in the progress of liver tumor	148
Lung cancer	MiR-21,miR-191,miR-210,miR-155,miR-205,miR-24-2,miR-212,miR-214,and miR-17-3 prec up MiR-126,miR-143,miR-192 prec.miR-224,miR-126,miR-30a-5 prec.miR-140,and miR-9down	Microarray, confirmed by real-time RT-PCR	miRNA expression profiles could be diagnostic and prognostic markers of lung cancer	149
Colorectal cancer	MiR-19a,miR-21,miR-29a,miR-92,miR-148a,and miR-200b up MiR-30c,miR-133a,and miR-145 down	Real-time PCR	miRNA profiles has relevance to the biological and clinical behavior of colorectal neoplasia	58

Table 2 (continued)

Tumors/Cells	miRNA profiles	Identified methods	Comments	References
Pituitary adenomas	MiR-26a,miR-26b, miR-197,miR-103,miR-103-2,miR-192,miR-149, and miR-24 up MiR-128a,miR-136,miR-132,miR-223,miR-7-3,let-7a-1,let-7f-1,miR-192-2/3,miR-9-3,miR-7-1,let-7e,miR-212,miR-164,miR-138-2,miR-7-3,and miR-100-1/2down	Microarray, confirmed by real-time RT-PCR	Several differentially expressed miRNAs are involved in cell proliferation and apoptosis	150
Pancreatic cancer	MiR-221,miR-424,miR-301,miR-100, miR-376a,miR-125b-1,miR-2, miR-16-1,miR-181, miR-92-1, miR-15b, miR-155,let-7f-1, miR-212,miR-107,miR-24,and let-7d up MiR-345,miR-142 prec,and miR-139 down	Real-time PCR, confirmed by northern blot	Differentially expressed miRNAs could be involved in tumorigenesis in pancreatic adenocarcinoma.	151
Thyroid anaplastic carcinomas	MiR-30d, miR-125b,miR-26a, and miR-30a-5 prec down	Microarray, confirmed by northern blot and real-time PCR	a miRNA signature is associated with ATC and suggest the miRNAs as an important event in thyroid cell transformation	152
Prostate cancer	Let-7a, b,c,d,g; miR-16; miR-23a,b; miR-26a, miR-92, miR-143,miR-145,miR-195,miR-199, miR-221, miR-222,miR-497,miR-99a, miR-103,and miR-125a,b; down MiR-202,miR-210,miR-296,miR-320,miR-370,miR-373,miR-498,and miR-503 up	Oligonucleotide array, confirmed by northern blot	Differentially expressed miRNAs could become a novel diagnostic and prognostic tools for prostate cancer	57
Ovarian cancer	MiR-200a,miR-141,miR-200c,and miR-200b up MiR-199a, miR-140, miR-145, and miR-125b1 down	Microarray, confirmed by northern blot and real-time PCR	miRNAs might play a role in the pathogenesis of human epithelial ovarian cancer.	56

Table 2 (continued)

Tumors/Cells	miRNA profiles	Identified methods	Comments	References
Kidney cancer	*MiR-28,miR-185,miR-27,* and *let-7f-2* up	Microarray, confirmed by northern blot and real-time PCR	Differently expressed miRNAs are involved in the development and progression of kidney cancer	153
Bladder cancer	*MiR-223, miR-26b, miR-221,miR-103-1,miR-185,miR-23b,miR-203,miR-17-5p,miR-23a,*and *miR-205* up *MiR-26b* down	Microarray, confirmed by northern blot and real-time PCR	Differently expressed miRNAs are involved in the development and progression of bladder cancer	153
Papillary thyroid carcinoma	*MiR-221,miR-222 ,*and *miR-146* up	Microarray, confirmed by northern blot	Upregulated miRNAs are involved in papillary thyroid carcinoma pathogenesis	154

profiles in cancer. Pallante et al. analyzed the genome-wide miRNA expression profile in human thyroid papillary carcinomas (PTCs) using a miRNACHIP microarray containing hundreds of human precursor and mature miRNA oligonucleotide probes [55]. Using this approach, they found an aberrant miRNA expression profile that clearly differentiates PTCs from normal thyroid tissues. In particular, a significant increase in *miR-221, miR-222*, and *miR-181b* was detected in PTCs in comparison with normal thyroid tissue. They also functionally studied the *miR-221*, and reported a miRNA signature associated with PTCs, and also suggested miRNA deregulation as an important event in thyroid cell transformation. Iorio et al. used microarray to identify miRNA profiles in human ovarian cancer and found that *miR-200a, miR-141, miR-200c*, and *miR-200b* were the most significantly overexpressed, whereas *miR-199a, miR-140, miR-145*, and *miR-125b1* were the most downmodulated miRNAs [56].

Unique miRNA signatures distinguishing between benign tumors and carcinoma tumors has also been established for prostate cancer. For example, Porkka et al. investigated differentially expressed miRNAs between prostate benign tumors and carcinomas tumors using an oligonucleotide array hybridization method. Fifty-one differentially expressed miRNAs were detected, 37 of them were downregulated while 14 miRNAs were upregulated in carcinoma tumors and indicated that those miRNAs could be significant in prostate cancer development and/or growth [57].

Bandrés et al. examined the expression of 156 mature miRNA in colorectal cancer by real-time PCR and the results suggested that miRNA expression profile could be relevant to the biological and clinical behavior of colorectal neoplasia [58]. Michael et al. identified 28 different miRNAs in a colonic adenocarcinoma and normal mucosa by using miRNA cloning and northern blotting. They also indicated that *miR-143* and *miR-145* are downregulated in cells derived from breast, prostate, cervical, and lymphoid cancers as well as colorectal tumors [59].

Because colorectal cancer develops through two differently pathological pathways, Lanza et al. used miRNA microarray chip to investigate different miRNA profiles of colorectal cancer between two differently pathological pathways. They reported the presence of 27 differently expressed gene, including 8 miRNAs and showed that their functions were most frequently associated with cell cycle, DNA replication, recombination, repair, gastrointestinal disease, and immune response [60].

Within a single developmental cell lineage such as acute lymphoblastic leukaemia, distinct patterns of miRNA expression can also be observed that represent different mechanisms of transformation [61]. Zanette et al. determined miRNA expression profile of chronic and acute lymphoblastic leukaemia (CCL and ALL) using TaqMan MicroRNA Assay Human Panel [62]. The five most highly expressed miRNAs were *miR-128b, miR-204, miR-218, miR-331*, and *miR-181b-1* in ALL, and *miR-331, miR-29a, miR-195, miR-34a*, and *miR-29c* in CLL [62]. Using cloning and quantitative real-time PCR, *miR-21* and *miR-155* have been confirmed to be highly overexpressed in the patients with CLL [63].

Taken together, miRNA expression profiles in cancer provides important clues for further understanding tumor development/metastases as well as for diagnosis and prognosis. The levels of some miRNAs are reduced in tumors with poor cell differentiation, reflecting the role of miRNAs in cell differentiation in cancer tissues. Conversely, the levels of some miRNAs are increased in tumors, potentially indicating the role of miRNAs as oncogenes. Consequently, investigation of miRNAs that are enriched in tumor but not normal tissues, or vice versa, may identify miRNA-regulated genes involved in human cancer. If the levels of miRNAs in cancer cells, relative to normal tissues, are different, it is important to identify those genes that are regulated by these miRNAs and to see how these altered expressions influence the development of malignancy. The study of tumor suppressor and oncogene miRNA targets using computational prediction softwares and carrying out experiments for validation, should further our understanding of tumor development or metastases. Given the number of miRNAs and genes, it remains to be determined whether each miRNA can target the exact genes and genetic pathways under miRNA control in tumorigenesis.

4.2 miRNA Roles in Tumorigenesis

With extensive investigation of miRNA profiles between cancer and normal tissues, specific miRNAs have been suggested to be associated with tumor initiation, promotion, and progression as called tumorigenesis. Some miRNAs involved in tumorigenesis are summarized in Table 3. *lin-4* and *let-7* which control the timing of fate specification of neuronal and hypodermal cells in *C. elegans* during larval development was the first evidence of miRNAs involvement in cell proliferation [21]. Human *let-7* shows diminished expression in lung tumors, whereas Ras is overexpressed, which is an oncogene regulated by *let-7*miRNA. Moreover, overexpression of *let-7* in lung cancer cell lines decreases growth rates [64]. Recently, a published study by Schultz et al. indicated that the members of *let-7* miRNA family are downregulated in primary melanomas and demonstrated that *let-7b* represses expression of cyclins D1, D3, Cdk4, and CyclinA and consequently effects cell-cycle progression and anchorage-independent growth [65]. Additionally, Shell et al. demonstrated that the expression of *let-7* can define two differentiation stages of cancer using ovarian cancer as a model [66], suggesting that *let-7* is involved in tumor development at the specific manner. It is interesting to note that *let-7* miRNA family can suppress non-small cell development in lung tumor [67], suggesting that *let-7* acts as a tumor suppressor. These studies further provide clear evidences to support that miRNAs regulate tumor development. Sempere et al. observed that the mammalian ortholog of *C. elegans lin-28*, which is downregulated by *lin-4* in worms, was also repressed during neuronal differentiation of mammalian embryonal carcinoma cells and indicated that

Table 3 Roles of some miRNAs in tumorigenesis

miRNA	Expressed patterns	Tumors	Target mRNAs	Functions/Observation	References
Let-7b	↓	Melanomas	Cyclin D1	*Let-7b* reduces cells cycle progress in primary melanomas	65
miR-378	↑	Numbers of tumors	SuFu and Fus-1	*miR-378* promotes cell survival, tumor growth and angiogenesis	155
miR-34b/34c	↓↑	Numbers of tumors	p53, E2F3 or MYCN	*miR-34b/34c* are targets of p53, E2F3, or MYCN and then inhibit cell proliferation, is also overexpressed in various type of human cancer	79,81,83,84
miR-15a/16-1	↓	Chronic lymphocytic leukemia	Bcl2	*miR-15a* and *miR-16-1* are natural antisense Bcl2 interactors	105
miR-372/373	↑	Testicular germ cell tumors	LATS2	*miR-372/373* are potential oncogenes in the development of human testicular germ cell tumors	98,156
miR-200 Family and *miR-205*	↓	MDCK cells with modification	ZEB1 and SIP1	*miR-200* family and *miR-205* downregulate tumor metastasis	157
miR-17-5p-92	↑	Neuroblastoma	p21 and BIM	The upmodulation of miR-17-5p mediates the oncogenic properties of *MYCN*, through a direct suppression of *p21* and *BIM* translation	131
miR-137	↓	Melanoma cell lines	MITF	*miR-137* downregulated MITF which is the master regulator of melanocyte development, survival, and functions	158

SuFu – suppressor of fused homolog; MYCN – MYC family of proto-oncogenes; Bcl2 – B-cell lymphoma 2 protein; MDCK – Madin Darby Canine Kidney; LAST2 – large tumor suppressor 2; ZEB1 – zinc finger E-box binding homeobox 1, SIP1 – survival of motor neuron protein interacting protein 1; BIM – Bcl 2 interacting mediator of cell death; MITF – micropthalmia-associated transcription factor.

mammalian *lin-28* messenger RNAs contain conserved predicted binding sites in their 3'-UTR regions for neuron-expressed *mir-125b, let-7a, mir-218* [68]. This result suggested miRNAs (*let-7, mir-125b, let-7a,* and *mir-218*) could be involved in tumor differentiation via binding to 3' untranslated regions of target gene. Recent evidence strongly suggests *miR-373* and *miR-520c* are involved in stimulating cancer cell migration and invasion, indicating that those miRNAs can promote cancer metastasis [27].

Apart from downregulated miRNAs, upregulated miRNAs are also associated with tumorigenesis. It is well established that *miR-17-92* polycistron is located in chromosome 13q31 that is amplified in human B-cell lymphomas. He et al. demonstrated that *miRNA-17-92* cluster can cooperate with oncogene gene c-Myc, which is a oncogenic transcription factor, to promote tumor development [69]. To further reveal mechanism behind this phenomenon, O'Donnell et al. also investigated the interaction between *miR-17-92* cluster with Myc [70]. They found that Myc directly binds to *miR-17-92* locus on chromosome 13 and activates expression of the miRNA cluster and also shows that two miRNAs from this cluster (*miR-17-5p* and *miR-20a*) negatively regulate expression of E2F1 transcription factor, which is an additional target of Myc that promotes cell-cycle progression. Further evidence provided by Chang and coworkers revealed that c-Myc can regulate a much broader set of miRNAs than previously anticipated and indicated that much of this repression is likely to be a direct result of Myc binding to miRNA promoters [71]. In addition, Hayashita et al. observed that the overexpression of *miR-17-92* is associated with the enhancement of cell proliferation in human lung cancers [72]. Wang et al. indicated that *miR-17-92* cluster can accelerate adipocyte differentiation by negatively regulating tumor-suppressor gene Rb2/p130 [73]. Recently published results indicated that *miR-17* polycistron (*miR-17-18-19-20-92*) with transcript factor Myc can synergistically contribute to tumor development, probably by repressing tumor-suppressor genes [74]. Using transgenic mice to overexpress *mir-17-92* cluster in embryonic lung epithelium, it has been observed that *mir-17-92* promotes the high proliferation and undifferentiated phenotype of lung epithelial progenitor cells [75]. Another well-characterized miRNA-*miR-21*, which is overexpressed in a wide variety of cancers, will be introduced in the section of miRNAs as oncogenes.

miR-34a has been demonstrated to target MYCN, which is commonly found to be amplified in neuroblastoma as well as brain tumor [76], breast tumor [77], and cervix cancer [78]. Wei and coworkers demonstrated that *miR-34a* causes significant decrease of cell growth through increased apoptosis and inhibited DNA synthesis [79], suggesting that *miR-34a* is a tumor-suppressor miRNA. Further studies indicated *miR-34, miR-34b,* and *miR-34c* can cooperate with p53 tumor suppressor in control of tumor growth and development [80, 81]. The expression of *miR-34a* could lead to cell apoptosis by p53-dependent pathway. Conversely, perturbation of *miR-34a* expression, as occurs in some human cancers, could contribute to tumorigenesis [82]. In addition, Welch et al. also demonstrated that *miR-34a* functions as a potential tumor suppressor by inducing apoptosis in neuroblastoma cell though targeting E2F3 protein, which is a potent transcriptional inducer of cell-cycle progression [83]. However, Dutta et al. indicated that the overexpression of *miR-34a* can also be observed in various types of human cancers such as mucinous adenocarcinoma and infiltrating papillary carcinoma, which is associated with cell proliferation [84]. Those results suggest that even one miRNA probably has different roles in different type of cancer.

So far, the main epigenetic alternations in cancer are aberrant DNA hypermethylation of tumor-suppressor genes, global genomic DNA hypomethylation, and disruption of the histone modification patterns, which result in inappropriate cellular proliferation and survival. The epigenetic modification could attribute to miRNA-mediated tumorigenesis due to the downregulated expression of miRNAs that are considered as tumor-suppressor gene [56, 85]. For example, *miR-127* and *miR-124a* are transcriptionally inactivated by CpG island hypermethylatin in colorectal cancer [86], whereas in lung cancer, the overexpression of miRNA with oncogenic function, *let-7a-3*, seems to be due to DNA hypomethylation [87].

Overall, the upregulated miRNAs with oncogenic function in caner could be considered oncogenic miRNAs, named as oncomirs. The downregulated miRNAs with tumor-suppressor function could be considered as tumor-suppressor miRNAs. We will discuss the most well-understood oncomirs and tumor-suppressor miRNAs in the following sections.

4.3 miRNAs as Oncogenes

miRNAs act as oncogenes by inhibiting the expression of tumor suppressors or by downregulating genes that inhibit the activity of known oncogenes [88]. Table 4 summarizes some well-characterized oncogenic miRNAs. *miR-155*, which is a product of the *BIC* transcript, was the first oncomir discovered and it has been shown to be upregulated in many solid tumors as well as in leukemias and lymphomas [89]. In an avian model, oncogenic cooperation between the *BIC* and the *MYC* genes in lymphomagenesis and erythroleukemogenesis has been observed, indicating that MYC and BIC might cooperate in human tumors [90]. Costinean and coworkers developed the first transgenic mouse that specifically overexpresses *miR-155* in B cells, thus modeling the human B-cell leukemia where the upregulation of *miR-155* is observed. The transgenic mice developed polyclonal pre-leukemia B-cell type followed by B-cell malignancy. However, the death of these mice is not an early event, suggesting that *miR-155* deregulation needs additional genetic alterations for the development of the fully malignant phenotype [91].

The best characterized oncogenic miRNA is *miR-17-92* cluster. This miRNA cluster is encoded by a polycistronic transcript from the chromosome 13 open reading frame 25. *miR-17-92* cluster interacts with c-myc, which is

Table 4 List of some miRNAs as oncogenes

miRNA	Tumors	Effect factors/proposed targets	Functions/Observation	References
miR-17-92 clusters	Human B-cell lymphomas	c-myc	miRNAs can modulate tumor formation	69
miR-373/520c	Testicular germ cell tumors	CD44	miRNAs stimulate cancer cell migration and invasion	27
miR-10b	Breast cancer	Twist	*miR-10b* positively regulates cell migration and invasion	92
miR-221/222	Prostate carcinoma	Kip1	The overexpression of these miRNAs probably contribute to the oncogenesis and progression of prostate carcinoma	97
miR-372/373	Testicular Germ Cell Tumors	LATS2	These miRNAs neutralize p53-mediated CDK inhibition	98
miR-21	Numbers of tumors	PTEN or TPM1	*miR-21* suppresses the expression of tumor-suppressor gene	93,95

LAST2 – large tumor suppressor 2; PTEN – phosphatase and tensin homolog; TPM1 – tumor-suppressor tropomyosin-1.

pathologically activated in many human cancers, to accelerate tumor development [69]. *miR-10b* has also been shown to positively regulate cells migration and invasion in breast cancer upon inducing by transcription factor twist [92]. Both the overexpression of *miR-17-92* and *miR-10b* results from the oncogenic transcript factors binding with genome and initiating mRNA transcript. *miR-21*, which is another well-characterized oncogenic miRNA, is overexpressed in a wide variety of cancer and has been demonstrated to be linked to cell proliferation, apoptosis, and cell migration. Knockdown of *miR-21* in cultured glioblastoma cells triggers activation of caspase activity, leading to increased apoptotic cell death. In addition, the disruption of *miR-21* affects the glioma growth in vivo. Si et al. demonstrated that *miR-21* can promote growth of the breast cancer cell line MCF-7 both in vitro and in vivo, which may be due to the ability of *miR-21* to suppress the expression of the tumor-suppressor PTEN and tropomyosin 1 (TPM1) [93–95]. *miR-21* can also target and downregulate the expression of sprouty 2 and inhibit the cell of outgrowth [96]. Galardi et al. indicated that *miR-221/222* can be a new family of oncogenes, directly targeting the tumor-suppressor p27(Kip1), and that their overexpression might be one of the factors contributing to the oncogenesis and progression of prostate carcinoma through p27(Kip1) downregulation [97].

Some oncogenic miRNAs control tumor development by mediating the expression of tumor-suppressor genes such as p53 and TPM1. For example, Voorhoeve et al. demonstrated that *miR-372/373* neutralize p53-mediated CDK inhibition and then potentially become novel oncogenes participating in the development of human testicular germ cell tumors [98]. On the other side, some miRNAs can also regulate tumor development by adjusting the activities of some kinases. For example, *miR-106-363* cluster potentially regulates homeodomain-interacting protein kinase 3 and then promotes cancer metastasis [99].

4.4 miRNAs as Tumor Suppressors

miRNAs function as tumor suppressors by inhibiting the expression of oncogenes and then blocking tumorigenesis as summarized in Table 5. miRNA-*let-7* has been shown to act as a tumor suppressor in extensive tumors including lung cancers [64], colorectal [100] and breast cancers [101], and leiomyoma [102]. Now it has been demonstrated that, *let-7* can regulate cell differentiation, proliferation, apoptosis, and transformation by suppressing the expression of Ras and high-mobility group A2 (HMGA2), which are kind of oncogenes [64, 102]. Disruption of the pairing between *let-7* and HMGA2 can enhance oncogenic transformation [103]. Furthermore, the introduction of *let-7* miRNA by intranasal administration can suppress the growth and formation of lung tumor in xenografts mice [104]. These observations suggest *let-7* miRNA may be useful as a therapeutic agent in cancer.

Table 5 List of some miRNAs as tumor suppressors

miRNA	Tumors	Target mRNA	Functions	References
miR-221/222	Glioblastomas	p27^{Kip1}	miR-221/222 inhibit tumor proliferation	159
miR-29	Cholangiocarcinoma cell line and lung cancer	Mcl-1, DM3a, and DM3b	miR-29 induces tumor cell apoptosis	106,109
Let-7	Numbers of cancers	Ras or HMGA	Let-7 inhibits tumor cell growths and proliferation	64,102,104
miR-15/16	Chronic lymphocytic leukemia	Bcl2	miR-15/16 induce apoptosis by targeting BCL2	105
miR-119a	Fibroblasts tumor	Met or ERK2	miR-199a may be effective in inhibiting cell proliferation and motility and invasive capabilities of tumor cells	107
miR-7	Glioblastoma	EGFR, Ras 1, or Ras2	miR-7 is a regulator of major cancer pathway	108

DM3a – DNA methyltransferase 3A; DM3b – DNA methyltransferase 3b; HMGA – HMAG, high mobility group A; BCL2 – B-cell lymphoma 2 protein; ERK2 – extracellular signal-regulated kinase 2; EGRF – epidermal growth factor receptor.

miRNAs can also downregulate the expression of antiapoptotic proteins or kinases in cancer by serving as tumor suppressors. For example, Cimmino et al. demonstrated that *miR-15* and *miR-16* can induce apoptosis by targeting anti-apoptotic B-cell lymphoma 2 protein (BCL2), which is a central player in the genetic program of eukaryotic cells favoring survival by inhibiting cell death in B-cell chronic lymphocytic leukemia [105]. *miR-29* can induce tumor cell apoptosis by negatively regulating Mcl-1 protein expression, which belongs to BCL2 protein family [105, 106]. Kim et al. documented that *miR-199a* regulates not only the Met-proto-oncogene but also the downstream extracellular signal-regulated kinase 2 (ERK2), leading to tumor cell apoptosis [107]. Recently, *miR-7* has been identified a new tumor suppressor by suppressing epidermal growth factor receptor expression (EGFR) and inhibiting the Akt pathway via targeting upstream regulators such as Ras 1 or Ras 2 [108].

miRNAs can also regulate the expression of enzymes involved DNA methylation and then control tumor development. For example, Fabbri et al. demonstrated that *miR-29* family including *miR-29a*, *b*, and *c*, which is downregulated in tumor cells line, target DNA methyltransferase 3A and 3B. The enforced expression of *miR-29* in lung tumor induces reexpression of methylation-silenced tumor-suppressor gene and inhibits tumorigensis both in vitro and in vivo [109].

5 miRNA for Diagnosis and Prognosis in Cancer Patients

miRNA expression profiling using bead-based flow cytometry, northern blot analyses, RT-PCR, and miRNA microarrays has been used to demonstrate distinct expressions of specific miRNAs in certain tumor tissues [49, 54, 110–113]. These characteristic miRNA signatures suggest that miRNAs have the potential to be used as diagnostic and prognostic tools, especially since they are more informative in distinguishing between cancer types and for determining cancer metastases when compared with traditional biomarkers. For example, Lu *et al.* used a novel bead-based flow cytometry miRNA expression profiling method to analyze the systematic expression of 217 mammalian miRNAs in normal and human cancer samples. Overall, they observed a downregulation of the miRNAs in tumors compared with normal tissues. Additionally, Lu and coworkers were able to classify poorly differentiated tumors using expression profiles of relatively few miRNA [54]. Furthermore, Chen et al. showed that miR-181, miR-223, and miR-142 s were overexpressed in hematopoietic tissues using northern blot analysis [25]. Using real-time PCR to analyze the expression of miR-21 in 37 gastric patients, Chan et al. found a 92% overexpression of miR-21 in tumor tissue, demonstrating the potential of miR-21 as diagnostic marker for gastric cancer [114]. With the application of oligonucleotide micro-chips, Croce's group observed unique miRNA signatures for human breast cancer, human megakaryocytopoiesis, and B-cell CLL [115, 116].

miRNA signatures can also provide useful information for determining prognosis in patients with cancer. For example, in ovarian cancer the expression of *let-7* and HMGA2 is a better predictor of disease progression than classical markers such as E-cadherin, vimentin, and snail [66]. Also, the high expression of *miR-21* has been linked with poor survival and therapeutic response in patients with colon adenocarcinoma [117]; while high expression of *miR-191* and *miR-199a* in acute myeloid leukemia patients correlated with poor prognosis compared with those with low expression [118]. Guo and coworkers have also shown that a high expression of *miR-103/107* leads to low survival in patients with esophageal cancer [119]. Another example of miRNA expression and cancer prognosis is the high *miR-155* expression and low *let-7a-2* expression resulting in poor survival in the patients with lung cancer.

It is important to note, that some miRNA signatures are efficient diagnostic markers but poor indicators of clinical prognosis. For example, Chan et al. used quantitative PCR to examine the expression level of *miR-21* in 37 patients with gastric cancer and found *miR-21* to be an efficient diagnostic marker, but a poor prognostic tool for gastric cancer [114]. Taken together, distinct miRNA signatures can be used as cancer diagnostics and to foretell prognosis. However, there is still a long way to adopt this technology clinically since the function of unique miRNAs differently expressed in different tumors should first be well understood.

6 Therapeutic Implication of miRNAs

Many cancer types are characterized by an aberrant expression of miRNAs and as such represent a potential therapeutic target for cancer therapy. Presently, two technologies adapted from gene therapy and RNAi technology may be used to alter the levels of expression of miRNAs. In the first approach, antisense oligonucleotides (ASOs) can be used to inhibit the effects of miRNA by specifically binding with target miRNA and then blocking its normal function, while in the second approach, cancer causing miRNAs can be replaced by vectors overexpressing a specific miRNA or by transiently transfected double-stranded miRNAs.

6.1 miRNA Inhibition

Inhibition of miRNA can be achieved by introducing antisense molecules targeting mature miRNA or introducing siRNA/shRNA to silence the various components involved in miRNA processing.

6.1.1 miRNA Inhibition Using Modified Antisense Oligonucleotide

ASO-based gene therapy has been clinically applied for human disease [120]. Now it also was extended for silencing miRNA. To the best of our knowledge, the first reported study on miRNAs silencing by using ASO was presented by Boutla et al. in 2003 [121]. In this study, the authors synthesized 11 DNA oligonucleotides complementary to 11 miRNAs and then injected them into *Drosophila* embryos, then a variety of developmental defects were observed, suggesting that these oligonucleotides inhibited miRNA activity and could become a potential target for treating cancer by inhibiting oncogenic miRNA.

To improve potency for the target nucleic acid, resistance to endogenous nuclease, or improved activation of RNase H or other protein involved in the terminating mechanism, several strategies have been applied to modify ASO for silencing a given gene [12]. The first generation of ASO was designed to resist nuclease attack by replacing one of the non-bridging oxygen atoms in the phosphate group of ASO with either sulfur or a methyl group [122]. However, this modification leads to several side effects due to unspecific interaction and poor solubility in water [123]. Then, sugars were also modified by adding *O*-methyl, fluro, *O*-propyl, *O*-allyl or other groups at the 2′ position to increase affinity for RNA and impart some nuclease stability, named as the second generation of ASO [124]. Additionally, 3′-hydroxyl group of the 2′-deoxyribose has been replaced with a 3′-amino group for ASO, named as N3′→P5′ phosphoramidates, and shown a very high-binding affinity to complementary DNA or RNA [125].

To date, phosphorothioate and/or 2′ sugar modified ASO has also been used to silence miRNA (Fig. 3). To the best of our knowledge, the first report to use

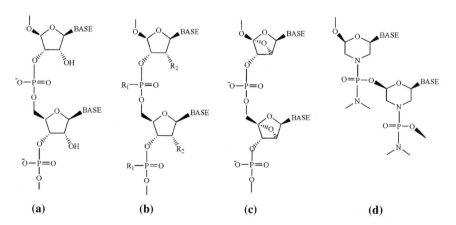

Fig. 3 Chemically modified ASOs that have been used for anti-miRNA. (**a**) Unmodified ASO. (**b**) Chemically modified ASO with phosphorothioate backbone (R1 position) and 2′ sugar modification such as 2′-*O*-methyl, 2′-*O*-methyoxyethyl, and 2′-flouro (R2 position). (**c**) Locked nucleic acid. (**d**) Morpholino

modified ASO to silence miRNA was presented by Hutvagner et al. and cow-orkers in 2004 [126]. They injected the 2′-O-methyl modified ASO, which is complementary to the miRNA *let-7*, leading to a *let-7* loss-of-function pheno-copy in *C. elegans* [126]. Davis et al. systematically evaluated the correlation between ASO with 2′-sugar and 2′-F modified backbone and its potency target-ing miRNA and demonstrated that ASO modification improve miRNA ASO activity by improving target affinity [127]. They also noted that the positioning of high-affinity modifications had dramatically different effects on miRNA activity. Locked nucleic acid (LNA) modified oligonucleotides have been used as sensitive and specific miRNA detection probes in northern blots due to its high efficiency for binding targeting sequence [128]. Then LNA modified nucleotide has been shown to have specific and long-lasting silencing effect on miRNA in cell lines [129, 130]. Fontana et al. used 2′-O-methyl modified antagomir targeting *miR-17-5p-92* and demonstrated that both in vitro and in vivo treatments with antagomir-*17-5p* abolishe the growth of *MYCN*-amplified and therapy-resistant neuroblastoma through p21 and BIM upmodulation, leading to cell-cycling blockade and activation of apoptosis, respectively [131]. As we mentioned above, *miR-21* has been found to be upregulated in variety of solid tumors. Transfection of breast cancer MCF-7 cells with anti-miR-21 oligonucleotide with 2′-O-methyl modification suppressed cell growth in vitro and tumor growth in the xenograft mouse model by increasing cell apoptosis and increasing cell proliferation [93]. All these data suggest that downregulation of *miR-21* in solid tumors might be a way for tumor regression. Apart from modified ASOs, which are targeting mature miRNAs, Morpholino has been shown to affect the processing of the pri-miRNA and pre-miRNA and then inhibit the activity of mature miRNA as presented by Kloosterman and coworkers [132]. In this study, they also observed that knockdown of *miR-375* causes morphological defect in pancreatic islets by using Morpholino [132].

To further improve potency for targeting miRNA in vivo, modified ASOs could be conjugated with delivery agents such as cholesterols or be formulated with lipid, polymer or peptide-based delivery system (Fig. 4). Krützfeldt et al. [133] used cholesterol to conjugate with a series of modified miRNA antisenses, named as 'antagomirs' and demonstrated that antagomirs are efficient and specific silencers of endogenous miRNAs in mice. Intravenous administration of antagomirs against *miR-16*, *miR-122*, *miR-192*, and *miR-194* resulted in a marked reduction of corresponding miRNA levels in most organ, suggesting that the silencing of endogenous miRNAs by this novel method is specific, efficient and long-lasting, and potentially toward therapeutic propose. They also noted that injection of unmodified single-stranded RNA targeting *miR-122* had no effect on level of *miR-122* in liver, whereas injection of unconjugated, but chemically modified, single-stranded RNAs with a partially modified or fully modified phosphorothioate backbone and 2′-OMe sugar modification led to an incomplete effect, suggesting that modified miRNA antisenses can sig-nificantly improve potency in vivo. Fontana et al. also used 2′-OMe modified,

Anti-miRNA ASO

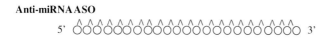

Anti-miRNA ASO with chemical modifications

◎ 2'-Sugar modification

＊ Backbone modification

Cholesterol-conjugated anti-miRNA ASO

◎ 2'-Sugar modification

＊ Backbone modification

cholesterol

Fig. 4 Scheme for improving ASO stability and silencing effect for miRNA. (**a**) Unmodified ASO. (**b**) 2′ Sugar and backbone modified ASO. (**c**) Cholesterol-conjugated ASO at 3′ end

phosphorothioate backbone, and cholesterol-conjugated ASO to target *miR-17-5p-92* cluster and demonstrated that the abrogation of *miR-17-5p-92* leads to cell-cycling blockade and activation of apoptosis [131]. Overall, modifications of different positions of ASO including 2′-hydroxyl group and backbone as well as conjugation with delivery agent could at most facilitate miRNA silencing effect.

Esau and coworkers also inhibited miR-122 in normal mice by intraperitoneally injecting an unconjugated 2′-MOE modified anti-miRNA oligonucleotide (AMO) [134]. This led to an increase in mRNA levels of miR-122 target genes and a decrease in plasma cholesterol. While the mechanism governing the reduction of miRNA by the AMOs is not clear, it is known that the AMO acts on the mature miRNAs since the levels of pre-miR-122 remain unchanged.

In spite of the potential therapeutic benefits of using AMOs for treating cancer, clinical application is presently inhibited due to a lack of effective delivery of AMOs into target sites. Possible approaches to delivering AMOs include complexing them with lipids or proteins; using cationic liposomes [135, 136] or conjugating AMOs with homing signals for site-specific delivery. Recently, Akinc et al. developed a new class of lipid-like delivery molecules, termed lipidoids, as delivery agent for RNAi therapeutics and reported that lipidoids facilitate high levels of specific silencing of miRNAs when formulated with single-strand antisense 2'-O-methyl oligoribonucleotides [137]. With progress in the development of better delivery vehicles, miRNA targeting will ultimately become commercially available as a therapeutic agent.

6.1.2 Targeting miRNAs Processing Using Antisense Oligonucleotide

Another approach for therapeutically inhibiting miRNA expression involves downregulating the various components in the miRNA biogenesis pathway to prevent the production of mature miRNA [138]. Small molecule drugs or RNAi interference can be used to achieve this by inhibiting *Drosha*, *Dicer*, and other miRNA pathway components [15, 18]. However, this therapeutic approach is often accompanied by pleiotropic effects which can be minimized by tightly controlling the expression of miRNA pathway components using a tetracycline-inducible shRNA for downregulation. Nevertheless, recent studies indicate that the inhibition of components involved in the miRNA biogenesis pathway has very little effect on miRNA levels possibly due to the slow turnover of mature miRNA [15, 16].

The application of RNAi interference for silencing various component of the miRNA pathway has historically been inhibited by the fact that the miRNA/RISC complex and the hairpin pre-miRNA are not easily accessible by siRNA. Furthermore, since siRNA is active in the cytoplasm, it cannot be used to target pri-miRNA which is located in the nucleus. In one study, Lee and coworkers used siRNA to target the loop region of a pre-miRNA in the cytoplasm and found it to be highly inefficient requiring a very high dose compared to other mRNA targets. Since then, developing ways to obtain long-term suppression of miRNA has been the subject of intense research.

One approach which may be used to target pri-miRNAs involves using ASOs utilizing the RNase H mechanism since their primary site of action is in the nucleus [139, 140]. This strategy may be valuable for inhibiting polycistronic pri-miRNAs where one ASO can be used to target the transcripts of pri-miRNAs and hence inhibit the processing of the mature miRNA; whereas multiple AMOs would be needed to target each miRNA individually.

6.2 *miRNA Replacement*

As mentioned above, the replacement of cancer causing miRNAs may be used as a therapy for various cancers. This may be done by transiently transfecting double-stranded miRNA mimetics or by using vectors overexpressing a particular miRNA. In both approaches, the goal is to re-establish the levels of miRNA expression occurring prior to the inception of cancer. The double-stranded miRNA mimetic introduced is equivalent to the *Dicer* product and analogous in its function on target mRNAs. Since double-stranded miRNA mimetics are analogous in structure to siRNAs they are subject to all the limitations associated with siRNA therapy, including the difficulty in systemic delivery to tissues and the need for modifications to enhance their stability and cellular uptake [141– 143]. An additional issue with this method is the transient nature of miRNA expression.

One way of addressing this limitation is to use a gene therapy approach that results in longer lasting miRNA expression. In this approach, a plasmid or viral vector driven by a pol II or III promoter upstream of short hairpin RNA (shRNA) is used to express a specific miRNA which is then loaded into RISC after being processed into mature miRNA by *Dicer*. The benefits associated with these constructs are their long-lasting silencing compared to double-stranded miRNA mimetics and their capacity to express multiple miRNAs from one transcript. Examples include the use of adeno-associated virus (AAV) virus vectors as therapeutics for miRNA delivery to the liver and brain [144, 145]. However, the eliciting of immune response and the possibility of insertional mutagenesis has limited clinical use of AAVs and lentiviruses, respectively.

7 Concluding Remarks

miRNAs are small non-coding RNAs of about 22 nt, which modulate gene expression in a sequence-specific manner. It has been established that miR-NAs play an important role in cell proliferation, differentiation, and apoptosis. Because cancer is a class of disease in which a group of cells display the trait of uncontrolled growth, invasion, and metastasis, accumulated evidence indicated that miRNAs act as an important regulator in tumorigenesis such as oncogenes, tumor-suppressor factor, or other effective factors. Unique miRNA signatures have provided useful information for diagnosis and prognosis in patients with cancer. Blockage of miRNAs with oncogenic function by ASO has been shown to inhibit tumor cell growth and proliferation. Several types of modified ASOs as well as conjugation with cholesterols or lipid-based delivery have been demonstrated to improve potency both in vitro and in vivo. Overexpression of tumor-suppressor miRNA by introducing plasmid encoding miRNA or infecting lentivirus encoding miRNAs can suppress tumor development.

Although miRNA therapeutic modulation is potentially attractive for treating cancer as well as diagnosis and prognosis, there is still a great need to deeply understand the roles of miRNA in tumorigenesis. It is also necessary to develop an effective and efficient method for delivering antagomirs in vivo. Finally, the inhibition of miRNAs in conjunction with other chemotherapy strategies could significantly improve the outcome of cancer patients.

References

1. Bartel DP 2004. MicroRNAs: genomics, biogenesis, mechanism, and function. Cell 116(2):281–297.
2. Pasquinelli AE, Ruvkun G 2002. Control of developmental timing by micrornas and their targets. Annu Rev Cell Dev Biol 18:495–513.
3. Lee RC, Feinbaum RL, Ambros V 1993. The C. elegans heterochronic gene lin-4 encodes small RNAs with antisense complementarity to lin-14. Cell 75(5):843–854.
4. Berezikov E, Guryev V, van de Belt J, Wienholds E, Plasterk RH, Cuppen E 2005. Phylogenetic shadowing and computational identification of human microRNA genes. Cell 120(1):21–24.
5. Lewis BP, Burge CB, Bartel DP 2005. Conserved seed pairing, often flanked by adenosines, indicates that thousands of human genes are microRNA targets. Cell 120(1):15–20.
6. Meltzer PS 2005. Cancer genomics: small RNAs with big impacts. Nature 435:745–746.
7. Cheng AM, Byrom MW, Shelton J, Ford LP 2005. Antisense inhibition of human miRNAs and indications for an involvement of miRNA in cell growth and apoptosis. Nucleic Acids Res 33(4):1290–1297.
8. He L, Hannon GJ 2004. MicroRNAs: small RNAs with a big role in gene regulation. Nat Rev Genet 5:522–531.
9. Ellington AD, Szostak JW 1990. In vitro selection of RNA molecules that bind specific ligands. Nature 346(6287):818–822.
10. Kumar SA, Beach TA, Dickerman HW 1980. Specificity of oligodeoxynucleotide binding of mouse uterine cytosol estradiol receptors. Proc Natl Acad Sci USA 77(6):3341–3345.
11. Fire A, Xu S, Montgomery MK, Kostas SA, Driver SE, Mello CC 1998. Potent and specific genetic interference by double-stranded RNA in Caenorhabditis elegans. Nature 391(6669):806–811.
12. Mahato RI, Cheng K, Guntaka RV 2005. Modulation of gene expression by antisense and antigene oligodeoxynucleotides and small interfering RNA. Expert Opin Drug Deliv 2(1):3–28.
13. Lee Y, Jeon K, Lee JT, Kim S, Kim VN 2002. MicroRNA maturation: stepwise oricessing and subcellular localization. Eur Mol Biol Organization J 21:4663–4670.
14. Denli AM, Tops BB, Plasterk RH, Ketting RF, Hannon GJ 2004. Processing of primary microRNAs by the Microprocessor complex. Nature 432:231–235.
15. Lee Y, Ahn C, Han J, Choi H, Kim J, Yim J, Lee J, Provost P, Radmark O, Kim S, Kim VN 2003. The nuclear RNase III Drosha initiates microRNA processing. Nature 425:415–419.
16. Yi R, Qin Y, Macara IG, Cullen BR 2003. Exportin-5 mediates the nuclear export of pre-microRNAs and short hairpin RNAs. Genes Dev 17(24):3011–3016.
17. Zeng Y, Cullen BR 2004. Structural requirements for pre-microRNA binding and nuclear export by Exportin 5. Nucleic Acids Res 32(16):4776–4785.
18. Lund E, Guttinger S, Calado A, Dahlberg JE, Kutay U 2004. Nuclear export of micro-RNA precursors. Science 303(5654):95–98.
19. Khvorova A, Reynolds A, Jayasena SD 2003. Functional siRNAs and miRNAs exhibit strand bias. Cell 115(2):209–216.
20. Guarnieri DJ, DiLeone RJ 2008. MicroRNAs: a new class of gene regulators. Ann Med 40(3):197–208.
21. Reinhart BJ, Slack FJ, Basson M, Pasquinelli AE, Bettinger JC, Rougvie AE, Horvitz HR, Ruvkun G 2000. The 21-nucleotide let-7 RNA regulates developmental timing in Caenorhabditis elegans. Nature 403(6772):901–906.
22. Wightman B, Ha I, Ruvkun G 1993. Posttranscriptional regulation of the heterochronic gene lin-14 by lin-4 mediates temporal pattern formation in C. elegans. Cell 75(5):855–862.
23. Johnston RJ, Hobert O 2003. A microRNA controlling left/right neuronal asymmetry in Caenorhabditis elegans. Nature 426(6968):845–849.

24. Brennecke J, Hipfner DR, Stark A, Russell RB, Cohen SM 2003. bantam encodes a developmentally regulated microRNA that controls cell proliferation and regulates the proapoptotic gene hid in Drosophila. Cell 113(1):25–36.
25. Chen CZ, Li L, Lodish HF, Bartel DP 2004. MicroRNAs modulate hematopoietic lineage differentiation. Science 303(5654):83–86.
26. Poy MN, Eliasson L, Krutzfeldt J, Kuwajima S, Ma X, Macdonald PE, Pfeffer S, Tuschl T, Rajewsky N, Rorsman P, Stoffel M 2004. A pancreatic islet-specific microRNA regulates insulin secretion. Nature 432(7014):226–230.
27. Huang Q, Gumireddy K, Schrier M, le Sage C, Nagel R, Nair S, Egan DA, Li A, Huang G, Klein-Szanto AJ, Gimotty PA, Katsaros D, Coukos G, Zhang L, Pure E, Agami R 2008. The microRNAs miR-373 and miR-520c promote tumour invasion and metastasis. Nat Cell Biol 10(2):202–210.
28. Lewis BP, Shih IH, Jones-Rhoades MW, Bartel DP, Burge CB 2003. Prediction of mammalian microRNA targets. Cell 115(7):787–798.
29. Enright AJ, John B, Gaul U, Tuschl T, Sander C, Marks DS 2003. MicroRNA targets in Drosophila. Genome Biol 5(1):R1.
30. John B, Enright AJ, Aravin A, Tuschl T, Sander C, Marks DS 2004. Human MicroRNA targets. PLoS Biol 2(11):e363.
31. Rehmsmeier M, Steffen P, Hochsmann M, Giegerich R 2004. Fast and effective prediction of microRNA/target duplexes. RNA 10(10):1507–1517.
32. Krek A, Grun D, Poy MN, Wolf R, Rosenberg L, Epstein EJ, MacMenamin P, da Piedade I, Gunsalus KC, Stoffel M, Rajewsky N 2005. Combinatorial microRNA target predictions. Nat Genet 37(5):495–500.
33. Yousef M, Jung S, Kossenkov AV, Showe LC, Showe MK 2007. Naive Bayes for microRNA target predictions – machine learning for microRNA targets. Bioinformatics 23(22):2987–2992.
34. Long D, Lee R, Williams P, Chan CY, Ambros V, Ding Y 2007. Potent effect of target structure on microRNA function. Nat Struct Mol Biol 14(4):287–294.
35. Betel D, Wilson M, Gabow A, Marks DS, Sander C 2008. The microRNA.org resource: targets and expression. Nucleic Acids Res 36(Database issue):D149–D153.
36. Griffiths-Jones S, Grocock RJ, van Dongen S, Bateman A, Enright AJ 2006. miRBase: microRNA sequences, targets and gene nomenclature. Nucleic Acids Res 34(Database issue):D140–D144.
37. Megraw M, Sethupathy P, Corda B, Hatzigeorgiou AG 2007. miRGen: a database for the study of animal microRNA genomic organization and function. Nucleic Acids Res 35(Database issue):D149–D155.
38. Shahi P, Loukianiouk S, Bohne-Lang A, Kenzelmann M, Kuffer S, Maertens S, Eils R, Grone HJ, Gretz N, Brors B 2006. Argonaute – a database for gene regulation by mammalian microRNAs. Nucleic Acids Res 34(Database issue):D115–D118.
39. Hsu PW, Huang HD, Hsu SD, Lin LZ, Tsou AP, Tseng CP, Stadler PF, Washietl S, Hofacker IL 2006. miRNAMap: genomic maps of microRNA genes and their target genes in mammalian genomes. Nucleic Acids Res 34(Database issue):D135–D139.
40. Landgraf P, Rusu M, Sheridan R, Sewer A, Iovino N, Aravin A, Pfeffer S, Rice A, Kamphorst AO, Landthaler M, Lin C, Socci ND, Hermida L, Fulci V, Chiaretti S, Foa R, Schliwka J, Fuchs U, Novosel A, Muller RU, Schermer B, Bissels U, Inman J, Phan Q, Chien M, Weir DB, Choksi R, De Vita G, Frezzetti D, Trompeter HI, Hornung V, Teng G, Hartmann G, Palkovits M, Di Lauro R, Wernet P, Macino G, Rogler CE, Nagle JW, Ju J, Papavasiliou FN, Benzing T, Lichter P, Tam W, Brownstein MJ, Bosio A, Borkhardt A, Russo JJ, Sander C, Zavolan M, Tuschl T 2007. A mammalian microRNA expression atlas based on small RNA library sequencing. Cell 129(7):1401–1414.
41. Burgler C, Macdonald PM 2005. Prediction and verification of microRNA targets by MovingTargets, a highly adaptable prediction method. BMC Genomics 6(1):88.

42. Kiriakidou M, Nelson PT, Kouranov A, Fitziev P, Bouyioukos C, Mourelatos Z, Hatzigeorgiou A 2004. A combined computational-experimental approach predicts human microRNA targets. Genes Dev 18(10):1165–1178.
43. Miranda KC, Huynh T, Tay Y, Ang YS, Tam WL, Thomson AM, Lim B, Rigoutsos I 2006. A pattern-based method for the identification of MicroRNA binding sites and their corresponding heteroduplexes. Cell 126(6):1203–1217.
44. Brennecke J, Stark A, Russell RB, Cohen SM 2005. Principles of microRNA-target recognition. PLoS Biol 3(3):e85.
45. Stark A, Brennecke J, Russell RB, Cohen SM 2003. Identification of Drosophila Micro-RNA targets. PLoS Biol 1(3):E60.
46. Stark A, Brennecke J, Bushati N, Russell RB, Cohen SM 2005. Animal MicroRNAs confer robustness to gene expression and have a significant impact on 3'UTR evolution. Cell 123(6):1133–1146.
47. Jones-Rhoades MW, Bartel DP 2004. Computational identification of plant microRNAs and their targets, including a stress-induced miRNA. Mol Cell 14(6):787–799.
48. Tian Z, Greene AS, Pietrusz JL, Matus IR, Liang M 2008. MicroRNA-target pairs in the rat kidney identified by microRNA microarray, proteomic, and bioinformatic analysis. Genome Res 18(3):404–411.
49. Lim LP, Lau NC, Garrett-Engele P, Grimson A, Schelter JM, Castle J, Bartel DP, Linsley PS, Johnson JM 2005. Microarray analysis shows that some microRNAs downregulate large numbers of target mRNAs. Nature 433(7027):769–773.
50. German MA, Pillay M, Jeong DH, Hetawal A, Luo S, Janardhanan P, Kannan V, Rymarquis LA, Nobuta K, German R, De Paoli E, Lu C, Schroth G, Meyers BC, Green PJ 2008. Global identification of microRNA-target RNA pairs by parallel analysis of RNA ends. Nat Biotechnol 26(8): 941–946.
51. Calin GA, Dumitru CD, Shimizu M, Bichi R, Zupo S, Noch E, Aldler H, Rattan S, Keating M, Rai K, Rassenti L, Kipps T, Negrini M, Bullrich F, Croce CM 2002. Frequent deletions and down-regulation of micro- RNA genes miR15 and miR16 at 13q14 in chronic lymphocytic leukemia. Proc Natl Acad Sci USA 99(24):15524–15529.
52. Castoldi M, Benes V, Hentze MW, Muckenthaler MU 2007. miChip: a microarray platform for expression profiling of microRNAs based on locked nucleic acid (LNA) oligonucleotide capture probes. Methods 43(2):146–152.
53. Liang RQ, Li W, Li Y, Tan CY, Li JX, Jin YX, Ruan KC 2005. An oligonucleotide microarray for microRNA expression analysis based on labeling RNA with quantum dot and nanogold probe. Nucleic Acids Res 33(2):e17.
54. Lu J, Getz G, Miska EA, Alvarez-Saavedra E, Lamb J, Peck D, Sweet-Cordero A, Ebert BL, Mak RH, Ferrando AA, Downing JR, Jacks T, Horvitz HR, Golub TR 2005. MicroRNA expression profiles classify human cancers. Nature 435(7043):834–838.
55. Pallante P, Visone R, Ferracin M, Ferraro A, Berlingieri MT, Troncone G, Chiappetta G, Liu CG, Santoro M, Negrini M, Croce CM, Fusco A 2006. MicroRNA deregulation in human thyroid papillary carcinomas. Endocr Relat Cancer 13(2):497–508.
56. Iorio MV, Visone R, Di Leva G, Donati V, Petrocca F, Casalini P, Taccioli C, Volinia S, Liu CG, Alder H, Calin GA, Menard S, Croce CM 2007. MicroRNA signatures in human ovarian cancer. Cancer Res 67(18):8699–8707.
57. Porkka KP, Pfeiffer MJ, Waltering KK, Vessella RL, Tammela TL, Visakorpi T 2007. MicroRNA expression profiling in prostate cancer. Cancer Res 67(13):6130–6135.
58. Bandres E, Cubedo E, Agirre X, Malumbres R, Zarate R, Ramirez N, Abajo A, Navarro A, Moreno I, Monzo M, Garcia-Foncillas J 2006. Identification by Real-time PCR of 13 mature microRNAs differentially expressed in colorectal cancer and non-tumoral tissues. Mol Cancer 5:29.
59. Michael MZ, SM OC, van Holst Pellekaan NG, Young GP, James RJ 2003. Reduced accumulation of specific microRNAs in colorectal neoplasia. Mol Cancer Res 1(12):882–891.

60. Lanza G, Ferracin M, Gafa R, Veronese A, Spizzo R, Pichiorri F, Liu CG, Calin GA, Croce CM, Negrini M 2007. mRNA/microRNA gene expression profile in microsatellite unstable colorectal cancer. Mol Cancer 6:54.

61. Zanette DL, Rivadavia F, Molfetta GA, Barbuzano FG, Proto-Siqueira R, Falcao RP, Zago MA, Silva-Jr WA 2007. miRNA expression profiles in chronic lymphocytic and acute lymphocytic leukemia. Braz J Med Biol Res 40(11):1435–1440.

62. Zanette DL, Rivadavia F, Molfetta GA, Barbuzano FG, Proto-Siqueira R, Silva-Jr WA 2007. miRNA expression profiles in chronic lymphocytic and acute lymphocytic leukemia. Braz J Med Biol Res 40(11):1435–1440.

63. Fulci V, Chiaretti S, Goldoni M, Azzalin G, Carucci N, Tavolaro S, Castellano L, Magrelli A, Citarella F, Messina M, Maggio R, Peragine N, Santangelo S, Mauro FR, Landgraf P, Tuschl T, Weir DB, Chien M, Russo JJ, Ju J, Sheridan R, Sander C, Zavolan M, Guarini A, Foa R, Macino G 2007. Quantitative technologies establish a novel microRNA profile of chronic lymphocytic leukemia. Blood 109(11):4944–4951.

64. Johnson SM, Grosshans H, Shingara J, Byrom M, Jarvis R, Cheng A, Labourier E, Reinert KL, Brown D, Slack FJ 2005. RAS is regulated by the let-7 microRNA family. Cell 120(5):635–647.

65. Schultz J, Lorenz P, Gross G, Ibrahim S, Kunz M 2008. MicroRNA let-7b targets important cell cycle molecules in malignant melanoma cells and interferes with anchorage-independent growth. Cell Res 18(5): 549–557.

66. Shell S, Park SM, Radjabi AR, Schickel R, Kistner EO, Jewell DA, Feig C, Lengyel E, Peter ME 2007. Let-7 expression defines two differentiation stages of cancer. Proc Natl Acad Sci USA 104(27):11400–11405.

67. Kumar MS, Erkeland SJ, Pester RE, Chen CY, Ebert MS, Sharp PA, Jacks T 2008. Suppression of non-small cell lung tumor development by the let-7 microRNA family. Proc Natl Acad Sci USA 105(10):3903–3908.

68. Sempere LF, Freemantle S, Pitha-Rowe I, Moss E, Dmitrovsky E, Ambros V 2004. Expression profiling of mammalian microRNAs uncovers a subset of brain-expressed microRNAs with possible roles in murine and human neuronal differentiation. Genome Biol 5(3):R13.

69. He L, Thomson JM, Hemann MT, Hernando-Monge E, Mu D, Goodson S, Powers S, Cordon-Cardo C, Lowe SW, Hannon GJ, Hammond SM 2005. A microRNA polycis-tron as a potential human oncogene. Nature 435(7043):828–833.

70. O'Donnell KA, Wentzel EA, Zeller KI, Dang CV, Mendell JT 2005. c-Myc-regulated microRNAs modulate E2F1 expression. Nature 435(7043):839–843.

71. Chang TC, Yu D, Lee YS, Wentzel EA, Arking DE, West KM, Dang CV, Thomas-Tikhonenko A, Mendell JT 2008. Widespread microRNA repression by Myc contributes to tumorigenesis. Nat Genet 40(1):43–50.

72. Hayashita Y, Osada H, Tatematsu Y, Yamada H, Yanagisawa K, Tomida S, Yatabe Y, Kawahara K, Sekido Y, Takahashi T 2005. A polycistronic microRNA cluster, miR-17-92, is overexpressed in human lung cancers and enhances cell proliferation. Cancer Res 65(21):9628–9632.

73. Wang Q, Li YC, Wang J, Kong J, Qi Y, Quigg RJ, Li X 2008. miR-17-92 cluster accelerates adipocyte differentiation by negatively regulating tumor-suppressor Rb2/p130. Proc Natl Acad Sci USA 105(8):2889–2894.

74. Tagawa H, Karube K, Tsuzuki S, Ohshima K, Seto M 2007. Synergistic action of the microRNA-17 polycistron and Myc in aggressive cancer development. Cancer Sci 98(9):1482–1490.

75. Lu Y, Thomson JM, Wong HY, Hammond SM, Hogan BL 2007. Transgenic over-expression of the microRNA miR-17-92 cluster promotes proliferation and inhibits differentiation of lung epithelial progenitor cells. Dev Biol 310(2):442–453.

76. Hashimoto N, Ichikawa D, Arakawa Y, Date K, Ueda S, Nakagawa Y, Horii A, Nakamura Y, Abe T, Inazawa J 1995. Frequent deletions of material from

chromosome arm 1p in oligodendroglial tumors revealed by double-target fluorescence in situ hybridization and microsatellite analysis. Genes Chromosomes Cancer 14(4):295–300.

77. Bieche I, Khodja A, Lidereau R 1998. Deletion mapping in breast tumor cell lines points to two distinct tumor-suppressor genes in the 1p32-pter region, one of deleted regions (1p36.2) being located within the consensus region of LOH in neuroblastoma. Oncol Rep 5(1):267–272.

78. Cheung TH, Lo KW, Yim SF, Poon CS, Cheung AY, Chung TK, Wong YF 2005. Clinicopathologic significance of loss of heterozygosity on chromosome 1 in cervical cancer. Gynecol Oncol 96(2):510–515.

79. Wei JS, Song YK, Durinck S, Chen QR, Cheuk AT, Tsang P, Zhang Q, Thiele CJ, Slack A, Shohet J, Khan J 2008. The MYCN oncogene is a direct target of miR-34a. Oncogene 27(39):5204–5213.

80. Bommer GT, Gerin I, Feng Y, Kaczorowski AJ, Kuick R, Love RE, Zhai Y, Giordano TJ, Qin ZS, Moore BB, MacDougald OA, Cho KR, Fearon ER 2007. p53-mediated activation of miRNA34 candidate tumor-suppressor genes. Curr Biol 17(15):1298–1307.

81. Corney DC, Flesken-Nikitin A, Godwin AK, Wang W, Nikitin AY 2007. MicroRNA-34b and MicroRNA-34c are targets of p53 and cooperate in control of cell proliferation and adhesion-independent growth. Cancer Res 67(18):8433–8438.

82. Raver-Shapira N, Marciano E, Meiri E, Spector Y, Rosenfeld N, Moskovits N, Bentwich Z, Oren M 2007. Transcriptional activation of miR-34a contributes to p53-mediated apoptosis. Mol Cell 26(5):731–743.

83. Welch C, Chen Y, Stallings RL 2007. MicroRNA-34a functions as a potential tumor suppressor by inducing apoptosis in neuroblastoma cells. Oncogene 26(34):5017–5022.

84. Dutta KK, Zhong Y, Liu YT, Yamada T, Akatsuka S, Hu Q, Yoshihara M, Ohara H, Takehashi M, Shinohara T, Masutani H, Onuki J, Toyokuni S 2007. Association of microRNA-34a overexpression with proliferation is cell type-dependent. Cancer Sci 98(12):1845–1852.

85. Lujambio A, Esteller M 2007. CpG island hypermethylation of tumor suppressor microRNAs in human cancer. Cell Cycle 6(12):1455–1459.

86. Toyota M, Suzuki H, Sasaki Y, Maruyama R, Imai K, Shinomura Y, Tokino T 2008. Epigenetic silencing of microRNA-34b/c and B-cell translocation gene 4 is associated with CpG island methylation in colorectal cancer. Cancer Res 68(11):4123–4132.

87. Brueckner B, Stresemann C, Kuner R, Mund C, Musch T, Meister M, Sultmann H, Lyko F 2007. The human let-7a-3 locus contains an epigenetically regulated microRNA gene with oncogenic function. Cancer Res 67(4):1419–1423.

88. Gartel AL, Kandel ES 2008. miRNAs: Little known mediators of oncogenesis. Semin Cancer Biol 18(2):103–110.

89. Tam W, Ben-Yehuda D, Hayward WS 1997. bic, a novel gene activated by proviral insertions in avian leukosis virus-induced lymphomas, is likely to function through its noncoding RNA. Mol Cell Biol 17(3):1490–1502.

90. Tam W, Hughes SH, Hayward WS, Besmer P 2002. Avian bic, a gene isolated from a common retroviral site in avian leukosis virus-induced lymphomas that encodes a noncoding RNA, cooperates with c-myc in lymphomagenesis and erythroleukemogenesis. J Virol 76(9):4275–4286.

91. Costinean S, Zanesi N, Pekarsky Y, Tili E, Volinia S, Heerema N, Croce CM 2006. Pre-B cell proliferation and lymphoblastic leukemia/high-grade lymphoma in E(mu)-miR155 transgenic mice. Proc Natl Acad Sci USA 103(18):7024–7029.

92. Ma L, Teruya-Feldstein J, Weinberg RA 2007. Tumour invasion and metastasis initiated by microRNA-10b in breast cancer. Nature 449(7163):682–688.

93. Si ML, Zhu S, Wu H, Lu Z, Wu F, Mo YY 2007. miR-21-mediated tumor growth. Oncogene 26(19):2799–2803.

94. Meng F, Henson R, Lang M, Wehbe H, Maheshwari S, Mendell JT, Jiang J, Schmittgen TD, Patel T 2006. Involvement of human micro-RNA in growth and response to chemotherapy in human cholangiocarcinoma cell lines. Gastroenterology 130(7):2113–2129.
95. Zhu S, Si ML, Wu H, Mo Y Y 2007. MicroRNA-21 targets the tumor suppressor gene tropomyosin 1 (TPM1). J Biol Chem 282(19):14328–14336.
96. Sayed D, Rane S, Lypowy J, He M, Chen IY, Vashistha H, Yan L, Malhotra A, Vatner D, Abdellatif M 2008. MicroRNA-21 targets sprouty2 and promotes cellular outgrowths. Mol Biol Cell 19(8):3272–3282.
97. Galardi S, Mercatelli N, Giorda E, Massalini S, Frajese GV, Ciafre SA, Farace MG 2007. miR-221 and miR-222 expression affects the proliferation potential of human prostate carcinoma cell lines by targeting p27Kip1. J Biol Chem 282(32): 23716–23724.
98. Voorhoeve PM, le Sage C, Schrier M, Gillis AJ, Stoop H, Nagel R, Liu YP, van Duijse J, Drost J, Griekspoor A, Zlotorynski E, Yabuta N, De Vita G, Nojima H, Looijenga LH, Agami R 2006. A genetic screen implicates miRNA-372 and miRNA-373 as oncogenes in testicular germ cell tumors. Cell 124(6):1169–1181.
99. Landais S, Landry S, Legault P, Rassart E 2007. Oncogenic potential of the miR-106-363 cluster and its implication in human T-cell leukemia. Cancer Res 67(12):5699–5707.
100. Akao Y, Nakagawa Y, Naoe T 2006. let-7 microRNA functions as a potential growth suppressor in human colon cancer cells. Biol Pharm Bull 29(5):903–906.
101. Yu F, Yao H, Zhu P, Zhang X, Pan Q, Gong C, Huang Y, Hu X, Su F, Lieberman J, Song E 2007. let-7 regulates self renewal and tumorigenicity of breast cancer cells. Cell 131(6):1109–1123.
102. Peng Y, Laser J, Shi G, Mittal K, Melamed J, Lee P, Wei JJ 2008. Antiproliferative effects by let-7 repression of high-mobility group A2 in uterine leiomyoma. Mol Cancer Res 6(4):663–673.
103. Mayr C, Hemann MT, Bartel DP 2007. Disrupting the pairing between let-7 and Hmga2 enhances oncogenic transformation. Science 315(5818):1576–1579.
104. Esquela-Kerscher A, Trang P, Wiggins JF, Patrawala L, Cheng A, Ford L, Weidhaas JB, Brown D, Bader AG, Slack FJ 2008. The let-7 microRNA reduces tumor growth in mouse models of lung cancer. Cell Cycle 7(6).
105. Cimmino A, Calin GA, Fabbri M, Iorio MV, Ferracin M, Shimizu M, Wojcik SE, Aqeilan RI, Zupo S, Dono M, Rassenti L, Alder H, Volinia S, Liu CG, Kipps TJ, Negrini M, Croce CM 2005. miR-15 and miR-16 induce apoptosis by targeting BCL2. Proc Natl Acad Sci USA 102(39):13944–13949.
106. Mott JL, Kobayashi S, Bronk SF, Gores GJ 2007. mir-29 regulates Mcl-1 protein expression and apoptosis. Oncogene 26(42):6133–6140.
107. Kim S, Lee UJ, Kim MN, Lee EJ, Kim JY, Lee MY, Choung S, Kim YJ, Choi YC 2008. MicroRNA miR-199A* regulates the Met proto-oncogene and the downstream extracellular signal-regulated kinase 2 (ERK2). J Biol Chem 283(26):18158–18166.
108. Kefas B, Godlewski J, Comeau L, Li Y, Abounader R, Hawkinson M, Lee J, Fine H, Chiocca EA, Lawler S, Purow B 2008. microRNA-7 inhibits the epidermal growth factor receptor and the Akt pathway and is down-regulated in glioblastoma. Cancer Res 68(10):3566–3572.
109. Fabbri M, Garzon R, Cimmino A, Liu Z, Zanesi N, Callegari E, Liu S, Alder H, Costinean S, Fernandez-Cymering C, Volinia S, Guler G, Morrison CD, Chan KK, Marcucci G, Calin GA, Huebner K, Croce CM 2007. MicroRNA-29 family reverts aberrant methylation in lung cancer by targeting DNA methyltransferases 3A and 3B. Proc Natl Acad Sci USA 104(40):15805–15810.
110. Lagos-Quintana M, Rauhut R, Meyer J, Borkhardt A, Tuschl T 2003. New microRNAs from mouse and human. RNA 9(2):175–179.
111. Liu CG, Calin GA, Meloon B, Gamliel N, Sevignani C, Ferracin M, Dumitru CD, Shimizu M, Zupo S, Dono M, Alder H, Bullrich F, Negrini M, Croce CM 2004. An

oligonucleotide microchip for genome-wide microRNA profiling in human and mouse tissues. Proc Natl Acad Sci USA 101(26):9740–9744.

112. Nelson PT, Baldwin DA, Scearce LM, Oberholtzer JC, Tobias JW, Mourelatos Z 2004. Microarray-based, high-throughput gene expression profiling of microRNAs. Nat Methods 1(2):155–161.

113. Babak T, Zhang W, Morris Q, Blencowe BJ, Hughes TR 2004. Probing microRNAs with microarrays: tissue specificity and functional inference. RNA 10(11):1813–1819.

114. Chan SH, Wu CW, Li AF, Chi CW, Lin WC 2008. miR-21 microRNA expression in human gastric carcinomas and its clinical association. Anticancer Res 28(2A):907–911.

115. Iorio MV, Ferracin M, Liu CG, Veronese A, Spizzo R, Sabbioni S, Magri E, Pedriali M, Fabbri M, Campiglio M, Menard S, Palazzo JP, Rosenberg A, Musiani P, Volinia S, Nenci I, Calin GA, Querzoli P, Negrini M, Croce CM 2005. MicroRNA gene expression deregulation in human breast cancer. Cancer Res 65(16):7065–7070.

116. Calin GA, Ferracin M, Cimmino A, Di Leva G, Shimizu M, Wojcik SE, Iorio MV, Visone R, Sever NI, Fabbri M, Iuliano R, Palumbo T, Pichiorri F, Roldo C, Garzon R, Sevignani C, Rassenti L, Alder H, Volinia S, Liu CG, Kipps TJ, Negrini M, Croce CM 2005. A MicroRNA signature associated with prognosis and progression in chronic lymphocytic leukemia. N Engl J Med 353(17):1793–1801.

117. Schetter AJ, Leung SY, Sohn JJ, Zanetti KA, Bowman ED, Yanaihara N, Yuen ST, Chan TL, Kwong DL, Au GK, Liu CG, Calin GA, Croce CM, Harris CC 2008. MicroRNA expression profiles associated with prognosis and therapeutic outcome in colon adenocarcinoma. JAMA 299(4):425–436.

118. Garzon R, Volinia S, Liu CG, Fernandez-Cymering C, Palumbo T, Pichiorri F, Fabbri M, Coombes K, Alder H, Nakamura T, Flomenberg N, Marcucci G, Calin GA, Kornblau SM, Kantarjian H, Bloomfield CD, Andreeff M, Croce CM 2008. MicroRNA signatures associated with cytogenetics and prognosis in acute myeloid leukemia. Blood 111(6):3183–3189.

119. Guo Y, Chen Z, Zhang L, Zhou F, Shi S, Feng X, Li B, Meng X, Ma X, Luo M, Shao K, Li N, Qiu B, Mitchelson K, Cheng J, He J 2008. Distinctive microRNA profiles relating to patient survival in esophageal squamous cell carcinoma. Cancer Res 68(1):26–33.

120. Patil SD, Rhodes DG, Burgess DJ 2005. DNA-based therapeutics and DNA delivery systems: a comprehensive review. Aaps J 7(1):E61–E77.

121. Boutla A, Delidakis C, Tabler M 2003. Developmental defects by antisense-mediated inactivation of micro-RNAs 2 and 13 in Drosophila and the identification of putative target genes. Nucleic Acids Res 31(17):4973–4980.

122. Opalinska JB, Gewirtz AM 2002. Nucleic-acid therapeutics: basic principles and recent applications. Nat Rev Drug Discov 1(7):503–514.

123. Tonkinson JL, Stein CA 1996. Antisense oligodeoxynucleotides as clinical therapeutic agents. Cancer Invest 14(1):54–65.

124. Verma S, Eckstein F 1998. Modified oligonucleotides: synthesis and strategy for users. Annu Rev Biochem 67:99–134.

125. Gryaznov SM, Winter H 1998. RNA mimetics: oligoribonucleotide N3'–>P5' phos-phoramidates. Nucleic Acids Res 26(18):4160–4167.

126. Hutvagner G, Simard MJ, Mello CC, Zamore PD 2004. Sequence-specific inhibition of small RNA function. PLoS Biol 2(4):E98.

127. Davis S, Lollo B, Freier S, Esau C 2006. Improved targeting of miRNA with antisense oligonucleotides. Nucleic Acids Res 34(8):2294–2304.

128. Valoczi A, Hornyik C, Varga N, Burgyan J, Kauppinen S, Havelda Z 2004. Sensitive and specific detection of microRNAs by northern blot analysis using LNA-modified oligonucleotide probes. Nucleic Acids Res 32(22):e175.

129. Naguibneva I, Ameyar-Zazoua M, Nonne N, Polesskaya A, Ait-Si-Ali S, Groisman R, Souidi M, Pritchard LL, Harel-Bellan A 2006. An LNA-based loss-of-function assay for micro-RNAs. Biomed Pharmacother 60(9):633–638.

130. Orom UA, Kauppinen S, Lund AH 2006. LNA-modified oligonucleotides mediate specific inhibition of microRNA function. Gene 372:137–141.
131. Fontana L, Fiori ME, Albini S, Cifaldi L, Giovinazzi S, Forloni M, Boldrini R, Donfrancesco A, Federici V, Giacomini P, Peschle C, Fruci D 2008. Antagomir-17-5p abolishes the growth of therapy-resistant neuroblastoma through p21 and BIM. PLoS ONE 3(5):e2236.
132. Kloosterman WP, Lagendijk AK, Ketting RF, Moulton JD, Plasterk RH 2007. Targeted inhibition of miRNA maturation with morpholinos reveals a role for miR-375 in pancreatic islet development. PLoS Biol 5(8):e203.
133. Krutzfeldt J, Rajewsky N, Braich R, Rajeev KG, Tuschl T, Manoharan M, Stoffel M 2005. Silencing of microRNAs in vivo with 'antagomirs'. Nature 438(7068):685–689.
134. Esau C, Davis S, Murray SF, Yu XX, Pandey SK, Pear M, Watts L, Booten SL, Graham M, McKay R, Subramaniam A, Propp S, Lollo BA, Freier S, Bennett CF, Bhanot S, Monia BP 2006. miR-122 regulation of lipid metabolism revealed by in vivo antisense targeting. Cell Metab 3(2):87–98.
135. Dass CR 2002. Liposome-mediated delivery of oligodeoxynucleotides in vivo. Drug Deliv 9(3):169–180.
136. Dritschilo A, Huang CH, Rudin CM, Marshall J, Collins B, Dul JL, Zhang C, Kumar D, Gokhale PC, Ahmad A, Ahmad I, Sherman JW, Kasid UN 2006. Phase I study of liposome-encapsulated c-raf antisense oligodeoxyribonucleotide infusion in combination with radiation therapy in patients with advanced malignancies. Clin Cancer Res 12(4):1251–1259.
137. Akinc A, Zumbuehl A, Goldberg M, Leshchiner ES, Busini V, Hossain N, Bacallado SA, Nguyen DN, Fuller J, Alvarez R, Borodovsky A, Borland T, Constien R, de Fougerolles A, Dorkin JR, Narayanannair Jayaprakash K, Jayaraman M, John M, Koteliansky V, Manoharan M, Nechev L, Qin J, Racie T, Raitcheva D, Rajeev KG, Sah DW, Soutschek J, Toudjarska I, Vornlocher HP, Zimmermann TS, Langer R, Anderson DG 2008. A combinatorial library of lipid-like materials for delivery of RNAi therapeutics. Nat Biotechnol 26(5):561–569.
138. Soifer HS, Rossi JJ, Saetrom P 2007. MicroRNAs in disease and potential therapeutic applications. Mol Ther 15(12):2070–2079.
139. Cerritelli SM, Frolova EG, Feng C, Grinberg A, Love PE, Crouch RJ 2003. Failure to produce mitochondrial DNA results in embryonic lethality in Rnaseh1 null mice. Mol Cell 11(3):807–815.
140. Wu H, Lima WF, Zhang H, Fan A, Sun H, Crooke ST 2004. Determination of the role of the human RNase H1 in the pharmacology of DNA-like antisense drugs. J Biol Chem 279(17):17181–17189.
141. Prakash TP, Allerson CR, Dande P, Vickers TA, Sioufi N, Jarres R, Baker BF, Swayze EE, Griffey RH, Bhat B 2005. Positional effect of chemical modifications on short interference RNA activity in mammalian cells. J Med Chem 48(13):4247–4253.
142. Chiu YL, Rana TM 2003. siRNA function in RNAi: a chemical modification analysis. RNA 9(9):1034–1048.
143. Czauderna F, Fechtner M, Dames S, Aygun H, Klippel A, Pronk GJ, Giese K, Kaufmann J 2003. Structural variations and stabilising modifications of synthetic siRNAs in mammalian cells. Nucleic Acids Res 31(11):2705–2716.
144. Xia H, Mao Q, Paulson HL, Davidson BL 2002. siRNA-mediated gene silencing in vitro and in vivo. Nat Biotechnol 20(10):1006–1010.
145. Uprichard SL, Boyd B, Althage A, Chisari FV 2005. Clearance of hepatitis B virus from the liver of transgenic mice by short hairpin RNAs. Proc Natl Acad Sci USA 102(3):773–778.
146. Calin GA, Liu CG, Sevignani C, Ferracin M, Felli N, Dumitru CD, Shimizu M, Cimmino A, Zupo S, Dono M, Dell'Aquila ML, Alder H, Rassenti L, Kipps TJ, Bullrich F, Negrini M, Croce CM 2004. MicroRNA profiling reveals distinct

signatures in B cell chronic lymphocytic leukemias. Proc Natl Acad Sci USA 101(32):11755–11760.

147. Ciafre SA, Galardi S, Mangiola A, Ferracin M, Liu CG, Sabatino G, Negrini M, Maira G, Croce CM, Farace MG 2005. Extensive modulation of a set of microRNAs in primary glioblastoma. Biochem Biophys Res Commun 334(4):1351–1358.

148. Murakami Y, Yasuda T, Saigo K, Urashima T, Toyoda H, Okanoue T, Shimotohno K 2006. Comprehensive analysis of microRNA expression patterns in hepatocellular carcinoma and non-tumorous tissues. Oncogene 25(17):2537–2545.

149. Yanaihara N, Caplen N, Bowman E, Seike M, Kumamoto K, Yi M, Stephens RM, Okamoto A, Yokota J, Tanaka T, Calin GA, Liu CG, Croce CM, Harris CC 2006. Unique microRNA molecular profiles in lung cancer diagnosis and prognosis. Cancer Cell 9(3):189–198.

150. Bottoni A, Zatelli MC, Ferracin M, Tagliati F, Piccin D, Vignali C, Calin GA, Negrini M, Croce CM, Degli Uberti EC 2007. Identification of differentially expressed microRNAs by microarray: a possible role for microRNA genes in pituitary adenomas. J Cell Physiol 210(2):370–377.

151. Lee EJ, Gusev Y, Jiang J, Nuovo GJ, Lerner MR, Frankel WL, Morgan DL, Postier RG, Brackett DJ, Schmittgen TD 2007. Expression profiling identifies microRNA signature in pancreatic cancer. Int J Cancer 120(5):1046–1054.

152. Visone R, Pallante P, Vecchione A, Cirombella R, Ferracin M, Ferraro A, Volinia S, Coluzzi S, Leone V, Borbone E, Liu CG, Petrocca F, Troncone G, Calin GA, Scarpa A, Colato C, Tallini G, Santoro M, Croce CM, Fusco A 2007. Specific microRNAs are downregulated in human thyroid anaplastic carcinomas. Oncogene 26(54):7590–7595.

153. Gottardo F, Liu CG, Ferracin M, Calin GA, Fassan M, Bassi P, Sevignani C, Byrne D, Negrini M, Pagano F, Gomella LG, Croce CM, Baffa R 2007. Micro-RNA profiling in kidney and bladder cancers. Urol Oncol 25(5):387–392.

154. He H, Jazdzewski K, Li W, Liyanarachchi S, Nagy R, Volinia S, Calin GA, Liu CG, Franssila K, Suster S, Kloos RT, Croce CM, de la Chapelle A 2005. The role of microRNA genes in papillary thyroid carcinoma. Proc Natl Acad Sci USA 102(52):19075–19080.

155. Lee DY, Deng Z, Wang CH, Yang BB 2007. MicroRNA-378 promotes cell survival, tumor growth, and angiogenesis by targeting SuFu and Fus-1 expression. Proc Natl Acad Sci USA 104(51):20350–20355.

156. Voorhoeve PM, le Sage C, Schrier M, Gillis AJ, Stoop H, Nagel R, Liu YP, van Duijse J, Drost J, Griekspoor A, Zlotorynski E, Yabuta N, De Vita G, Nojima H, Looijenga LH, Agami R 2007. A genetic screen implicates miRNA-372 and miRNA-373 as oncogenes in testicular germ cell tumors. Adv Exp Med Biol 604:17–46.

157. Gregory PA, Bert AG, Paterson EL, Barry SC, Tsykin A, Farshid G, Vadas MA, Khew-Goodall Y, Goodall GJ 2008. The miR-200 family and miR-205 regulate epithelial to mesenchymal transition by targeting ZEB1 and SIP1. Nat Cell Biol 10(5): 593–601.

158. Bemis LT, Chen R, Amato CM, Classen EH, Robinson SE, Coffey DG, Erickson PF, Shellman YG, Robinson WA 2008. MicroRNA-137 targets microphthalmia-associated transcription factor in melanoma cell lines. Cancer Res 68(5):1362–1368.

159. le Sage C, Nagel R, Egan DA, Schrier M, Mesman E, Mangiola A, Anile C, Maira G, Mercatelli N, Ciafre SA, Farace MG, Agami R 2007. Regulation of the p27(Kip1) tumor suppressor by miR-221 and miR-222 promotes cancer cell proliferation. Embo J 26(15):3699–3708.

Targeted Therapies for Malignant Brain Tumors

Matthew A. Tyler, Adam Quasar Sugihara, Ilya V. Ulasov,
and Maciej S. Lesniak

1 Introduction

Battling aggressive brain tumors represents a struggle endeavored by scientists
and physicians across many different disciplines. The molecular and physiological abnormalities that accompany this fatal disease render malignant brain
tumors arguably one of the most difficult pathologies to treat. For this reason,
the efforts to combat this fatal disease are represented by a plethora of research.
This chapter is organized to illustrate common themes in drug targeting for the
treatment of brain tumors. Each section is organized based on the therapeutic
approach: small molecules, local drug delivery, or biological therapy. In each
subsection we discuss the rationale that has ushered each development to the
'center stage' in brain tumor therapy and provide illustrative examples using the
most relevant and heretofore advanced developments. In this way, we hope to
provide a discussion of brain tumor therapy that is all-encompassing yet
detailed enough to give the reader a broad understanding of how researchers
and clinicians attempt to improve the outcome of patients diagnosed with this
debilitating disease.

Conventional therapy for malignant brain tumors involves a combination of
surgery, radiation therapy, and chemotherapy. Radiation therapy originally
directed at whole brain has become progressively focused, currently delivered
in many places in the form of intensity-modulated radiotherapy (IMRT).
Chemotherapy has relied largely on alkylating agents; however, chemotherapy
for the treatment of brain tumors remains a controversial topic of debate.
Despite these gains, the overall prognosis remains poor and recurrence remains
the norm. Recurrence is thought to be driven by diffuse micro-infiltration of
tumor cells into normal brain. Eliminating these micro-metastases remains a
challenge because of the risk of damaging surrounding normal brain and the
accompanying disability that may ensue.

M.S. Lesniak (✉)
Section of Neurosurgery, The University of Chicago Pritzker School of Medicine, 5841
South Maryland Ave, MC 3026, Chicago, IL 60637, USA
e-mail: mlesniak@surgery.bsd.uchicago.edu

Y. Lu, R.I. Mahato (eds.), *Pharmaceutical Perspectives of Cancer Therapeutics*,
DOI 10.1007/978-1-4419-0131-6_15, © Springer Science+Business Media, LLC 2009

2 Current and Novel Chemotherapies for Brain Tumors

Chemotherapy for the treatment of brain tumors varies depending on the origin of the tumor and the indication for the treatment. Each subclass of malignant CNS tumors carries a different prognosis; as such, conventional chemotherapeutic treatments can include the use of synthetically derived alkylating agents, anti-metabolites, pro-drugs, and DNA synthesis/mitotic inhibitors. These types of drugs can have multiple and overlapping actions on cells with overactive metabolic pathways – i.e., quickly growing tumor cells. Many of the commonly used chemotherapy agents generated in the last 30–40 years were the result of NCI-funded research and multi-billion dollar cooperative research and development agreements (CRADAs) between NCI and research and development companies. Below, we discuss, by drug class, some representative chemotherapeutics that are commonly used to treat brain tumors.

Alkylating agents: Alkylating agents are not specific for any one pathway in particular, however, researchers have identified that some of these agents act to functionally inhibit proteins that are vital to cellular replication. Alkylation of important cellular DNA/proteins will effectively make certain cellular molecules/proteins inert and dysfunctional, causing disruption of metabolic pathways and eventually cell death. It is not uncommon for a physician to prescribe multiple alkylating agents to a patient, as their cancers may develop 'cross-resistance' to similar classes of drugs which share overlapping mechanisms of cytotoxicity.

Temozolomide and carmustine (BCNU) are the most commonly used alkylating agents for primary CNS malignancies, such as anaplastic astrocytoma and glioblastoma multiforme (GBM). In a recent landmark study by Stupp and colleagues, the authors elucidated that the methylation status of the O-6-methylguanine-DNA methyltransferase (MGMT) gene served a prognostic factor in the anti-tumor efficacy of temozolomide-based therapies [1, 2]. It was shown that patients containing epigenetic silencing of the MGMT promoter, as detected by methylation-specific PCR, when treated with temozolomide and radiation therapy, resulted in increased median survival (21.7 months when MGMT promoter is methylated; 15.3 months when MGMT promoter is not methylated) when compared to patients receiving only radiation therapy without concomitant temozolomide [1, 2]. The studies conducted by Stupp resulted in the FDA's approval of temozolomide for the treatment of high-grade glioma. Continued studies are investigating the potential of temozolomide in combination with other chemotherapies.

Anti-metabolites: Anti-metabolites are drugs that 'gunk up' metabolic pathways such as cellular respiration and nucleotide metabolism. Commonly, anti-metabolites are chemical analogues of endogenous metabolites and they act to oppose metabolic processes; in doing so, they cause irreparable damage and eventually cell death. Methotrexate is a water-soluble drug commonly used by oncologists to treat primary CNS lymphoma. Methotrexate inhibits folic acid synthesis by reversibly binding dihydrofolate reductase, an enzyme that cata-lyzes the formation of tetrahydrofolate from dihydrofolate. Folic acid is a crucial molecule involved in nucleotide and protein synthesis and inhibiting its formation results in cell death.

DNA synthesis/mitotic inhibitors: Irinotecan: Irinotecan is a drug that has been studied more recently within the context of malignant CNS tumors, especially in concert with bevicizumab (discussed below). Irinotecan is a semi-synthetic derivative of camptothecin, a topoisomerase I inhibitor. Irinotecan binds and stabilizes topoisomerase-DNA complexes, preventing the unwinding of DNA, thereby causing irreparable DNA double-strand breaks and even-tually cell death.

Conventional chemotherapies have shown some efficacy in brain tumors because it is likely they target multiple pathways in cells exhibiting high meta-bolic rates and high mitotic indices. However, the exact mechanism of action of these agents is still largely unknown, as is the reason why certain agents work in certain types of tumors and not others. Because of this lack of information, researchers continue to unravel how these compounds exert their toxic effects in tumor cells and in specific types of cancers. With regard to CNS malignancies, oligodendrogliomas have offered hope in identifying subclasses of tumors (and patients) that respond favorably to certain chemotherapies. For instance, the 1p19q loss of function mutation in these tumors is predictive of a patient's response to chemotherapy [3, 4]. Discoveries such as these offer the hope to develop novel chemotherapies that are specific to different molecular patho-geneses of brain tumors.

2.1 Targeting Growth Factor Signaling Axes in Brain Tumors

Just like studies unraveling the details involved in mitosis yielded a generation of chemotherapies that were to target mitotic pathways, so has recent under-standing of the biochemistry of signal transduction cascades allowed scientific researchers to develop a new generation of chemotherapies that target signaling cascades in cancer. We have come to understand the processes of cell growth, migration, and angiogenesis as a cascade of signals which are transmitted from the cell surface to the nucleus and this has allowed researchers to identify some of the crucial regulators involved in cell growth and tissue regeneration. Many researchers and clinicians believe that identifying molecular abnormalities of brain tumors on a patient-to-patient basis will allow a physician to prescribe a chemotherapy regimen that will have the best benefit for the individual patient.

The bulk of the novel chemotherapies have now become known as the small-molecule inhibitors (of growth factor cascades). Many of these agents are inhibitors of receptor tyrosine kinases (RTKs), a group of cell membrane-spanning receptors that contain intracellular tyrosine kinase domains. The intracellular tyrosine kinase domains of multiple RTK receptor subtypes represent a major integration point of signaling cascades involved in cell growth, differentiation, and increased metabolic activity. Catalytically active RTKs are 'docking stations' upon which many intracellular effectors (i.e., Ras, Raf, PI3K) converge to transmit signals received at the cell surface into an amplified intracellular response, and many times, a whole tissue response. Much of the aggressive cancerous growth of malignant brain tumors has been associated with overactive RTK-associated signal transduction pathways. Inhibiting these pathways will likely halt cellular growth and tissue regeneration. In this section, we discuss three principle targets of novel therapies within the context of brain tumor treatments: cell proliferation and the epidermal growth factor receptor, EGFR; angiogenesis and the vascular endothelial growth factor, VEGFR; and the intracellular effectors where both of these pathways can converge. Because there are new studies involved with similar agents surfacing every day, we limit our discussion to some of the most studied agents tested in brain tumors.

2.1.1 Targeting Cell Proliferation: EGFR Axis

The epidermal growth factor receptor (EGFR) is an RTK, a member of the Her/Erb family of proteins (EGFR is also known as Erb1 or Her1 [5]). EGFR is amplified in 40–60% of glioblastomas and approximately 30–50% of these tumors also possess the EGFRvIII mutation in which coding regions in the extracellular ligand domain (exons 2–7) are absent [6, 7]. EGFR plays an integral role in the malignant phenotype of malignant brain tumors and it is a common hope amongst researchers and clinicians that functional inhibition of EGFR-mediated signaling will slow tumor growth [8].

A randomized phase II trial compared the efficacy of temozolomide or BCNU versus the small-molecule EGFR tyrosine kinase inhibitor, erlotinib, in patients with recurrent glioblastoma multiforme [9] (GBM). The 6-month progression-free survival (PFS-6) was 12% for erlotinib and 24% for temozolomide or BCNU. Further, the response to erlotinib could not be correlated to EGFR expression, amplification, or EGFRvIII mutation. Nonetheless, responses were noted and continued studies with EGFR RTK inhibitors in malignant glioma seek to define a correlation between patient response and EGFR-associated molecular aberrations. A molecular analysis was performed in tissue sets compiled from a multicenter phase I/II trial performed through the North American Brain Tumor Consortium (NATBC) [10]. The authors showed that erlotinib/gefitinib does not effect EGFR signaling (phosphorylation) in vivo and there was no correlation between deletion/amplification of EGFR and sensitivity to these EGFR inhibitors, yet, the authors hint at an association between decreased Akt/PI3K activity (phosphorylation) and response to erlotinib and gefitinib in two patients. Of note, there were no tissue sets which demonstrated the EGFRvIII mutation. Another study conducted by Mellinghoff et al. performed a molecular analysis in tissue sets from patients receiving gefitinib or erlotinib treatments for glioblastoma [11]. Their investigation supported previous reports which failed to find a correlation between EGFR amplification and polysomy and a response to EGFR inhibitors ($p < 0.001$). However, in this study, the authors were able to draw a strong correlation between EGFRvIII, PTEN and tumor sensitivity to EGFR kinase inhibitors. The authors found that 50% (6/12) of tumors expressing EGFRvIII were responsive to EGFR kinase inhibitors while only 1 of 14 non-responding patients expressed EGFRvIII ($p = 0.03$). The authors also observed that 7 of 13 responding patients were PTEN-positive while no non-responding patients were missing the PTEN locus ($p = 0.005$). The greatest predictor of response to EGFR kinase inhibitors in this tissue set was coexpression of EGFRvIII and PTEN ($p<0.001$). These findings indicate a molecular basis for patients' response to such therapies and will most likely have an impact on whether or not EGFR kinase inhibitors are for patient-specific treatment.

2.1.2 Targeting Angiogenesis: VEGFR Axis

Vascular proliferation and neoangiogenesis are trademarks of aggressive brain tumors. The extent of neovascularization in primary brain tumors, such as malignant glioma, has often been associated with a poor patient prognosis. Angiogenesis in both healthy and diseased tissue involves complex signaling cascades involving molecules such as VEGF-A, VEGFRs1-3, PDGF, and a/bFGF, to name a few among many [12]. One of the more thoroughly investigated signaling pathways are the ones that associate with VEGF and its receptors VEGFRs1-3. VEGF is over-secreted in malignant glial tumors and regulates paracrine and autocrine loops along with endothelial cells, resulting in vascular recruitment, vascular permeability, cell proliferation, tumor cell invasion and migration. Researchers have developed small-molecule inhibitors as well as monoclonal antibodies (bevacizumab, discussed below) to target important mediators involved in the so-called, 'angiogenic switch' signaling that is often associated with VEGF and related molecules [13, 14].

There are ongoing trials which seek to identify the potential of small-molecule inhibitors, including RTK inhibitors, such as Vandetanib (Zactima, ZD6474; AstraZeneca). Vandetanib is currently being evaluated as a dual VEGFR and EGFR inhibitor. While a report on efficacy remains to be published, participating institutions in a phaseI/II trial conducted by the NIH Neuro-Oncology branch report that this drug is well tolerated and its administration has produced significant radiographic responses in patients diagnosed with high-grade recurrent gliomas [15].

2.1.3 Intracellular Effectors in Growth Cascades

The loss of function deletion/mutation in the phosphatase and tensin homolog (*PTEN*) tumor-suppressor locus is found to occur in 30–40% of GBM patients [16, 17]. PTEN is a regulator of the pro-growth kinases, PI3K and AKT. Phosphorylation of these proteins can activate pro-growth/pro-survival pathways while dephosphorylation by PTEN phosphatase activity negatively regulates the kinase activity mediated by PI3K and AKT. mTOR (*m*ammalian *T*arget of *R*apamycin) is a downstream target of PI3K and AKT activity and also a crucial integrative regulatory kinase involved with the following meta-bolic transduction proteins: T-cell proliferation through interaction with immu-nophilin FKBP-12, p70s6 kinase activity, eukaryotic initiation factor 4E-bind-ing protein 1 [18– 25]. All of these regulatory proteins integrate key cell growth and survival signals important in normal cell and tumor cell growth. Functional inhibition of pathways involving these molecules has been achieved using the small-molecule inhibitors, Sirolimus (rapamycin) and its ester analog, temsir-olimus (CCI-779), which have been shown to inhibit mTOR-regulated path-ways. Pre-clinical models have demonstrated a sensitivity of PTEN-deficient tumors to mTOR inhibition using these agents [26, 27].

A recent phase II study conducted by Gulanis et al. tested the efficacy of Temsirolimus (CCI-779) in 65 patients with recurrent GBM [22]. Twenty patients showed radiographic responses, as determined by a decreased T2-weighted MRI signal. However, the progression-free survival was only 7.8% at 6 months for patients receiving Temsirolimus treatment and no objective response was observed. The authors noted a correlation between radiographic response and p70s6 kinase phosphorylation in baseline tumor samples, although, there was no association with radiographic response and EGFR amplification/expression, PTEN deletion/expression, or AKT phosphorylation.

3 Barriers in the CNS and Novel Approaches in Delivering Drugs to Brain Tumors

The blood–brain barrier refers to a physiological state in which the brain is protected from an array of potentially dangerous insults that circulate in the blood. The protective physiological landscape that describes the blood–brain barrier is represented by both physical and molecular properties, the combina-tion of which provides very selective uptake and filtering of key agents impor-tant for optimal brain function.

There are two barrier systems in the normal adult brain: the blood–brain barrier (BBB) and the blood cerebrospinal fluid barrier (BCSFB). The BBB is composed of three cell types, all of which play an important role in BBB integrity and regulation: endothelial cells of the cerebral vasculature, astrocytes, and pericytes (Fig. 1). Pericytes of BBB localize to the capillary basement membrane, sandwiched next to endothelial vessel cells by astrocytic end feet, which form very extensive and intimate bundles around both pericytes and endothelial vessel cells (Fig. 1). Specific characteristics of the BBB are believed to be maintained and induced by the astrocytic processes [28– 30]. The endothe-lial cells of the cerebral vasculature differ from their counterparts in peripheral systems in that they lack fenestrations [31– 33], demonstrate little to no

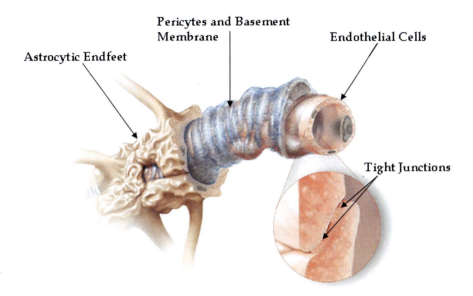

Pericytes and Basement Membrane

Astrocytic Endfeet

Endothelial Cells

Tight Junctions

Fig. 1 **Anatomical makeup of the blood–brain barrier**. Endothelial cells of the cerebral capillaries are tightly joined by complexes of tight junctions. Pericytes are found surrounding the capillary endothelium and are continuous with the basement membrane of the endothelium. The astrocytic endfeet are wrapped tightly around both pericytes and endothelial cells. Together, these cells work together to tightly regulate the influx/efflux and metabolism of molecules important for optimal brain function. Figure was reprinted, with permission [243]

pinocytic activity [34– 36], possess a high content of tight junctions (TJ) [37, 38], and maintain a characteristically elevated metabolic activity [34, 35]. The anatomical characteristics of the BBB and their molecular 'building blocks' function to prevent paracellular and transcellular transport of blood-borne substances, including cells and hydrophilic substances, both large and small (>180 Da). Thus, transport through the BBB is limited to miniscule, lipophilic entities and substances that are transported using molecular transport mechanisms. The molecular transport systems in the CNS are highly coordinated to regulate the influx and efflux of important molecules from brain parenchyma, thereby maintaining CNS homeostasis. These transport systems include organic anion and organic cation transporters (OATs and OCTs), ATP-dependent transporters (i.e., p-glycoprotein), nucleoside transporters, amino acid transporters, and receptor-mediated transporters [39– 46]. The most cited transport system of the BBB is represented by members of the multidrug-resistance protein family (MDR), the most popular being p-glycoprotein.

The BCSFB constitutes an additional compartment in the CNS which drugs must traverse. The BCSFB is comprised of the choroid plexus and arachnoid membranes which consist of choroid and arachnoid epithelium, respectively, as their major cell constituents. These structures interface with nearly all major brain structures in the CNS, particularly the ventricular cavities and outer cerebral cortex structures [47]. The major role of the epithelial cells of the BCSFB is to secrete cerebrospinal fluid, a cocktail of micronutrients, electrolytes, neuropeptides, and proteins which immerse major CNS structures and related capillary endothelium. The epithelial cells of the choroid plexus represent major regulators of homeostasis and bulk flow in the CNS (Fig. 2). As

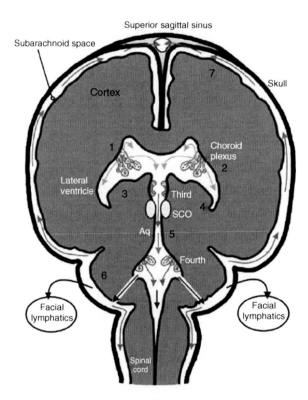

Fig. 2 CSF flow pathways in the adult. Nearly all major brain structures interface with the CSF system. This coronal section of the posterior CNS captures all the ventricles: lateral, third, and fourth. CSF originates from the choroid plexuses of the lateral and third ventricles and percolates downward through the narrow cerebral aqueduct (Aq). The bottom of the Aq empties into the fourth ventricle, to the roof of which is attached more choroidal tissue. CSF flows out of the fourth ventricle though foramina into the cisterna magna and other nearby large basal cisterns. From the cisterns, the CSF is convicted posteriorly downward around the spinal cord (subarachnoid space) as well as upward over the convexities of the cerebral hemispheres. At more distal sites in the subarachnoid system, the CSF flows outward though the arachnoid villi into venous blood of the superior sagittal sinus. *Arrows* depict the general patterns of CSF flow from the interior of the brain to various exterior loci in the spinal cord and hemispheres. SCO, subcommissural organ. Some CSF drains directly into lymphatic glands. 1 – Caudate; 3 – centrum ovale (white matter); 3 – thalamus; 4 – hippocampus; 5 – periaqueductal gray; 6 – cerebellum; 7 – cerebral motor cortex. Figure and corresponding text were reprinted, with permission [47]

such, the BCSFB has been known to be a drug sink, in that it can draw drugs out of the CNS interstitium, into the CSF, and into venous circulation [47, 48].

The BBB and BCSFB signify major hurdles in drug delivery to the CNS, and especially to brain tumors. Malignant brain tumors have been known to proliferate around cerebral vasculature with intact BBB in addition to demonstrating neovascularization, which are less predictable in nature than intact BBB and CSF-structures. Together, the barrier pathophysiology which describes blood flow in CNS malignancies has been referred to as the blood–brain tumor barrier (BBTB). Malignant CNS tumors demonstrate tortuous vascular pathologies, along with enhanced drug efflux capabilities. Given this pathological landscape, the interstitial pressures in different areas of the tumor can vary greatly, making it extremely difficult for a drug to reach high intratumoral concentrations. To overcome these obstacles in delivering drugs to the brain, researchers have devised novel invasive and non-invasive mechanisms in an attempt to achieve high drug concentrations within the brain and the brain tumor for sustained periods of time. Whether a drug is delivered systemically or locally, the rationale for each approach is the same: maintenance of high concentrations of the cytotoxic compound within the brain tumor/CNS.

3.1 Inhibiting Drug Transporters

Recent discoveries involving the molecular underpinnings of chemotherapy efflux in the brain have drawn researcher's attention toward manipulating these transport systems to achieve high concentrations of an anti-tumor agent within the brain. In particular, the p-glycoprotein transporters of the multidrug-resistant protein family are documented as playing a central role in the efflux of xenobiotic agents away from the CNS. P-glycoprotein is not a discriminatory transport protein; this is substantiated with studies showing that many current chemotherapy compounds are substrates for p-glycoprotein-mediated efflux [49]. Clinical researchers have hypothesized that inhibiting the transport function of p-glyco-protein in the BBB may expose brain tumors to elevated levels of anti-tumor agents for sustained periods of time [43]. Results from clinical trials were at first promising, but advanced studies revealed disappointing results [50]. The major limitation of this approach is obvious: while p-glycoprotein expression may be higher intratumorally and in CNS barrier structures, it is not unique to these organs. Inhibition of p-glycoprotein leads to systemic toxicities in the liver, kidney, and pancreas, all of which express p-glycoprotein as a functional transport protein.

3.2 Invasive Drug Delivery to Brain Tumors

Because the CNS barriers limit the amount of cytotoxic agent that can access the brain, invasive drug delivery methods have been developed to bypass CNS barriers. Invasive drug delivery to brain tumors can describe a variety of methods, depending on the type of brain tumor and its exact location within the CNS. Typically, invasive methods for drug delivery can include intratumoral/intracavitary delivery, intra-arterial delivery, and delivery using CSF compartments.

3.2.1 CSF Delivery

Delivery of chemotherapies and other drugs using the cerebrospinal compartments represents a way to achieve sustained concentrations of drug in the brain (Reviewed in [47]). Unlike capillary endothelium of the BBB, endothelial vessels of choroid plexus villi demonstrate multiple sites of fenestration. In addition, choroid epithelia are less restrictive in their paracellular transport capacity, as demonstrated by their ability to allow paracellular transport of intravascular administrations of mannitol ($M_w = 182$), inulin polysaccharide ($M_w \sim 5000$), and other hydrophilic substances [51– 54]. Indeed, CSF is the preferred route for the delivery of hydrophilic anti-cancer agents, such as methotrexate [49]. Because CSF interfaces most of the brain's superficial structures, CSF-drug delivery has shown efficacy for tumors localized to leptomeningeal structures, ependymal structures, and the periventricular compartments. The Ommaya reservoir was developed to harness these features of CSF-mediated delivery. With an Ommaya reservoir, an implantable pump is placed into CSF-structures – such as the ventricular compartments and subarachnoid spaces – and drugs are delivered over a sustained period of time. This technique has been used to deliver chemotherapies such as methotrexate and BCNU, and biological agents such as IL-2 and IFN-γ [55– 59]. The CSF route for drug delivery may also represent a feasible delivery platform using cell-based and recombinant protein-based anti-tumor therapies [47]. The major limitations involved in utilizing CSF compartments for drug delivery include bulk flow of CSF compartments, laborious and potentially dangerous procedures, and diffusion limitations. Bulk flow in CSF is difficult to monitor and the influx/efflux patterns between CSF compartments, ependyma, capillary endothelium, and brain parenchyma is difficult to anticipate, especially in heterogeneous CNS malignancies. Infection and morbidity are always potential complications associated with this type of drug administration. Lastly, the amount of brain surface area exposed to CSF compartment is considerably less than BBB structures and in many cases diffusion of a particular drug to brain parenchyma can drop with the square of the diffusion distance [60]. This is a significant hurdle in using this route to deliver drugs to CNS tumors that reside beyond superficial areas of the brain.

3.2.2 Blood–Brain Barrier Disruption and Intra-Arterial Delivery

Intra-arterial drug (IA) delivery to brain tumors involves the use of cerebral arteries for the local delivery of anti-tumor agents. With IA drug delivery, a catheter is placed in an artery in close proximity to the lesion(s) (left or right carotid artery versus left or right vertebral artery). After the catheter has been placed in a predetermined artery, a drug is infused into the artery for a sustained period of time. IA drug delivery for the treatment of malignant brain tumors has experienced a re-awakening with advent of blood–brain barrier disruption (BBBD) agents, such as the hyperosmotic agent, mannitol, and the bradykinin analog, RMP-7. The use of these agents effectively shrinks cerebral capillary endothelium and creates a transient opening of the BBB (15 minutes–2 hours) [61, 62], allowing transcellular passage of chemotherapy agents that would normally not have access to brain parenchyma without BBBD. While the use of this technique for the delivery of drugs is somewhat controversial given its laborious procedure, there exists an international consortium devoted to IA and BBBD drug delivery (the International BBBD Consortium) paradigms in treating CNS tumors. Researchers from this consortium have found that this method of drug delivery is both feasible and promising. While a phase III randomized trial has yet to be conducted, this is mostly because of a need for multi-disciplinary expertise to carry out such a study. Thus, patient stratification and powerful analysis has been limited in past studies. However, studies conducted in patients with primary CNS lymphoma, metastatic lesions, and malignant glioma have demonstrated the potential promise of IA and BBBD drug delivery approaches [49, 63– 66].

3.2.3 Intratumoral and Intracavitary Delivery

For many current experimental forms of brain tumor therapy, delivering drugs directly into the tumor mass or the tumor resection cavity represents a very common and promising method for drug delivery. Intracavitary delivery of drugs to brain tumors allows the neurosurgeon to visually map out the desired target and deliver an agent. This method of delivery has the ability to circumvent CNS barrier structures and is indeed the method of choice for delivering experimental therapeutics, such as vector therapies (discussed below) and other novel therapies. Below, we discuss some of the most commonly referenced investigations which employed intracavitary drug delivery approaches, namely, intracavitary depositing of polymer-laden drugs and convection-enhanced delivery (CED). From this point on, we will refer to intratumoral/intracavitary drug delivery as 'local delivery', for simplicity.

Polymer-Laden Drug Delivery

Many drugs that have showed promise for the treatment of the most aggressive brain tumors are not feasible for delivery by the IV or oral route because systemic toxicities are a significant problem. This was the case for carmustine (1,3-bis(2-chloroethyl)-1-nitrosurea; BCNU). Carmustine is an alkylating agent that was approved in 1977 to treat malignant gliomas because it was proven to be one of the first effective therapies in treating this most aggressive subclass of malignant brain tumors [67– 69]. However, the IV use of BCNU was hampered because of systemic toxicities, including severe myelosuppression, pulmonary fibrosis, and secondary acute leukemia [70– 74].

Given these disappointing findings, Dr. Henry Brem at Johns Hopkins and Dr. Robert Langer at MIT developed the idea of embedding BCNU in a polymer matrix to achieve sustained drug delivery to malignant glioma [75]. The final BCNU–polymer matrix used in clinical trials was composed of a poly(carboxyphenoxy-propane/sebacic acid) matrix loaded with carmustine, also known as Gliadel[R]. Phase III clinical trials used a 3.5% BCNU loading per 200 mg of polymer matrix and wafers were placed in regions lining the resection cavity (Fig. 3). This method of drug delivery allows for an in vivo release period of 21 days, with much of the drug release taking place over the first 5–7 days after implantation and complete degradation was noted at 6–8 weeks after implantation [76– 80]. Most importantly, this method of drug delivery demonstrates little to no systemic toxicities. A meta-analysis reported the results from two phase III trials which tested the effect of BCNU wafers and radiation versus placebo wafers and radiation in patients with newly diagnosed malignant glioma [81– 83]. This meta-analysis found a 13.1 month median survival in patients receiving Gliadel[R] and a 10.9 month median survival in patients receiving placebo wafers ($p = 0.031$). The results from this meta-analysis led to the FDA approval of Gliadel for newly diagnosed malignant glioma patients in 2003. While these findings may seem somewhat modest, they have provided a framework for developing polymer-laden drugs for local delivery to brain tumors. Polymer-based drug delivery represents a method to achieve sustained drug activity in the brain and new developments in local delivery to brain tumors continue to investigate the use of such delivery platforms using other drugs. Similar to carmustine, other agents such as methotrexate, which demonstrate considerable anti-tumor toxicity but limited clinical application in gliomas because of poor penetrability of brain parenchyma, are being investigated for their potential to be delivered using polymer platforms.

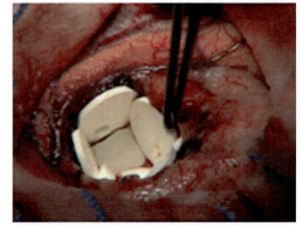

Fig. 3 Polymer-laden drug delivery. Following resection of a malignant glioma, up to eight carmustine (BCNU)-polymer wafers are placed within the tumor cavity. As the wafers dissolve, they release BCNU locally and provide direct delivery of chemotherapy to the tumor cavity. Figure and text were reprinted, with permission [57]

Convection-Enhanced Delivery

When delivered locally within the brain, the concentration of a drug traveling by diffusion drops exponentially from the site of administration. This becomes more of a burden with micrometastases and infiltrative satellites that are commonly seen in the most aggressive type of brain tumor, malignant glioma, where it is difficult for a drug to reach intraparenchymal regions of the brain beyond the resection cavity and especially in 'eloquent' areas of the brain. With this in mind, researchers at NIH developed convection-enhanced delivery (CED) as a novel way to deliver drugs over a large volume of tissue. With CED, a catheter(s) is placed in a predetermined area of the brain using standard imaging techniques (i.e., postoperative MRI scans and computed tomography scans) and a drug is infused over a period of hours to days. A constant pressure gradient created by an infusion pump permits the drug infusate to be delivered homogenously to circumscribed areas of brain tissue without causing significant tissue damage. This method of delivery has especially become relevant in drug delivery to brain tumors because it bypasses the BBB and reduces systemic toxicities. Moreover, it allows for the local delivery of macromolecules, such as viruses, liposomes, targeted antibodies and protein moieties to large areas of brain parenchyma.

One of the first clinical trials to evaluate the application of convection-enhanced delivery in brain tumors involved studies with cintredekin besudotox (CB), a recombinant protein toxin consisting of the IL-13 ligand conjugated to a truncated form of *Pseudomonas* exotoxin. CB targets the IL13 receptor $\alpha 2$ commonly over-expressed in malignant glioma. This recombinant cytotoxin demonstrated potent anti-tumor activity in vitro and in vivo, with 50% inhibitory concentrations of 0.1–30 ng/ml [84–86]. The first clinical studies assessing the CED-mediated delivery of CB were in patients with recurrent malignant glioma [87]. These studies established the dose-limiting toxicity (0.5 µg/ml), infusion dose (6 days of infusion well tolerated) as well as the importance of catheter placement in outcome efficacy. A follow-up study was conducted with CB in patients with newly diagnosed malignant gliomas. Twenty-two patients undergoing gross total resection of their mass received 96-hour infusions of CB (0.25 or 0.5 µg/ml), followed by external beam radiation and temozolomide or no temozolomide treatment [88]. The majority of treatment-related adverse events recorded were either grade 1 or 2, which related to catheter placement and CB. Unfortunately, a recent phase III study comparing the efficacy of IL13-*Pseudomonas* exotoxin therapy versus Gliadel wafers failed to show any benefit over Gliadel alone.

In a recent phase I trial conducted by Sampson et al., the authors utilized CED to infuse an EGFR-targeted toxin, TP-38, to patients diagnosed with recurrent malignant brain tumors [89]. TP-38 is a recombinant protein consisting of a genetic fusion of TGF-α and a modified form of *Pseudomonas* exotoxin. In this study, the authors infused TP-38 at a flow rate of 0.4 ml/h/catheter over a period of 50 hours, for a total volume of 40 ml. The study investigated the toxicity and response of three doses: 25 ng/ml, 50 ng/ml, and 100 ng/ml. There were little dose-limiting toxicities associated with the study, and no systemic toxicities were reported. The overall median time to progression was 14.9 weeks. Of note, 2 of 15 patients with residual tumor at the time of therapy demonstrated radiographic response and were alive at the time of report. One patient diagnosed with multirecurrent bifrontal GBM treated at the 25-ng/ml level had a nearly complete response that persisted for 198 weeks without progression. Another patient diagnosed with GBM showed nearly complete response and remained (alive for >260 weeks).

What was interesting about this phase I study was that the authors conducted SPECT (Single-Photon Emission Computed Tomography) imaging to monitor the distribution of drug infusate (Fig. 4). Usually, the infusate is

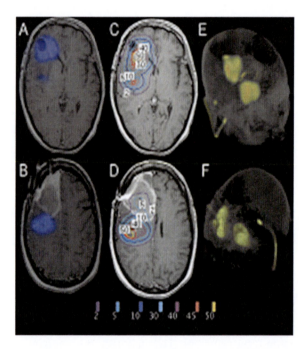

Fig. 4 CED of the targeted toxin, TP-38. (**A**) Single-photon emission computed tomography (SPECT) image of TP-38 distribution co-registered with axial MR image for anterior catheter positioned *below* the resection cavity. SPECT imaging was obtained by coinfusing ^{123}I-albumin in the same volume of infusate (**B**) SPECT image of ^{123}I-albumin distribution co-registered with axial MR image for catheter positioned *behind* the resection cavity. (**C,D**) Corresponding SPECT-derived isodose contours co-registered with axial T1-weighted MR images located at the tip of each catheter in the right frontal lobe of the brain. Isodose lines show the percent concentration of 123I-albumin relative to the infused concentration (0.25 mg/ml) such that at the 50% isodose line the concentration of albumin is 0.125 mg/ml and at the 10% isodose line the concentration of albumin is 0.025 mg/ml (**E,F**) Oblique reconstructions of complete SPECT imaging showing areas covered and not covered by the infusion. Figure and text were reprinted, with permission [89]

co-administered with albumin, which serves as a carrier protein for the infused drug. In its place, the authors used ^{123}I-labeled albumin coinfused in the same volume with TP-38, and subsequently, they were allowed to observe the drug distribution properties mediated by CED. This method allows for a better interpretation of the clinical efficacy of TP-38. Their results and those from other groups revealed one of the major obstacles encountered in CED – the need to optimize drug delivery parameters using CED. Many times, the area in which a catheter is placed (i.e., white matter versus gray matter) can effect the distribution of a particular drug. The drug may enter areas of lower resistance (i.e., ventricular compartments, CSF) rather than the intended target. Such findings illustrate a requisite need to employ state-of-the art imaging systems to track drug distribution. These findings also underscore the need to better understand the parameters in the diseased brain which dictate the distribution of a particular drug [90].

4 Targeted Biological Therapy for Brain Tumors

4.1 Antibody-Based Drugs and Recombinant Proteins: Active Targeting of Brain Tumors

Scientific researchers are consumed with the idea of identifying the 'magic bullet,' as Paul Ehrlich once hypothesized, which will one day successfully treat the most devastating cancers; malignant brain tumors are no exception. The development of monoclonal antibodies against cancer targets symbolizes a principle manifestation of Ehrlich's concept. The rationale for developing antibody-based mechanisms to target brain tumors is obvious. With the advent of hybridoma technology, antibodies can be generated against any conceivable target on the tumor cell surface or the tumor interstitium (i.e., secreted ligands). This is especially relevant in the case of cancer, where the restricted expression of so-called 'tumor-associated antigens' (TAA) can readily be identified using modern biotechnological screenings.

Monoclonal antibodies are engineered to elicit their anti-tumor responses in three putative fashions: (i) conveying toxins in the form of chemical conjugation to the antibody, aka immunoconjugates, immunotoxins; (ii) inhibiting activation of pivotal signal transduction proteins involved in cell growth and tissue regeneration; and (iii) activation of the immune system [91– 93]. Currently, antibodies have been engineered according to three basic classifications, namely, chimeric (mouse + human), human (entirely human), and humanized (mouse complementary determining region (CDR) + human). The most well-known examples of antibody-based drug delivery in brain tumors refer to studies with the mAb, bevacizumab (Avastin®). Bevacizumab is a humanized IgG_1 mAb engineered to bind secreted VEGF protein, preventing its interaction with cognate receptors and the downstream signals that eventually result in tumor angiogenesis. Bevacizumab has been approved to treat patients diagnosed with metastatic colorectal cancer, and since then, it has been evaluated in the treatment of patients with malignant glial tumors. Trials investigating the potential utility of bevacizumab in combination with the topoisomerase I inhibitor, irinotecan, have yielded astonishing results. In a trial conducted by Vredenburgh et al. at Duke University, patients with recurrent GBM were treated with 10 mg/kg bevacizumab plus irinotecan every 2 weeks [94]. Twenty out of the 35 patients treated had at least a partial response, using a greater than 50% decrease in contrast-enhanced MRI signal as a criterion for partial response. The overall 6-month PFS was 46% (95% CI, 32–66%) and the 6-month overall survival was 77% (95% CI, 64–92%). These results are extremely promising, given the poor prognosis of patients diagnosed with recurrent GBM. It has been speculated that antagonizing VEGF activity helps to reduce the tortuous vasculature associated with GBM pathogenesis by reducing vascular permeability and interstitial pressures within the tumor mass, making it easier for drugs like irinotecan to penetrate the tumor bulk [94, 95]. These speculations pose another intriguing question: Are the radiographic responses reported due to the reduced vascular permeability, or a result of a bevacizumab-mediated anti-tumor response? Questions like these underscore a need for new radiographic criteria to be developed to better assess the anti-tumor effect of novel agents. There are currently 22 active and approved clinical trials (mostly phase II) that are assessing the activity of bevacizumab against malignant CNS tumors. The results from these studies are awaited with interest.

In addition to the uses described above, antibodies and recombinant proteins/peptides have been engineered to target membrane proteins of the BBB and tumor surface to achieve delivery of cytotoxic agents to tumor parenchyma [41, 96]. This approach was developed based on our current knowledge of receptor-mediated transcytosis (RMT) mechanisms in BBB endothelial cells. The BBB contains multiple receptor types that utilize RMT to ferry metabolites from the BBB luminal surface, through the cell cytoplasm to the abluminal surface and brain interstitium. With this in mind, monoclonal antibodies and recombinant proteins have been engineered to target receptors of the BBB, such as LDL receptors, the transferrin receptor (TfR), and IGF receptor [39, 85]. More recently, these antibody systems and recombinant proteins have been engineered and used to 'decorate' polymeric nanoparticles such as PEG, liposomes, and others in an attempt to actively target the brain parenchyma through the vascular delivery route. For instance, Hallahan et al. showed that a fibrinogen ligand could be conjugated to liposomes and albumin nanoparticles and could effectively target radiation-induced integrin expression in tumor vasculature when delivered intravenously [97]. Polymeric 'bioconjugates', or nanoparticles, consisting of a polymer, encapsulated drug, and recombinant protein targeting moiety represent a novel and active area of research. Formulations have been innovated using chemotherapies such as methotrexate, cisplatin, paclitaxel with targeting moieties against EGFR and TfR. Although, these studies are still in their infancy and relevant pre-clinical studies have yet to become prevalent. The antibody/protein density that is used to decorate polymeric nanoparticles is a critical factor in affecting good delivery and stability of the devised nanocarrier and a researcher must engineer the protein so as not to compete with endogenous ligand. These systems represent a somewhat novel yet exciting delivery approach for brain tumor therapy and it is likely that these systems will enter 'center stage' in the near future.

4.2 Vector Therapy

Vector therapies for the treatment of brain tumors represent a significant research interest in the realm of experimental brain tumor therapies. Because the brain represents an area of 'immune privilege' (discussed below), the local delivery of allogenic agents directly into the tumor cavity is both a feasible and a logical approach to achieve selective anti-tumor therapy. Vector therapy refers to a type of gene therapy in which nucleic acid, whether it is DNA or RNA, is targeted to a specific cell type, cancer cells in our case. Upon vector delivery, the gene of interest is expressed (or, knocked down in the case of siRNA/miRNA) and tumor cell cytotoxicity is concomitant with gene delivery. Similar to antibody development strategies, the potential targets are left to the researcher's imagination; however, the range of cancer targets is more extensive with vector therapy than with antibody-based therapy. With vector therapies, the cancer target is not limited to cell surface or interstitial expression. For this reason, vector therapies all differ in their particular genetic construction and choice of cancer target, but can still be classified based on the method of delivery: (i) viral vector delivery and (ii) non-viral vector delivery. Up until now, the gene of interest has included oncolytic viral genes (aka, virotherapy), suicide genes (e.g., v-tk), cytokine gene transfer, and tumor-suppressor gene transfer [98, 99]. In any case, the goal of any gene therapy approach is as such: targeted gene expression *throughout* the tumor tissue.

4.2.1 Non-Viral Vector Delivery

Non-viral vector delivery has been characterized largely by the use of cell-based and liposomal-based gene delivery systems. In the earliest malignant brain tumor clinical trials which assessed the efficacy of cell-based gene delivery systems, researchers employed a murine fibroblast cell line to transduce tumor cells with the HSV thymidine kinase gene (HSV-*tk*) [100]. In a phase III study conducted by the GL1328 international study group, patients with previously untreated GBM received 30–50 single intracavitary injections of vector producing cells (VPC) in a mean volume of 9.1 ml (range 4.0–12.6 ml at 1×10^8 VPC/ml), after which, the thymidine kinase inhibitor, ganciclovir (GCV) was administered IV (5 mg/kg over 1 hour period) 2 weeks after VPC injection for a period of 2 weeks. The median time to progression for the gene therapy treatment arm was 180 days, while the control groups, which received standard fractionated radiotherapy was 183 days. The median survival was 365 days and 354 days, and the 12-month survival rates were 50 and 55% for the gene therapy and control groups, respectively. While this treatment proved safe and feasible, there clearly was no benefit when compared to standard therapy. Researchers believe that the lack of success was most likely due to limited gene delivery resulting from the non-motile murine fibroblast and the MLV vector. Since then, researchers have entered into an age where the use of bone marrow-derived progenitor cells and neural stem cells has become the cell of choice for targeted gene delivery to brain tumors. These cells demonstrate a characteristic tropism for CNS pathology, regardless of whether the tumor originated within the CNS or metastasized from another organ system [101]. Stem cells are commonly engineered using retroviral-based expression cassettes, in which, a retroviral vector is used to insert a specific gene of interest into the tumor-tropic stem cell. Theoretically, the genetically engineered cell should express the gene of interest once inserted. Upon expression of inserted gene into the tumor region, tumor cell toxicity results. More commonly, lentiviral-based retroviral vectors have become the favorite vector for stem cell engineering, because these viruses have a higher rate of gene insertion into the host genome, most likely because lentiviral insertion is not dependent on the stage of the host's cell cycle, unlike MLV vectors employed in first generation trials. Aboody and colleagues have conducted extensive studies showing the suitability of neural stem cells (NSC) in delivering suicide genes, such as cytosine deaminase, in effecting tumor reduction [102– 106]. These researchers have documented their observations to the extent that the development of a NSC-based clinical trial is currently under development. In addition to the pioneering studies such as those of the Aboody group, researchers have engineered stem cells to express siRNA to 'knock-down' cancerous gene expression, immunogenic cytokines, etc. Other cell-based strategies that fall within the category of 'immunotherapy' are relevant under a gene therapy context. These strategies, however, are discussed in more detail below, under immunotherapy approaches.

The half-life of nucleic acid, when delivered in its 'naked' form, is very low. Liposomal-mediated delivery of genes represents a way of shuttling genes to tumor tissues in the brain and protecting them from host nucleases. In addition, liposomes are relatively easy to manufacture and they possess no inherent toxic or immunogenic characteristics at the doses used. In a recent study, cationic liposomes were employed to deliver the suicide gene, HSV-*tk*, to patients afflicted with GBM [107]. In this study, researchers used PET imaging and CED to deliver the HSV-*tk* suicide gene. While the study included only eight patients, one of the patients demonstrated sites of necrosis correlating to GCV activity by PET [107]. The use of liposomes has been argued to be non-specific in activity, however, novel studies have shown that liposomes can be functionalized with specific peptides/antibodies which can mediate specific gene delivery based on the expression of characteristic tumor cell surface proteins [108, 109].

4.2.2 Viral Vector Delivery

Viruses have evolved to achieve robust gene expression within a host's cell. For this reason, viral gene delivery represents a substantial amount of current gene therapy research, and so far, the best way to deliver a gene to a desired cell type. Viral vector delivery to brain tumors has been investigated using different types of viruses, including adenovirus (Ad), herpes simplex virus (HSV), retrovirus (RV), measles virus, adeno-associated virus (AAV), Newcastle disease virus (NDV), Semliki Forest virus, vaccinia virus, and reovirus [110]. The most commonly used viruses represented in experimental brain tumor therapies are the HSV and Ad viruses.

Replication-deficient viral vectors have been used in early clinical trials for patients with recurrent GBM to deliver the HSV-*tk* gene, with some promise [111– 114]. After a phase I trial established that adenovirus-mediated HSV-*tk* therapy significantly improved survival (15.0 months) of malignant glioma patients when compared to retrovirus-mediated HSV-*tk* gene delivery (7.4 months; $p<0.012$), a randomized controlled study by Immonen et al. was undertaken in patients with primary and recurrent gliomas [111]. Patients in the active treatment group received intracavitary injections of 3×10^{10} PFUs of the ADvHSV-*tk* vector in aliquots of 0.1–0.3 ml for a total volume of 10 ml. The treatment was tolerated well; anti-Ad antibodies could be detected in 6 out of 17 patients receiving the active treatment without any particularly adverse effects. Most importantly, patients in the active treatment group demonstrated significantly longer mean survival time (70.6 +/– 52.9 weeks) than a historical control group (62.4 +/– 30.9 weeks; $p<0.0017$, log rank regression). The results from these clinical trials have led researchers to investigate the role of Ad's ability to deliver other anti-tumor genes, such as the cytokine IFN-β.

IFN-β is a pleiotropic cytokine with anti-proliferative and immunomodulatory activities. Pre-clinical studies evaluating the anti-tumor activity of Ad-delivered IFN-β in murine models (hIFN-β) demonstrated that administration could affect complete tumor regression, $CD8^+$ activation and long-term resistance to re-challenge in an intraperitoneal tumor model [115]. Chiocca et al. recently published a phase I trial which investigated safety and potential efficacy of Ad-delivered human IFN-β (Ad.hIFN-β) in patients with malignant glioma [116]. A total of 11 patients in the active treatment group were subdivided into 3 treatment cohorts based on vector dose (2×10^{10}, 6×10^{10}, 2×10^{11} viral particles). Patients received two separate injections of Ad.hIFN-β; on day 1, patients received five stereotactic injections directly into the tumor mass. Four to eight days after the first injection, the tumor was removed and a total of 10 vector injections (1.0 ml total volume) were administered by free hand directly into the tumor resection cavity. Biological response to vector delivery was analyzed by measuring serum Il-6 and IL-10 concentrations, hIFN-β levels in resected tissue and CSF samples, anti-Ad antibodies, vector biodistribution, serum neopterin concentration, and histopathological analysis. Histological analysis of brain tumor tissue indicated a dose-related induction in apoptosis which was consistent with inflammatory infiltrates with populations of neutro-phils, macrophages, and monocytes. Intratumoral Ad.hIFN-β DNA was detected in 10 out of 11 patients receiving active treatment. The authors noted a variable yet dose-related increase in anti-Ad titers (1/6 in low and intermediate groups versus 4/5 in high-dose treatment group). There was one patient who experienced grade 4 dose-limiting toxicity of confusion which was associated with treatment administration. The authors posited that this may have been due to extravasation of the vector into CSF fluids.

The use of replication-deficient vectors prevents promiscuous and poten-tially hazardous viral replication; however, it also limits the extent of gene delivery. For this reason, virotherapy (virotherapy = VIRal Oncolytic THER-APY) has been developed. With virotherapy, researchers hope to exploit the lytic replication cycle of a virus to achieve a sustained anti-tumor infection. Commonly, a replication-competent viral vector is engineered to specifically transduce and replicate in tumor tissue, thereby lysing tumor cells in a specific fashion. There exist a number of genetic engineering strategies in which researchers modify the virus genome so that a replicating virus specifically kills tumors cells. First generation viral vectors possessed deletion mutations which attenuated viral replication and restricted cell lysis to cells with over-active metabolisms, i.e., rapidly dividing tumor cells. Viral vectors falling under this category include ONYX-015, a human Ad type 5 vector missing the 55 kDa E1B protein; and G207, a HSV-1 vector containing deletion modifications in regions of its genome corresponding to $\gamma_1 34.5$ and $U_L 39$ coding regions [117, 118]. The initial phase I trials assessing the dose-limiting toxicities of these agents show that there is little toxicity resulting from local administration of these agents [117, 118]. A clinical study conducted by the New Approaches to Brain Tumor Therapy CNS Consortium (NABTT) with the ONYX-015 vector found that the replicating Ad was well tolerated, with no serious adverse events related to treatment. Further, no maximum tolerated dose was achieved (max. dose: 10^{10} PFUs). The median time to progression after treatment was 46 days. Three patients remained alive with more than 19 months of follow-up and one patient had not progressed at the time of report. These studies have provided a logistical framework for the use of replicating viral vectors in patients with aggressive brain tumors. Given the somewhat low toxicity profile of these agents, additional studies will need to evaluate the efficacy of these approaches.

In addition to deletion modifications which render these attenuated viruses more specific, researchers have recently made use of tissue-specific promoters (TSPs) and transductional modifications to achieve efficient tumor-specific cell lysis. Continued studies with ONYX-015 and G207 showed that these viruses do not transduce the tumor tissue to an extent that would produce observable therapeutic benefits. The use of TSPs that control the expression of viral replication proteins is a useful strategy and has been documented by several groups [119– 124]. Transductional modifications also increase gene transfer to tumor cells. The incorporation of the RGD (Arg-Gly-Asp) peptide motif into the Ad type 5 virus has been shown to improve viral transduction to malignant glioma cells by targeting $\alpha_v\beta_3$ and $\alpha_v\beta_5$ integrins [125– 128].

Most experimental strategies investigating the potential of anti-tumor viral vectors utilize local intratumoral/intracavitary injections to deliver a viral agent. This bears several limitations, namely, gene expression is limited to areas surrounding the injection tract. In addition, despite the fact that patients with CNS malignancies are severely immunocomprimised, clearance of the viral agent by local immune cell populations has been documented [129, 130]. It is likely that the use of an additional agent, such as stem cells [131], polymer systems [132], and immunosuppressants [133] will increase the residence of these viral particles within the brain, permitting adequate gene amplification and tumor toxicity. Also, with the advent and promise demonstrated with CED systems, viral delivery may be significantly enhanced when administered using CED platforms. It is also likely that these virolytic agents will show promise when combined with other treatment modalities. Pre-clinical studies assessing the use of oncolytic viral agents in combination with chemotherapies and radiotherapies have shown promise [134– 137] and it is likely that in the future the efficacy of oncolytic agents will be assessed when combined with different therapies, such as temozolomide and radiotherapy.

4.3 Immunotherapy

Multiple forms of immunotherapy are being explored both as an adjuvant and as an alternative treatment. However the effectiveness of these approaches is limited by the immune privileged status of the brain. The concept of immune privilege grew out of experiments by Peter B. Medawar showing that unlike the rest of the body, the brain did not immediately reject foreign transplanted tissue. Once thought to be a result of the immune system's 'ignorance' of what transpired within the brain [138], over time the concept of immune privilege has been challenged and refined as increasing evidence suggests that the immune system is functional within the CNS, albeit in a finely regulated manner [139].

'Immune Privilege' in the CNS: The immune system is thought of comprising two arms, an afferent or immune sensing arm that detects the presence of pathogens or altered self cells and primes or activates the efferent arm, tasked with killing or neutralizing the invader [140]. Both of these arms are limited or otherwise restricted within the brain in ways which limit the immune system's ability to respond to glioma.

Dendritic cells (DC) are a critical component of the afferent arm, but their function is restricted within the brain. In other organ systems of the body, DC serve as the most effective of the professional antigen presenting cells (APC), sentinels that phagocytose or otherwise absorb intruders and then travel through the lymphatic system to draining lymph nodes where they present foreign antigen to B and T cells of the efferent arm to activate the immune response. The CNS lacks a conventional lymphatic system and DC are not present in non-inflamed brain parenchyma [141]. Furthermore, in experiments in which DC were injected into parenchyma, they did not home to draining lymph nodes, supporting the theory that DC do not patrol the parenchyma where glioma develop [142]. Instead, afferent sensing within the parenchyma works through drainage of soluble antigen along perivascular spaces of capillaries and arteries into lymph nodes [143]. Although there are no DC in normal parenchyma, DC are present in cerebrospinal fluid (CSF; CSF-DC) and do home to lymph nodes when stimulated there. However, both CSF-DC and soluble antigen draining appear to skew the efferent arm away from generating a Th-1 Cytotoxic T-cell (CTL) response thought to be most effective against tumor toward a Th-2 humoral response more suited to targeting a bacterial infection.

The efferent arm, once thought to be largely intact in the CNS, has proven to be highly regulated as well. Entry of potential effector cells, T cells, B cells, and monocytes, is tightly controlled by the blood–brain barrier physiology in a two-step process, each one requiring different activation steps. First, cells must pass through the vascular endothelium of the post capillary venule into the Virchow–Robin space. Second, they then must penetrate the glia limitans to finally reach the parenchyma [144]. Molecular impediments to T-cell function in the CNS include widespread expression of Fas ligand, which induces apoptosis in Fas positive immune cells [144], low expression of MHC in the non-inflamed state [145], which impedes T-cell activation and constitutive expression of B7-H1 on the surface of microglia, which downregulates T-cell activation and cytokine production [146].

Immune system–Glioma interactions: In spite of the efferent and afferent barriers to immune activation, there is some evidence of an immune-mediated anti-tumor response against glioma. Most glioma have tumor infiltrating lymphocytes (TIL), however, the prognostic significance of this is still controversial, with some studies showing a survival benefit associated with increased infiltration [146– 148] and others showing no significant benefit [149, 150]. Furthermore, tumor-specific CD8$^+$ T cells have been detected in the peripheral blood of patients with GBM [151]. These cells produce IFN-γ when incubated with autologous tumor cells as well as with DC pulsed with the U118 GBM tumor line, but not with unstimulated DC alone or U118 alone. The limited activation of the immune response versus GBM supports the theory that the tumor is actively escaping or impeding immune surveillance.

The most commonly cited mechanisms of glioma immune escape include impaired tumor–T-cell binding, resistance to T-cell-mediated killing, production of immunomodulatory surface molecules, factors, and cytokines, and recruitment/generation of regulatory T cells (Treg) [152]. Impaired tumor-T-cell binding can be mediated through glycosaminoglycan coats that directly block cell–cell binding [153]; decreased expression of cell–cell binding proteins such as intracellular adhesion molecule (ICAM-1) [154]; and decreased expression of proteins involved in antigen processing and presentation such as transporter associated with antigen processing-1 and human leukocyte antigen-1 (HLA-1) [155].

Mechanisms of direct resistance to T–cell-mediated killing include downregulation of Fas [156] and production of soluble decoy receptor for Fas ligand [157], increased production of anti-apoptotic proteins resulting from constitutive activation of signal transducer and activator of transcription 3 (STAT-3). Immunomodulatory surface molecules include B7-H1, which binds PD-1 to inhibit T-cell activation and cytokine secretion [158], Fas ligand, which allows the tumor to kill activated immune cells [159], and ectopic HLA-G which binds to an inhibitory receptor on both NK cells and cytotoxic lymphocytes [160].

Secretion of immunosuppressive factors such as TGF-β2, IL-10, and prostaglandin E2 plays an important role in suppressing T-cell activation and facilitating glioma immune escape. TGF-β2 acts to suppress immune response in numerous ways: it inhibits T-cell activation and proliferation [161, 162]; downregulates MHC II expression [163]; inhibits function of mononuclear phagocytes and microglial cells [164]; and inhibits function of cytotoxic lymphocytes through inhibiting production of perforin, granzyme A and B, IFN-γ, and Fas ligand [165, 166]. IL-10 inhibits the immune system by impairing maturation, activation and function of antigen presenting cells [167] as well as T-cell proliferation in response to IL-2 [168]. Prostaglandin E2 blocks the pro-inflammatory action of cyclooxygenase [169], inhibits T-cell and NK-cell activation and shifts the T-cell repertoire toward a Th-2, B cell, antibody-mediated immunity instead of Th-1, CTL-mediated immunity [169].

Treg are a subset of CD4$^+$ T cells that have been shown to suppress immune responses by rendering conventional CD4$^+$ T cells (Tconv) anergic, i.e., unable to trigger an immune response when presented with their cognate antigen [170]. Our lab and others have demonstrated increased Treg infiltration into glioma tumors [171, 172] and that this infiltration correlates with tumor grade [173].

Immunotherapy in Glioma: Immunmotherapeutic strategies rely on the immune system's ability to mount a clearance of foreign entities based on the recognition of specific antigens. Thus, much of the research in cancer immunotherapy aims at sensitizing the host's immune system to cancer antigens, or boosting the host's immune system, in an attempt to generate a host immune reaction to the resident tumor, and, ideally, a sustained and 'learned' anti-tumor immune response. Therapies fall into three major categories: immune priming strategies, adoptive immunotherapy, and immunomodulation. Immune priming strategies seek to correct the defects of the afferent arm through vaccination with tumor-specific antigens as well as transfer of dendritic cells loaded with tumor antigens. Adoptive immunotherapy works through the efferent arm of the immune system by transferring sensitized immune cells in the hope that they will attack the tumor directly. Immunomodulatory strategies seek to recalibrate the regulatory networks that have been subverted by the glioma in an attempt to generate anti-tumor immune reactivity. Because these strategies share many overlapping features, we have chosen to organize immunotherapy approaches according to cell-based and non-cell-based approaches, both of which constitute major areas in cancer immunotherapy.

4.3.1 Non-Cell-Based Immunotherapy

Generating Tumor-Specific Immunity: Peptide Vaccines

One of the most promising approaches to overcoming immune suppression has been the use of peptide vaccines derived from tumor antigens to prime the immune system to respond to the tumor. Just as vaccines are engineered to generate immune protection in anticipation of pathogen infection, so are they generated to combat tumor recurrence and progression. Potential tumor antigens fall into two categories, namely, 'tumor associated', which are expressed in other tissues, but over-expressed within the tumors; and, 'tumor specific', composed of antigens that are only found within the tumor. These antigens are generated by somatic mutation of normal proteins that would otherwise be considered 'tumor associated' if it were not for the existence of a somatic mutation in clonal populations of tumor cells. Tumor-specific antigens are greatly preferred because of the consequences of collateral damage with the brain are particularly grave given its vulnerability to inflammation and inability to regenerate. Vaccines can be screened using techniques such as 'reverse immunogenetics'. With reverse immunogenetics, peptides – whether endogenous or genetically engineered – can be eluted from MHC-class peptide clefts and screened for their ability to generate classic immune responses in vitro, such as T-cell proliferation, cytokine production, humoral immune response (antibody production), and others. Vaccines with high immunogenecity are used in vivo by themselves, or with cellular co-administrations, such as DC (discussed below). We discuss in detail the generation of a peptide generated to mount an immune response against the EGFRvIII peptide.

As mentioned above, EGFRvIII is an attractive target because it is not expressed in normal tissues but is expressed in a wide number of malignancies including breast, lung, colon, and ovarian cancers [174– 176] as well as between 31 and 50% of malignant gliomas [177, 178]. Initial pre-clinical studies targeting EGFRvIII in rodents were promising; a peptide vaccine developed targeting the novel EGFRvIII epitope was successful in raising antibodies, stimulating a CTL response and extending survival [179– 181]. The success of these pre-clinical studies led to several human trials that have also produced promising results.

VICTORI was the first Phase I human trial of the EGFRvIII keyhole limpet vaccine (PEPvIII-KLH). The vaccine was well tolerated and showed promise [182]. The Duke-based study enrolled 20 patients with a WHO grade III or IV glioma who had undergone gross resection and radiotherapy. Qualified patients ($n = 16$) received three intradermal administrations of the vaccine at 2 week intervals via PEPvIII-KLH-pulsed autologous dendritic cells. The vaccine was successful in stimulating cellular immunity; post-vaccination restimulation with the peptide alone gave rise to a delayed hypersensitivity response in 5 of 13 patients and a positive in vitro proliferation response from samples of 10 of 13 patients. The clinical results were also promising; no major adverse effects was reported and among grade III patients, 2 of 3 had stable disease at 66 and 123 months, while among the 13 GBM patients, mean time of progression was 46.9 weeks and median survival was 110.8 weeks. For the phase II trial of ACTIVATE, the study was expanded to include MD Anderson and the protocol was simplified to eliminate autologous DC and instead deliver the PEPvIII-KLH peptide vaccine along with GM-CSF to stimulate DC maturation in situ. Preliminary results indicate the vaccine was well tolerated and ex vivo studies have demonstrated humoral and cellular immunity; final results have not yet been reported [182]. A phase III comparing EGFRvIII vaccine and GM-CSF versus the alkylating agent, temozolomide (TMZ), on the basis of progression-free survival for 6 months, overall survival, and immune response, is underway and expected to be completed in the near future (NCT00458601).

One of the potential problems facing tumor vaccine researchers is the possibility of immunoediting, in which targeting a specific peptide merely selects for variants that lack that peptide. This was observed in the original murine experiments investigating the EGFRvIII peptide vaccine [175] in which recurrent tumors that were EGFRvIII negative developed in 15% of the surviving mice. One approach to avoid immunoediting is to target multiple peptides in a tumor, either through autologous whole tumor vaccines or personalized peptide vaccines. The personal peptide vaccine approach screens patient peripheral blood mononuclear cells (PBMC) for reactivity against a panel of tumor associated and specific peptides and then inoculates them with the best matches. In a 2005 phase I trial 25 patients (8 with AA and 17 with GBM) were screened and treated with up to four peptide vaccines [183]. The vaccine was well tolerated and the majority showed increased cellular and humoral responses. Clinical results were moderately favorable with 5 of 21 showing partial radiographic response, 8 of 21 showing stable disease, and 8 of 21 showing progressive disease. Median survival among GBM patients was 622 days. Other tumor vaccine targets under investigation include cytochrome p450 [184], telomerase [185], GALT3 [186], survivin [187], tenascin [188], glycoprotein 240 [189], and SART1 [190].

Immunomodulatory Strategies

Attempts to counteract the inherent immunosuppressive activities of malignant glioma have focused primarily on changing the cytokine environment. This has involved either seeking to replace or supplement immuno-activating cytokines, such as IL-2, that are missing or otherwise present at low levels in the tumor micro-environment, or, conversely, to counteract immunosuppressive cytokines such as transforming growth factor beta 2 (TGF-β2) that are present at abnormally high levels. In addition, recent pre-clinical research has revealed a role for Treg in immune escape and new studies are focusing on depleting or otherwise counteracting these cells. TGF-β2 is known to be one of the most potent immunosuppressive molecules produced in the body and is commonly over-expressed in glioma. It is capable of interfering with both the afferent arm by downregulating MHC expression [191] and the efferent arm by directly inhibiting effector cells [192– 194].

Fakhri and colleagues sought to block TGF-β2 in order to make a more effective vaccine [195]. They injected six GBM patients with a whole cell vaccine comprised of tumor cells genetically modified with a TGF-β2 anti-sense transgene. This blocked tumor cells' ability to produce TGF-β2 and thereby improved the immune system's ability to raise both CTL and humoral immune responses. Most importantly, median survival was increased when compared to historical controls (68 weeks versus 47 weeks). In a phase I/II trial of 24 patients with malignant glioma, Hau and colleagues tested anti-sense oligonucleotides to directly block production of TGF-β1 [196]. Results were very encouraging. Two AA patients experienced complete remissions and overall survival times in both AA and GBM patients, 146.6 weeks and 44 weeks, respectively, were increased relative to historical controls.

Targeting Treg to limit glioma immunosuppression is supported by preclinical data from murine models. It is reasonable to suggest that a population of lymphocytes exist in the tumor mass to sequester pro-inflammatory cytokines. Data from our lab indicate that depleting Treg with anti-CD25 antibodies (PC61) prolongs survival without inducing autoimmunity [197]. Other labs have achieved similar results with both anti-CD25 [198] and anti-CTLA-4 [199] antibodies. Finally, there is data to suggest that temozolomide may decrease tumor progression of the Treg chemoattractant CCL2 [200]. Data from Grauer suggest that depleting Treg prior to vaccination with tumor lysate-pulsed DC greatly increased the efficacy of the vaccine [201]. Recent data from the Castro lab suggest that the timing of Treg depletion is critical. When glioma-bearing mice were treated with PC61 antibody early on in disease course, Treg were depleted and the adenoviral tumor vectors were more effective in inducing a CTL response [202]. However, when the mice were treated later in the disease course, the PC61 antibody also affected $CD4^+$ and $CD8^+$ effector cells and weakened the immune response. Although there is not yet any published data on Treg and human glioma, a clinical trial at Duke is currently recruiting patients for Treg depletion with Daclizumab, an anti-CD25 alpha antibody accompanied by TMZ and an RNA-pulsed DC vaccine [203].

Immunomodulatory therapy, particularly interventions that target Treg and TGF-β2 , represents one of the most exciting developments in glioma therapeutics. It offers the possibility of reversing glioma immunosuppression, which has been a major unseen obstacle to the efficacy of other immunotherapies, and as such, it brings new hope for achieving the potential benefits that have been so difficult to realize in the transition from murine to human experiments.

4.3.2 Cell-Based Immunotherapy

Dendritic Cell-Based Strategies

Dendritic cell (DC)-based strategies seek to leverage the critical role DC play in the afferent arm of the immune system. DC are the most potent APC and are capable of presenting antigen on both MHC I and MHC II. With their ability to stimulate a variety of afferent and efferent immune cell types, DC represent a crucial integrative regulator between the innate and adaptive immune arms. Because of these qualities, it was thought that DC would be more effective at overcoming tumor immunosuppression than directly injected peptide vaccines. Thus much of the recent work involving anti-tumor vaccines have focused on DC as a main component in the development of tumor vaccines. Typically DC are harvested from bone marrow (i.e., from the patient or a partially matched donor), expanded ex vivo with GM-CSF, IL-4, and TNF-a, then pulsed with either known tumor antigens, patient-derived tumor lysates, or RNA, and then re-infused. This process is technically challenging and this has led some investigators, such as in the ACTIVATE study described above, to turn back to alternatives such as direct injection of tumor vaccines and cytokine adjuvants to activate local DC at the injection site. Although DC have been tested with individual peptides targeting specific tumor antigens, notably EGFRvIII and survivin, a major part of their appeal is that they can be used with whole tumor lysates or peptides eluted from tumor MHC I that would presumably target multiple tumor antigens, preventing tumor immunoediting and recurrence of tumor cells lacking that specific antigen. The main concern with the tumor lysate and related approaches is that they run the risk of breaking self-tolerance and inducing an auto-immune encephalitis. However, this risk remains theoretical and to date no such reactions have been reported.

In HGG-IMMUNO, one of the largest DC studies to date, De Vleeschouwer's group treated 56 recurrent GBM patients with autologous early mature DC pulsed with autologous tumor lysates [204]. Patients were divided into three cohorts that each received between two and five induction vaccinations followed by either booster vaccinations or tumor lysates every 4 weeks. Although the majority of adverse reactions were mild, there was one grade IV neurotoxicity reaction and several grade II hematological reactions. Clinical response was mixed, although median progression-free survival and overall survival were not impressive at 3 and 9.6 months, respectively, overall survival at 24 and 36 months was encouraging at 14.8 and 11.1%. While the differences between treatment arms were not statistically significant, there was a trend supporting longer overall survival in Cohort C which received 4 weekly induction vaccinations followed by boosters of tumor lysates only.

Although the results from HGG-IMMUNO are disappointing, multiple human trials investigating the use of autologous DC pulsed with autologous tumor lysates in glioma are ongoing or recently completed. Results from these trials are expected to clarify the value of such strategies. These include two dose escalation trials at UCLA in pediatric patients by Lasky and Liau [205, 206], a phase II trial at Cedars Sinai by Yu which is expected to be completed in 2008 [207], and a phase II trial comparing patients treated with conventional therapy (including TMZ) and tumor lysates pulsed DC with historical controls which was recently completed by Fadul at Dartmouth and is awaiting publication [208]. Finally a large multi-institutional randomized placebo-controlled phase II study evaluating DCVax, a commercial tumor lysate-pulsed DC preparation, is underway [209]. Other alternatives to tumor lysates include apoptotic bodies and whole tumor RNA. Although neither is in glioma clinical trials, the early data from animal experiments are promising. The Pollack lab showed increased survival in a rat model using DC that were cocultured with apoptotic tumor cells [210]. The Kobayashi group pulsed DC from five GBM patients with tumor mRNA and was able to raise a strong tumor-specific CTL response [211]. Peptide-pulsed DC approaches under study include hyaluronan mRNA [212] and SART-1 [213]. The Jadus lab recently published a proof of principle paper showing that allogenic partially HLA-matched tumor lines could be used to generate peptides for vaccine generation or pulsing dendritic cells [214].

The great potential suggested by pre-clinical trials of DC vaccines remains unrealized. While a small minority of patients seem to have benefited in certain trials, for the majority, concrete benefits are elusive. Significant work remains to be done in optimizing protocols and identifying those most likely to respond. It remains to be determined which is the most effective DC subtype, method of generation, loading protocol, dose and route of administration. The Sloan lab sought to begin answering these questions by directly comparing four of the most common whole tumor DC-based therapies [215]. Working with patient-derived PMBC, they compared DC fused with MHC-matched glioma cells (Fusion), DC pulsed with apoptotic tumor cells (DC/APO), DC pulsed with total tumor ribonucleic acid (DC/RNA), and DC pulsed with tumor lysates (DC/Lys). They found that none of the preparations produced significantly more mature DC than any other and that both DC/RNA and DC/APO were better at inducing CTL from PBMC than Fusion or DC/Lys. However, DC/APO also produced significantly more NKT cells which could potentially lyse glioma cells in a non-MHC I-dependent fashion. On this basis they judged DC/APO superior.

Adoptive Transfer Immunotherapy

Adoptive therapy attempts to overcome blocks to the efferent arm of the immune system by harvesting immune cells from the patient, manipulating them to activate them or otherwise increase their effectiveness and then re-infusing them to target the tumor. Classically, the cell types used have included peripheral blood mononuclear cells (PBMC), lymphokine-activated killer cells (LAK), tumor infiltrating lymphocytes (TIL), and cytotoxic lymphocytes (CTL).

Lymphokine-Activated Killer Cells

Interest in lymphokine-activated killer (LAK) cells followed Rosenberg's pilot treatment of four lung or liver cancer patients with LAK cells [216] and in vitro experiments demonstrating LAK lysed 36 of the 41 tumor samples tested but did not attack allogenic non-tumor tissue [217]. Unfortunately, the majority of studies that used LAK in glioma did not live up the initial high hopes surrounding the therapy, although many showed clinical or radiographic improvements, most failed to show any survival benefit [218–223].

The most positive reports came from Hayes and colleagues in a phase I study in which 19 patients with recurrent disease (15 GBM and 4 AA) were treated with surgery followed by intratumoral LAK and IL-2 [224]. This study differed from previous studies in their explicit restrictions on steroid use during immunotherapy. Steroids were reduced or eliminated when possible, although they were available as bolus treatments for acute symptoms of IL-2 toxicity. CNS toxicities related to IL-2 occurred and were dose related; they included transient cerebral edema, confusion, and decreased alertness. All toxicities resolved with a steroid bolus. Results were very encouraging among GBM patients; there were two partial radiographic responses and one complete response that occurred 17 months after treatment. One of the four AA patients had a complete response. Most impressively, the median survival for GBM patients was 53 weeks post-reoperation, with 53% alive after 1 year, while a contemporary control group treated with chemotherapy alone had a median survival of 25.5 weeks and only 6% were alive after 1 year. Hayes reported that as of 1999 both complete response patients were still alive [225].

The largest study of intratumoral LAK therapy was conducted by Dillman and colleagues and comprised 40 patients who were reoperated on for recurrent GBM [226]. IL-2 was given to 23 of the patients at infusion, but dose and schedule were not specified. However, receipt of IL-2 did not have a significant effect on survival ($p = 0.24$). Adverse effects were not described. Median survival among the 31 patients who had a consistent diagnosis of GBM at both initial presentation and re-operation was significantly higher than comparable historical controls, 17.5 months versus 13.6 months ($p = 0.012$). Survival at 6 months and 2 years were superior as well, at 69 and 31%, respectively. Median survival also compared favorably with reports in the literature which ranges from 4.3 [227] to 8.6 months [228].

Work from the Ohno lab indicated that tumor infiltrating lymphocytes (TIL) could be harvested from patient tumors and that they had significantly greater lytic activity than LAK on a per cell basis [229]. Quattrocchi and colleagues reported results from a phase I trial using TIL and IL-2. Six patients with recurrent glioma (3 AA and 3 GBM) were treated with 1×10^9 autologous TIL and IL-2 [230]. Adverse effects were mild, one patient complained of transient low grade fevers and two developed asymptomatic hydrocephalus. All patients developed transient cerebral edema but none required steroids. Clinical outcomes were encouraging, at 3 and 6 months three patients showed partial radiographic response. Two died at 12 months and one at 18 months post-immunotherapy. At 45 months 3 of 6 patients were still alive. Despite this, interest in TIL was supplanted by interest in antigen-specific cytotoxic lymphocytes.

Interest in using tumor-specific cytotoxic lymphocytes grew out of evidence of the immunological deficiencies present in studies using TIL and the belief that enhancing specificity for tumor would increase efficacy. Although TIL were able to lyse glioma cells, they displayed two log lower proliferative capacity, even when stimulated with strong reagents such as phytohemagglutinin (PHA) [231]. TIL, particularly the CD4+ fraction, produced less IL-2 upon stimulation and had lower IL-2 receptor expression than control lymphocytes [232, 233]. Experiments by researchers working in a melanoma model demonstrated that it was possible to produce tumor-specific CTL from lymph nodes of immunized patients [234]. Furthermore, CTL were shown to home to tumor sites and were shown to reject tumors in animal models of glioma [235].

Kitahara and colleagues demonstrated that tumor-specific CTL could be generated from peripheral blood without prior immunization with tumor [236]. Five patients with malignant glioma were treated with intratumoral autologous tumor-specific CTL. One patient with GBM showed temporary regression for 20 weeks prior to recurrence, while three others recurred quickly and died. One patient with primary mixed AA-GBM, had near complete tumor regression on CT at 104 weeks remained healthy and without neural deficits. Several studies followed seeking to build on Kitahara's results by using adjuvants such as Bacillus of Calmette and Guerin (BCG) injections prior to PBMC harvest, IL-2 and GM-CSF prior to PBMC harvest in order to increase CTL yield and efficacy. In a follow-up study of nine patients with grade III or IV malignant glioma, anti-CD3 antibody and IL-2 were used in place of autologous tumor cells and IL-2 for post-vaccination restimulation of PMBCs [237]. Adverse effects from infusion were minor and transient and were limited to fever, chills, and nausea. Clinical results were mixed. The response among patients with grade III disease was very encouraging. Two patients had complete or near complete radiographic tumor regression and were alive and disease free at 4 and 5 years post-recurrence, while a third showed partial regression with no effect on survival. Among the GBM patients there were no signs of regression and no effect on survival. Median survival post-recurrence in this group was 6 months.

Plautz and colleagues also pursued an autologous tumor immunization model to raise tumor-specific CTL but replaced BCG with GM-CSF and harvested lymphocytes from draining lymph nodes instead of from peripheral blood [238]. Ten patients, two with progressive primary and eight with recurrent GBM, were treated. Adverse effects were minor, with fever the most common. There were no serious toxicities. Clinical effects were mixed. There were two patients that showed 6 months radiographic regression and one that had stable disease for 17 months but the remainder had progressive disease. The most encouraging result of the trial was that of the 8 patients with recurrent GBM, half were still alive 1 year after the re-operation and immunotherapy.

In a 2000 follow-up study, Plautz and colleagues sought to confirm their findings using a group of 12 newly diagnosed patients, two with grade II astrocytoma, four with AA, and six with GBM [239]. Patients were free of corticosteroids during immunotherapy and were preconditioned with cyclophosphamide and acetaminophen. Clinical results included partial radiographic regression in four of eight patients with visible residual disease following initial surgery. Among the patients with GBM, four had gross residual disease post surgery and two showed partial regression that occurred several months after treatment. Survival statistics were not calculated because of small sample size and heterogeneity, but among the patients with GBM, median time to progression was 11 months, with the two who showed partial radiographic response at 14 months and greater than 29 months.

While adoptive transfer immunotherapy techniques have produced some scattered clinical successes and shown glimmers of promise, results from over 30 years of research remain unsatisfactory. Much of the initial interest has waned as attention has shifted to other techniques such as tumor vaccination and dendritic cell vaccination. However, recent findings have the potential to re-invigorate the field. Among the most interesting is work from the Agur lab in creating a mathematical model of glioma–immune system interactions [240]. The model takes into account adoptively transferred CTL, the patients own CTL, tumor size, growth rate, MHC-class I and II expression, and the cytokine microenvironment. The model was then tested against clinical trial data and model predictions were compared with actual trial results. In the case of results from Kruse's group [241], the model predicted both the treatment success of the AA patients and the failure of the GBM patients. Based on predictions from the model and the biological differences between tumor types, Agur predicts that the number of CTL used in protocols needs to be increased by 20-fold. These conclusions are supported by recent data re-evaluating the role of age as a prognostic factor. Wheeler and colleagues found that the number of recent thymic emigrant $CD8^+$ T cells in peripheral blood was a better predictor of clinical outcome than age in vaccine trials [242]. This suggests that decreasing capacity for thymic production of new $CD8^+$ T cells may play an important role in glioma immune escape. Taken together with the data from the Agur lab, it suggests that adoptive CTL therapies at higher doses merit further investigation.

5 Conclusions

Malignant brain tumors represent a group of cancers that have eluded successful treatment strategies since they were first described. Indeed, the heterogeneous nature of malignant brain tumors and complex physiology of the CNS have stumped researchers' and physicians' attempts at treating this disease for many years. However, the rapid evolution in our understanding of the molecular underpinnings and complex physiologies of brain tumors have allowed researchers to develop novel treatment approaches which have changed the once devastating nature of this disease. The research that has gone into these developments has warranted the application of some of the most sophisticated and innovative approaches in experimental therapeutics. Translating these developments into successful clinical application will rely on the development of novel technologies in diagnostics and an improved understanding of the complex physiology of CNS tumors.

While not discussed in this chapter, the development of novel imaging technologies that better define a brain tumor's pathogenic characteristics will greatly enhance the development and application of targeted therapeutics. Markers that are capable of mapping molecular and physical traits responsible for the aggressive and drug-resistant nature of brain tumors will allow the application of targeted therapies and delivery paradigms, such as CED and IA delivery, to reach their full potential. While CED is still a novel delivery approach, it possesses vast potential. When we understand the parameters which dictate fluid flow in the cancerous brain tissue, CED can most effectively be applied to deliver experimental agents such as cells, viruses, liposome, and polymer formulations. In addition, state-of-the-art imaging developments will allow for the development of novel and improved non-invasive approaches for brain tumor targeting strategies.

Like many translational approaches in medicine, improved therapeutic application in brain tumors will arise with relevant discoveries in the basic sciences. Our understanding of how certain proteins and receptors partake in aberrant signal transduction cascades is still somewhat limited in scope. A greater understanding of the role of specific proteins in cellular physiology will allow the proper application of targeted molecular therapies, such as growth factor inhibitors and gene therapy. In addition, a more detailed understanding of how genetic and molecular aberrations contribute to the cancer pathology *as a tissue* will do much to improve novel applications. Understanding the role of different tissue compartments in the tumor, such as the tumor stroma, will speed these developments. Immunotherapy for brain tumor therapies symbolizes a very promising and exciting treatment strategy for brain tumors and cancer in general. An understanding of the immune system's role in the healthy and diseased brain will enhance the development of sophisticated protocols that can lead to most optimal treatment outcome using these approaches. The physiological barriers in the CNS still continue to confound researchers' efforts to deliver drugs to the brain. A greater understanding of the BBB in health and disease will do much to optimize drug delivery to brain tumors. In summary, these understandings may one day lead to treatment algorithms which can include a combination of different treatment approaches and delivery strategies more extensive and effective than those used today, to the extent that the goals of molecular medicine come to fruition.

References

1. Stupp R, Hegi ME, van den Bent MJ, Mason WP, Weller M, Mirimanoff RO et al. Changing paradigms – an update on the multidisciplinary management of malignant glioma. *Oncologist* 2006; **11**: 165–180.
2. Hegi ME, Diserens AC, Gorlia T, Hamou MF, de Tribolet N, Weller M et al. MGMT gene silencing and benefit from temozolomide in glioblastoma. *N Engl J Med* 2005; **352**: 997–1003.

3. Sonabend AM, Lesniak MS. Oligodendrogliomas: clinical significance of 1p and 19q chromosomal deletions. *Expert Rev Neurother* 2005; **5**: S25–S32.
4. Cairncross JG, Ueki K, Zlatescu MC, Lisle DK, Finkelstein DM, Hammond RR et al. Specific genetic predictors of chemotherapeutic response and survival in patients with anaplastic oligodendrogliomas. *J Natl Cancer Inst* 1998; **90**: 1473–1479.
5. Citri A, Yarden Y. EGF-ERBB signalling: towards the systems level. *Nat Rev Mol Cell Biol* 2006; **7**: 505–516.
6. Humphrey PA, Wong AJ, Vogelstein B, Friedman HS, Werner MH, Bigner DD et al. Amplification and expression of the epidermal growth factor receptor gene in human glioma xenografts. *Cancer Res* 1988; **48**: 2231–2238.
7. Pelloski CE, Ballman KV, Furth AF, Zhang L, Lin E, Sulman EP et al. Epidermal growth factor receptor variant III status defines clinically distinct subtypes of glioblastoma. *J Clin Oncol* 2007; **25**: 2288–2294.
8. Sarkaria JN, Yang L, Grogan PT, Kitange GJ, Carlson BL, Schroeder MA et al. Identification of molecular characteristics correlated with glioblastoma sensitivity to EGFR kinase inhibition through use of an intracranial xenograft test panel. *Mol Cancer Ther* 2007; **6**: 1167–1174.
9. Van den Bent MJ, Brandes A, Rampling R, Kouwenhoven M, Kros JM, Carpentier A et al. Randomized phase II trial of erlotinib (E) versus temozolomide (TMZ) or BCNU in recurrent glioblastoma multiforme (GBM): EORTC 26034. *2007 ASCO Annual Meeting J Clin Oncol* 2007, 18S.
10. Lassman AB, Rossi MR, Raizer JJ, Abrey LE, Lieberman FS, Grefe CN et al. Molecular study of malignant gliomas treated with epidermal growth factor receptor inhibitors: tissue analysis from North American Brain Tumor Consortium Trials 01-03 and 00-01. *Clin Cancer Res* 2005; **11**: 7841–7850.
11. Mellinghoff IK, Wang MY, Vivanco I, Haas-Kogan DA, Zhu S, Dia EQ et al. Molecular determinants of the response of glioblastomas to EGFR kinase inhibitors. *N Engl J Med* 2005; **353**: 2012–2024.
12. Hanahan D, Folkman J. Patterns and emerging mechanisms of the angiogenic switch during tumorigenesis. *Cell* 1996; **86**: 353–364.
13. Sipos EP, Brem H. Local anti-angiogenic brain tumor therapies. *J Neurooncol* 2000; **50**: 181–188.
14. Weingart JD, Laterra JJ, Brem H. Cerebral gliomas. Growth factors and angiogenesis. *Baillieres Clin Neurol* 1996; **5**: 307–318.
15. Fine HA. Promising new therapies for malignant gliomas. *Cancer J* 2007; **13**: 349–354.
16. Rajaraman P, Wang SS, Rothman N, Brown MM, Black PM, Fine HA et al. Polymorphisms in apoptosis and cell cycle control genes and risk of brain tumors in adults. *Cancer Epidemiol Biomarkers Prev* 2007; **16**: 1655–1661.
17. Wang SI, Puc J, Li J, Bruce JN, Cairns P, Sidransky D et al. Somatic mutations of PTEN in glioblastoma multiforme. *Cancer Res* 1997; **57**: 4183–4186.
18. Boluyt MO, Li ZB, Loyd AM, Scalia AF, Cirrincione GM, Jackson RR. The mTOR/p70S6K signal transduction pathway plays a role in cardiac hypertrophy and influences expression of myosin heavy chain genes in vivo. *Cardiovasc Drugs Ther* 2004; **18**: 257–267.
19. Brunn GJ, Fadden P, Haystead TA, Lawrence JC, Jr. The mammalian target of rapamycin phosphorylates sites having a (Ser/Thr)-Pro motif and is activated by antibodies to a region near its COOH terminus. *J Biol Chem* 1997; **272**: 32547–32550.
20. Brunn GJ, Hudson CC, Sekulic A, Williams JM, Hosoi H, Houghton PJ et al. Phosphorylation of the translational repressor PHAS-I by the mammalian target of rapamycin. *Science* 1997; **277**: 99–101.
21. Chang SM, Wen P, Cloughesy T, Greenberg H, Schiff D, Conrad C et al. Phase II study of CCI-779 in patients with recurrent glioblastoma multiforme. *Invest New Drugs* 2005; **23**: 357–361.

22. Galanis E, Buckner JC, Maurer MJ, Kreisberg JI, Ballman K, Boni J et al. Phase II trial of temsirolimus (CCI-779) in recurrent glioblastoma multiforme: a North Central Cancer Treatment Group Study. *J Clin Oncol* 2005; **23**: 5294–5304.
23. Molnar-Kimber KL. Mechanism of action of rapamycin (Sirolimus, Rapamune). *Transplant Proc* 1996; **28**: 964–969.
24. Sehgal SN. Rapamune (Sirolimus, rapamycin): an overview and mechanism of action. *Ther Drug Monit* 1995; **17**: 660–665.
25. Sehgal SN. Rapamune (RAPA, rapamycin, sirolimus): mechanism of action immunosuppressive effect results from blockade of signal transduction and inhibition of cell cycle progression. *Clin Biochem* 1998; **31**: 335–340.
26. Neshat MS, Mellinghoff IK, Tran C, Stiles B, Thomas G, Petersen R et al. Enhanced sensitivity of PTEN-deficient tumors to inhibition of FRAP/mTOR. *Proc Natl Acad Sci USA* 2001; **98**: 10314–10319.
27. Podsypanina K, Lee RT, Politis C, Hennessy I, Crane A, Puc J et al. An inhibitor of mTOR reduces neoplasia and normalizes p70/S6 kinase activity in Pten +/– mice. *Proc Natl Acad Sci USA* 2001; **98**: 10320–10325.
28. Gaillard PJ, van der Sandt IC, Voorwinden LH, Vu D, Nielsen JL, de Boer AG et al. Astrocytes increase the functional expression of P-glycoprotein in an in vitro model of the blood-brain barrier. *Pharm Res* 2000; **17**: 1198–1205.
29. Janzer RC, Raff MC. Astrocytes induce blood-brain barrier properties in endothelial cells. *Nature* 1987; **325**: 253–257.
30. Rubin LL, Staddon JM. The cell biology of the blood-brain barrier. *Annu Rev Neurosci* 1999; **22**: 11–28.
31. Fenstermacher J, Gross P, Sposito N, Acuff V, Pettersen S, Gruber K. Structural and functional variations in capillary systems within the brain. *Ann N Y Acad Sci* 1988; **529**: 21–30.
32. Fenstermacher J, Kaye T. Drug 'diffusion" within the brain. *Ann N Y Acad Sci* 1988; **531**: 29–39.
33. Hutson SM, Fenstermacher D, Mahar C. Role of mitochondrial transamination in branched chain amino acid metabolism. *J Biol Chem* 1988; **263**: 3618–3625.
34. Ciechanover A. Proteolysis: from the lysosome to ubiquitin and the proteasome. *Nat Rev Mol Cell Biol* 2005; **6**: 79–87.
35. el-Bacha RS, Minn A. Drug metabolizing enzymes in cerebrovascular endothelial cells afford a metabolic protection to the brain. *Cell Mol Biol (Noisy-le-grand)* 1999; **45**: 15–23.
36. Sedlakova R, Shivers RR, Del Maestro RF. Ultrastructure of the blood-brain barrier in the rabbit. *J Submicrosc Cytol Pathol* 1999; **31**: 149–161.
37. Kniesel U, Wolburg H. Tight junctions of the blood-brain barrier. *Cell Mol Neurobiol* 2000; **20**: 57–76.
38. Liebner S, Kniesel U, Kalbacher H, Wolburg H. Correlation of tight junction morphology with the expression of tight junction proteins in blood-brain barrier endothelial cells. *Eur J Cell Biol* 2000; **79**: 707–717.
39. Borst P, Evers R, Kool M, Wijnholds J. The multidrug resistance protein family. *Biochim Biophys Acta* 1999; **1461**: 347–357.
40. Cordon-Cardo C, O'Brien JP, Casals D, Rittman-Grauer L, Biedler JL, Melamed MR et al. Multidrug-resistance gene (P-glycoprotein) is expressed by endothelial cells at blood-brain barrier sites. *Proc Natl Acad Sci USA* 1989; **86**: 695–698.
41. de Boer AG, Gaillard PJ. Drug targeting to the brain. *Annu Rev Pharmacol Toxicol* 2007; **47**: 323–355.
42. de Boer AG, van der Sandt IC, Gaillard PJ. The role of drug transporters at the blood-brain barrier. *Annu Rev Pharmacol Toxicol* 2003; **43**: 629–656.
43. Deeken JF, Loscher W. The blood-brain barrier and cancer: transporters, treatment, and Trojan horses. *Clin Cancer Res* 2007; **13**: 1663–1674.

44. Lee G, Dallas S, Hong M, Bendayan R. Drug transporters in the central nervous system: brain barriers and brain parenchyma considerations. *Pharmacol Rev* 2001; **53**: 569–596.
45. Loscher W, Potschka H. Role of drug efflux transporters in the brain for drug disposition and treatment of brain diseases. *Prog Neurobiol* 2005; **76**: 22–76.
46. Schinkel AH, Wagenaar E, van Deemter L, Mol CA, Borst P. Absence of the mdr1a P-Glycoprotein in mice affects tissue distribution and pharmacokinetics of dexamethasone, digoxin, and cyclosporin A. *J Clin Invest* 1995; **96**: 1698–1705.
47. Johanson CE, Duncan JA, Stopa EG, Baird A. Enhanced prospects for drug delivery and brain targeting by the choroid plexus-CSF route. *Pharm Res* 2005; **22**: 1011–1037.
48. Groothuis DR. The blood-brain and blood-tumor barriers: a review of strategies for increasing drug delivery. *Neuro Oncol* 2000; **2**: 45–59.
49. Muldoon LL, Soussain C, Jahnke K, Johanson C, Siegal T, Smith QR et al. Chemotherapy delivery issues in central nervous system malignancy: a reality check. *J Clin Oncol* 2007; **25**: 2295–2305.
50. Bates SF, Chen C, Robey R, Kang M, Figg WD, Fojo T. Reversal of multidrug resistance: lessons from clinical oncology. *Novartis Found Symp* 2002; **243**: 83–96; discussion 96–102, 180–105.
51. Johanson CE. Permeability and vascularity of the developing brain: cerebellum vs cerebral cortex. *Brain Res* 1980; **190**: 3–16.
52. Johanson CE, Woodbury DM. Uptake of [14C]urea by the in vivo choroid plexus–cerebrospinal fluid–brain system: identification of sites of molecular sieving. *J Physiol* 1978; **275**: 167–176.
53. Murphy VA, Johanson CE. Adrenergic-induced enhancement of brain barrier system permeability to small nonelectrolytes: choroid plexus versus cerebral capillaries. *J Cereb Blood Flow Metab* 1985; **5**: 401–412.
54. Parandoosh Z, Johanson CE. Ontogeny of blood-brain barrier permeability to, and cerebrospinal fluid sink action on, [14C]urea. *Am J Physiol* 1982; **243**: R400–R407.
55. Boiardi A, Eoli M, Pozzi A, Salmaggi A, Broggi G, Silvani A. Locally delivered chemotherapy and repeated surgery can improve survival in glioblastoma patients. *Ital J Neurol Sci* 1999; **20**: 43–48.
56. Boiardi A, Silvani A, Milanesi I, Munari L, Broggi G, Botturi M. Local immunotherapy (beta-IFN) and systemic chemotherapy in primary glial tumors. *Ital J Neurol Sci* 1991; **12**: 163–168.
57. Lesniak MS, Brem H. Targeted therapy for brain tumours. *Nat Rev Drug Discov* 2004; **3**: 499–508.
58. Lesniak MS, Langer R, Brem H. Drug delivery to tumors of the central nervous system. *Curr Neurol Neurosci Rep* 2001; **1**: 210–216.
59. Morantz RA, Kimler BF, Vats TS, Henderson SD. Bleomycin and brain tumors. A review. *J Neurooncol* 1983; **1**: 249–255.
60. Pardridge WM. Blood-brain barrier biology and methodology. *J Neurovirol* 1999; **5**: 556–569.
61. Neuwelt EA. Mechanisms of disease: the blood-brain barrier. *Neurosurgery* 2004; **54**: 131–140; discussion 141–132.
62. Neuwelt EA, Barnett PA, McCormick CI, Remsen LG, Kroll RA, Sexton G. Differential permeability of a human brain tumor xenograft in the nude rat: impact of tumor size and method of administration on optimizing delivery of biologically diverse agents. *Clin Cancer Res* 1998; **4**: 1549–1555.
63. Fortin D, Desjardins A, Benko A, Niyonsega T, Boudrias M. Enhanced chemotherapy delivery by intraarterial infusion and blood-brain barrier disruption in malignant brain tumors: the Sherbrooke experience. *Cancer* 2005; **103**: 2606–2615.
64. Fortin D, Gendron C, Boudrias M, Garant MP. Enhanced chemotherapy delivery by intraarterial infusion and blood-brain barrier disruption in the treatment of cerebral metastasis. *Cancer* 2007; **109**: 751–760.

65. Hall WA, Doolittle ND, Daman M, Bruns PK, Muldoon L, Fortin D et al. Osmotic blood-brain barrier disruption chemotherapy for diffuse pontine gliomas. *J Neurooncol* 2006; **77**: 279–284.
66. Kraemer DF, Fortin D, Doolittle ND, Neuwelt EA. Association of total dose intensity of chemotherapy in primary central nervous system lymphoma (human non-acquired immunodeficiency syndrome) and survival. *Neurosurgery* 2001; **48**: 1033–1040; discussion 1040–1031.
67. Chang CH, Horton J, Schoenfeld D, Salazer O, Perez-Tamayo R, Kramer S et al. Comparison of postoperative radiotherapy and combined postoperative radiotherapy and chemotherapy in the multidisciplinary management of malignant gliomas. A joint Radiation Therapy Oncology Group and Eastern Cooperative Oncology Group study. *Cancer* 1983; **52**: 997–1007.
68. Green SB, Byar DP, Walker MD, Pistenmaa DA, Alexander E, Jr, Batzdorf U et al. Comparisons of carmustine, procarbazine, and high-dose methylprednisolone as additions to surgery and radiotherapy for the treatment of malignant glioma. *Cancer Treat Rep* 1983; **67**: 121–132.
69. Selker RG, Shapiro WR, Burger P, Blackwood MS, Arena VC, Gilder JC et al. The Brain Tumor Cooperative Group NIH Trial 87-01: a randomized comparison of surgery, external radiotherapy, and carmustine versus surgery, interstitial radiotherapy boost, external radiation therapy, and carmustine. *Neurosurgery* 2002; **51**: 343–355; discussion 355–347.
70. Cohen RJ, Wiernik PH, Walker MD. Acute nonlymphocytic leukemia associated with nitrosourea chemotherapy: report of two cases. *Cancer Treat Rep* 1976; **60**: 1257–1261.
71. Crittenden D, Tranum BL, Haut A. Pulmonary fibrosis after prolonged therapy with 1,3-bis (2-chloroethyl)-1-nitrosourea. *Chest* 1977; **72**: 372–373.
72. De Vita VT, Carbone PP, Owens AH, Jr, Gold GL, Krant MJ, Edmonson J. Clinical trials with 1,3-bis(2-chloroethyl)-1-nitrosourea, NSC-409962. *Cancer Res* 1965; **25**: 1876–1881.
73. Litam JP, Dail DH, Spitzer G, Vellekoop L, Verma DS, Zander AR et al. Early pulmonary toxicity after administration of high-dose BCNU. *Cancer Treat Rep* 1981; **65**: 39–44.
74. Michels SD, McKenna RW, Arthur DC, Brunning RD. Therapy-related acute myeloid leukemia and myelodysplastic syndrome: a clinical and morphologic study of 65 cases. *Blood* 1985; **65**: 1364–1372.
75. Brem H, Piantadosi S, Burger PC, Walker M, Selker R, Vick NA et al. Placebo-controlled trial of safety and efficacy of intraoperative controlled delivery by biodegradable polymers of chemotherapy for recurrent gliomas. The Polymer-brain Tumor Treatment Group. *Lancet* 1995; **345**: 1008–1012.
76. Bota DA, Desjardins A, Quinn JA, Affronti ML, Friedman HS. Interstitial chemotherapy with biodegradable BCNU (Gliadel) wafers in the treatment of malignant gliomas. *Ther Clin Risk Manag* 2007; **3**: 707–715.
77. Dang W, Daviau T, Brem H. Morphological characterization of polyanhydride biodegradable implant gliadel during in vitro and in vivo erosion using scanning electron microscopy. *Pharm Res* 1996; **13**: 683–691.
78. Domb AJ, Rock M, Perkin C, Yipchuck G, Broxup B, Villemure JG. Excretion of a radiolabelled anticancer biodegradable polymeric implant from the rabbit brain. *Biomaterials* 1995; **16**: 1069–1072.
79. Grossman SA, Reinhard C, Colvin OM, Chasin M, Brundrett R, Tamargo RJ et al. The intracerebral distribution of BCNU delivered by surgically implanted biodegradable polymers. *J Neurosurg* 1992; **76**: 640–647.
80. Judy KD, Olivi A, Buahin KG, Domb A, Epstein JI, Colvin OM et al. Effectiveness of controlled release of a cyclophosphamide derivative with polymers against rat gliomas. *J Neurosurg* 1995; **82**: 481–486.

81. Meldorf MG, Riddle VD, Group GMT, Agarwal S. Long-term efficacy of local chemotherapy with biodegradable carmustine implants (Gliadel) in high-grade malignant gliomas. *American Association of Neurological Surgeons*. American Association of Neurological Surgeons (ASSN), 2003.

82. Valtonen S, Timonen U, Toivanen P, Kalimo H, Kivipelto L, Heiskanen O et al. Interstitial chemotherapy with carmustine-loaded polymers for high-grade gliomas: a randomized double-blind study. *Neurosurgery* 1997; **41**: 44–48; discussion 48–49.

83. Westphal M, Hilt DC, Bortey E, Delavault P, Olivares R, Warnke PC et al. A phase 3 trial of local chemotherapy with biodegradable carmustine (BCNU) wafers (Gliadel wafers) in patients with primary malignant glioma. *Neuro Oncol* 2003; **5**: 79–88.

84. Debinski W, Obiri NI, Powers SK, Pastan I, Puri RK. Human glioma cells overexpress receptors for interleukin 13 and are extremely sensitive to a novel chimeric protein composed of interleukin 13 and pseudomonas exotoxin. *Clin Cancer Res* 1995; **1**: 1253–1258.

85. Husain SR, Puri RK. Interleukin-13 receptor-directed cytotoxin for malignant glioma therapy: from bench to bedside. *J Neurooncol* 2003; **65**: 37–48.

86. Kioi M, Husain SR, Croteau D, Kunwar S, Puri RK. Convection-enhanced delivery of interleukin-13 receptor-directed cytotoxin for malignant glioma therapy. *Technol Cancer Res Treat* 2006; **5**: 239–250.

87. Kunwar S, Prados MD, Chang SM, Berger MS, Lang FF, Piepmeier JM et al. Direct intracerebral delivery of cintredekin besudotox (IL13-PE38QQR) in recurrent malignant glioma: a report by the Cintredekin Besudotox Intraparenchymal Study Group. *J Clin Oncol* 2007; **25**: 837–844.

88. Vogelbaum MA, Sampson JH, Kunwar S, Chang SM, Shaffrey M, Asher AL et al. Convection-enhanced delivery of cintredekin besudotox (interleukin-13-PE38QQR) followed by radiation therapy with and without temozolomide in newly diagnosed malignant gliomas: phase 1 study of final safety results. *Neurosurgery* 2007; **61**: 1031–1037; discussion 1037–1038.

89. Sampson JH, Akabani G, Archer GE, Berger MS, Coleman RE, Friedman AH et al. Intracerebral infusion of an EGFR-targeted toxin in recurrent malignant brain tumors. *Neuro Oncol* 2008; **10**: 320–329.

90. Vogelbaum MA. Convection enhanced delivery for treating brain tumors and selected neurological disorders: symposium review. *J Neurooncol* 2007; **83**: 97–109.

91. Adams GP, Weiner LM. Monoclonal antibody therapy of cancer. *Nat Biotechnol* 2005; **23**: 1147–1157.

92. Imai K, Takaoka A. Comparing antibody and small-molecule therapies for cancer. *Nat Rev Cancer* 2006; **6**: 714–727.

93. Reichert JM, Valge-Archer VE. Development trends for monoclonal antibody cancer therapeutics. *Nat Rev Drug Discov* 2007; **6**: 349–356.

94. Vredenburgh JJ, Desjardins A, Herndon JE, 2nd, Marcello J, Reardon DA, Quinn JA et al. Bevacizumab plus irinotecan in recurrent glioblastoma multiforme. *J Clin Oncol* 2007; **25**: 4722–4729.

95. Schiff D, Purow B. Bevacizumab in combination with irinotecan for patients with recurrent glioblastoma multiforme. *Nat Clin Pract Oncol* 2008; **5**: 186–187.

96. Beduneau A, Saulnier P, Benoit JP. Active targeting of brain tumors using nanocarriers. *Biomaterials* 2007; **28**: 4947–4967.

97. Hallahan D, Geng L, Qu S, Scarfone C, Giorgio T, Donnelly E et al. Integrin-mediated targeting of drug delivery to irradiated tumor blood vessels. *Cancer Cell* 2003; **3**: 63–74.

98. Barzon L, Zanusso M, Colombo F, Palu G. Clinical trials of gene therapy, virotherapy, and immunotherapy for malignant gliomas. *Cancer Gene Ther* 2006; **13**: 539–554.

99. Pulkkanen KJ, Yla-Herttuala S. Gene therapy for malignant glioma: current clinical status. *Mol Ther* 2005; **12**: 585–598.

100. Rainov NG. A phase III clinical evaluation of herpes simplex virus type 1 thymidine kinase and ganciclovir gene therapy as an adjuvant to surgical resection and radiation in

adults with previously untreated glioblastoma multiforme. *Hum Gene Ther* 2000; **11**: 2389–2401.

101. Aboody KS, Najbauer J, Danks MK. Stem and progenitor cell-mediated tumor selective gene therapy. *Gene Ther* 2008; **15**: 739–752.

102. Aboody KS, Brown A, Rainov NG, Bower KA, Liu S, Yang W et al. Neural stem cells display extensive tropism for pathology in adult brain: evidence from intracranial gliomas. *Proc Natl Acad Sci USA* 2000; **97**: 12846–12851.

103. Kim SK, Kim SU, Park IH, Bang JH, Aboody KS, Wang KC et al. Human neural stem cells target experimental intracranial medulloblastoma and deliver a therapeutic gene leading to tumor regression. *Clin Cancer Res* 2006; **12**: 5550–5556.

104. Kim SU. Human neural stem cells genetically modified for brain repair in neurological disorders. *Neuropathology* 2004; **24**: 159–171.

105. Shimato S, Natsume A, Takeuchi H, Wakabayashi T, Fujii M, Ito M et al. Human neural stem cells target and deliver therapeutic gene to experimental leptomeningeal medulloblastoma. *Gene Ther* 2007; **14**: 1132–1142.

106. Tang Y, Shah K, Messerli SM, Snyder E, Breakefield X, Weissleder R. In vivo tracking of neural progenitor cell migration to glioblastomas. *Hum Gene Ther* 2003; **14**: 1247–1254.

107. Jacobs A, Voges J, Reszka R, Lercher M, Gossmann A, Kracht L et al. Positron-emission tomography of vector-mediated gene expression in gene therapy for gliomas. *Lancet* 2001; **358**: 727–729.

108. Maclachlan I. siRNAs with guts. *Nat Biotechnol* 2008; **26**: 403–405.

109. Peer D, Park EJ, Morishita Y, Carman CV, Shimaoka M. Systemic leukocyte-directed siRNA delivery revealing cyclin D1 as an anti-inflammatory target. *Science* 2008; **319**: 627–630.

110. Sonabend AM, Ulasov IV, Lesniak MS. Gene therapy trials for the treatment of high-grade gliomas. *Gene Ther Mol Biol* 2007; **11**: 79–92.

111. Immonen A, Vapalahti M, Tyynela K, Hurskainen H, Sandmair A, Vanninen R et al. AdvHSV-tk gene therapy with intravenous ganciclovir improves survival in human malignant glioma: a randomised, controlled study. *Mol Ther* 2004; **10**: 967–972.

112. Sandmair AM, Loimas S, Puranen P, Immonen A, Kossila M, Puranen M et al. Thymidine kinase gene therapy for human malignant glioma, using replication-deficient retroviruses or adenoviruses. *Hum Gene Ther* 2000; **11**: 2197–2205.

113. Sandmair AM, Vapalahti M, Yla-Herttuala S. Adenovirus-mediated herpes simplex thymidine kinase gene therapy for brain tumors. *Adv Exp Med Biol* 2000; **465**: 163–170.

114. Trask TW, Trask RP, Aguilar-Cordova E, Shine HD, Wyde PR, Goodman JC et al. Phase I study of adenoviral delivery of the HSV-tk gene and ganciclovir administration in patients with current malignant brain tumors. *Mol Ther* 2000; **1**: 195–203.

115. Odaka M, Sterman DH, Wiewrodt R, Zhang Y, Kiefer M, Amin KM et al. Eradication of intraperitoneal and distant tumor by adenovirus-mediated interferon-beta gene therapy is attributable to induction of systemic immunity. *Cancer Res* 2001; **61**: 6201–6212.

116. Chiocca EA, Smith KM, McKinney B, Palmer CA, Rosenfeld S, Lillehei K et al. A phase I trial of Ad.hIFN-beta gene therapy for glioma. *Mol Ther* 2008; **16**: 618–626.

117. Chiocca EA, Abbed KM, Tatter S, Louis DN, Hochberg FH, Barker F et al. A phase I open-label, dose-escalation, multi-institutional trial of injection with an E1B-Attenuated adenovirus, ONYX-015, into the peritumoral region of recurrent malignant gliomas, in the adjuvant setting. *Mol Ther* 2004; **10**: 958–966.

118. Markert JM. Biologic warfare for a good cause: HSV-1 anti-tumor therapy. *Clin Neurosurg* 2004; **51**: 73–80.

119. Fueyo J, Gomez-Manzano C, Yung WK, Liu TJ, Alemany R, Bruner JM et al. Suppression of human glioma growth by adenovirus-mediated Rb gene transfer. *Neurology* 1998; **50**: 1307–1315.

120. Lamfers ML, Grill J, Dirven CM, Van Beusechem VW, Geoerger B, Van Den Berg J et al. Potential of the conditionally replicative adenovirus Ad5-Delta24RGD in the treatment of malignant gliomas and its enhanced effect with radiotherapy. *Cancer Res* 2002; **62**: 5736–5742.
121. Stolarek R, Gomez-Manzano C, Jiang H, Suttle G, Lemoine MG, Fueyo J. Robust infectivity and replication of Delta-24 adenovirus induce cell death in human medulloblastoma. *Cancer Gene Ther* 2004; **11**: 713–720.
122. Ulasov IV, Rivera AA, Nettelbeck DM, Rivera LB, Mathis JM, Sonabend AM et al. An oncolytic adenoviral vector carrying the tyrosinase promoter for glioma gene therapy. *Int J Oncol* 2007; **31**: 1177–1185.
123. Ulasov IV, Rivera AA, Sonabend AM, Rivera LB, Wang M, Zhu ZB et al. Comparative evaluation of survivin, midkine and CXCR4 promoters for transcriptional targeting of glioma gene therapy. *Cancer Biol Ther* 2007; **6**: 679–685.
124. Ulasov IV, Zhu ZB, Tyler MA, Han Y, Rivera AA, Khramtsov A et al. Survivin-driven and fiber-modified oncolytic adenovirus exhibits potent antitumor activity in established intracranial glioma. *Hum Gene Ther* 2007; **18**: 589–602.
125. Gomez-Manzano C, Yung WK, Alemany R, Fueyo J. Genetically modified adenoviruses against gliomas: from bench to bedside. *Neurology* 2004; **63**: 418–426.
126. Jiang H, Gomez-Manzano C, Aoki H, Alonso MM, Kondo S, McCormick F et al. Examination of the therapeutic potential of Delta-24-RGD in brain tumor stem cells: role of autophagic cell death. *J Natl Cancer Inst* 2007; **99**: 1410–1414.
127. Tyler MA, Sonabend AM, Ulasov IV, Lesniak MS. Vector therapies for malignant glioma: shifting the clinical paradigm. *Expert Opin Drug Deliv* 2008; **5**: 445–458.
128. Tyler MA, Ulasov IV, Borovjagin A, Sonabend AM, Khramtsov A, Han Y et al. Enhanced transduction of malignant glioma with a double targeted Ad5/3-RGD fiber-modified adenovirus. *Mol Cancer Ther* 2006; **5**: 2408–2416.
129. Kurozumi K, Hardcastle J, Thakur R, Yang M, Christoforidis G, Fulci G et al. Effect of tumor microenvironment modulation on the efficacy of oncolytic virus therapy. *J Natl Cancer Inst* 2007; **99**: 1768–1781.
130. Lamfers ML, Fulci G, Gianni D, Tang Y, Kurozumi K, Kaur B et al. Cyclophosphamide increases transgene expression mediated by an oncolytic adenovirus in glioma-bearing mice monitored by bioluminescence imaging. *Mol Ther* 2006; **14**: 779–788.
131. Sonabend AM, Ulasov IV, Tyler MA, Rivera AA, Mathis JM, Lesniak MS. Mesenchymal stem cells effectively deliver an oncolytic adenovirus to intracranial glioma. *Stem Cells* 2008; **26**: 831–841.
132. Wang C, Pham PT. Polymers for viral gene delivery. *Expert Opin Drug Deliv* 2008; **5**: 385–401.
133. Chiocca EA. The host response to cancer virotherapy. *Curr Opin Mol Ther* 2008; **10**: 38–45.
134. Alonso MM, Gomez-Manzano C, Jiang H, Bekele NB, Piao Y, Yung WK et al. Combination of the oncolytic adenovirus ICOVIR-5 with chemotherapy provides enhanced anti-glioma effect in vivo. *Cancer Gene Ther* 2007; **14**: 756–761.
135. Alonso MM, Jiang H, Yokoyama T, Xu J, Bekele NB, Lang FF et al. Delta-24-RGD in combination with RAD001 induces enhanced anti-glioma effect via autophagic cell death. *Mol Ther* 2008; **16**: 487–493.
136. Cascallo M, Alonso MM, Rojas JJ, Perez-Gimenez A, Fueyo J, Alemany R. Systemic toxicity-efficacy profile of ICOVIR-5, a potent and selective oncolytic adenovirus based on the pRB pathway. *Mol Ther* 2007; **15**: 1607–1615.
137. Nandi S, Ulasov IV, Tyler MA, Sugihara AQ, Molinero L, Han Y et al. Low-dose radiation enhances survivin-mediated virotherapy against malignant glioma stem cells. *Cancer Res* 2008; **68**: 5778–5784.
138. Medawar P. Immunity to homologous grafted skin. *Brit J Exp Path* 1948; **28**.

139. Galea I, Bechmann I, Perry VH. What is immune privilege (not)? *Trends Immunol* 2007; **28**: 12–18.
140. Carpentier AF, Meng Y. Recent advances in immunotherapy for human glioma. *Curr Opin Oncol* 2006; **18**: 631–636.
141. Matyszak MK, Perry VH. The potential role of dendritic cells in immune-mediated inflammatory diseases in the central nervous system. *Neuroscience* 1996; **74**: 599–608.
142. Hatterer E, Davoust N, Didier-Bazes M, Vuaillat C, Malcus C, Belin MF et al. How to drain without lymphatics? Dendritic cells migrate from the cerebrospinal fluid to the B-cell follicles of cervical lymph nodes. *Blood* 2006; **107**: 806–812.
143. Harling-Berg CJ, Park TJ, Knopf PM. Role of the cervical lymphatics in the Th2-type hierarchy of CNS immune regulation. *J Neuroimmunol* 1999; **101**: 111–127.
144. Bechmann I, Galea I, Perry VH. What is the blood-brain barrier (not)? *Trends Immunol* 2007; **28**: 5–11.
145. Perry VH. A revised view of the central nervous system microenvironment and major histocompatibility complex class II antigen presentation. *J Neuroimmunol* 1998; **90**: 113–121.
146. Ridley A, Cavanagh JB. Lymphocytic infiltration in gliomas: evidence of possible host resistance. *Brain* 1971; **94**: 117–124.
147. Brooks WH, Markesbery WR, Gupta GD, Roszman TL. Relationship of lymphocyte invasion and survival of brain tumor patients. *Ann Neurol* 1978; **4**: 219–224.
148. Palma L, Di Lorenzo N, Guidetti B. Lymphocytic infiltrates in primary glioblastomas and recidivous gliomas. Incidence, fate, and relevance to prognosis in 228 operated cases. *J Neurosurg* 1978; **49**: 854–861.
149. Burger PC, Vogel FS, Green SB, Strike TA. Glioblastoma multiforme and anaplastic astrocytoma. Pathologic criteria and prognostic implications. *Cancer* 1985; **56**: 1106–1111.
150. Rossi ML, Hughes JT, Esiri MM, Coakham HB, Brownell DB. Immunohistological study of mononuclear cell infiltrate in malignant gliomas. *Acta Neuropathol* 1987; **74**: 269–277.
151. Tang J, Flomenberg P, Harshyne L, Kenyon L, Andrews DW. Glioblastoma patients exhibit circulating tumor-specific CD8+ T cells. *Clin Cancer Res* 2005; **11**: 5292–5299.
152. Gomez GG, Kruse CA. Mechanisms of malignant glioma immune resistance and sources of immunosuppression. *Gene Ther Mol Biol* 2006; **10**: 133–146.
153. Dick SJ, Macchi B, Papazoglou S, Oldfield EH, Kornblith PL, Smith BH et al. Lymphoid cell-glioma cell interaction enhances cell coat production by human gliomas: novel suppressor mechanism. *Science* 1983; **220**: 739–742.
154. Schiltz PM, Gomez GG, Read SB, Kulprathipanja NV, Kruse CA. Effects of IFN-gamma and interleukin-1beta on major histocompatibility complex antigen and intercellular adhesion molecule-1 expression by 9L gliosarcoma: relevance to its cytolysis by alloreactive cytotoxic T lymphocytes. *J Interferon Cytokine Res* 2002; **22**: 1209–1216.
155. Facoetti A, Nano R, Zelini P, Morbini P, Benericetti E, Ceroni M et al. Human leukocyte antigen and antigen processing machinery component defects in astrocytic tumors. *Clin Cancer Res* 2005; **11**: 8304–8311.
156. Bodey B, Bodey B, Jr, Siegel SE, Kaiser HE. Fas (Apo-1, CD95) receptor expression in childhood astrocytomas. Is it a marker of the major apoptotic pathway or a signaling receptor for immune escape of neoplastic cells? *In Vivo* 1999; **13**: 357–373.
157. Chen TC, Hinton DR, Sippy BD, Hofman FM. Soluble TNF-alpha receptors are constitutively shed and downregulate adhesion molecule expression in malignant gliomas. *J Neuropathol Exp Neurol* 1997; **56**: 541–550.
158. Rahaman SO, Harbor PC, Chernova O, Barnett GH, Vogelbaum MA, Haque SJ. Inhibition of constitutively active Stat3 suppresses proliferation and induces apoptosis in glioblastoma multiforme cells. *Oncogene* 2002; **21**: 8404–8413.

159. Husain N, Chiocca EA, Rainov N, Louis DN, Zervas NT. Co-expression of Fas and Fas ligand in malignant glial tumors and cell lines. *Acta Neuropathol* 1998; **95**: 287–290.

160. Wiendl H, Mitsdoerffer M, Hofmeister V, Wischhusen J, Bornemann A, Meyermann R et al. A functional role of HLA-G expression in human gliomas: an alternative strategy of immune escape. *J Immunol* 2002; **168**: 4772–4780.

161. Gorelik L, Flavell RA. Abrogation of TGFbeta signaling in T cells leads to spontaneous T cell differentiation and autoimmune disease. *Immunity* 2000; **12**: 171–181.

162. Ranges GE, Figari IS, Espevik T, Palladino MA, Jr. Inhibition of cytotoxic T cell development by transforming growth factor beta and reversal by recombinant tumor necrosis factor alpha. *J Exp Med* 1987; **166**: 991–998.

163. Czarniecki CW, Chiu HH, Wong GH, McCabe SM, Palladino MA. Transforming growth factor-beta 1 modulates the expression of class II histocompatibility antigens on human cells. *J Immunol* 1988; **140**: 4217–4223.

164. Suzumura A, Sawada M, Yamamoto H, Marunouchi T. Transforming growth factor-beta suppresses activation and proliferation of microglia in vitro. *J Immunol* 1993; **151**: 2150–2158.

165. Smyth MJ, Strobl SL, Young HA, Ortaldo JR, Ochoa AC. Regulation of lymphokine-activated killer activity and pore-forming protein gene expression in human peripheral blood CD8 + T lymphocytes. Inhibition by transforming growth factor-beta. *J Immunol* 1991; **146**: 3289–3297.

166. Thomas DA, Massague J. TGF-beta directly targets cytotoxic T cell functions during tumor evasion of immune surveillance. *Cancer Cell* 2005; **8**: 369–380.

167. Hishii M, Nitta T, Ishida H, Ebato M, Kurosu A, Yagita H et al. Human glioma-derived interleukin-10 inhibits antitumor immune responses in vitro. *Neurosurgery* 1995; **37**: 1160–1166; discussion 1166–1167.

168. Grutz G. New insights into the molecular mechanism of interleukin-10-mediated immunosuppression. *J Leukoc Biol* 2005; **77**: 3–15.

169. Wang D, Dubois RN. Prostaglandins and cancer. *Gut* 2006; **55**: 115–122.

170. Takahashi T, Kuniyasu Y, Toda M, Sakaguchi N, Itoh M, Iwata M et al. Immunologic self-tolerance maintained by CD25 + CD4 + naturally anergic and suppressive T cells: induction of autoimmune disease by breaking their anergic/suppressive state. *Int Immunol* 1998; **10**: 1969–1980.

171. El Andaloussi A, Lesniak MS. An increase in CD4 + CD25 + FOXP3 + regulatory T cells in tumor-infiltrating lymphocytes of human glioblastoma multiforme. *Neuro Oncol* 2006; **8**: 234–243.

172. Fecci PE, Mitchell DA, Whitesides JF, Xie W, Friedman AH, Archer GE et al. Increased regulatory T-cell fraction amidst a diminished CD4 compartment explains cellular immune defects in patients with malignant glioma. *Cancer Res* 2006; **66**: 3294–3302.

173. El Andaloussi A, Lesniak MS. CD4 + CD25 + FoxP3 + T-cell infiltration and heme oxygenase-1 expression correlate with tumor grade in human gliomas. *J Neurooncol* 2007; **83**: 145–152.

174. Garcia de Palazzo IE, Adams GP, Sundareshan P, Wong AJ, Testa JR, Bigner DD et al. Expression of mutated epidermal growth factor receptor by non-small cell lung carcinomas. *Cancer Res* 1993; **53**: 3217–3220.

175. Moscatello DK, Holgado-Madruga M, Godwin AK, Ramirez G, Gunn G, Zoltick PW et al. Frequent expression of a mutant epidermal growth factor receptor in multiple human tumors. *Cancer Res* 1995; **55**: 5536–5539.

176. Wikstrand CJ, Hale LP, Batra SK, Hill ML, Humphrey PA, Kurpad SN et al. Monoclonal antibodies against EGFRvIII are tumor specific and react with breast and lung carcinomas and malignant gliomas. *Cancer Res* 1995; **55**: 3140–3148.

177. Ekstrand AJ, James CD, Cavenee WK, Seliger B, Pettersson RF, Collins VP. Genes for epidermal growth factor receptor, transforming growth factor alpha, and epidermal

growth factor and their expression in human gliomas in vivo. *Cancer Res* 1991; **51**: 2164–2172.

178. Heimberger AB, Hlatky R, Suki D, Yang D, Weinberg J, Gilbert M et al. Prognostic effect of epidermal growth factor receptor and EGFRvIII in glioblastoma multiforme patients. *Clin Cancer Res* 2005; **11**: 1462–1466.

179. Ciesielski MJ, Kazim AL, Barth RF, Fenstermaker RA. Cellular antitumor immune response to a branched lysine multiple antigenic peptide containing epitopes of a common tumor-specific antigen in a rat glioma model. *Cancer Immunol Immunother* 2005; **54**: 107–119.

180. Heimberger AB, Crotty LE, Archer GE, Hess KR, Wikstrand CJ, Friedman AH et al. Epidermal growth factor receptor VIII peptide vaccination is efficacious against established intracerebral tumors. *Clin Cancer Res* 2003; **9**: 4247–4254.

181. Moscatello DK, Ramirez G, Wong AJ. A naturally occurring mutant human epidermal growth factor receptor as a target for peptide vaccine immunotherapy of tumors. *Cancer Res* 1997; **57**: 1419–1424.

182. Sampson JH, Archer GE, Mitchell DA, Heimberger AB, Bigner DD. Tumor-specific immunotherapy targeting the EGFRvIII mutation in patients with malignant glioma. *Semin Immunol* 2008; **20**: 267–275.

183. Yajima N, Yamanaka R, Mine T, Tsuchiya N, Homma J, Sano M et al. Immunologic evaluation of personalized peptide vaccination for patients with advanced malignant glioma. *Clin Cancer Res* 2005; **11**: 5900–5911.

184. Barnett JA, Urbauer DL, Murray GI, Fuller GN, Heimberger AB. Cytochrome P450 1B1 expression in glial cell tumors: an immunotherapeutic target. *Clin Cancer Res* 2007; **13**: 3559–3567.

185. Komata T, Kanzawa T, Kondo Y, Kondo S. Telomerase as a therapeutic target for malignant gliomas. *Oncogene* 2002; **21**: 656–663.

186. Tsuda N, Nonaka Y, Shichijo S, Yamada A, Ito M, Maeda Y et al. UDP-Gal: betaGlc-NAc beta1, 3-galactosyltransferase, polypeptide 3 (GALT3) is a tumour antigen recognised by HLA-A2-restricted cytotoxic T lymphocytes from patients with brain tumour. *Br J Cancer* 2002; **87**: 1006–1012.

187. Yamada Y, Kuroiwa T, Nakagawa T, Kajimoto Y, Dohi T, Azuma H et al. Transcriptional expression of survivin and its splice variants in brain tumors in humans. *J Neurosurg* 2003; **99**: 738–745.

188. Ventimiglia JB, Wikstrand CJ, Ostrowski LE, Bourdon MA, Lightner VA, Bigner DD. Tenascin expression in human glioma cell lines and normal tissues. *J Neuroimmunol* 1992; **36**: 41–55.

189. Kurpad SN, Zhao XG, Wikstrand CJ, Batra SK, McLendon RE, Bigner DD. Tumor antigens in astrocytic gliomas. *Glia* 1995; **15**: 244–256.

190. Imaizumi T, Kuramoto T, Matsunaga K, Shichijo S, Yutani S, Shigemori M et al. Expression of the tumor-rejection antigen SART1 in brain tumors. *Int J Cancer* 1999; **83**: 760–764.

191. Zuber P, Kuppner MC, De Tribolet N. Transforming growth factor-beta 2 down-regulates HLA-DR antigen expression on human malignant glioma cells. *Eur J Immunol* 1988; **18**: 1623–1626.

192. Kehrl JH, Roberts AB, Wakefield LM, Jakowlew S, Sporn MB, Fauci AS. Transforming growth factor beta is an important immunomodulatory protein for human B lymphocytes. *J Immunol* 1986; **137**: 3855–3860.

193. Kehrl JH, Wakefield LM, Roberts AB, Jakowlew S, Alvarez-Mon M, Derynck R et al. Production of transforming growth factor beta by human T lymphocytes and its potential role in the regulation of T cell growth. *J Exp Med* 1986; **163**: 1037–1050.

194. Rook AH, Kehrl JH, Wakefield LM, Roberts AB, Sporn MB, Burlington DB et al. Effects of transforming growth factor beta on the functions of natural killer cells:

depressed cytolytic activity and blunting of interferon responsiveness. *J Immunol* 1986; **136**: 3916–3920.

195. Fakhrai H, Mantil JC, Liu L, Nicholson GL, Murphy-Satter CS, Ruppert J et al. Phase I clinical trial of a TGF-beta antisense-modified tumor cell vaccine in patients with advanced glioma. *Cancer Gene Ther* 2006; **13**: 1052–1060.

196. Hau P, Jachimczak P, Schlingensiepen R, Schulmeyer F, Jauch T, Steinbrecher A et al. Inhibition of TGF-beta2 with AP 12009 in recurrent malignant gliomas: from preclinical to phase I/II studies. *Oligonucleotides* 2007; **17**: 201–212.

197. El Andaloussi A, Han Y, Lesniak MS. Prolongation of survival following depletion of CD4 + CD25 + regulatory T cells in mice with experimental brain tumors. *J Neurosurg* 2006; **105**: 430–437.

198. Fecci PE, Sweeney AE, Grossi PM, Nair SK, Learn CA, Mitchell DA et al. Systemic anti-CD25 monoclonal antibody administration safely enhances immunity in murine glioma without eliminating regulatory T cells. *Clin Cancer Res* 2006; **12**: 4294–4305.

199. Fecci PE, Ochiai H, Mitchell DA, Grossi PM, Sweeney AE, Archer GE et al. Systemic CTLA-4 blockade ameliorates glioma-induced changes to the CD4 + T cell compartment without affecting regulatory T-cell function. *Clin Cancer Res* 2007; **13**: 2158–2167.

200. Jordan JT, Sun W, Hussain SF, DeAngulo G, Prabhu SS, Heimberger AB. Preferential migration of regulatory T cells mediated by glioma-secreted chemokines can be blocked with chemotherapy. *Cancer Immunol Immunother* 2008; **57**: 123–131.

201. Grauer OM, Sutmuller RP, van Maren W, Jacobs JF, Bennink E, Toonen LW et al. Elimination of regulatory T cells is essential for an effective vaccination with tumor lysate-pulsed dendritic cells in a murine glioma model. *Int J Cancer* 2008; **122**: 1794–1802.

202. Curtin JF, Candolfi M, Fakhouri TM, Liu C, Alden A, Edwards M et al. Treg depletion inhibits efficacy of cancer immunotherapy: implications for clinical trials. *PLoS ONE* 2008; **3**: e1983.

203. Mitchell DA. REGULATory T-Cell Inhibition With Daclizumab (Zenapax®) During Recovery From Therapeutic Temozolomide-Induced Lymphopenia During Antitumor Immunotherapy Targeted Against Cytomegalovirus in Patients With Newly-Diagnosed Glioblastoma Multiforme [REGULATe], 2008. URL: http://clinicaltrials.gov/ct/show/NCT00626483.

204. De Vleeschouwer S, Fieuws S, Rutkowski S, Van Calenbergh F, Van Loon J, Goffin J et al. Postoperative adjuvant dendritic cell-based immunotherapy in patients with relapsed glioblastoma multiforme. *Clin Cancer Res* 2008; **14**: 3098–3104.

205. Lasky, J. Phase I Dose Escalation Study of Autologous Tumor Lysate-Pulsed Dendritic Cell Immunotherapy for Malignant Gliomas in Pediatric Patients, 2005.

206. Liau LM. Phase I Dose Escalation Study of Autologous Tumor Lysate-Pulsed Dendritic Cell Immunotherapy for Malignant Gliomas. National Library of Medicine, 2003.

207. Yu JS. Phase II Trial of Tumor Lysate-Pulsed Dendritic Cell Immunotherapy for Patients With Atypical or Malignant, Primary or Metastatic Brain Tumors of the Central Nervous System, 2001.

208. Fadul C. DMS-0536: A Phase II Feasibility Study of Adjuvant Intra-Nodal Autologous Dendritic Cell Vaccination for Newly Diagnosed Glioblastoma Multiforme, 2006.

209. Ferstenberg L. A Phase II Clinical Trial Evaluating DCVax®-Brain, Autologous Dendritic Cells Pulsed With Tumor Lysate Antigen For The Treatment Of Glioblastoma Multiforme (GBM), 2002.

210. Witham TF, Erff ML, Okada H, Chambers WH, Pollack IF. 7-Hydroxystaurosporine-induced apoptosis in 9L glioma cells provides an effective antigen source for dendritic cells and yields a potent vaccine strategy in an intracranial glioma model. *Neurosurgery* 2002; **50**: 1327–1334; discussion 1334–1325.

211. Kobayashi T, Yamanaka R, Homma J, Tsuchiya N, Yajima N, Yoshida S et al. Tumor mRNA-loaded dendritic cells elicit tumor-specific CD8(+) cytotoxic T cells in patients with malignant glioma. *Cancer Immunol Immunother* 2003; **52**: 632–637.

212. Amano T, Kajiwara K, Yoshikawa K, Morioka J, Nomura S, Fujisawa H et al. Antitumor effects of vaccination with dendritic cells transfected with modified receptor for hyaluronan-mediated motility mRNA in a mouse glioma model. *J Neurosurg* 2007; **106**: 638–645.

213. Yoshida S, Tanaka R. Generation of a human leukocyte antigen-A24-restricted antitumor cell with the use of SART-1 peptide and dendritic cells in patients with malignant brain tumors. *J Lab Clin Med* 2004; **144**: 201–207.

214. Zhang JG, Eguchi J, Kruse CA, Gomez GG, Fakhrai H, Schroter S et al. Antigenic profiling of glioma cells to generate allogeneic vaccines or dendritic cell-based therapeutics. *Clin Cancer Res* 2007; **13**: 566–575.

215. Parajuli P, Mathupala S, Sloan AE. Systematic comparison of dendritic cell-based immunotherapeutic strategies for malignant gliomas: in vitro induction of cytolytic and natural killer-like T cells. *Neurosurgery* 2004; **55**: 1194–1204.

216. Rosenberg SA. Immunotherapy of cancer by systemic administration of lymphoid cells plus interleukin-2. *J Biol Response Mod* 1984; **3**: 501–511.

217. Rayner AA, Grimm EA, Lotze MT, Chu EW, Rosenberg SA. Lymphokine-activated killer (LAK) cells. Analysis of factors relevant to the immunotherapy of human cancer. *Cancer* 1985; **55**: 1327–1333.

218. Barba D, Saris SC, Holder C, Rosenberg SA, Oldfield EH. Intratumoral LAK cell and interleukin-2 therapy of human gliomas. *J Neurosurg* 1989; **70**: 175–182.

219. Blancher A, Roubinet F, Grancher AS, Tremoulet M, Bonate A, Delisle MB et al. Local immunotherapy of recurrent glioblastoma multiforme by intracerebral perfusion of interleukin-2 and LAK cells. *Eur Cytokine Netw* 1993; **4**: 331–341.

220. Boiardi A, Silvani A, Ruffini PA, Rivoltini L, Parmiani G, Broggi G et al. Loco-regional immunotherapy with recombinant interleukin-2 and adherent lymphokine-activated killer cells (A-LAK) in recurrent glioblastoma patients. *Cancer Immunol Immunother* 1994; **39**: 193–197.

221. Jacobs SK, Wilson DJ, Kornblith PL, Grimm EA. Interleukin-2 or autologous lymphokine-activated killer cell treatment of malignant glioma: phase I trial. *Cancer Res* 1986; **46**: 2101–2104.

222. Merchant RE, Grant AJ, Merchant LH, Young HF. Adoptive immunotherapy for recurrent glioblastoma multiforme using lymphokine activated killer cells and recombinant interleukin-2. *Cancer* 1988; **62**: 665–671.

223. Sankhla SK, Nadkarni JS, Bhagwati SN. Adoptive immunotherapy using lymphokine-activated killer (LAK) cells and interleukin-2 for recurrent malignant primary brain tumors. *J Neurooncol* 1996; **27**: 133–140.

224. Hayes RL, Koslow M, Hiesiger EM, Hymes KB, Hochster HS, Moore EJ et al. Improved long term survival after intracavitary interleukin-2 and lymphokine-activated killer cells for adults with recurrent malignant glioma. *Cancer* 1995; **76**: 840–852.

225. Hayes RL, Arbit E, Odaimi M, Pannullo S, Scheff R, Kravchinskiy D et al. Adoptive cellular immunotherapy for the treatment of malignant gliomas. *Crit Rev Oncol Hematol* 2001; **39**: 31–42.

226. Dillman RO, Duma CM, Schiltz PM, DePriest C, Ellis RA, Okamoto K et al. Intracavitary placement of autologous lymphokine-activated killer (LAK) cells after resection of recurrent glioblastoma. *J Immunother* 2004; **27**: 398–404.

227. Sipos L, Afra D. Re-operations of supratentorial anaplastic astrocytomas. *Acta Neurochir (Wien)* 1997; **139**: 99–104.

228. Salcman M, Scholtz H, Kaplan RS, Kulik S. Long-term survival in patients with malignant astrocytoma. *Neurosurgery* 1994; **34**: 213–219; discussion 219–220.

229. Tsurushima H, Liu SQ, Tsuboi K, Yoshii Y, Nose T, Ohno T. Induction of human autologous cytotoxic T lymphocytes against minced tissues of glioblastoma multiforme. *J Neurosurg* 1996; **84**: 258–263.

230. Quattrocchi KB, Miller CH, Cush S, Bernard SA, Dull ST, Smith M et al. Pilot study of local autologous tumor infiltrating lymphocytes for the treatment of recurrent malignant gliomas. *J Neurooncol* 1999; **45**: 141–157.

231. Miescher S, Whiteside TL, de Tribolet N, von Fliedner V. In situ characterization, clonogenic potential, and antitumor cytolytic activity of T lymphocytes infiltrating human brain cancers. *J Neurosurg* 1988; **68**: 438–448.

232. Elliott LH, Brooks WH, Roszman TL. Cytokinetic basis for the impaired activation of lymphocytes from patients with primary intracranial tumors. *J Immunol* 1984; **132**: 1208–1215.

233. Elliott LH, Brooks WH, Roszman TL. Inability of mitogen-activated lymphocytes obtained from patients with malignant primary intracranial tumors to express high affinity interleukin 2 receptors. *J Clin Invest* 1990; **86**: 80–86.

234. Chang AE, Yoshizawa H, Sakai K, Cameron MJ, Sondak VK, Shu S. Clinical observations on adoptive immunotherapy with vaccine-primed T-lymphocytes secondarily sensitized to tumor in vitro. *Cancer Res* 1993; **53**: 1043–1050.

235. Holladay FP, Heitz T, Chen YL, Chiga M, Wood GW. Successful treatment of a malignant rat glioma with cytotoxic T lymphocytes. *Neurosurgery* 1992; **31**: 528–533.

236. Kitahara T, Watanabe O, Yamaura A, Makino H, Watanabe T, Suzuki G et al. Establishment of interleukin 2 dependent cytotoxic T lymphocyte cell line specific for autologous brain tumor and its intracranial administration for therapy of the tumor. *J Neurooncol* 1987; **4**: 329–336.

237. Wood GW, Holladay FP, Turner T, Wang YY, Chiga M. A pilot study of autologous cancer cell vaccination and cellular immunotherapy using anti-CD3 stimulated lymphocytes in patients with recurrent grade III/IV astrocytoma. *J Neurooncol* 2000; **48**: 113–120.

238. Plautz GE, Barnett GH, Miller DW, Cohen BH, Prayson RA, Krauss JC et al. Systemic T cell adoptive immunotherapy of malignant gliomas. *J Neurosurg* 1998; **89**: 42–51.

239. Plautz GE, Miller DW, Barnett GH, Stevens GH, Maffett S, Kim J et al. T cell adoptive immunotherapy of newly diagnosed gliomas. *Clin Cancer Res* 2000; **6**: 2209–2218.

240. Kronik N, Kogan Y, Vainstein V, Agur Z. Improving alloreactive CTL immunotherapy for malignant gliomas using a simulation model of their interactive dynamics. *Cancer Immunol Immunother* 2008; **57**: 425–439.

241. Kruse CA, Cepeda L, Owens B, Johnson SD, Stears J, Lillehei KO. Treatment of recurrent glioma with intracavitary alloreactive cytotoxic T lymphocytes and interleukin-2. *Cancer Immunol Immunother* 1997; **45**: 77–87.

242. Wheeler CJ, Black KL, Liu G, Ying H, Yu JS, Zhang W et al. Thymic CD8+ T cell production strongly influences tumor antigen recognition and age-dependent glioma mortality. *J Immunol* 2003; **171**: 4927–4933.

243. Miller G. Drug targeting. Breaking down barriers. *Science* 2002; **297**: 1116–1118.

The Complexity of the HIF-1-Dependent Hypoxic Response in Breast Cancer Presents Multiple Avenues for Therapeutic Intervention

Tiffany N. Seagroves

Abstract A critical aspect of tumor physiology is the sensation of oxygen in the microenvironment. The oxygen-responsive Hypoxia-Inducible Factor (HIF)-1α protein is a master transcriptional regulator of the hypoxic response, controlling expression of a variety of genes related to metabolism, glucose transport, cell cycle progression, cell migration, multidrug resistance, and angiogenesis. Several studies have demonstrated that over-expression HIF-1α protein in breast cancer correlates with poor prognosis, increased risk of metastasis and decreased survival. Moreover, hypoxic regions of tumors are believed to be the source of tumor cells that are resistant to radiation and chemotherapy. More recently, it has also been proposed that hypoxia stimulates expansion of normal and cancer stem cells. Despite a complete understanding of how HIF-1α impacts breast cancer progression and metastasis, the HIF-1α pathway is ideal for targeting drug design since interfering with a master regulator of the hypoxic response could disrupt multiple downstream processes essential to tumor cell self-renewal, expansion, dissemination, and metastatic colonization.

1 Introduction to the HIF-1α Pathway and Its Relevance to Breast Cancer

1.1 Relevance of Hypoxia to Tumorigenesis

In response to hypoxia, or low oxygen levels, cells try to restore homeostasis through regulation of cellular metabolism, erythropoiesis, angiogenesis, and balancing decisions between survival and cell death [1]. As part of adaptation to their local microenvironment, most solid tumors have bypassed the normal cellular controls that regulate these processes [2]. The hypoxia-inducible factor (HIF)-1α transcription factor is a master regulator of the hypoxic response in

T.N. Seagroves (✉)
Center for Cancer Research, Department of Pathology and Laboratory Medicine,
University of Tennessee Health Science Center, Memphis, TN 38163, USA
e-mail: tseagro1@utmem.edu

Y. Lu, R.I. Mahato (eds.), *Pharmaceutical Perspectives of Cancer Therapeutics*,
DOI 10.1007/978-1-4419-0131-6_16, © Springer Science+Business Media, LLC 2009

multiple cell types, directly and indirectly controlling activation and repression of hundreds of genes [3–5]. Zhong et al. first reported in 1999 that HIF-1α protein, detected by immunohistochemistry, was over-expressed in the majority of solid tumors that had originated in multiple tissue types (13/19 tissues), including the breast. In fact, HIF-1α was over-expressed in 29% of primary late-stage breast carcinomas and perhaps more significantly, 69% of metastases from the breast [6]. As expected, HIF-1α protein was also detected in layers of cells immediately surrounding necrotic areas of tumors, however, no expression was detectable within "normal" breast tissue adjacent to tumors [6].

A study of breast cancers by Bos et al. followed in 2001, in which high levels of HIF-1α immunostaining were found to be positively correlated with other clinical prognostic factors including high proliferation rates, increased tumor grade, and positive staining for human epidermal growth factor receptor 2 (HER2)/Neu [7], also known as ERBB2. In this study, a majority of well-differentiated (11/20) and poorly differentiated (17/20) ductal carcinoma in situ (DCIS) samples over-expressed HIF-1α, whereas over-expression was noted in all (20/20) tumors classified as poorly differentiated invasive carcinomas [7]. Moreover, several clinical studies have demonstrated that over-expression of HIF-1α in breast cancer patients correlates with aggressiveness, and ultimately, poor prognosis and decreased survival [8–11]. In fact, in a large retrospective study on patients who had surgery from 1986 to 1995 without chemotherapy or hormone therapy prior to surgery, *HIF-1α* expression *independently* correlated with high risk of metastasis and with an increased chance of relapse [12].

Hypoxia also impacts the clinical response to therapy. Hypoxic regions of tumors in which HIF-1α is abundant are resistant to therapeutic interventions, including ionizing radiation and a variety of chemotherapeutics, as reviewed in [13, 14]. Moreover, hypoxic induction of HIF-1α is a potent mechanism to down-regulate ERα protein in breast cancer cells [15], suggesting that chronic hypoxia may contribute to tamoxifen resistance in breast cancer as only ER+ patients respond to tamoxifen therapy. Finally, it has also been proposed that hypoxia stimulates renewal and expansion of normal and cancer stem cells (CSCs) [16]. This concept is highly relevant to breast cancer patients since studies have demonstrated that the population of breast tumor cells that have the ability to self-renew are enriched with the ability to initiate tumorigenesis in vivo [17–21]. Moreover, breast cancer cells that exhibit properties of CSCs are the most resistant to therapeutic intervention, including radiation and DNA damaging drugs [20, 22, 23]. These topics will be discussed in further detail later in this chapter.

According to American Cancer Society, the 5-year survival rate drops from 98% for women who are diagnosed with localized breast tumors to 80% for women with regional metastasis and 26% for women with distant metastases [24]. Therefore, understanding the contribution of the hypoxic response to breast cancer is of critical significance not only for designing treatment for primary tumors that contain hypoxic regions resistant to intervention but also for preventing metastasis since HIF-1α may control a metastatic switch. Despite a complete understanding of how HIF-1α impacts breast epithelial cell tumorigenesis and metastasis, the HIF-1α pathway is ideal for targeted drug design since interfering with a master regulator of the hypoxic response could disrupt multiple downstream processes essential to tumor cell expansion and dissemination.

1.2 Overview of the HIF-1 Pathway

HIF-1α is the oxygen-responsive partner of the HIF-1 heterodimer, which functions as a transcription factor, and binds to the hypoxic response elements (HREs) in target gene promoters; the HRE consensus site is 5′-RCGTG-3′ [25]. There are also two other HIF-α isoforms in mammals, HIF-2α and HIF-3α, which bind to the same HRE consensus. HIF-1 controls transcription of multiple gene families including glycolytic metabolism, glucose transport, cell cycle progression, growth factors, cell migration and adhesion, multidrug resistance, and angiogenesis [4, 5]. As shown in Fig. 1, HIF-1α levels are regulated primarily at the post-translational level via proteosome-dependent protein stability. Hypoxic exposure induces and stabilizes HIF-1α protein accumulation, although the oxygen tensions at which HIF-1α is stabilized are tissue-type dependent [26]. More importantly, up to 50% of locally advanced breast cancers exhibit heterogenous regions of hypoxia that correspond to 0.1–1% O_2 [27], which is in the range of oxygen exposure commonly used to model tissue hypoxia in vitro. In contrast, HIF-1α's partner, the aryl hydrocarbon receptor nuclear translocator (ARNT) protein (or HIF-1β), is expressed constitutively and can heterodimerize with multiple other bHLH partners [25].

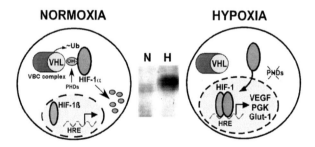

Fig. 1 Oxygen-dependent stabilization of HIF-1α. (Left) At 21% O_2, HIF prolyl hydroxylase domain (PHD) enzymes hydroxylate HIF-1α on two key proline resides, permitting physical interaction with the von Hippel-Lindau (VHL) tumor suppressor protein, which in conjunction with a Cullin2/Skp1/Elongin-B/C (VBC) complex, functions as a E3 ubiquitin ligase, leading to rapid HIF-1α proteolytic degradation. **(Right)** Under hypoxic stress, PHD activity is reduced, HIF-1α is stabilized and partners with ARNT (orange oval) to form the HIF-1 heterodimer, which binds HREs within target gene promoters. Classic direct target genes include vascular endothelial growth factor (*VEGF*), glucose transporter-1 (*SLC2A1*), and phosphoglycerate kinase-1 (*PGK1*). **(Center)** Western blot: Strong hypoxic induction of HIF-1α protein in primary mammary murine epithelial cells cultured overnight at 0.5% O_2

The basic helix-loop-helix (bHLH) and Per-Arnt-Sim (PAS) domains of HIF-1α, which mediate DNA-binding and HIF-1β interactions, respectively, are located at the N-terminus, whereas the C-terminal half of HIF-1α contains three important domains: the oxygen-dependent degradation (ODD) domain, a nuclear translocation signal, and two transactivation domains (N-terminal, N-TAD and C-terminal, C-TAD). The ODD domain is comprised of the region that binds to the tumor suppressor protein von Hippel-Lindau (VHL) as well as the N-TAD. The ODD contains two key proline residues (Pro^{402} and Pro^{564}) that are hydroxylated by a family of HIF prolyl hydroxylase domain (PHD) enzymes, PHD 1-3 [2]. Activity of the PHDs depends on the presence of oxygen, iron, and 2-oxoglutarate as co-factors [28]. The consequence of PDH-mediated hydroxylation is rapid, 26S proteosome-dependent degradation of HIF-1α, reliant upon its interaction with VHL, which is part of a larger Cullin2/EloginB/C protein complex (VBC) that functions as an E3 ubiquitin ligase. The necessity for tight control of the HIFα subunits' stability via VHL is clear from observation of tumors that develop in patients with VHL disease, which are characterized by high levels of expression of the HIFα subunits, and downstream HIF target genes, as reviewed in [29]. In addition, it has been shown that breast cancer cells that express lower VHL levels have higher levels of HIF-1α, as would be expected [30]. More recently, a novel E3 ubiquitin ligase, hypoxia-associated factor (HAF), has been reported to target HIF-1α, but not HIF-2α, for proteolytic degradation independent of oxygen tension[31]. Over-expression of HAF led to decreased HIF-1α expression and decreased tumor growth. HIF-1α is also hydroxylated on Asn^{803} in the C-TAD by the asparaginyl hydroxylase, factor inhibiting HIF-1 (or FIH-1). FIH-1-mediated hydroxylation inhibits the recruitment of the transcriptional co-activator p300/CBP to HIF-1α, thereby inhibiting downstream gene transcription [32]. In sum, in response to hypoxia, there is a dramatic increase in HIF-1α protein expression, as well as enhancement of its transcriptional activity.

The potential redundancy in transcriptional regulation between HIF-1α and HIF-2α is an area of intense investigation. Although HIF-1α and HIF-2α are closely related proteins, they have been shown to regulate different target gene sets depending on the cell type and microenvironment context [33–39]. Although HIF-2α was originally reported to be highly enriched in the vasculature, is also expressed in multiple other tissues [40], and it has been shown to have an essential role in promoting renal clear cell carcinoma[41]. HIF-3α lacks critical TADs conserved in HIF-1α and HIF-2α, and therefore may act as a dominant-negative inhibitor [42].

In addition to HIF-1α, breast cancer cells also express HIF-2α. However, in a study of a panel of breast cancer cell lines, HIF-2α expression was low to undetectable, suggesting that HIF-1α is the primary regulator of the hypoxic response in the breast [43]. This was later confirmed using siRNAs to either *HIF-1α* or *HIF-2α* and analyzing mRNA expression of key HIFα target genes [36]. However, a recent study that characterized expression of HIF-1α and HIF-2α immunostaining in breast cancers identified HIF-2α as the predominant HIFα subunit that independently predicted survival [44]. Therefore, there is still controversy regarding whether HIF-1α or HIF-2α is the predominant player in predicting breast cancer survival, although it is clear that the HIF-dependent hypoxic response pathway is a key mediator of breast cancer pathology. Furthermore, a large-scale microarray profiling screen has recently identified a 123-gene "hypoxic signature" that functions as an independent predictor of prognosis and survival in breast cancer patients, which exhibited more predictive power than the previously described "wound" signature in breast cancer [3].

1.3 Use of Mouse Models to Understand HIF-1 Function

1.3.1 Conditional Knockout of HIF-1α During Normal Mammary Gland Development

Due to embryonic lethality associated with global knockout of *HIF-1α* [45], the use of genetic mouse models to understand HIF-1α function in various tissues and cell types has focused on the Cre/*loxP* conditional gene deletion strategy [46], as reviewed in [47]. Deletion of both *HIF-1α* "*floxed*" (flanked by *loxP*) alleles [48] in the mammary epithelium is accomplished using transgenic mice that express Cre recombinase under control of the long terminal repeat (LTR) of the MTMV promoter [49, 50]. Using this approach, it was demonstrated that HIF-1α expression is critical for differentiation, but not proliferation, of the mammary gland during pregnancy and for milk production and secretion at lactation [51]. The first stage at which the glands lacking *HIF-1α* in the differed by histology was at day 15 of pregnancy (15-P). This time point represents a period of mammary gland development that is well into the period termed "secretory differentiation," which is characterized by expression of milk protein genes, such as β-casein and α-lactalbumin, markers of the casein, and whey fractions of milk, respectively [52]. In addition, by 15-P there was accumulation of large cytoplasmic lipid droplets (CLDs) and proteinaceous material within the wild-type alveoli, whereas the HIF-1α null alveoli did not exhibit any evidence of differentiation and remained "collapsed," and devoid of CLDs. mRNA expression of two markers associated with the milk lipid globule, xanthine oxioreductase (*Xor*) and adipophilin (*Adph*), was also reduced by over 50% in response to *HIF-1α* deletion [51]. These phenotypes, evidence of a failure to differentiate, were maintained through the remainder of pregnancy, as shown in Fig. 2.

Regulation of these markers by HIF-1α is of interest since *ADPH* mRNA expression is directly regulated by HIF-1α in MCF-7 cells [53] and deletion of a single copy of *Xor* gene recapitulates the phenotype observed in HIF-1α null-lactating glands [54]. Moreover, expression of ADPH appears to be required to form CLDs [55]. Therefore, HIF-1α is essential for differentiation of the mammary gland in preparation for lactation by regulating cellular metabolism. Moreover, the results from these studies suggest that although HIF-1α is not detectable by immunostaining of the normal human breast, low levels of HIF-1α present in normal murine breast tissue are necessary to regulate breast

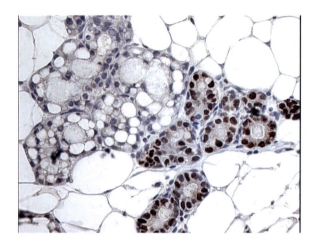

Fig. 2 Heterogenous expression of Cre recombinase in the MMTV-Cre (line A) transgenic mouse during pregnancy. Mammary tissue harvested from a HIF "double-*floxed*" (DF); MMTV-Cre transgenic mouse at day 18 of pregnancy was immunostained with a polyclonal antibody to Cre recombinase (Novagen) (brown, nuclear stain) and counterstained with hematoxylin (200× magnification). The Cre-negative alveoli exhibited evidence of milk precursor production, such as CLDs, whereas the Cre-positive staining alveoli did not, as in [51]

physiology. Therefore, it must be considered that inhibitors of the HIF pathway may have adverse effects in the normal breast or in tissue adjacent to tumors.

1.3.2 Conditional Knockout of HIF-1α in a Mouse Model of Breast Cancer Reveals that HIF-1α Is a Key Mediator of Metastasis

There are a variety of well-characterized transgenic mice that reproducibly develop mammary tumors; in these models, an oncogene, such as *ras, polyoma middle T* (PyMT), *Neu* (the rat homologue of *HER2/ERBB2*), or *c-Myc* is expressed under control of the MMTV minimal promoter. Overall, these models mimic the pathology observed in human breast cancers [56, 57], and more importantly, they have a subset of the same molecular lesions to those found in breast cancer patients [58, 59]. The Neu and Myc transgenic models also mimic human cancer in several ways: (1) *MYC* and *ERBB2* are amplified in 17 and 30% of human breast cancer patients, respectively [60], and (2) the tumors exhibit stages of progression in vivo and have a pathology similar to human DCIS and lobular carcinoma [61, 62].

Recently we crossed the MMTV-Cre *HIF-1α floxed* conditional deletion model to the MMTV-PyMT transgenic mouse. This model was chosen since tumors produced by the MMTV-PyMT model have been shown to faithfully mimic the pathology of breast cancers [63], and more recently, the luminal subtype of breast cancer [64]. In addition, all nulliparous PyMT transgenic females develop mammary tumors with a high incidence of lung metastases[63] within 3 months, in contrast to the MMTV-Myc and MMTV-Neu models, which must be bred to exhibit mammary tumors within 4–6 months of age. As shown by the staining for the tissue hypoxia marker hypoxyprobe-1 in Fig. 3, there are large waves of intratumor hypoxia present in murine mammary tumors, as has been documented in breast cancer patients in which oxygen tension was directly measured using an electrode [27].

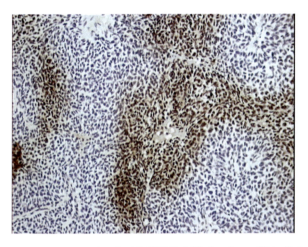

Fig. 3 Mammary tumors originating in MMTV-PyMT females exhibit distinct regions of hypoxia. Two hours prior to sacrifice, a PyMT+ female transgenic mouse bearing a late-stage mammary carcinoma was injected i.p. with hypoxyprobe-1 (NPI, Inc.), which binds to DNA and protein adducts created by hypoxic exposure[228]. Tumor sections were probed with anti-hypoxyprobe-1 antibodies (brown staining) and counterstained with hematoxylin (200× magnification)

We found that deletion of *HIF-1α* in tumor cells expressing the MMTV-PyMT oncogene delayed the time to palpable tumor onset and decreased cellular proliferation and tumor microvessel density during early carcinoma stages at 10 weeks of age. However, tumor wet weight and volume were equivalent at study end point in late-stage carcinomas at 14 weeks of age. Perhaps the most striking effect was that deletion of *HIF-1α* significantly prolonged survival, likely due to dramatically reduced size and number of metastases to the lung [65] as shown in Fig. 4.

1.3.3 Limitations of Animal Models

Although gene deletion models have been useful to confirm that *HIF-1α* is a critical regulator of breast cancer growth and metastasis, these animal models do not mimic what is actually observed in the clinic, which is over-expression of HIF-1α. Generation of novel transgenic mouse models in which HIF-1α is

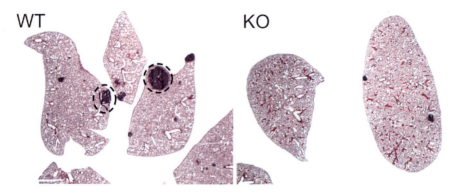

Fig. 4 Conditional deletion of *HIF-1α in MMTV-PyMT mammary tumors reduces the number of lung metastases, particularly macromets*. Lungs were harvested from MMTV-PyMT transgenic females bearing late-stage mammary carcinomas by inflating with 10% formalin followed by fixation and paraffin embedding. Sections were prepared at every 100 microns through the lung and then stained with H&E to reveal metastatic lesions, as in[65]. The presence of macrometastases (*dashed circle*) visible to the naked eye prior to sectioning the lung were only observed in mice bearing *HIF-1α* wild-type tumors

over-expressed in the MECs would be a useful resource to address this deficiency. Alternatively, stable over-expression of HIF-1α could also be achieved through viral transduction of normal or breast cancer cell lines and transplantation of these cells into the cleared mammary fat pad. Furthermore, the molecular analysis of HIF-1α function in breast epithelium has largely been performed in immortalized human breast cancer cell lines cultured in vitro in monolayer on plastic and/or in xenografted immunocompromised mouse models that lack an intact immune response, thereby eliminating the critical influence of the local tissue microenvironment on evaluating the hypoxic response. The mechanisms by which HIF-1α impacts breast cancer growth, aggressiveness, and therapeutic response are highly complex and likely involve multiple interacting pathways that are microenvironment and cell type-context specific. Moreover, the specific contribution of HIF-1α in the breast tumor epithelial cells versus myoepithelial cells versus stromal cells (including endothelial cells) versus recruited immune cells, such as tumor-associated macrophages, remains undefined, although the tissue-specific Cre transgenic mouse models reagents to execute these studies are available [47].

1.4 Oxygen-Independent, Growth Factor Receptor Tyrosine Kinase Regulation of HIF-1: A Key Role for the EGFR Family?

Although hypoxia rapidly stabilizes HIF-1α protein, oxygen-independent mechanisms have also been demonstrated to increase/stabilize HIF-1α protein expression, as reviewed in [66]. For example, HIF-1α stability can be induced by oncogene activation through Src and Ras, or via activation of a variety of growth factor tyrosine kinase receptors (RTKs), resulting in increased protein synthesis of HIF-1α. This regulation is independent of oxygen or HIF-1α's interactions with VHL [66]. For example, in PC3 prostate cancer cells treated with insulin, IGF-I, IGF-II, or platelet-derived growth factor (PDGF) [67], HIF-1α was stabilized via either the mitogen-activated protein kinase (MAPK) or phosphatidylinositol 3-kinase (PI3K)/Akt/mammalian target of rapamycin (mTOR) signaling pathways [4]. In MCF-7 cells, over-expression of the HER2 tyrosine kinase receptor or treatment with the ligand heregulin (which binds ERBB3/ERBB4 receptors) was reported to stimulate HIF-1α protein synthesis in a PI3K-dependent manner [68]. Supporting the relevance of these in vitro observations, studies in a mouse model of hepatocellular carcinoma model have shown that the *hypoxia-independent* over-expression of HIF-1α is an early event in cancer progression, occurring at the hyperplasia stage prior to development of decreased oxygen tensions [69]. Therefore, regulation of HIF-1α expression is not restricted to cells undergoing hypoxic stress, thereby adding an additional layer of complexity to the role of the hypoxic response in cancer.

It is also becoming increasingly clear that there are strong interactions between the members of the EGFR family (EGFR/ERBB1, ERBB2, ERBB3, ERRB4) of RTKs and HIF-1α in tumor cells. These relationships are highly relevant to breast cancer since over-expression of EGFR and HER2 is commonly observed in patients [70]. Constitutive activation of RTKs in breast cancers would likely synergize with tumor hypoxia to further increase HIF-1α stability/expression. For example, in a panel of breast cancer cell lines cultured in the presence of EGF, the levels of HIF-1α protein expressed at normoxia were increased, and HIF-1α synergized with EGFR to regulate survivin expression through the Akt pathway [71]. More recent studies have demonstrated that EGFR expression, independent of its kinase activity, is critical for tumor cell survival. Even a kinase dead EGFR construct prevented tumor cell autophagy through stabilization of the Na+/ glucose co-transporter 1 SGLT1[72], which facilitated tumor cell survival in low glucose conditions, and is a hypoxia-inducible transcriptional target gene [73]. Moreover, it has been shown that the EGFR tyrosine kinase inhibitor (TKI) gefitinib (Iressa) decreased HIF-1α protein expression in head and neck squamous cell carcinomas through decreased translation mediated through the PI3K/ Akt pathway [74]. High levels of HIF-1α expression in A431 squamous vulvar carcinoma cells have also been shown to contribute to resistance to both gefitinib and the EGFR-blocking antibody cetuximab (C225) [75]. Finally, activation of the EGFR by the ligand-transforming growth factor (TGF)α, which is upregulated in VHL null renal clear cell carcinomas, stimulates RCC proliferation, whereas this was blocked with treatment with the EGFR inhibitor PD153035 [76]. Together, these observations suggest that combining therapies to block the EGFR and HIF pathways would synergize to kill tumor cells, a strategy that has been previously recommended in an excellent review of HIF-1 inhibitors as anticancer agents [77].

1.5 HIF-1α and Angiogenesis

Hypoxia resulting from limited diffusion of oxygen from distant or local, but immature, blood vessels is a common feature of solid tumors. Hypoxia is a well-characterized inducer of tumor neo-angiogenesis and VEGF-regulated blood vessel growth, as reviewed in [78]. However, tumor vasculature is distinctly different that normal vasculature, often forming a poorly organized vascular network consisting of primarily immature, tortuous vessels that are leaky, collapsed, or have arterial to venous shunts, creating areas of hypoxic stress, as reviewed in [14]. Ultimately, compromised vessel function and tissue hypoxia leads to resistance to both ionizing radiation and chemotherapy [1].

1.5.1 VEGF Therapies and Intratumor Hypoxia

The connection between the hypoxic response and the angiogenic switch is also clear from pathology of tumors arising in patients with VHL disease; these tumors are characterized by hypervascularity and extremely elevated levels of VEGF expression [79]. VEGF has been shown in animal models of pancreatic cancer to be a key mediator of the angiogenic switch [80]. The demonstrated critical role for VEGF in regulation of tumor neo-angiogenesis and vascular function in a variety of tumor types led the push in the 1990s to develop anti-VEGF blocking anti-bodies, such as Avastin (bevacizumab), which are currently being used as adjuvant therapies in metastatic breast cancer [81]. One drawback of anti-angiogenesis therapy has been the reported rapid re-growth of the vasculature following drug withdrawal. Studies in animal models have postulated that this is perhaps due to tracks of basement membrane and pericytes that remain upon destruction of immature endothelial cells, since new vessels developed rapidly along these "tracks" upon withdrawal of anti-VEGF therapy [82, 83]. Vessel "normalization" as a means to improve therapeutic response has also become a hot topic [84]. It has been observed that use of VEGF blocking antibodies in conjunction with chemotherapy increases the clinical response and reduces intratumor hypoxia, as reviewed in [85], possibly through pruning immature vessels, allowing better tumor perfusion by the more organized, mature vessels.

1.5.2 Relevance of Angiogenesis to Breast Cancer

Several studies have noted correlations between high microvessel density (MVD) and poor prognosis in breast cancer patients [86–89]. More specifically, HIF-1α over-expression in breast cancer has been associated with increased MVD, increased expression of pro-angiogenic factors, including VEGF and basic fibro-blast growth factor (bFGF), and ultimately, poor prognosis [90]. Interestingly, the dual EGFR/VEGFR family kinase inhibitor AEE788 when combined with ionizing radiation was effective in improving tumor oxygenation by reducing intratumor hypoxia and reducing expression of the classic HIF-1α target gene, glucose transporter-1 (Glut-1) in tumors derived from the MMTV-Neu (murine HER2 homologue) transgenic model of breast cancer [91].

1.5.3 Role of HIF-1α in Angiogenesis Is Microenvironment-Context Specific

In teratocarcinomas derived from global *HIF-1α* null embryonic stem (ES) cells, tumor vascularization was dramatically decreased [45, 92]. This finding was in contrast to data generated in fibrosarcomas in which *HIF-1α* had been conditionally deleted; these tumors exhibited a relatively small decrease in MVD in spite of consistently reduced tumor mass [48]. In PyMT-derived mammary tumors, deletion of *HIF-1α* resulted in a decrease in MVD within early-stage carcinomas, but no difference in MVD was noted in late-stage carcinomas at the study end point [65]. Finally, deletion of *HIF-1α* in the normal mammary epithelium had neither an effect upon *Vegf* mRNA production at 15-P nor resulted in changes in MVD or gross vessel branching by the end of pregnancy prior to parturition [51]. Although mice conditionally deleted for *Vegf* in the mammary epithelium were reported to also exhibit lactation defects similar to the conditional *HIF-1α* model [93], it is possible that in the normal tissue setting, other factors besides HIF-1α can substitute for regulation of VEGF activity, including estrogen and progesterone, whereas HIF-1α may be required for neo-angiogenesis in breast cancers. Together, these data indicate that the pro-angiogenic effect of HIF-1α is highly sensitive to context-specific differences in the microenvironment.

1.6 HIF-1α and Tumor Metabolism

As tumors enlarge, they exhibit changes in energy metabolism relative to untransformed cells [1]. In the presence of O_2 normal tissues primarily utilize oxidative phosphorylation to form ATP from glucose. However, in response to hypoxia, cells switch to a glycolytic metabolism, producing only a fraction of the ATP generated under aerobic conditions. Although glycolysis is less efficient than oxidative phosphorylation to produce ATP, in the presence of sufficient glucose, glycolysis can sustain ATP production due to increases in the activity of the glycolytic enzymes. Many regions within solid tumors adapt to hypoxia by permanently relying on glycolysis to survive, regardless of subsequent exposure to normoxic oxygen levels (i.e., "aerobic glycolysis"). This phenomenon is referred to as the "Warburg effect" [94], which also correlates with a higher constitutive level of glycolytic enzyme expression. It is not surprising, therefore, that cancer therapies that inhibit the glycolytic pathway, such as 2-deoxyglucose, decrease the rate of proliferation of transformed cells [95].

1.6.1 HIF-1α Is a Key Regulator of Glycolytic Energy Production

We have previously demonstrated that HIF-1α is a critical regulator of hypoxic glycolytic metabolism and production of ATP in primary and transformed fibroblasts [96]. Although *HIF-1α* null cells grown in high-glucose medium at 21% O_2 grow at the same rate as wild-type cells during log-phase, at hypoxia (1% O_2), exponential growth of *HIF-1α* null cells was severely impaired. The total amount of free ATP produced under hypoxia by either primary or transformed *HIF-1α* null MEFs was also approximately half that of wild-type cells [96]. Similar results have been obtained in endothelial cells and macrophages in which *HIF-1α* has been conditionally deleted [97, 98]. Therefore, HIF-1α expression is critical to regulate the metabolism and the proliferative potential of oxygen-depleted cells.

1.6.2 Importance of Glycolysis in the Breast

HIF-1α's role in glycolytic metabolism is also relevant in the breast. HIF-1α protein is stabilized even under normoxic conditions in the metastatic, ERα-negative breast cancer cell lines MDA-MD-435 and MDA-MB-231, but not in $ERα^+$ MCF-7 cells. Furthermore, glycolytic activity at normoxia was elevated in the MDA-MB-435 cells compared to MCF-7 cells [99]. More recently, Robey et al. have demonstrated that in 10 of 12 low-passage breast cell lines derived from patients, there were significant correlations between glycolytic rate and phosphorylated c-Myc and HIF-1α levels [100]. In addition, HIF-1α expression has been shown to be responsible for resistance of HeLa cells to the glycolysis inhibitor 2-deoxyglucose (2-DG) as HeLa cells in which HIF-1α had been knocked down were more cytotoxic following 2-DG treatment compared to control cells [101]. Moreover, regulation of glycolysis is also critical in the lactating normal mammary gland, a time of a coordinated upregulation of glycolytic enzyme activity due to the increased demands for energy to produce and secrete milk [102]. For example, the level of lactate dehydrogenase (LDH) activity increases from 52,500 mUnits/g wet weight in pregnant mice to 81,400 mU/g wet weight in lactating mice, and the activity of pyruvate kinase (PK) increases from 43,500 to 102,000 mU/g, respectively [102].

1.7 HIF-1α and Metastasis

Metastasis is the primary cause of death for breast cancer patients. A large body of evidence supports the hypothesis that hypoxia, in general, and HIF-1α specifically, plays a critical role in cancer metastasis, as reviewed in [103]. For example, as discussed, HIF-1α has been found to be over-expressed in a high percentage of metastatic lesions from the breast [6], HIF-1α over-expression correlates with decreased disease-free survival and is an independent marker of poor prognosis in breast cancer patients [8, 12], and in orthotopic animal model of breast cancer, deletion of *HIF-1α* strongly impairs metastasis to the lung [65].

In addition, it is of note that *HIF-1α* was found to be significantly upregulated in a screen of breast cancer patients that had bone marrow (BM) micrometastases compared to BM-metastases negative patients [104]. The presence of disseminated breast cancer cells in the BM of patients has been shown previously to predict unfavorable outcome [105].

1.7.1 HIF-1α Targets Are Key Mediators of Metastasis

Some of the genes that have been connected to HIF-1α that regulate breast cancer metastasis include the ligand/chemokine receptor *CXCL12* (*SDF-1*)/ *CXCR4*, lysyl oxidase (*LOX*), *Twist*, *Snail*, and osteopontin (*Spp1*). The CXCL12/CXCR4 pathway is a critical regulator of breast cancer cell metastasis, as reviewed in [106]. The CXCR4 receptor is expressed by breast cancer cells and corresponding metastases, whereas high levels of CXCL12/SDF-1 are found in organs that are common sites of breast metastasis, including the lymph nodes, bone, lung, and liver [107]. Activation of CXCR4 in response to exposure to CXCL12/SDF-1 also increases breast cancer cell motility and invasion, whereas over-expression of CXCR4 in breast tumor cells increases lung and bone metastases in vivo and downregulation of CXCR4 decreases metastasis[106]. The breast tumor stroma also expresses CXCL12. In fact, carcinoma-associated fibroblasts (CAFs) expressing CXCL12 have been shown to participate in recruitment of endothelial progenitors from the circulation to the primary tumor [108].

Both *CXCR4* and *CXCL12/SDF-1* are induced by hypoxic exposure and are direct-HIF-1α transcriptional target genes [109, 110]. Moreover, the CXCL12/CXCR4 axis is a key player in stem cell homing to target tissues as well as maintenance of the stem cell niche since CXCR4 is expressed by many embryonic and adult stem cells that either migrate toward an SDF-1 signal or remain in their respective niche due to high expression of SDF-1, as occurs in hematopoietic stem cells (HSCs) in the bone marrow [111]. Finally, inhibitors to CXCR4, originally developed to target HIV-1 infection, have shown promise in blocking metastasis in animal models of breast cancer [112, 113].

Lysyl oxidase (LOX) is a catalytic extracellular matrix remodeling enzyme that was found in vitro to be upregulated at the mRNA level in invasive breast cancer cell lines and to be upregulated in invasive breast cancer cells relative to primary tumors [114]. *LOX* has also been shown to be a direct HIF-1α transcriptional target [115]. Furthermore, breast cancer patients with high LOX-expressing tumors have poor survival, and secreted LOX has been found to be a key player in hypoxia-induced metastasis since blocking *LOX* expression in MDA-MB-231 cells using a short hairpin RNA (shRNA) significantly reduced the number of metastases to the lung following orthotopic injection of tumor cells into the mammary fat pads of nude mice [116].

1.7.2 Role of HIF-1α in EMT

Acquiring the ability to mobilize to distant sites in the body may be regulated in part by the epithelial–mesenchymal transition (EMT) in which epithelial cells lose polarity, exhibit a decrease in E-cadherin, and acquire markers of expressed by stromal fibroblasts, such as vimentin, as reviewed in [117]. A key mediator of this pathway is Twist, a basic-helix-loop helix transcription factor that has been shown to promote EMT and to mediate metastasis [118], and is also a direct HIF-1α-regulated gene [119]. Snail, a zinc-finger transcriptional repressor, also promotes EMT and invasion and metastasis in multiple cancer types [120] and is regulated by the hypoxic response pathway via the VHL/HIF axis [121]. For example, elevated levels of HIF-1α resulting from loss of VHL in renal cell carcinomas downregulates E-cadherin expression through regulation of Snail and the sphingosine-1-phopsphate receptor sub-type 1 (S1P1) [121]. Interestingly, when Yang et al. knocked down *Snail* in conjunction with over-expression of Twist or when *Lox* was knocked down in conjunction with *Twist*, Twist over-expression could not completely restore migration and invasion, suggesting that Snail, Lox, and Twist may regulate distinct pathways critical for metastasis [119]. Given the direct role of HIF-1α in mediating expression of each of these genes, HIF-1α may influence EMT and metastasis through multiple molecular mechanisms.

1.7.3 HIF-1α and Osteopontin Regulation, a Plasma Biomarker of Poor Prognosis

Finally, in multiple cell types, hypoxia induces expression of secreted phospho-protein 1 (Spp1), also known as osteopontin, (OPN) [122, 123], which is believed to be indirect since no functional HREs have been confirmed to exist in the OPN promoter. OPN is a glycoprotein highly expressed in multiple cell types, including immune cells and osteocytes of the bone, as reviewed in [124]. OPN is also over-expressed in a variety of cancers, including breast cancer, as well as the infiltrating inflammatory immune cells present in cancers [124]. Expression of OPN by tumor cells, or high levels of circulating OPN, correlates with a poor prognosis in head and neck cancer and breast cancer patients [124]. Moreover, studies of mice xenografted with MDA-MB-231 cells via intracardiac injection that had formed osteolytic lesions and were further selected in vivo for bone metastasis, identified both CXCR4 and OPN as highly enriched in 231 cells with high rates of metastasis to bone [125]. More recently, work from the Weinberg laboratory has elegantly demonstrated that secretion of OPN by subcutaneous implantation of "instigator," or tumorigenic, invasive human breast tumor cells (BPLER or MDA-MB-231) into mice promoted growth and metastasis of normally weakly tumorigenic breast cancer cells (the "indolent" or responder cells, human mammary epithelial cell line with hygro-H-*ras*V12, HMLER-HR) [126]. OPN secreted by the instigating primary tumor was shown to activate the bone marrow and to then mobilize mesenchymal precursor cells into circulation, which resulted in induction of rapid growth of the HMLER-HR cells into large tumors. In addition, knockdown of *OPN* in the instigator population completely blocked formation of lung macrometastases. Although the influence of tissue hypoxia was not investigated in these studies, it is of note that HSCs reside in the most hypoxic regions of the bone and that hypoxia has been recently implicated in recruitment of mesenchymal stem cells from bone marrow to sites of tissue injury [127] and in regulation of stem cell biology, which will be discussed in detail in the following section.

1.8 Hypoxia, HIF-1, and Cancer Stem Cells

1.8.1 Impact of Hypoxia/HIF-1 on Cancer Stem Cells

The HIF-1 pathway has been proposed to impose a stem cell (SC) identity on more differentiated transformed cells [16]. This complements popular theory that tumors contain a rare fraction of cancer stem cells (CSCs), which have been defined as similar to normal SCs in that they can (1) self-renew, (2) form tumors upon serial transplantation into host mice, and (3) recapitulate the phenotype of the parental cancer [128]. CSCs were first described in acute myeloid leukemia using antibodies to specific cell surface markers and fluorescence-activated cell sorting (FACS), which isolated a small fraction of cells capable of self-renewal and tumor formation when transplanted to the bone marrow of immunocompromised mice [129]. By using a similar strategy, a population of tumor-initiating cells (TICs) has also been identified from a variety of solid tumors, including breast cancer [130]. The characterization of breast TICs or CSCs, and the genes and pathways that control their self-renewal, survival, and expansion is essential in order to design therapies that preferentially target the relatively rare fraction of CSCs present in a breast tumor. This is particularly true in light of increasing evidence that suggests that the CSC population represents the fraction of tumor cells resistant to radiation and chemotherapy, as reviewed in [131, 132]. To date, the specific contribution of hypoxia, generally, or HIF-1α specifically, to tumor-initiating ability (TIA) and CSC self-renewal and during breast tumor progression or to chemotherapy resistance mediated by CSCs remains largely undefined.

1.8.2 Connections Between Hypoxia, HIF, and Cancer Stem Cell Behavior

There are several connections between hypoxia and control of normal stem cell biology. For example, hematopoietic stem cells (HSCs) are enriched in hypoxic regions of bone [133], expansion of HSCs ex vivo is more efficient under hypoxic conditions [134], and neurosphere formation is also enhanced at 3% O_2 [135]. In addition, it has been suggested that CSCs exist in a hypoxic environment and that hypoxia stimulates expansion of CSCs, as reviewed in [16]. For example, the local microenvironment of the stem cell niche may influence the ability of CSCs to metastasize [136] and also likely strongly impacts therapeutic response [14, 132]. It has been recently reported that most of the tumor cells detected in the bone marrow of breast cancer patients have a stem cell phenotype, which suggests there is selective pressure for their dissemination [137]. Of additional interest, two of the four genes (*Klf4*, *Sox2*, *Oct-4*, and *c-Myc*) recently demonstrated to convert normal murine fibroblasts to cells with embryonic stem cell activity, *Oct-4* and *c-Myc*, are modulated directly by the HIFα subunits, reviewed in [16].

1.8.3 Overview of Profiling for Breast Cancer Stem Cells

Several laboratories have purified and characterized putative normal SCs and breast CSCs using cell surface markers in which bone marrow lineage-depleted (Lin⁻) mammary epithelial cells are sorted for sub-populations that express cell surface markers that then correlate with self-renewal, regeneration, and/or TIA. However, there is still controversy regarding whether breast CSCs may express different cell surface markers than normal breast SCs, whether the same markers that are described for human samples will also define SCs in a mouse mammary gland, and whether CSC markers may vary among tumors arising from different tissues types. For example, in human breast cancer samples, Al-Hajj et al. found that, in eight of nine patients, the $CD44^+/CD24^{-/low}$ sub-population of cells of breast tumors had high TIA in nude mice [138]. In contrast, in the normal gland, single β1-integrin $(CD29)^{hi}/CD24^+$ cells are able to reconstitute an entire functional mammary gland [139]. More recent studies in transgenic murine models of breast cancer have shown that in the *p53* null mammary tumor model, the $CD29^+/CD24^+$ population defines the population with enriched TIA. TIA was not observed in $CD24^+/CD29^-$ population, which constituted the bulk of tumor cells, or with $CD44^+$ tumor cells [140]. β3-integrin (CD61) has also been shown in the normal mammary gland to define the more committed "luminal" progenitor population that is responsive to Gata-3; when *Gata-3* was deleted, an increase in CD61 + luminal progenitor cells is observed [141]. Similarly, enriched TIA was recently described for the $CD61^+$ population of tumor cells in the MMTV-Wnt1 and p53 + /- mouse tumor models of breast cancer, although this population did not define TIA in the more well-differentiated MMTV-Neu tumor model [19]. In contrast, in the MMTV-Neu model, the $CD24^+$ and stem cell antigen (Sca-1)$^+/CD24^+$ populations have enriched TIA [18]. And, in MMTV-PyMT tumors [63], the $CD24^+/CD29^+$ or $CD29^+/CD61^+$ sub-populations were increasingly enriched during the course of tumor progression from a hyperplasia to early to late carcinomas [17]. Finally, use of CD133 (Prominin-1) as a surface marker of TICs has been well described for brain, prostate, and colon cancers [142]. In *Brca1* null breast tumor cells, the $CD133^+$ sub-population defined the cell population with enhanced TIA [20]. Although there is controversy regarding whether CD133 + is a stable CSC marker [143], or whether changes in CD133 are merely related to the cell cycle [144], it is of heightened interest that CD133 was recently described to be a hypoxia-inducible, oxygen-responsive gene [145].

1.8.4 Relevance of Notch and Wnt/β -Catenin Pathways in Stem Cell Biology

The Notch and canonical Wnt pathways are known regulators of HSCs, and Notch is required for Wnt to maintain undifferentiated HSCs [146]. The Notch and Wnt pathways also cross talk during tumorigenesis [147]. As reviewed in [148], Notch receptors (Notch-1-4 in mammals) undergo a series of proteolytic cleavages in response to activation by DSL [Delta, Serrate (Jagged in mammals), and Lag-2] ligands presented by neighboring cells. This leads to translocation of the Notch intracellular domain (NICD) to the nucleus, where it interacts with the DNA-binding protein CSL (also known as RBP-Jk or CBF-1, or Suppressor of Hairless [Su(H)] in *Drosophila*). In the canonical Wnt pathway, in the absence of Wnt ligand, β-catenin is degraded by the proteosome following its phosphorylation by the kinase glycogen synthase kinase (GSK)-3β. In the presence of ligand, GSK3-β activity is repressed, allowing β-catenin accumulation, and its binding to the LEF/TCF family of transcription factors to upregulate Wnt target genes, including *c-Myc*, which has been shown to interface with HIF-1α to regulate cellular metabolism [149].

1.8.5 Interactions Between NOTCH, HIF-1α, and FIH-1 in Cancer Cells

There are several lines of evidence that the Notch pathway is a key player in breast CSC biology. Aberrant Notch activation transforms human breast and murine MECs and mammary stem cells are enriched for Notch activity (reviewed in [150]). In addition, elevated *Notch1* and *Jagged-1* mRNA levels correlate with poor prognosis in breast cancer patients [151] and Notch-4 promotes self-renewal of mammary stem cells [152], *Notch-3* is upregulated 3-fold in normal breast cells grown as mammospheres in suspension culture [153], and over-expression of the Notch-3 ICD in transgenic mice causes precocious alveolar development in pregnancy and produces mammary tumors [154]. Furthermore, it has been shown that when MS isolated from the normal human breast are exposed to hypoxia, expression of Shc [p66Shc [155]] increases, which is required to induce Notch-3 and that blocking *Notch-3* using short-hairpin RNA (shRNA) reduces both primary and secondary MS formation as well as the expression of *carbonic anhydrase IX (CAIX)* [156]. Of note, *CAIX* is direct HIF-1α target gene for which expression negatively correlates with disease-free survival in breast cancer patients [9].

Observations in P19 neuronal stem cells and C2C12 myogenic cells that hypoxia increases the transcriptional activity of the Notch1 intracellular domain (N1ICD), increases N1ICD expression and that HIF-1α and N1ICD physically interact to mediate repression of differentiation [157] have directly connected HIF-1α to the Notch pathway. Hypoxia potentiates Notch signaling in multiple tumor cell lines, leading to increased transcriptional expression of several Notch target genes, including *Hey1*, as well as *Delta-like 1 (Dll1)*, a Notch ligand [115]. There are also connections between the hypoxia/Notch and the epithelial–mesenchymal transition (EMT) in cancer cells. In SKVO-3 ovarian carcinoma cells and MCF-7 breast cancer cells, hypoxia promoted EMT [115]. Transient expression of the N1ICD in SKVO-3 cells promotes tumor cell invasion and migration through Notch-dependent upregulation of *Snail*. Furthermore, HIF-1α was recruited to the *Snail* promoter only under stimulation from both hypoxia and Notch ligand [115]. In addition, FIH-1 has recently been shown to hydroxylate the ankryin (Ank) 1–7 repeat of the NICD in Notch-1, Notch-2, and Notch-3, but not Notch-4, resulting in decreased Notch transactivation and acceleration of myogenic and neuronal differentiation in C2C12 and P19 cells [158].

Recent studies have suggested that ER-negative, but not ERα+, breast cancers become "addicted" to Notch signaling through upregulation of *survivin*, which leads to therapeutic resistance [159]. In addition, expression of cytoplasmic FIH-1 has been reported to be an independent factor that negatively correlates with disease-free survival in invasive breast cancer patients, whereas nuclear expression of FIH-1 correlated with decreased tumor grade and recurrence [160]. As FIH-1 directly represses both HIF-1α and Notch transcriptional activity, it may be an attractive candidate for targeting the eradication of breast CSCs.

1.8.6 The Wnt/β -Catenin Pathway in Breast Cancer and Interactions Between HIF-1α and β -Catenin in Hypoxic Cancer Cells

Direct connections between HIF-1α and the Wnt/β-catenin pathway in the breast are less well defined, although it has been clear for some time that dysregulation of the Wnt pathway leads to breast cancer. For example, transgenic MMTV-Wnt-1 and MMTV-DN89β-catenin (a stabilized β-catenin) mice develop mammary hyperplasias/tumors [161]. In addition, mammary tumors that originate in either MMTV-Wnt-1 or MMTV-Myc mice contain an expansion of MECs that express Sca-1, whereas this is not observed in MMTV-Neu tumors [162]. In contrast, when a dominant-negative chimera of β-catenin known as β-engrailed is expressed in the mammary gland, which suppresses β-catenin signaling without affecting cell–cell adhesion, cell survival of lobuloalveolar progenitors is decreased [163]. Finally, when murine preneoplastic COMMA-D β-geo cells are engineered to express a stabilized version of β-catenin, there is an enrichment of MS formation efficiency (MSFE), whereas expression of β-engrailed repressed MSFE [22]. It has been shown in HepG2 and renal carcinoma cells that GSK3β directly phosphorylates HIF-1α on three Ser/Thr residues, leading to its degradation by the proteosome independent of VHL [164]. In contrast, hypoxic exposure blocked GSK-3β activity, permitting HIF-1α to accumulate as well as presumably β-catenin. Direct physical interactions between β-catenin and HIF-1α proteins were also recently observed in colon carcinoma cells *only under hypoxic stress* [165]. VHL also plays a direct role in downregulation of β-catenin stability through its interaction with a previously identified VHL-interacting protein, Jade-1. Chitalia et al. found that Jade-1 functioned as a single subunit E3 ubiquitin ligase that targeted both phosphorylated and non-phosphorylated β-catenin for proteolytic degradation, thereby establishing a pathway in which VHL can repress Wnt-on or Wnt-off signaling [166].

2 HIF-1 and Therapeutic Resistance in Breast Cancer

A direct role for HIF-1α in mediating resistance to radiation and chemotherapy has been confirmed in a variety of cell types since downregulation of HIF-1α at least partially restored sensitivity to therapy [167–173]. If one accepts the CSC concept as highly relevant to cancer control and that HIF-1α is a key regulator of CSC behavior, then the HIF-1 pathway must be critical for the survival of the CSCs after radiation or chemotherapy. If this relationship could be firmly established, it would have a significant impact on breast cancer clinical outcomes since it is believed that the CSCs remaining post-therapy are the fraction capable of tumor cell regeneration.

2.1 HIF-1α and Radiation Resistance

Elegant studies by Moeller et al. in the Balb/C-derived 4T1 murine mammary cancer model have demonstrated that HIF-1α promotes tumor radioresistance in part by upregulating expression of VEGF and bFGF during the period of re-oxygenation following single-dose irradiation, stabilizing the tumor vasculature [174]. However, animal studies such as these may not reflect what is observed in the clinic since most patients receive fractionated irradiation, in which radiotherapy is provided in multiple doses over a course of a few weeks. It has been shown that immediately after a large, single dose of IR, most of the cells in a tumor will be hypoxic, but after several hours of recovery, previously hypoxic regions of tumors can be re-oxygenated [13]. This type of intermittent hypoxia has been shown to enhance the survival of the tumor endothelial cells in a HIF-1α-dependent manner in a liver xenograft mouse model [175]. In head and neck cancers, the level of pimonidazole binding (which detects tissue hypoxia) has been shown to correlate with the ability to predict treatment outcome [176], although similar studies failed to find the same relationship between the staining for CAIX and the ability to predict outcome [177]. An excellent review that clearly outlines the potential role of CSCs in radioresistance has been recently published [178].

Using FACS-based methods to sort for breast tumor cells with enriched CSC activity, studies have shown that the breast CSC population for a particular cell line is more radioresistant than its parental cell line. For example, MCF-7 and MDA-MD-231 cells that were enriched for a $CD24^{-/lo}/CD44^{+}$ profile and grown as mammospheres were more radioresistant than parental monolayer-cultured cells [179]. In MCF-7 cells exposed to increasing doses of IR, the Sca-1+ and $CD24^{+}/CD29^{+}$ sub-populations increased, whereas the Sca-1− or $CD24^{-}/CD29^{-}$ population decreased. There were increases in γH2AX, a marker of DNA damage in the Sca1− versus the Sca-1+ population [23]. Independent studies have shown in normal MECs that the Sca-1+ progenitor population is highly resistant to radiation, that Sca-1+ cells contain less DNA damage than Sca1− cells, and that active β-catenin mediates self-renewal of

Sca-1 + cells, possibly through induction of *survivin* [22]. By testing for the role of *HIF-1α* versus *HIF-2α* in these model systems using stable-hairpin RNA (shRNA) knockdown, or by using genetic models of *HIFα* subunit deletion, it will be possible to test for a direct role of HIF-1 or HIF-2 in mediating radiation resistance in CSCs. In order to maintain the pertinent microenvironment and to preserve the potentially hypoxic CSC niche in vivo, these studies should also be conducted in transgenic models of breast cancer, which develop spontaneous tumors, which are then subjected to radiation therapy at particular stages of tumor progression.

2.2 HIF-1α and Chemotherapy Resistance

There are several mechanisms by which hypoxia, and thereby HIF-1α expression, within solid tumors may regulate resistance to chemotherapy [14]. First, the limited and disorganized vasculature in tumors results in poor perfusion and delivery of nutrients, which could lead to reduced proliferation in hypoxic regions, and therefore, poor clinical response, since most chemotherapeutic agents are most effective in highly proliferating cells. Second, it has been proposed that doxorubicin (DOX) relies on generation of superoxide from oxygen for cytotoxicity [180], therefore DOX would be expected to be less effective in hypoxic regions of tumors. HIF-1α has also been shown to regulate expression of two proteins that control drug efflux, the multidrug resistance gene (*MDR1*) [167] and the ABC transporter breast cancer resistance protein (*BCRP/ABCG2*) [181]. Of note, ABCG2 effluxes Hoechst 33342 dye, which has been used to enrich the "side-population" of cells with stem-like features in multiple tissues, including the breast [182, 183].

2.3 HIF-1α and the Estrogen Receptor

Interestingly, hypoxic exposure downregulates estrogen receptor (ER)α protein through HIF-1-dependent proteolytic degradation, suggesting that hypoxia may contribute to tamoxifen resistance [15, 184]. Several recent studies have noted an association between HIF-1α and decreased expression of ERα in breast tumors [184–186]. This is an important finding since ERα-negative tumors are associated with an increase risk of progression to metastasis and ERα is reduced in the majority of tamoxifen-resistant tumors [187]. Because ERα *represses* up to 70% of its 400 target genes in MCF-7 cells [188], it is possible that HIF-1α may function to relieve repression of a subset of ERα targets in the breast. They may be cancer-associated candidate genes that are co-regulated by HIF-1α and ERα that could be exploited in the future to treat breast cancer patients.

3 Therapeutic Strategies That Modulate HIF-1α

3.1 Overview of HIF-1α Inhibitors

Several reviews have highlighted the benefit of targeting tumor hypoxia, generally, and the HIF-1 pathway, specifically, in treating solid tumors [13, 77, 189]. Therefore, I will focus on those pathways and inhibitors that have been tested in vitro in breast cancer cell lines, that have been tested for efficacy in animal models of cancer, or that have been used successfully in clinical trials to treat solid tumors.

3.1.1 Inhibitors of Receptor Tyrosine Kinases and the PI3K/Akt/mTOR Pathway

As discussed previously, constitutive RTK activation and/or the downstream PI3K-AKT-mTOR pathway can stabilize HIF-1α independent of oxygen and result in upregulation of HIF-1α target genes, such as VEGF. Therefore, it is not surprising that various inhibitors of these pathways have been shown to result in decreased HIF-1α expression and transcriptional activity. For example, treatment of cancer cells with small molecule inhibitors of EGFR, such as gefitinib (Iressa) or erlotinib (Tarceva), or with monoclonal-antibody based therapy, such as cetuximab/C225, reduces HIF-1α expression [74, 190]. Inhibitors of mTOR also reduce HIF-1α synthesis and therefore, transcriptional activity. For example, rapamycin (sirolimus), temsirolimus, and everolimus/RAD-001 can each reduce tumor growth, in part through reducing VEGF-dependent tumor angiogenesis [191]. Rapamycin treatment of transgenic MMTV-Neu female mice resulted in decreased tumor progression through decreased tumor cell proliferation and increased apoptosis, albeit without significant changes in MVD [192]. In MDA-MB-231 cells, when RAD-001 was combined with radiation therapy, this strategy enhanced reduction in colony formation post-irradiation, although the effect on HIF-1α expression was not evaluated in this study [193]. The inhibition of PI3K by LY294002 also resulted in decreased HIF-1α expression in a panel of breast cancer cell lines [194].

Currently, there are several pending clinical trials to investigate the efficacy of combinatorial therapies targeting various RTK-activated pathways in treating metastatic and inflammatory breast cancer [195]. The rationale for these types of trials is supported by pre-clinical studies that have shown that therapies combining anti-EGFR family inhibitors and mTOR inhibitors are synergistic in killing MDA-MB-468 cultured cells and Calu6 non-small cell lung cancer tumors in the xenograft setting [196]. With respect to breast cancer, treatment of transgenic mice with MMTV-Neu mammary tumors with rapamycin and Herceptin (trastuzumab), which targets HER2 receptors, is also synergistic, resulting in enhanced tumor apoptosis [197]. It also should be considered that at least part of the therapeutic response may be due to the repression of HIF-1α and its downstream target genes.

3.1.2 DNA Modification Inhibitors

It is becoming increasingly appreciated that tissue hypoxia represents a potent epigenetic modifier to regulate gene expression in tumors [198]. Various histone deacetylase (HDAC) inhibitors have been shown to reduce HIF-1α expression and tumor angiogenesis, likely due to the ability of HIF-1α to physically interact with various HDAC enzymes [199]. For example, HDAC inhibitors FK228 and LAQ824 have been shown to inhibit HIF-1α protein accumulation and transcriptional activation in Lewis lung carcinoma and renal carcinoma cells [200, 201].

Topotecan (TPT) is a molecule discovered in a HIF-1-targeted high-throughput screen of the NCI Diversity Set and is a topoisomerase I inhibitor. TPT acts by inhibiting the hypoxic induction of HIF-1α protein and interferes with its ability to bind DNA [202]. However, in a phase I/II clinical study of patients with metastatic breast cancer, TPT therapy was found to have limited efficacy and deemed not appropriate as a first-line therapy for breast cancer[203]. Several clinical trials are currently recruiting women with locally advanced or metastatic breast cancer to test efficacy of these types of inhibitors in combination therapy [195].

3.1.3 Inhibitors of Hsp90

Heat shock protein 90 (HSP90) is a molecular chaperone over-expressed in multiple cancers that has multiple signal transduction proteins as substrates for stabilization, folding, and maturation including ERBB2, Akt, and HIF-1α [204]. Therefore, although HSP90 inhibitors are not specific to a particular pathway, they are advantageous for killing tumor cells in that they are capable of blocking multiple, signaling pathways in the cell that are often nodes for signaling cross talk. In addition, it has been demonstrated by comparison of normal and tumor cells of breast and colon cancer that the HSP90 inhibitor 17-allylamino-17-demethoxy-geldanamycin (17-AAG), a derivative of geldanamycin, preferentially targets tumor cells since in tumor cells, HSP90 is found in multiprotein complexes with high ATPase activity, whereas HSP90 in normal cells is uncomplexed [205]. The ability of the 17-AAG to interact with HIF-1α and then target it for proteosomal degradation independent of oxygen or VHL[206] has been found to be dependent upon interactions with receptor of activated protein C kinase (RACK1) [207].

17-AAG has been tested in phase I clinical trials in patients with progressive solid tumor malignancies, with hepatotoxicity as the primary dose-limiting factor [208]. In addition, there is a lot of excitement regarding the ability of Hsp90 inhibitors to suppress the ability of breast cancer cells to develop resistance to small molecules TKIs [209], particularly in women with HER2 + breast cancers [210]. Several clinical trials are in the recruitment phase to test the ability of 17-AAG in combination therapies to treat locally advanced and metastatic breast cancer [195]. Novel synthetic Hsp90 inhibitors that are more bioavailable, such as SNX-2112, or its prodrug SNX-5542, have also been developed and shown in cultured cells as well as xenografted tumor models to have potent inhibition of Hsp90 at least equivalent to 17-AAG [211]. A Phase I clinical trial is in the recruitment phase to test the safety and maximum tolerated dose of SNX-5542 in refractory lymphoma or in patients with solid tumors [195].

3.1.4 Other Small Molecule HIF Inhibitors

YC-1, 3-(5'-hydroxymethyl-2'-furyl)-1-benzylindazole, a soluble guanylyl cyclase stimulator, has been shown in several xenograft cancer models to inhibit HIF-1α protein expression and to have anti-angiogenic activity [212]. In addition, in an animal model of metastasis, YC-1 treatment dramatically reduced cell migration and metastatic burden [213]. Likewise, YC-1 treatment has been shown to decrease bone metastases derived from MDA-MD-231 breast cancer cells that were introduced into animals by intracardiac injection [214]. YC-1 was recently reported in a human lung cancer cell line to also reduce cell proliferation to block activation of matrix metalloproteinases (MMP-2 and MMP-9) and to reduce cyclin D1 expression [215]. However, to date no clinical trials using YC-1 have been initiated.

Another small molecule inhibitor of HIF-1α that has also been shown to have potent antitumor activity is PX-478 (S-2-amino-3-[4'-N,N,-bis(chloroethyl)amino]phenyl propionic acid N-oxide dihydrochloride) [216]. The primary mechanism of action of PX-478 is to block translation-dependent accumulation of HIF-1α independent of VHL in addition to decreasing HIF-1α mRNA levels and reducing deubiquitination[217]. A phase I trial is in recruitment to test PX-478 safety in patients with a secondary focus of evaluating its impact on the HIF-1α pathway [195].

Olenyuk et al. have developed a novel approach to HIF inhibition through the rationale development and characterization of DNA sequence-specific synthetic, cell-permeable polyamides [218]. The strategy for blocking HIF-1α-mediated transcriptional regulation was based on a FITC-conjugated polyamide that blocked HIF-α/HIF-1β from binding to the HRE located at −947 to −939 of the VEGF promoter (polyamide 1) [219]. It later demonstrated that whereas delivery of siRNA to HIF-1α or treatment with the HIF inhibitor echinomycin, a DNA-binding natural product, modulated nearly every known target gene of the HIF-1 pathway, that polyamide 1 was more restricted in its regulation of the HIF-1 response [220].

3.1.5 Glycolytic Inhibitors

Because of the HIF-1α-dependent Warburg effect observed in tumors, inhibition of the glycolytic pathway, which has been proposed in the literature for decades [221], is an attractive therapeutic approach. Clinical studies in glioma patients have shown that administration of 2-deoxyglucose (2DG) was well tolerated in combination with radiotherapy [222]. In animal models, some groups have reported a synergy of 2DG with chemotherapy or radiation and others have reported that 2DG reduced therapeutic effect. For example, in an animal model of pancreatic cancer, combination of 2DG with radiotherapy sensitized tumor cells to radiation [223] and 2DG in combination with cisplatin-enhanced therapeutic response in cultured FaDu head and neck cancer cells [224]. In contrast, in human monocytic leukemia U937 cells, 2DG blocked etoposide-induced apoptosis [225]. In addition, in pancreatic cancer cells, combining geldanamycin and the hexokinase II inhibitor 3-broma-pyruvate (3BrPA) was synergistic in reducing xenograft tumor growth [21]. Currently, two clinical trials are recruiting patients with advanced solid tumors or prostate cancer to evaluate 2DG as safe therapy for these patients. In addition, several prospective clinical trials are ongoing in which 18 fluoro-2-deoxyglucose (18 FDG)-based PTE scanning will be used to evaluate tumor metabolism as a key future clinical parameter in refining treatment of a variety of tumor types, including breast cancer [195].

3.2 Limitations of Current Anti-HIF Therapies

Key limitations of current anti-HIF therapies are that they do not exclusively inhibit HIF-1 and the likelihood that, given the high number of genes that HIF-1 regulates, there will be adverse side effects in normal cells. Moreover, HIF-1α not only activates but also represses target genes. And, the magnitude of HIF-1-dependent regulation is highly cell specific. As an example, HIF-1α induces expression of pro-survival genes as well as genes that are pro-apoptotic, therefore the overall microenvironment context will be important for pushing tumor cells to decide between survival and death. In addition, since HIF-1α can be stabilized under normoxic conditions due to activation of oncogenes, activation of RTKs or deletion of tumor suppressors such as VHL, strategies that do not solely rely on the presence of hypoxia for blocking HIF-1α transcriptional activity must also be considered.

4 Summary: Challenges for the Future

The major challenge in applying new anti-HIF clinical regimens that will improve breast cancer patient survival is how to select for patients that will best respond to HIF inhibitors. For example, it is reasonable that patients with a HIF hypoxic response signature score [3] or that have tumors with a large hypoxic fraction or that have elevated glucose metabolism detected by 18 FDG imaging will benefit most from anti-HIF strategies. In addition, as new combinatorial approaches are evaluated in clinical trials that include pathway inhibitors to target the HIFα subunits, it will be critical to consider which therapies will best synergize with anti-HIF therapies and in what order they should be administered to patients. For example, the Dewhirst laboratory has demonstrated using colon HT116 xenografts that "radiation-first" strategies were most effective compared to "anti-HIF-first" approaches in combination therapy [168] and that the combined therapy was highly synergistic. This observation was explained in part due to the destabilization of the tumor vasculature in response to *HIF-1α* deletion. As another example, in a xenograft study of HeLa cells that expressed a pro-caspase3 construct under control of the HIF ODD delivered systemically through the protein-transduction domain of HIV-1 tat protein (TOP3 model), tumors from mice that had received combination therapy of ionizing radiation and TOP3 had synergistically reduced decreased tumor volume. In contrast, treatment with TOP3 alone only temporarily reduced tumor growth [226].

Another challenge in breast cancer treatment is to block metastasis. Since accumulating data strongly suggest that HIF-1α may regulate a metastatic switch in breast cancer by promoting EMT, cell invasion, homing, and coloni-zation, screens for compounds that limit HIF-1α-dependent steps of metastasis could have significant clinical impact. As reviewed in [227], a focus on blocking metastatic spread could perhaps be the most clinically relevant approach to cure breast cancer.

One way screening for efficacy of novel anti-HIF compounds that are also dependent on HIFα function could be accomplished is to subject cultured breast cancer cells, in which *HIF-1α* or *HIF-2α* is over-expressed (compared to the parental cell line), to high-throughput cell invasion assays in the presence or absence of drug. Drugs that block invasion in a HIFα-dependent manner could then be tested in pre-clinical transgenic or xenografted animal models in which breast cancer cells are known to metastasize. Some of the systems that could be utilized include mammary tumor cells derived from the PyMT mouse, which our laboratory is developing, the murine 4T1 transplant system or by xenografting MDA-MB-231 cells into the cleared mammary fat pad. In addi-tion, to quantitate the effect of novel HIF inhibitors on primary tumor growth and metastasis, the routine use of bio-imaging modalities in mice over the course of the experiment, such as with the Xenogen bio-imaging system, will facilitate observation of the potency of HIF inhibitors on these processes. In addition, if cells are first dually labeled with both a fluorophore and a luciferase reporter, then it would also be possible to determine if the mammary tumor cells are still alive (fluorophore + ; luciferase +), or if a therapy has killed the tumor cells (fluorophore + only). This is because activity of luciferase, visualized by injection of D-luciferin into the animal, depends on ATP production, which would only occur in live cells, whereas a fluorophore signal may still be detected if the dead cells have not yet been cleared by the host, as in the case of necrotic areas.

In conclusion, there are multiple avenues by which anti-HIF therapies may be beneficial to breast cancer patients. A more complete understanding of the role that HIF-1α plays in the various cell types that are involved in breast cancer progression and metastasis, in addition to fine dissection of the HIF-1α-regu-lated downstream pathways that may be preferentially up- or downregulated during specific stages of progression and metastasis, will be key to further refining therapies. The ultimate goal of such studies would be to tailor ther-apeutics to those breast cancer patients that are most likely to benefit from therapeutic regimens designed to block HIF-1α activity.

References

1. Brown JM, Giaccia AJ. The unique physiology of solid tumors: opportunities (and problems) for cancer therapy. *Cancer Res* 1998; **58**: 1408–1416.
2. Semenza GL. HIF-1 and human disease: one highly involved factor. *Genes Dev* 2000; **14**: 1983–1991.
3. Chi JT, Wang Z, Nuyten DS, Rodriguez EH, Schaner ME, Salim A, Wang Y, Kristensen GB, Helland A, Borresen-Dale AL, Giaccia A, Longaker MT, Hastie T, Yang GP, van de Vijver MJ, Brown PO. Gene expression programs in response to hypoxia: cell type specificity and prognostic significance in human cancers. *PLoS Med* 2006; **3**: e47.
4. Goonewardene TI, Sowter HM, Harris AL. Hypoxia-induced pathways in breast cancer. *Microsc Res Tech* 2002; **59**: 41–48.
5. Greijer AE, van der Groep P, Kemming D, Shvarts A, Semenza GL, Meijer GA, van de Wiel MA, Belien JA, van Diest PJ, van der Wall E. Up-regulation of gene expression by hypoxia is mediated predominantly by hypoxia-inducible factor 1 (HIF-1). *J Pathol* 2005; **206**: 291–304.
6. Zhong H, De Marzo AM, Laughner E, Lim M, Hilton DA, Zagzag D, Buechler P, Issacs WB, Semenza GL, Simons JW. Overexpression of hypoxia-inducible factor 1α in common human cancers and their metastases. *Cancer Res* 1999; **59**: 5830–5835.
7. Bos R, Zhong H, Hanrahan CF, Mommers E, Semenza GL, Pinedo HM, Abeloff MD, Simons JW, van Diest PJ, van der Wall E. Levels of hypoxia-inducible factor-1α during breast carcinogenesis. *J Natl Cancer Inst* 2001; **93**: 309–314.
8. Bos R, van der Groep P, Greijer AE, Shvarts A, Meijer S, Pinedo HM, Semenza GL, van Diest PJ, van der Wall E. Levels of hypoxia-inducible factor-1alpha independently predict prognosis in patients with lymph node negative breast carcinoma. *Cancer* 2003; **97**: 1573–1581.
9. Generali D, Berruti A, Brizzi MP, Campo L, Bonardi S, Wigfield S, Bersiga A, Allevi G, Milani M, Aguggini S, Gandolfi V, Dogliotti L, Bottini A, Harris AL, Fox SB. Hypoxia-inducible factor-1alpha expression predicts a poor response to primary chemoendocrine therapy and disease-free survival in primary human breast cancer. *Clin Cancer Res* 2006; **12**: 4562–4568.
10. Gruber G, Greiner RH, Hlushchuk R, Aebersold DM, Altermatt HJ, Berclaz G, Djonov V. Hypoxia-inducible factor 1 alpha in high-risk breast cancer: an independent prognostic parameter? *Breast Cancer Res* 2004; **6**: R191–R198.
11. Yamamoto Y, Ibusuki M, Okumura Y, Kawasoe T, Kai K, Iyama K, Iwase H. Hypoxia-inducible factor 1alpha is closely linked to an aggressive phenotype in breast cancer. *Breast Cancer Res Treat* 2008; **110**: 465–475.
12. Dales JP, Garcia S, Meunier-Carpentier S, Andrac-Meyer L, Haddad O, Lavaut MN, Allasia C, Bonnier P, Charpin C. Overexpression of hypoxia-inducible factor HIF-1alpha predicts early relapse in breast cancer: retrospective study in a series of 745 patients. *Int J Cancer* 2005; **116**: 734–739.
13. Brown JM. Tumor hypoxia in cancer therapy. *Methods Enzymol* 2007; **435**: 297–321.
14. Tredan O, Galmarini CM, Patel K, Tannock IF. Drug resistance and the solid tumor microenvironment. *J Natl Cancer Inst* 2007; **99**: 1441–1454.
15. Stoner M, Saville B, Wormke M, Dean D, Burghardt R, Safe S. Hypoxia induces proteasome-dependent degradation of estrogen receptor alpha in ZR-75 breast cancer cells. *Mol Endocrinol* 2002; **16**: 2231–2242.
16. Keith B, Simon MC. Hypoxia-inducible factors, stem cells, and cancer. *Cell* 2007; **129**: 465–472.
17. Kouros-Mehr H, Bechis SK, Slorach EM, Littlepage LE, Egeblad M, Ewald AJ, Pai SY, Ho IC, Werb Z. GATA-3 links tumor differentiation and dissemination in a luminal breast cancer model. *Cancer Cell* 2008; **13**: 141–152.

18. Liu JC, Deng T, Lehal RS, Kim J, Zacksenhaus E. Identification of tumorsphere- and tumor-initiating cells in HER2/Neu-induced mammary tumors. *Cancer Res* 2007; **67**: 8671–8681.

19. Vaillant F, Asselin-Labat ML, Shackleton M, Forrest NC, Lindeman GJ, Visvader JE. The mammary progenitor marker CD61/beta3 integrin identifies cancer stem cells in mouse models of mammary tumorigenesis. *Cancer Res* 2008; **68**: 7711–7717.

20. Wright MH, Calcagno AM, Salcido CD, Carlson MD, Ambudkar SV, Varticovski L. Brca1 breast tumors contain distinct CD44 + /CD24- and CD133 + cells with cancer stem cell characteristics. *Breast Cancer Res* 2008; **10**: R10.

21. Cao X, Bloomston M, Zhang T, Frankel WL, Jia G, Wang B, Hall NC, Koch RM, Cheng H, Knopp MV, Sun D. Synergistic antipancreatic tumor effect by simultaneously targeting hypoxic cancer cells with HSP90 inhibitor and glycolysis inhibitor. *Clin Cancer Res* 2008; **14**: 1831–1839.

22. Chen MS, Woodward WA, Behbod F, Peddibhotla S, Alfaro MP, Buchholz TA, Rosen JM. Wnt/beta-catenin mediates radiation resistance of Sca1 + progenitors in an immortalized mammary gland cell line. *J Cell Sci* 2007; **120**: 468–477.

23. Woodward WA, Chen MS, Behbod F, Alfaro MP, Buchholz TA, Rosen JM. WNT/beta-catenin mediates radiation resistance of mouse mammary progenitor cells. *Proc Natl Acad Sci USA* 2007; **104**: 618–623.

24. Cancer facts and figures, 2008. American Cancer Society: Atlanta, 2008.

25. Semenza GL. Hypoxia-inducible factor 1: master regulator of O_2 homeostasis. *Curr Opin Genet Dev* 1998; **8**: 588–594.

26. Stroka DM, Burkhardt T, Desbaillets I, Wenger RH, Neil DA, Bauer C, Gassmann M, Candinas D. HIF-1 is expressed in normoxic tissue and displays an organ-specific regulation under systemic hypoxia. *Faseb J* 2001; **15**: 2445–2453.

27. Vaupel P, Hockel M, Mayer A. Detection and characterization of tumor hypoxia using pO_2 histography. *Antioxid Redox Signal* 2007; **9**: 1221–1235.

28. Kenneth NS, Rocha S. Regulation of gene expression by hypoxia. *Biochem J* 2008; **414**: 19–29.

29. Maynard MA, Ohh M. Von Hippel-Lindau tumor suppressor protein and hypoxia-inducible factor in kidney cancer. *Am J Nephrol* 2004; **24**: 1–13.

30. Zia MK, Rmali KA, Watkins G, Mansel RE, Jiang WG. The expression of the von Hippel-Lindau gene product and its impact on invasiveness of human breast cancer cells. *Int J Mol Med* 2007; **20**: 605–611.

31. Koh MY, Darnay BG, Powis G. HAF, a novel E3-ubiquitin ligase, binds and ubiquitinates HIF-1{alpha} leading to its oxygen-independent degradation. *Mol Cell Biol* 2008.

32. Metzen E, Ratcliffe PJ. HIF hydroxylation and cellular oxygen sensing. *Biol Chem* 2004; **385**: 223–230.

33. Hu CJ, Iyer S, Sataur A, Covello KL, Chodosh LA, Simon MC. Differential regulation of the transcriptional activities of hypoxia-inducible factor 1 alpha (HIF-1alpha) and HIF-2alpha in stem cells. *Mol Cell Biol* 2006; **26**: 3514–3526.

34. Hu CJ, Sataur A, Wang L, Chen H, Simon MC. The N-terminal transactivation domain confers target gene specificity of hypoxia-inducible factors HIF-1alpha and HIF-2alpha. *Mol Biol Cell* 2007; **18**: 4528–4542.

35. Hu CJ, Wang LY, Chodosh LA, Keith B, Simon MC. Differential roles of hypoxia-inducible factor 1alpha (HIF-1alpha) and HIF-2alpha in hypoxic gene regulation. *Mol Cell Biol* 2003; **23**: 9361–9374.

36. Sowter HM, Raval RR, Moore JW, Ratcliffe PJ, Harris AL. Predominant role of hypoxia-inducible transcription factor (Hif)-1alpha versus Hif-2alpha in regulation of the transcriptional response to hypoxia. *Cancer Res* 2003; **63**: 6130–6134.

37. Wang V, Davis DA, Haque M, Huang LE, Yarchoan R. Differential gene up-regulation by hypoxia-inducible factor-1alpha and hypoxia-inducible factor-2alpha in HEK293T cells. *Cancer Res* 2005; **65**: 3299–3306.

38. Warnecke C, Weidemann A, Volke M, Schietke R, Wu X, Knaup KX, Hackenbeck T, Bernhardt W, Willam C, Eckardt KU, Wiesener MS. The specific contribution of hypoxia-inducible factor-2alpha to hypoxic gene expression in vitro is limited and modulated by cell type-specific and exogenous factors. *Exp Cell Res* 2008; **314**: 2016–2027.

39. Warnecke C, Zaborowska Z, Kurreck J, Erdmann VA, Frei U, Wiesener M, Eckardt KU. Differentiating the functional role of hypoxia-inducible factor (HIF)-1alpha and HIF-2alpha (EPAS-1) by the use of RNA interference: erythropoietin is a HIF-2alpha target gene in Hep3B and Kelly cells. *Faseb J* 2004; **18**: 1462–1464.

40. Wiesener MS, Jurgensen JS, Rosenberger C, Scholze CK, Horstrup JH, Warnecke C, Mandriota S, Bechmann I, Frei UA, Pugh CW, Ratcliffe PJ, Bachmann S, Maxwell PH, Eckardt KU. Widespread hypoxia-inducible expression of HIF-2alpha in distinct cell populations of different organs. *Faseb J* 2003; **17**: 271–273.

41. Seagroves T, Johnson RS. Two HIFs may be better than one. *Cancer Cell* 2002; **1**: 211–213.

42. Maynard MA, Qi H, Chung J, Lee EH, Kondo Y, Hara S, Conaway RC, Conaway JW, Ohh M. Multiple splice variants of the human HIF-3 alpha locus are targets of the von Hippel-Lindau E3 ubiquitin ligase complex. *J Biol Chem* 2003; **278**: 11032–11040.

43. Blancher C, Moore JW, Talks KL, Houlbrook S, Harris AL. Relationship of hypoxia-inducible factor (HIF)-1alpha and HIF-2alpha expression to vascular endothelial growth factor induction and hypoxia survival in human breast cancer cell lines. *Cancer Res* 2000; **60**: 7106–7113.

44. Helczynska K, Larsson A-M, Mengelbier L, Bridges E, Fredlund E, Borgquist S, Landberg G, Pahlman S, Jirstrom K. Hypoxia-Inducible Factor-2alpha correlates to distant recurrence and poor outcome in invasvive breast cancer. *Cancer Res* 2008; **68**: 9212–9220.

45. Ryan HE, Lo J, Johnson RS. HIF-1 alpha is required for solid tumor formation and embryonic vascularization. *Embo J* 1998; **17**: 3005–3015.

46. Nagy A. Cre recombinase: the universal reagent for genome tailoring. *Genesis* 2000; **26**: 99–109.

47. Doedens A, Johnson RS. Transgenic models to understand hypoxia-inducible factor function. *Methods Enzymol* 2007; **435**: 87–105.

48. Ryan HE, Poloni M, McNulty W, Elson D, Gassmann M, Arbeit JM, Johnson RS. Hypoxia-inducible factor-1alpha is a positive factor in solid tumor growth. *Cancer Res* 2000; **60**: 4010–4015.

49. Wagner KU, Wall RJ, St-Onge L, Gruss P, Wynshaw-Boris A, Garrett L, Li M, Furth PA, Hennighausen L. Cre-mediated gene deletion in the mammary gland. *Nucleic Acids Res* 1997; **25**: 4323–4330.

50. Wagner KU, McAllister K, Ward T, Davis B, Wiseman R, Hennighausen L. Spatial and temporal expression of the Cre gene under the control of the MMTV-LTR in different lines of transgenic mice. *Transgenic Res* 2001; **10**: 545–553.

51. Seagroves TN, Hadsell D, McManaman J, Palmer C, Liao D, McNulty W, Welm B, Wagner KU, Neville M, Johnson RS. HIF1alpha is a critical regulator of secretory differentiation and activation, but not vascular expansion, in the mouse mammary gland. *Development* 2003; **130**: 1713–1724.

52. Anderson SM, Rudolph MC, McManaman JL, Neville MC. Key stages in mammary gland development. Secretory activation in the mammary gland: it's not just about milk protein synthesis! *Breast Cancer Res* 2007; **9**: 204.

53. Saarikoski ST, Rivera SP, Hankinson O. Mitogen-inducible gene 6 (MIG-6), adipophilin and tuftelin are inducible by hypoxia. *FEBS Lett* 2002; **530**: 186–190.

54. Vorbach C, Scriven A, Capecchi MR. The housekeeping gene xanthine oxidoreductase is necessary for milk fat droplet enveloping and secretion: gene sharing in the lactating mammary gland. *Genes Dev* 2002; **16**: 3223–3235.

55. Russell TD, Palmer CA, Orlicky DJ, Fischer A, Rudolph MC, Neville MC, McManaman JL. Cytoplasmic lipid droplet accumulation in developing mammary epithelial cells: roles of adipophilin and lipid metabolism. *J Lipid Res* 2007; **48**: 1463–1475.

56. Cardiff RD. Validity of mouse mammary tumour models for human breast cancer: comparative pathology. *Microsc Res Tech* 2001; **52**: 224–230.
57. Wagner KU. Models of breast cancer: quo vadis, animal modeling? *Breast Cancer Res* 2004; **6**: 31–38.
58. Desai KV, Xiao N, Wang W, Gangi L, Greene J, Powell JI, Dickson R, Furth P, Hunter K, Kucherlapati R, Simon R, Liu ET, Green JE. Initiating oncogenic event determines gene-expression patterns of human breast cancer models. *Proc Natl Acad Sci USA* 2002; **99**: 6967–6972.
59. Qiu TH, Chandramouli GV, Hunter KW, Alkharouf NW, Green JE, Liu ET. Global expression profiling identifies signatures of tumor virulence in MMTV-PyMT-transgenic mice: correlation to human disease. *Cancer Res* 2004; **64**: 5973–5981.
60. Barnes DM, Bartkova J, Camplejohn RS, Gullick WJ, Smith PJ, Millis RR. Overexpression of the c-erbB-2 oncoprotein: why does this occur more frequently in ductal carcinoma in situ than in invasive mammary carcinoma and is this of prognostic significance? *Eur J Cancer* 1992; **28**: 644–648.
61. Cardiff RD, Wagner U, Hennighausen L. Mammary cancer in humans and mice: a tutorial for comparative pathology. *Vet Pathol* 2001; **38**: 357–358.
62. Rosner A, Miyoshi K, Landesman-Bollag E, Xu X, Seldin DC, Moser AR, MacLeod CL, Shyamala G, Gillgrass AE, Cardiff RD. Pathway pathology: histological differences between ErbB/Ras and Wnt pathway transgenic mammary tumors. *Am J Pathol* 2002; **161**: 1087–1097.
63. Lin EY, Jones JG, Li P, Zhu L, Whitney KD, Muller WJ, Pollard JW. Progression to malignancy in the polyoma middle T oncoprotein mouse breast cancer model provides a reliable model for human diseases. *Am J Pathol* 2003; **163**: 2113–2126.
64. Herschkowitz JI, Simin K, Weigman VJ, Mikaelian I, Usary J, Hu Z, Rasmussen KE, Jones LP, Assefnia S, Chandrasekharan S, Backlund MG, Yin Y, Khramtsov AI, Bastein R, Quackenbush J, Glazer RI, Brown PH, Green JE, Kopelovich L, Furth PA, Palazzo JP, Olopade OI, Bernard PS, Churchill GA, Van Dyke T, Perou CM. Identification of conserved gene expression features between murine mammary carcinoma models and human breast tumors. *Genome Biol* 2007; **8**: R76.
65. Liao D, Corle C, Seagroves TN, Johnson RS. Hypoxia-inducible factor-1alpha is a key regulator of metastasis in a transgenic model of cancer initiation and progression. *Cancer Res* 2007; **67**: 563–572.
66. Bilton RL, Booker GW. The subtle side to hypoxia inducible factor (HIFalpha) regulation. *Eur J Biochem* 2003; **270**: 791–798.
67. Feldser D, Agani F, Iyer NV, Pak B, Ferreira G, Semenza GL. Reciprocal positive regulation of hypoxia-inducible factor 1alpha and insulin-like growth factor 2. *Cancer Res* 1999; **59**: 3915–3918.
68. Laughner E, Taghavi P, Chiles K, Mahon PC, Semenza GL. HER2 (neu) signaling increases the rate of hypoxia-inducible factor 1alpha (HIF-1alpha) synthesis: novel mechanism for HIF-1-mediated vascular endothelial growth factor expression. *Mol Cell Biol* 2001; **21**: 3995–4004.
69. Tanaka H, Yamamoto M, Hashimoto N, Miyakoshi M, Tamakawa S, Yoshie M, Tokusashi Y, Yokoyama K, Yaginuma Y, Ogawa K. Hypoxia-independent overexpression of hypoxia-inducible factor 1alpha as an early change in mouse hepatocarcinogenesis. *Cancer Res* 2006; **66**: 11263–11270.
70. Gort EH, Groot AJ, Derks van de Ven TL, van der Groep P, Verlaan I, van Laar T, van Diest PJ, van der Wall E, Shvarts A. Hypoxia-inducible factor-1alpha expression requires PI 3-kinase activity and correlates with Akt1 phosphorylation in invasive breast carcinomas. *Oncogene* 2006; **25**: 6123–6127.
71. Peng XH, Karna P, Cao Z, Jiang BH, Zhou M, Yang L. Cross-talk between epidermal growth factor receptor and hypoxia-inducible factor-1alpha signal pathways increases resistance to apoptosis by up-regulating survivin gene expression. *J Biol Chem* 2006; **281**: 25903–25914.

72. Weihua Z, Tsan R, Huang WC, Wu Q, Chiu CH, Fidler IJ, Hung MC. Survival of cancer cells is maintained by EGFR independent of its kinase activity. *Cancer Cell* 2008; **13**: 385–393.
73. Vega C, R. Sachleben L J, Gozal D, Gozal E. Differential metabolic adaptation to acute and long-term hypoxia in rat primary cortical astrocytes. *J Neurochem* 2006; **97**: 872–883.
74. Pore N, Jiang Z, Gupta A, Cerniglia G, Kao GD, Maity A. EGFR tyrosine kinase inhibitors decrease VEGF expression by both hypoxia-inducible factor (HIF)-1-independent and HIF-1-dependent mechanisms. *Cancer Res* 2006; **66**: 3197–3204.
75. Lu Y, Liang K, Li X, Fan Z. Responses of cancer cells with wild-type or tyrosine kinase domain-mutated epidermal growth factor receptor (EGFR) to EGFR-targeted therapy are linked to downregulation of hypoxia-inducible factor-1alpha. *Mol Cancer* 2007; **6**: 63.
76. de Paulsen N, Brychzy A, Fournier MC, Klausner RD, Gnarra JR, Pause A, Lee S. Role of transforming growth factor-alpha in von Hippel–Lindau (VHL)(-/-) clear cell renal carcinoma cell proliferation: a possible mechanism coupling VHL tumor suppressor inactivation and tumorigenesis. *Proc Natl Acad Sci USA* 2001; **98**: 1387–1392.
77. Semenza GL. Evaluation of HIF-1 inhibitors as anticancer agents. *Drug Discov Today* 2007; **12**: 853–859.
78. Giordano F, Johnson R. Angiogenesis: the role of the microenvironment in flipping the switch. *Curr Opin Genet Dev* 2001; **11**: 35–40.
79. Krek W. VHL takes HIF's breath away. *Nat Cell Biol* 2000; **2**: E121–E123.
80. Inoue M, Hager JH, Ferrara N, Gerber HP, Hanahan D. VEGF-A has a critical, nonredundant role in angiogenic switching and pancreatic beta cell carcinogenesis. *Cancer Cell* 2002; **1**: 193–202.
81. Bando H. Vascular endothelial growth factor and bevacitumab in breast cancer. *Breast Cancer* 2007; **14**: 163–173.
82. Inai T, Mancuso M, Hashizume H, Baffert F, Haskell A, Baluk P, Hu-Lowe DD, Shalinsky DR, Thurston G, Yancopoulos GD, McDonald DM. Inhibition of vascular endothelial growth factor (VEGF) signaling in cancer causes loss of endothelial fenestrations, regression of tumor vessels, and appearance of basement membrane ghosts. *Am J Pathol* 2004; **165**: 35–52.
83. Mancuso MR, Davis R, Norberg SM, O'Brien S, Sennino B, Nakahara T, Yao VJ, Inai T, Brooks P, Freimark B, Shalinsky DR, Hu-Lowe DD, McDonald DM. Rapid vascular regrowth in tumors after reversal of VEGF inhibition. *J Clin Invest* 2006; **116**: 2610–2621.
84. Jain RK. Normalization of tumor vasculature: an emerging concept in antiangiogenic therapy. *Science* 2005; **307**: 58–62.
85. Fukumura D, Jain RK. Tumor microvasculature and microenvironment: targets for anti-angiogenesis and normalization. *Microvasc Res* 2007; **74**: 72–84.
86. Gasparini G, Toi M, Gion M, Verderio P, Dittadi R, Hanatani M, Matsubara I, Vinante O, Bonoldi E, Boracchi P, Gatti C, Suzuki H, Tominaga T. Prognostic significance of vascular endothelial growth factor protein in node-negative breast carcinoma. *J Natl Cancer Inst* 1997; **89**: 139–147.
87. Gasparini G, Toi M, Verderio P, Ranieri G, Dante S, Bonoldi E, Boracchi P, Fanelli M, Tominaga T. Prognostic significance of p53, angiogenesis, and other conventional features in operable breast cancer: subanalysis in node-positive and node-negative patients. *Int J Oncol* 1998; **12**: 1117–1125.
88. Koukourakis MI, Manolas C, Minopoulos G, Giatromanolaki A, Sivridis E. Angiogenesis relates to estrogen receptor negativity, c-erbB-2 overexpression and early relapse in node-negative ductal carcinoma of the breast. *Int J Surg Pathol* 2003; **11**: 29–34.
89. Tsutsui S, Kume M, Era S. Prognostic value of microvessel density in invasive ductal carcinoma of the breast. *Breast Cancer* 2003; **10**: 312–319.
90. Bos R, van Diest PJ, de Jong JS, van der Groep P, van der Valk P, van der Wall E. Hypoxia-inducible factor-1alpha is associated with angiogenesis, and expression of bFGF, PDGF-BB, and EGFR in invasive breast cancer. *Histopathology* 2005; **46**: 31–36.

91. Oehler-Janne C, Jochum W, Riesterer O, Broggini-Tenzer A, Caravatti G, Vuong V, Pruschy M. Hypoxia modulation and radiosensitization by the novel dual EGFR and VEGFR inhibitor AEE788 in spontaneous and related allograft tumor models. *Mol Cancer Ther* 2007; **6**: 2496–2504.

92. Carmeliet P, Dor Y, Herbert J, Fukumura D, Brusselmans K, Dewerchin M, Neeman M, Bono F, Abramovitch R, Maxwell P, Koch CJ, Ratcliffe P, Moons L, Jain RK, Collen D, Keshet E. Role of HIF-1alpha in hypoxia mediated apoptosis, cell proliferation and tumour angiogenesis. *Nature* 1998; **394**: 485–490.

93. Rossiter H, Barresi C, Ghannadan M, Gruber F, Mildner M, Fodinger D, Tschachler E. Inactivation of VEGF in mammary gland epithelium severely compromises mammary gland development and function. *Faseb J* 2007; **21**: 3994–4004.

94. Warburg O. *The Metabolism of Tumours*. Constable & Co., Ltd.: London, 1930.

95. Hamilton E, Fennell M, Stafford DM. Modification of tumour glucose metabolism for therapeutic benefit. *Acta Oncol* 1995; **34**: 429–433.

96. Seagroves T, Ryan HE, Lu H, Wouters BG, Knapp AM, Thibault P, Laderoute KR, Johnson RS. The transcription factor HIF-1 is a necessary mediator of the Pasteur effect in mammalian cells. *Mol Cell Biol* 2001; **21**: 3436–3444.

97. Cramer T, Yamanishi Y, Clausen BE, Forster I, Pawlinski R, Mackman N, Haase VH, Jaenisch R, Corr M, Nizet V, Firestein GS, Gerber HP, Ferrara N, Johnson RS. HIF-1alpha is essential for myeloid cell-mediated inflammation. *Cell* 2003; **112**: 645–657.

98. Tang N, Wang L, Esko J, Giordano FJ, Huang Y, Gerber HP, Ferrara N, Johnson RS. Loss of HIF-1alpha in endothelial cells disrupts a hypoxia-driven VEGF autocrine loop necessary for tumorigenesis. *Cancer Cell* 2004; **6**: 485–495.

99. Robey IF, Lien AD, Welsh SJ, Baggett BK, Gillies RJ. Hypoxia-inducible factor-1alpha and the glycolytic phenotype in tumors. *Neoplasia* 2005; **7**: 324–330.

100. Robey IF, Stephen RM, Brown KS, Baggett BK, Gatenby RA, Gillies RJ. Regulation of the Warburg effect in early-passage breast cancer cells. *Neoplasia* 2008; **10**: 745–756.

101. Maher JC, Wangpaichitr M, Savaraj N, Kurtoglu M, Lampidis TJ. Hypoxia-inducible factor-1 confers resistance to the glycolytic inhibitor 2-deoxy-D-glucose. *Mol Cancer Ther* 2007; **6**: 732–741.

102. Mazurek S, Weisse G, Wust G, Schafer-Schwebel A, Eigenbrodt E, Friis RR. Energy metabolism in the involuting mammary gland. *In Vivo* 1999; **13**: 467–478.

103. Gupta GP, Massague J. Cancer metastasis: building a framework. *Cell* 2006; **127**: 679–695.

104. Woelfle U, Cloos J, Sauter G, Riethdorf L, Janicke F, van Diest P, Brakenhoff R, Pantel K. Molecular signature associated with bone marrow micrometastasis in human breast cancer. *Cancer Res* 2003; **63**: 5679–5684.

105. Pierga JY, Bonneton C, Magdelenat H, Vincent-Salomon A, Nos C, Pouillart P, Thiery JP. Clinical significance of proliferative potential of occult metastatic cells in bone marrow of patients with breast cancer. *Br J Cancer* 2003; **89**: 539–545.

106. Luker KE, Luker GD. Functions of CXCL12 and CXCR4 in breast cancer. *Cancer Lett* 2006; **238**: 30–41.

107. Kucia M, Reca R, Miekus K, Wanzeck J, Wojakowski W, Janowska-Wieczorek A, Ratajczak J, Ratajczak MZ. Trafficking of normal stem cells and metastasis of cancer stem cells involve similar mechanisms: pivotal role of the SDF-1-CXCR4 axis. *Stem Cells* 2005; **23**: 879–894.

108. Orimo A, Gupta PB, Sgroi DC, Arenzana-Seisdedos F, Delaunay T, Naeem R, Carey VJ, Richardson AL, Weinberg RA. Stromal fibroblasts present in invasive human breast carcinomas promote tumor growth and angiogenesis through elevated SDF-1/CXCL12 secretion. *Cell* 2005; **121**: 335–348.

109. Ceradini DJ, Kulkarni AR, Callaghan MJ, Tepper OM, Bastidas N, Kleinman ME, Capla JM, Galiano RD, Levine JP, Gurtner GC. Progenitor cell trafficking is regulated by hypoxic gradients through HIF-1 induction of SDF-1. *Nat Med* 2004; **10**: 858–864.

110. Staller P, Sulitkova J, Lisztwan J, Moch H, Oakeley EJ, Krek W. Chemokine receptor CXCR4 downregulated by von Hippel-Lindau tumour suppressor pVHL. *Nature* 2003; **425**: 307–311.

111. Sugiyama T, Kohara H, Noda M, Nagasawa T. Maintenance of the hematopoietic stem cell pool by CXCL12-CXCR4 chemokine signaling in bone marrow stromal cell niches. *Immunity* 2006; **25**: 977–988.

112. Kim SY, Lee CH, Midura BV, Yeung C, Mendoza A, Hong SH, Ren L, Wong D, Korz W, Merzouk A, Salari H, Zhang H, Hwang ST, Khanna C, Helman LJ. Inhibition of the CXCR4/CXCL12 chemokine pathway reduces the development of murine pulmonary metastases. *Clin Exp Metastasis* 2008; **25**: 201–211.

113. Smith MC, Luker KE, Garbow JR, Prior JL, Jackson E, Piwnica-Worms D, Luker GD. CXCR4 regulates growth of both primary and metastatic breast cancer. *Cancer Res* 2004; **64**: 8604–8612.

114. Payne SL, Fogelgren B, Hess AR, Seftor EA, Wiley EL, Fong SF, Csiszar K, Hendrix MJ, Kirschmann DA. Lysyl oxidase regulates breast cancer cell migration and adhesion through a hydrogen peroxide-mediated mechanism. *Cancer Res* 2005; **65**: 11429–11436.

115. Sahlgren C, Gustafsson MV, Jin S, Poellinger L, Lendahl U. Notch signaling mediates hypoxia-induced tumor cell migration and invasion. *Proc Natl Acad Sci USA* 2008; **105**(17): 6392–6397.

116. Erler JT, Bennewith KL, Nicolau M, Dornhofer N, Kong C, Le QT, Chi JT, Jeffrey SS, Giaccia AJ. Lysyl oxidase is essential for hypoxia-induced metastasis. *Nature* 2006; **440**: 1222–1226.

117. Tse JC, Kalluri R. Mechanisms of metastasis: epithelial-to-mesenchymal transition and contribution of tumor microenvironment. *J Cell Biochem* 2007; **101**: 816–829.

118. Yang J, Mani SA, Donaher JL, Ramaswamy S, Itzykson RA, Come C, Savagner P, Gitelman I, Richardson A, Weinberg RA. Twist, a master regulator of morphogenesis, plays an essential role in tumor metastasis. *Cell* 2004; **117**: 927–939.

119. Yang MH, Wu MZ, Chiou SH, Chen PM, Chang SY, Liu CJ, Teng SC, Wu KJ. Direct regulation of TWIST by HIF-1alpha promotes metastasis. *Nat Cell Biol* 2008; **10**: 295–305.

120. Peinado H, Olmeda D, Cano A. Snail, Zeb and bHLH factors in tumour progression: an alliance against the epithelial phenotype? *Nat Rev Cancer* 2007; **7**: 415–428.

121. Evans AJ, Russell RC, Roche O, Burry TN, Fish JE, Chow VW, Kim WY, Saravanan A, Maynard MA, Gervais ML, Sufan RI, Roberts AM, Wilson LA, Betten M, Vandewalle C, Berx G, Marsden PA, Irwin MS, Teh BT, Jewett MA, Ohh M. VHL promotes E2 box-dependent E-cadherin transcription by HIF-mediated regulation of SIP1 and snail. *Mol Cell Biol* 2007; **27**: 157–169.

122. Zhu Y, Denhardt DT, Cao H, Sutphin PD, Koong AC, Giaccia AJ, Le QT. Hypoxia upregulates osteopontin expression in NIH-3T3 cells via a Ras-activated enhancer. *Oncogene* 2005; **24**: 6555–6563.

123. Sodhi CP, Phadke SA, Batlle D, Sahai A. Hypoxia stimulates osteopontin expression and proliferation of cultured vascular smooth muscle cells: potentiation by high glucose. *Diabetes* 2001; **50**: 1482–1490.

124. Tuck AB, Chambers AF, Allan AL. Osteopontin overexpression in breast cancer: knowledge gained and possible implications for clinical management. *J Cell Biochem* 2007; **102**: 859–868.

125. Kang Y, Siegel PM, Shu W, Drobnjak M, Kakonen SM, Cordon-Cardo C, Guise TA, Massague J. A multigenic program mediating breast cancer metastasis to bone. *Cancer Cell* 2003; **3**: 537–549.

126. McAllister SS, Gifford AM, Greiner AL, Kelleher SP, Saelzler MP, Ince TA, Reinhardt F, Harris LN, Hylander BL, Repasky EA, Weinberg RA. Systemic endocrine instigation of indolent tumor growth requires osteopontin. *Cell* 2008; **133**: 994–1005.

127. Rochefort GY, Delorme B, Lopez A, Herault O, Bonnet P, Charbord P, Eder V, Domenech J. Multipotential mesenchymal stem cells are mobilized into peripheral blood by hypoxia. *Stem Cells* 2006; **24**: 2202–2208.
128. Huntly BJ, Gilliland DG. Leukaemia stem cells and the evolution of cancer-stem-cell research. *Nat Rev Cancer* 2005; **5**: 311–321.
129. Bonnet D, Dick JE. Human acute myeloid leukemia is organized as a hierarchy that originates from a primitive hematopoietic cell. *Nat Med* 1997; **3**: 730–737.
130. Al-Hajj M, Wicha MS, Benito-Hernandez A, Morrison SJ, Clarke MF. Prospective identification of tumorigenic breast cancer cells. *Proc Natl Acad Sci USA* 2003; **100**: 3983–3988.
131. Morrison BJ, Schmidt CW, Lakhani SR, Reynolds BA, Lopez JA. Breast cancer stem cells: implications for therapy of breast cancer. *Breast Cancer Res* 2008; **10**: 210.
132. Rich JN. Cancer stem cells in radiation resistance. *Cancer Res* 2007; **67**: 8980–8984.
133. Parmar K, Mauch P, Vergilio JA, Sackstein R, Down JD. Distribution of hematopoietic stem cells in the bone marrow according to regional hypoxia. *Proc Natl Acad Sci USA* 2007; **104**: 5431–5436.
134. Piccoli C, D'Aprile A, Ripoli M, Scrima R, Boffoli D, Tabilio A, Capitanio N. The hypoxia-inducible factor is stabilized in circulating hematopoietic stem cells under normoxic conditions. *FEBS Lett* 2007; **581**: 3111–3119.
135. Yang Z, Levison SW. Hypoxia/ischemia expands the regenerative capacity of progenitors in the perinatal subventricular zone. *Neuroscience* 2006; **139**: 555–564.
136. Li F, Tiede B, Massague J, Kang Y. Beyond tumorigenesis: cancer stem cells in metastasis. *Cell Res* 2007; **17**: 3–14.
137. Balic M, Lin H, Young L, Hawes D, Giuliano A, McNamara G, Datar RH, Cote RJ. Most early disseminated cancer cells detected in bone marrow of breast cancer patients have a putative breast cancer stem cell phenotype. *Clin Cancer Res* 2006; **12**: 5615–5621.
138. Al-Hajj M, Clarke MF. Self-renewal and solid tumor stem cells. *Oncogene* 2004; **23**: 7274–7282.
139. Shackleton M, Vaillant F, Simpson KJ, Stingl J, Smyth GK, Asselin-Labat ML, Wu L, Lindeman GJ, Visvader JE. Generation of a functional mammary gland from a single stem cell. *Nature* 2006; **439**: 84–88.
140. Zhang M, Behbod F, Atkinson RL, Landis MD, Kittrell F, Edwards D, Medina D, Tsimelzon A, Hilsenbeck S, Green JE, Michalowska AM, Rosen JM. Identification of tumor-initiating cells in a p53-null mouse model of breast cancer. *Cancer Res* 2008; **68**: 4674–4682.
141. Asselin-Labat ML, Sutherland KD, Barker H, Thomas R, Shackleton M, Forrest NC, Hartley L, Robb L, Grosveld FG, van der Wees J, Lindeman GJ, Visvader JE. Gata-3 is an essential regulator of mammary-gland morphogenesis and luminal-cell differentiation. *Nat Cell Biol* 2007; **9**: 201–209.
142. Soeda A, Inagaki A, Oka N, Ikegame Y, Aoki H, Yoshimura S, Nakashima S, Kunisada T, Iwama T. Epidermal growth factor plays a crucial role in mitogenic regulation of human brain tumor stem cells. *J Biol Chem* 2008; **283**: 10958–10966.
143. Mizrak D, Brittan M, Alison MR. CD133: molecule of the moment. *J Pathol* 2008; **214**: 3–9.
144. Bidlingmaier S, Zhu X, Liu B. The utility and limitations of glycosylated human CD133 epitopes in defining cancer stem cells. *J Mol Med* 2008; **86**: 1025–1032.
145. Platet N, Liu SY, Atifi ME, Oliver L, Vallette FM, Berger F, Wion D. Influence of oxygen tension on CD133 phenotype in human glioma cell cultures. *Cancer Lett* 2007; **258**: 286–290.
146. Duncan AW, Rattis FM, DiMascio LN, Congdon KL, Pazianos G, Zhao C, Yoon K, Cook JM, Willert K, Gaiano N, Reya T. Integration of Notch and Wnt signaling in hematopoietic stem cell maintenance. *Nat Immunol* 2005; **6**: 314–322.
147. Katoh M. Networking of WNT, FGF, Notch, BMP, and Hedgehog signaling pathways during carcinogenesis. *Stem Cell Rev* 2007; **3**: 30–38.

148. Bray SJ. Notch signalling: a simple pathway becomes complex. *Nat Rev Mol Cell Biol* 2006; **7**: 678–689.
149. Gordan JD, Thompson CB, Simon MC. HIF and c-Myc: sibling rivals for control of cancer cell metabolism and proliferation. *Cancer Cell* 2007; **12**: 108–113.
150. Farnie G, Clarke RB. Mammary stem cells and breast cancer–role of Notch signalling. *Stem Cell Rev* 2007; **3**: 169–175.
151. Reedijk M, Odorcic S, Chang L, Zhang H, Miller N, McCready DR, Lockwood G, Egan SE. High-level coexpression of JAG1 and NOTCH1 is observed in human breast cancer and is associated with poor overall survival. *Cancer Res* 2005; **65**: 8530–8537.
152. Dontu G, Jackson KW, McNicholas E, Kawamura MJ, Abdallah WM, Wicha MS. Role of Notch signaling in cell-fate determination of human mammary stem/progenitor cells. *Breast Cancer Res* 2004; **6**: R605–R615.
153. Dontu G, Abdallah WM, Foley JM, Jackson KW, Clarke MF, Kawamura MJ, Wicha MS. In vitro propagation and transcriptional profiling of human mammary stem/progenitor cells. *Genes Dev* 2003; **17**: 1253–1270.
154. Hu C, Dievart A, Lupien M, Calvo E, Tremblay G, Jolicoeur P. Overexpression of activated murine Notch1 and Notch3 in transgenic mice blocks mammary gland development and induces mammary tumors. *Am J Pathol* 2006; **168**: 973–990.
155. Migliaccio E, Mele S, Salcini AE, Pelicci G, Lai KM, Superti-Furga G, Pawson T, Di Fiore PP, Lanfrancone L, Pelicci PG. Opposite effects of the p52shc/p46shc and p66shc splicing isoforms on the EGF receptor-MAP kinase-fos signalling pathway. *Embo J* 1997; **16**: 706–716.
156. Sansone P, Storci G, Giovannini C, Pandolfi S, Pianetti S, Taffurelli M, Santini D, Ceccarelli C, Chieco P, Bonafe M. p66Shc/Notch-3 interplay controls self-renewal and hypoxia survival in human stem/progenitor cells of the mammary gland expanded in vitro as mammospheres. *Stem Cells* 2007; **25**: 807–815.
157. Gustafsson MV, Zheng X, Pereira T, Gradin K, Jin S, Lundkvist J, Ruas JL, Poellinger L, Lendahl U, Bondesson M. Hypoxia requires notch signaling to maintain the undifferentiated cell state. *Dev Cell* 2005; **9**: 617–628.
158. Zheng X, Linke S, Dias JM, Zheng X, Gradin K, Wallis TP, Hamilton BR, Gustafsson M, Ruas JL, Wilkins S, Bilton RL, Brismar K, Whitelaw ML, Pereira T, Gorman JJ, Ericson J, Peet DJ, Lendahl U, Poellinger L. Interaction with factor inhibiting HIF-1 defines an additional mode of cross-coupling between the Notch and hypoxia signaling pathways. *Proc Natl Acad Sci USA* 2008; **105**: 3368–3373.
159. Lee CW, Raskett CM, Prudovsky I, Altieri DC. Molecular dependence of estrogen receptor-negative breast cancer on a notch-survivin signaling axis. *Cancer Res* 2008; **68**: 5273–5281.
160. Tan EY, Campo L, Han C, Turley H, Pezzella F, Gatter KC, Harris AL, Fox SB. Cytoplasmic location of factor-inhibiting hypoxia-inducible factor is associated with an enhanced hypoxic response and a shorter survival in invasive breast cancer. *Breast Cancer Res* 2007; **9**: R89.
161. Imbert A, Eelkema R, Jordan S, Feiner H, Cowin P. Delta N89 beta-catenin induces precocious development, differentiation, and neoplasia in mammary gland. *J Cell Biol* 2001; **153**: 555–568.
162. Li Y, Welm B, Podsypanina K, Huang S, Chamorro M, Zhang X, Rowlands T, Egeblad M, Cowin P, Werb Z, Tan LK, Rosen JM, Varmus HE. Evidence that transgenes encoding components of the Wnt signaling pathway preferentially induce mammary cancers from progenitor cells. *Proc Natl Acad Sci USA* 2003; **100**: 15853–15858.
163. Tepera SB, McCrea PD, Rosen JM. A beta-catenin survival signal is required for normal lobular development in the mammary gland. *J Cell Sci* 2003; **116**: 1137–1149.
164. Flugel D, Gorlach A, Michiels C, Kietzmann T. Glycogen synthase kinase 3 phosphorylates hypoxia-inducible factor 1alpha and mediates its destabilization in a VHL-independent manner. *Mol Cell Biol* 2007; **27**: 3253–3265.

165. Kaidi A, Williams AC, Paraskeva C. Interaction between beta-catenin and HIF-1 promotes cellular adaptation to hypoxia. *Nat Cell Biol* 2007; **9**: 210–217.
166. Chitalia VC, Foy RL, Bachschmid MM, Zeng L, Panchenko MV, Zhou MI, Bharti A, Seldin DC, Lecker SH, Dominguez I, Cohen HT. Jade-1 inhibits Wnt signalling by ubiquitylating beta-catenin and mediates Wnt pathway inhibition by pVHL. *Nat Cell Biol* 2008; **10**: 1208–1216.
167. Comerford KM, Wallace TJ, Karhausen J, Louis NA, Montalto MC, Colgan SP. Hypoxia-inducible factor-1-dependent regulation of the multidrug resistance (MDR1) gene. *Cancer Res* 2002; **62**: 3387–3394.
168. Moeller BJ, Dreher MR, Rabbani ZN, Schroeder T, Cao Y, Li CY, Dewhirst MW. Pleiotropic effects of HIF-1 blockade on tumor radiosensitivity. *Cancer Cell* 2005; **8**: 99–110.
169. Williams KJ, Telfer BA, Xenaki D, Sheridan MR, Desbaillets I, Peters HJ, Honess D, Harris AL, Dachs GU, van der Kogel A, Stratford IJ. Enhanced response to radiotherapy in tumours deficient in the function of hypoxia-inducible factor-1. *Radiother Oncol* 2005; **75**: 89–98.
170. Song X, Liu X, Chi W, Liu Y, Wei L, Wang X, Yu J. Hypoxia-induced resistance to cisplatin and doxorubicin in non-small cell lung cancer is inhibited by silencing of HIF-1alpha gene. *Cancer Chemother Pharmacol* 2006; **58**: 776–784.
171. Hussein D, Estlin EJ, Dive C, Makin GW. Chronic hypoxia promotes hypoxia-inducible factor-1alpha-dependent resistance to etoposide and vincristine in neuroblastoma cells. *Mol Cancer Ther* 2006; **5**: 2241–2250.
172. Zeng L, Kizaka-Kondoh S, Itasaka S, Xie X, Inoue M, Tanimoto K, Shibuya K, Hiraoka M. Hypoxia inducible factor-1 influences sensitivity to paclitaxel of human lung cancer cell lines under normoxic conditions. *Cancer Sci* 2007; **98**: 1394–1401.
173. Hao J, Song X, Song B, Liu Y, Wei L, Wang X, Yu J. Effects of lentivirus-mediated HIF-1alpha knockdown on hypoxia-related cisplatin resistance and their dependence on p53 status in fibrosarcoma cells. *Cancer Gene Ther* 2008; **15**: 449–455.
174. Moeller BJ, Cao Y, Li CY, Dewhirst MW. Radiation activates HIF-1 to regulate vascular radiosensitivity in tumors: role of reoxygenation, free radicals, and stress granules. *Cancer Cell* 2004; **5**: 429–441.
175. Martinive P, Defresne F, Bouzin C, Saliez J, Lair F, Gregoire V, Michiels C, Dessy C, Feron O. Preconditioning of the tumor vasculature and tumor cells by intermittent hypoxia: implications for anticancer therapies. *Cancer Res* 2006; **66**: 11736–11744.
176. Kaanders JH, Wijffels KI, Marres HA, Ljungkvist AS, Pop LA, van den Hoogen FJ, de Wilde PC, Bussink J, Raleigh JA, van der Kogel AJ. Pimonidazole binding and tumor vascularity predict for treatment outcome in head and neck cancer. *Cancer Res* 2002; **62**: 7066–7074.
177. Eriksen JG, Overgaard J. Lack of prognostic and predictive value of CA IX in radiotherapy of squamous cell carcinoma of the head and neck with known modifiable hypoxia: an evaluation of the DAHANCA 5 study. *Radiother Oncol* 2007; **83**: 383–388.
178. Baumann M, Krause M, Hill R. Exploring the role of cancer stem cells in radioresistance. *Nat Rev Cancer* 2008; **8**: 545–554.
179. Phillips TM, McBride WH, Pajonk F. The response of CD24(-/low)/CD44+ breast cancer-initiating cells to radiation. *J Natl Cancer Inst* 2006; **98**: 1777–1785.
180. Wardman P. Electron transfer and oxidative stress as key factors in the design of drugs selectively active in hypoxia. *Curr Med Chem* 2001; **8**: 739–761.
181. Krishnamurthy P, Ross DD, Nakanishi T, Bailey-Dell K, Zhou S, Mercer KE, Sarkadi B, Sorrentino BP, Schuetz JD. The stem cell marker Bcrp/ABCG2 enhances hypoxic cell survival through interactions with heme. *J Biol Chem* 2004; **279**: 24218–24225.
182. Welm BE, Tepera SB, Venezia T, Graubert TA, Rosen JM, Goodell MA. Sca-1(pos) cells in the mouse mammary gland represent an enriched progenitor cell population. *Dev Biol* 2002; **245**: 42–56.
183. Zhou S, Schuetz JD, Bunting KD, Colapietro AM, Sampath J, Morris JJ, Lagutina I, Grosveld GC, Osawa M, Nakauchi H, Sorrentino BP. The ABC transporter Bcrp1/

ABCG2 is expressed in a wide variety of stem cells and is a molecular determinant of the side-population phenotype. *Nat Med* 2001; **7**: 1028–1034.

184. Cooper C, Liu GY, Niu YL, Santos S, Murphy LC, Watson PH. Intermittent hypoxia induces proteasome-dependent down-regulation of estrogen receptor alpha in human breast carcinoma. *Clin Cancer Res* 2004; **10**: 8720–8727.

185. Kurebayashi J, Otsuki T, Moriya T, Sonoo H. Hypoxia reduces hormone responsiveness of human breast cancer cells. *Jpn J Cancer Res* 2001; **92**: 1093–1101.

186. Kronblad A, Helczynska K, Nielsen NH, Pahlman E, Emdin S, Pahlman S, Landberg G. Regional cyclin D1 overexpression or hypoxia correlate inversely with heterogeneous oestrogen receptor-alpha expression in human breast cancer. *In Vivo* 2003; **17**: 311–318.

187. Johnston SR, Saccani-Jotti G, Smith IE, Salter J, Newby J, Coppen M, Ebbs SR, Dowsett M. Changes in estrogen receptor, progesterone receptor, and pS2 expression in tamoxifen-resistant human breast cancer. *Cancer Res* 1995; **55**: 3331–3338.

188. Frasor J, Danes JM, Komm B, Chang KC, Lyttle CR, Katzenellenbogen BS. Profiling of estrogen up- and down-regulated gene expression in human breast cancer cells: insights into gene networks and pathways underlying estrogenic control of proliferation and cell phenotype. *Endocrinology* 2003; **144**: 4562–4574.

189. Diaz-Gonzalez JA, Russell J, Rouzaut A, Gil-Bazo I, Montuenga L. Targeting hypoxia and angiogenesis through HIF-1alpha inhibition. *Cancer Biol Ther* 2005; **4**: 1055–1062.

190. Luwor RB, Lu Y, Li X, Mendelsohn J, Fan Z. The antiepidermal growth factor receptor monoclonal antibody cetuximab/C225 reduces hypoxia-inducible factor-1 alpha, leading to transcriptional inhibition of vascular endothelial growth factor expression. *Oncogene* 2005; **24**: 4433–4441.

191. Del Bufalo D, Ciuffreda L, Trisciuoglio D, Desideri M, Cognetti F, Zupi G, Milella M. Antiangiogenic potential of the Mammalian target of rapamycin inhibitor temsirolimus. *Cancer Res* 2006; **66**: 5549–5554.

192. Mosley JD, Poirier JT, Seachrist DD, Landis MD, Keri RA. Rapamycin inhibits multiple stages of c-Neu/ErbB2 induced tumor progression in a transgenic mouse model of HER2-positive breast cancer. *Mol Cancer Ther* 2007; **6**: 2188–2197.

193. Albert JM, Kim KW, Cao C, Lu B. Targeting the Akt/mammalian target of rapamycin pathway for radiosensitization of breast cancer. *Mol Cancer Ther* 2006; **5**: 1183–1189.

194. Blancher C, Moore JW, Robertson N, Harris AL. Effects of ras and von Hippel-Lindau (VHL) gene mutations on hypoxia-inducible factor (HIF)-1alpha, HIF-2alpha, and vascular endothelial growth factor expression and their regulation by the phosphatidylinositol 3′-kinase/Akt signaling pathway. *Cancer Res* 2001; **61**: 7349–7355.

195. http://clinicaltrials.gov

196. Buck E, Eyzaguirre A, Brown E, Petti F, McCormack S, Haley JD, Iwata KK, Gibson NW, Griffin G. Rapamycin synergizes with the epidermal growth factor receptor inhibitor erlotinib in non-small-cell lung, pancreatic, colon, and breast tumors. *Mol Cancer Ther* 2006; **5**: 2676–2684.

197. Wang LH, Chan JL, Li W. Rapamycin together with herceptin significantly increased anti-tumor efficacy compared to either alone in ErbB2 over expressing breast cancer cells. *Int J Cancer* 2007; **121**: 157–164.

198. Johnson AB, Denko N, Barton MC. Hypoxia induces a novel signature of chromatin modifications and global repression of transcription. *Mutat Res* 2008; **640**: 174–179.

199. Okazaki K, Maltepe E. Oxygen, epigenetics and stem cell fate. *Regen Med* 2006; **1**: 71–83.

200. Mie Lee Y, Kim SH, Kim HS, Jin Son M, Nakajima H, Jeong Kwon H, Kim KW. Inhibition of hypoxia-induced angiogenesis by FK228, a specific histone deacetylase inhibitor, via suppression of HIF-1alpha activity. *Biochem Biophys Res Commun* 2003; **300**: 241–246.

201. Qian DZ, Kachhap SK, Collis SJ, Verheul HM, Carducci MA, Atadja P, Pili R. Class II histone deacetylases are associated with VHL-independent regulation of hypoxia-inducible factor 1 alpha. *Cancer Res* 2006; **66**: 8814–8821.

202. Rapisarda A, Uranchimeg B, Sordet O, Pommier Y, Shoemaker RH, Melillo G. Topoisomerase I-mediated inhibition of hypoxia-inducible factor 1: mechanism and therapeutic implications. *Cancer Res* 2004; **64**: 1475–1482.

203. Wolff AC, O'Neill A, Kennedy MJ, Stewart JA, Gradishar WJ, Lord RS, 3rd, Davidson NE, Wood WC. Single-agent topotecan as first-line chemotherapy in women with metastatic breast cancer: final results of eastern cooperative oncology group trial E8193. *Clin Breast Cancer* 2005; **6**: 334–339.

204. Neckers L. Heat shock protein 90: the cancer chaperone. *J Biosci* 2007; **32**: 517–530.

205. Kamal A, Thao L, Sensintaffar J, Zhang L, Boehm MF, Fritz LC, Burrows FJ. A high-affinity conformation of Hsp90 confers tumour selectivity on Hsp90 inhibitors. *Nature* 2003; **425**: 407–410.

206. Isaacs JS, Jung YJ, Mimnaugh EG, Martinez A, Cuttitta F, Neckers LM. Hsp90 regulates a von Hippel Lindau-independent hypoxia-inducible factor-1 alpha-degradative pathway. *J Biol Chem* 2002; **277**: 29936–29944.

207. Liu YV, Baek JH, Zhang H, Diez R, Cole RN, Semenza GL. RACK1 competes with HSP90 for binding to HIF-1alpha and is required for O(2)-independent and HSP90 inhibitor-induced degradation of HIF-1alpha. *Mol Cell* 2007; **25**: 207–217.

208. Solit DB, Ivy SP, Kopil C, Sikorski R, Morris MJ, Slovin SF, Kelly WK, DeLaCruz A, Curley T, Heller G, Larson S, Schwartz L, Egorin MJ, Rosen N, Scher HI. Phase I trial of 17-allylamino-17-demethoxygeldanamycin in patients with advanced cancer. *Clin Cancer Res* 2007; **13**: 1775–1782.

209. Sawai A, Chandarlapaty S, Greulich H, Gonen M, Ye Q, Arteaga CL, Sellers W, Rosen N, Solit DB. Inhibition of Hsp90 down-regulates mutant epidermal growth factor receptor (EGFR) expression and sensitizes EGFR mutant tumors to paclitaxel. *Cancer Res* 2008; **68**: 589–596.

210. Pashtan I, Tsutsumi S, Wang S, Xu W, Neckers L. Targeting Hsp90 prevents escape of breast cancer cells from tyrosine kinase inhibition. *Cell Cycle* 2008; **7**: 2936–2941.

211. Chandarlapaty S, Sawai A, Ye Q, Scott A, Silinski M, Huang K, Fadden P, Partdrige J, Hall S, Steed P, Norton L, Rosen N, Solit DB. SNX2112, a synthetic heat shock protein 90 inhibitor, has potent antitumor activity against HER kinase-dependent cancers. *Clin Cancer Res* 2008; **14**: 240–248.

212. Yeo EJ, Chun YS, Cho YS, Kim J, Lee JC, Kim MS, Park JW. YC-1: a potential anticancer drug targeting hypoxia-inducible factor 1. *J Natl Cancer Inst* 2003; **95**: 516–525.

213. Shin DH, Kim JH, Jung YJ, Kim KE, Jeong JM, Chun YS, Park JW. Preclinical evaluation of YC-1, a HIF inhibitor, for the prevention of tumor spreading. *Cancer Lett* 2007; **255**: 107–116.

214. Hiraga T, Kizaka-Kondoh S, Hirota K, Hiraoka M, Yoneda T. Hypoxia and hypoxia-inducible factor-1 expression enhance osteolytic bone metastases of breast cancer. *Cancer Res* 2007; **67**: 4157–4163.

215. Chen CJ, Hsu MH, Huang LJ, Yamori T, Chung JG, Lee FY, Teng CM, Kuo SC. Anticancer mechanisms of YC-1 in human lung cancer cell line, NCI-H226. *Biochem Pharmacol* 2008; **75**: 360–368.

216. Welsh S, Williams R, Kirkpatrick L, Paine-Murrieta G, Powis G. Antitumor activity and pharmacodynamic properties of PX-478, an inhibitor of hypoxia-inducible factor-1alpha. *Mol Cancer Ther* 2004; **3**: 233–244.

217. Koh MY, Spivak-Kroizman T, Venturini S, Welsh S, Williams RR, Kirkpatrick DL, Powis G. Molecular mechanisms for the activity of PX-478, an antitumor inhibitor of the hypoxia-inducible factor-1alpha. *Mol Cancer Ther* 2008; **7**: 90–100.

218. Dervan PB, Doss RM, Marques MA. Programmable DNA binding oligomers for control of transcription. *Curr Med Chem Anticancer Agents* 2005; **5**: 373–387.

219. Olenyuk BZ, Zhang GJ, Klco JM, Nickols NG, Kaelin WG, Jr, Dervan PB. Inhibition of vascular endothelial growth factor with a sequence-specific hypoxia response element antagonist. *Proc Natl Acad Sci USA* 2004; **101**: 16768–16773.

220. Nickols NG, Jacobs CS, Farkas ME, Dervan PB. Modulating hypoxia-inducible transcription by disrupting the HIF-1-DNA interface. *ACS Chem Biol* 2007; **2**: 561–571.
221. Black MM, Kleiner IS, Bolker H. Glycolytic enzyme inhibitor therapy in human malignant neoplasia. *Cancer Res* 1949; **9**: 314–319.
222. Mohanti BK, Rath GK, Anantha N, Kannan V, Das BS, Chandramouli BA, Banerjee AK, Das S, Jena A, Ravichandran R, Sahi UP, Kumar R, Kapoor N, Kalia VK, Dwarakanath BS, Jain V. Improving cancer radiotherapy with 2-deoxy-D-glucose: phase I/II clinical trials on human cerebral gliomas. *Int J Radiat Oncol Biol Phys* 1996; **35**: 103–111.
223. Coleman MC, Asbury CR, Daniels D, Du J, Aykin-Burns N, Smith BJ, Li L, Spitz DR, Cullen JJ. 2-deoxy-D-glucose causes cytotoxicity, oxidative stress, and radiosensitization in pancreatic cancer. *Free Radic Biol Med* 2008; **44**: 322–331.
224. Simons AL, Ahmad IM, Mattson DM, Dornfeld KJ, Spitz DR. 2-Deoxy-D-glucose combined with cisplatin enhances cytotoxicity via metabolic oxidative stress in human head and neck cancer cells. *Cancer Res* 2007; **67**: 3364–3370.
225. Haga N, Naito M, Seimiya H, Tomida A, Dong J, Tsuruo T. 2-Deoxyglucose inhibits chemotherapeutic drug-induced apoptosis in human monocytic leukemia U937 cells with inhibition of c-Jun N-terminal kinase 1/stress-activated protein kinase activation. *Int J Cancer* 1998; **76**: 86–90.
226. Harada H, Kizaka-Kondoh S, Li G, Itasaka S, Shibuya K, Inoue M, Hiraoka M. Significance of HIF-1-active cells in angiogenesis and radioresistance. *Oncogene* 2007; **26**(54): 7508–7516.
227. Perret GY, Crepin M. New pharmacological strategies against metastatic spread. *Fundam Clin Pharmacol* 2008; **22**: 465–492.
228. Raleigh JA, Koch CJ. Importance of thiols in the reductive binding of 2-nitroimidazoles to macromolecules. *Biochem Pharmacol* 1990; **40**: 2457–2464.

Cancer Stem Cells: Potential Mediators of Therapeutic Resistance and Novel Targets of Anti-cancer Treatments

Hong Yan, Jichao Qin, and Dean G. Tang

1 Introduction

Over the last decade, anti-cancer therapies (chemotherapy and radiation, hormonal, neoadjuvant, and combinatorial therapies) have prolonged the lives of cancer patients. However, present cancer therapies fail in a high percentage of cases due to an incomplete elimination of the tumor cells, resulting in relapse and metastasis of the tumor. The vast majority of cancer-related deaths are due to metastatic tumor growth that impairs the function of vital organ(s). Thus, cancer relapse and metastasis are the major challenges in fighting cancer.

Metastasis is an inefficient process in that <1% of the disseminated cancer cells are able to form clinically relevant macrometastases [1]. At present, this inefficiency is mostly explained in terms of the need for cancer cells to find the proper microenvironment. However, a hypothesis used to explain tumor formation, i.e., the cancer stem cell (CSC) hypothesis, might provide an alternative explanation for this inefficiency [2–5]. Application of the CSC hypothesis to metastasis suggests that this rare subset of cells within a primary tumor that are capable of re-initiating growth and forming metastasis in distant sites may in fact be CSCs.

Cancer relapse and metastasis often appear in patients after apparent successful initial therapy and recovery or after a long disease-free period. In some cases, the disease-free period is termed as "cancer dormancy," which is defined as the long latency period that occurs in some patients between initial treatment and clinical evidence of relapse and metastasis [6]. Clinically, cancer dormancy may be one of the major reasons of tumor recurrence and metastasis.

D.G. Tang (✉)

Department of Carcinogenesis, University of Texas M.D Anderson Cancer Center, Science Park-Research Division, 1808 Park Rd. 1C, Smithville, TX 78957; Program in Molecular Carcinogenesis, Graduate School of Biomedical Sciences (GSBS), The University of Texas Health Science Center, Houston, TX 77030, USA e-mail: dtang@mdanderson.org

Y. Lu, R.I. Mahato (eds.), *Pharmaceutical Perspectives of Cancer Therapeutics*, DOI 10.1007/978-1-4419-0131-6_17, © Springer Science+Business Media, LLC 2009

Two possible mechanisms may contribute to tumor dormancy. One is cancer mass dormancy in which some tumor cells proliferate while others undergo apoptosis, resulting in a clinically undetectable tumor mass for a long time [7, 8]. The other mechanism is attributable to the residual cancer cells that have undergone cell-cycle arrest, quiescence, or cell dormancy [9]. Normal adult stem cells (SCs) generally proliferate slowly and are even kept quiescent (or dormant) in their niche but can be "awaken" to contribute to tissue regeneration [10–12]. CSCs, responsible for initiating tumor and maintaining tumor homeostasis, might be endowed with some properties of their normal counterparts [13, 14]. That is to say, CSCs may also proliferate slowly or are kept quiescent in their niche although solid data are still absent. Collectively, CSCs may be the culprits of cancer dormancy that leads to relapse and metastasis.

In this chapter, we review the current definition of CSCs and several methods that can be used to prospectively identify putative CSCs and study their niche requirement. Then we present traditional view of chemoresistance and review newly emerged evidence that CSCs may be naturally resistant to therapy. Finally, novel potential therapeutic strategies targeting CSCs and their niches are introduced.

2 Cancer Stem Cells

2.1 Definition

In 1937, Furth and Kahn provided the first quantitative assessment of the frequency of the malignant cells in leukemia cell lines that could maintain the hematopoietic tumor in mice and the results indicated that not all of the cells could initiate tumor. Thus, the CSC principle was first introduced. Several studies in 1960s and 1970s elegantly showed the functional heterogeneity in tumors in that only a small subset of tumor cells can re-initiate tumor in vivo, and these studies officially introduced the CSC concept [15–18].

Studies in leukemia first provided compelling evidence for the existence of a putative CSC subpopulation or a hierarchical model of cancer [19]. By now, putative CSCs have been reported in multiple solid tumors including breast cancer, medulloblastoma, glioblastoma, colon cancer, pancreatic cancer, liver cancer, melanoma, and ovarian cancer (see Table 1). The observations that leukemic SCs appear to display a similar cell surface phenotype to the normal hematopoietic SCs (HSCs) suggest that CSCs may originate from their normal counterpart [20]. Emerging data show that CSCs may also derive from committed progenitors and even differentiated cells [21–23]. Together, CSCs may derive from stem cells that have acquired tumorigenic capacity or from committed progenitors or even differentiated cells that have acquired self-renewal and tumorigenic properties.

Table 1 CSC studies in human solid tumors (2003–2008)

Tumor type	Samples	Marker	Mice	Transplantation	Results	References
Breast cancer	9 (1 primary; 8 met.)	CD44+CD24−/to ESA+ FACS	NOD/SCID mice pretreated with VP16	Mammary fat pad	>50-fold enrichment	1
Breast cancer	4 xenotransplants (2 primary; 2 met.)	ALDH+ FACS	NOD/SCID mice	Humanized mammary fat pad	500 ALDH+ cells generate T; 20 ALDH+CD44+CD24− Lin− cells	2
Brain tumors	7 primary tumors	CD133+ (MACS)	6–8 wk NOD/SCID	Intracranial injection	CD133+ more tumorigenic	3
Prostate cancer	7 primary tumors	CD44+ α2β1hi CD133+ (MACS)	No in vivo tumor	Experiments were done	Positive cells are more clonogenic	4
Colon cancer	17 (6 primary, 10 liver, and 1 retroperitoneal met.)	CD133+ (double MACS)	8 wk NOD/SCID irradiated	Renal capsule	1 CSC/57,000 T. cells 1 CSC/262 CD133+ cells	5
Colon cancer	19 primary (5 Dukes A)	CD133+ (FACS or MACS)	SCID	Subcutaneous	3000 CD133+ cells generate T	6
Colon cancer	21 primary CRC	CD133+ (double MACS)	5–6 wk nude mice	Subcutaneous	2500 CD133+ cells generate T 25 CD133+-derived spheres generate T	7
Colon cancer	2 primary CRC, 6 xeno	EpCAMCD166+CD44+ (FACS)	6–8 wk NOD/SCID	Subcutaneous	150 EpCAMCD166+CD44+ cells generate T	8
Pancreatic cancer	10 (2 primary; 2 met.)	CD44+CD24-ESA+ (FACS)	NOD/SCID	Subcutaneous + orthotopic	>100-fold enrichment	9
Pancreatic cancer	11 (6 met.); sorting for L3.6pl metastatic line	CD133+ (MACS) CD133+CXCR4+ (FACS)	8–12 wk nude mice	Orthotopic	500 CD133+ cells generate T The CD133+CXCR4+ pop. Mediates met.	10
Head and Neck	25 primary (sorting for 9, 3 recurrences)	CD44+Lin−(FACS)	NOD/SCID and Rag2 mice	Subcutaneous	5,000 CD44+Lin− cells generate T	11

Table 1 (continued)

Tumor type	Samples	Marker	Mice	Transplantation	Results	References
Melanoma	7 (1 primary; 4 LN, and 2 visceral met.)	ABCB5$^+$ (MACS)	NOD/SCID mice	Subcutaneous	1 MMIC/1 million bulk T cells; 1st xeno: 1 MMIC/160,000 ABCB5$^+$ cells, 2^{ary} xeno: 1 MMIC/120,000 ABCB5$^+$ cells	12
Lung cancer	19 (18 primary, 1, met)	CD133$^+$ (FACS)	4 wk SCID or nude mice	Subcutaneous	10^4 CD133$^+$ cells generate T	13
Liver cancer	30 primary (2 pre-cancerous)	CD133$^-$CD90$^+$ (MACS)	SCID/Beige mice	Orthotopic	CD45$^-$ CD90$^+$ more tumorigenic	14
Ovarian cancer	2 xenograft (from sphere) B primary (1 fresh 2 cultured to spheroid)	CD44$^+$ CD117$^+$ (FACS)	3–4 wk nude mice	Subcutaneous	CD44$^+$ CD117$^+$ more tumorigenic	15

1. Al-Hajj M, et al. PNAS 2003; 100:3983–8.
2. Ginestier C et al. Cell Stom cell 2007; 1:555–67.
3. Singh SK, et al. Nature 2004; 432:396–401.
4. Collins AT, et al. Cancer Res 2005; 65:10946–51.
5. O' Brien CA, et al. Cells Stem Cell 2007; 1:389–402.
6. Ricci-vitiani L, et al. Nature 2007; 445:111–5.
7. Todaro M et al. Cell Stem Cell 2007: 1–389–402.
8. Dalerba P et al. PNAS 2007; 104:10158–63.
9. Li C et al. Cancer Res. 2007; 67:1030–7.
10. Hemann PC et al. Cell 2007; 1:313–32.
11. Prince ME et al. PNAS 2007; 104:973–8.
12. Schatton T, et al. Nature 2008; 451:345–9.
13. Eramo A et al. Cell Death Differ, 2008; 15:504–14.
14. Yang ZF et al. Cancer Cell 2008; 13:153–66.
15. Zhang S et al. Cancer Res. 2008; 68:4311–20.

How should a CSC be defined? A CSC is a cell within a tumor that possesses the capacity to self-renew and to cause the heterogeneous lineages of cancer cells that comprise the tumor, and the regenerated tumors can be serially xenotransplanted [20, 24]. Strictly speaking, none of the CSCs thus far reported can be truly classified as CSCs and should, more appropriately, be called "tumor-reinitiating cells," "tumorigenic cells," or "putative CSCs." In reality, it will be very difficult to identify a tumorigenic cell that can fulfill the strict definition of CSCs mentioned above. First, a tumor, especially a solid tumor, is made of numerous cell types. To expect one cell or even a population of cells, when transplanted into a foreign host (i.e., mice) in an exotic environment, to fully reconstitute an original patient tumor in its complete composition begs tremendous imagination and will be essentially impossible to prove. Second, when such experiments are actually done, the best one can do is to co-inject the putative tumorigenic cell population with stromal cells (e.g., fibroblasts) in an extracellular matrix (e.g., matrigel or collagen gel) into an "orthotopic" animal site such as brain, mammary fat pad, or prostate lobes. These so-called orthotopic sites are considerably different from their human counterparts and tumor establishment would inevitably require the recruitment of various host (i.e., mouse) cells by the tumor-reinitiating cells. One can be certain that such "reconstituted" tumors could never be the same as the original patient tumors. Third, during the purification process, the majority of cells are often discarded to obtain marker-positive and marker-negative populations. These discarded cells would be important in the original tumor composition but they would be very difficult to reconstitute in tumor development assays. Altogether, one can say, at the best, that the experimental tumor reconstituted from the presumptive CSCs histologically "resembles" the patient tumor [24].

2.2 Identification

2.2.1 Marker-Based Analysis

This is the most widely used and also the most practical approach. A variety of adult tissue SCs are found to express relatively specific markers, which can be cell surface or intracellular (e.g., nuclear and cytoskeletal). Interestingly, CSCs seem to express various cell surface markers such as CD44 and/or CD133 that identify their normal counterparts [25], which allows a relatively simple enrichment procedure by utilizing either flow cytometry-based cell sorting or microbeads-based affinity purification. For intracellular markers such as a nuclear or cytoskeletal protein, a gene promoter-driven reporter construct such as GFP-tagged retroviral or lentiviral vector system can be developed to track down and purify putative (cancer) SCs [26]. Alternatively, transgenic animal models can be made by knocking in the gene promoter-driven reporter (GFP, LacZ, etc.) followed by further flow cytometry purification [27]. The disadvantages associated with using predetermined marker(s) to identify CSCs include that the marker proteins frequently change during cell development in vivo and cell preparation in vitro and that in many cases the functions of these markers in both normal SCs and stem-like cancer cells are unclear.

2.2.2 Side Population (SP) Analysis

Mouse HSCs are found to preferentially express multidrug resistance (MDR) family proteins such as MDR1 and other membrane transporters such as ABCG2 (also called breast cancer resistance protein (BCRP)) [28]. This property allows the HSCs, in an experimental setting, to pump out the Hoechst 33342 dye. Therefore, on dual-wavelength flow cytometry, the CSC-enriched cell population is identified as a side or tail Hoechst^{dim} population at the lower left quadrant of the histogram. By contrast, the major population of cells is displayed as Hoechst^{hi} cells called as non-SP or main population [29, 30]. Recent work reveals that multiple adult tissue SCs can also be enriched by the SP protocol and that the SP from several cancer types are also enriched in stem-like cancer cells [31, 32]. The major advantage of this technique when used to identify putative CSCs is its simplicity and independence of predetermined markers. The potential problems associated with the technique are that chronic accumulation of Hoechst dye in non-SP cells may be cytotoxic (thus invalidating suitable controls) and that SP cells isolated from some normal tissues or tumors seem to be enriched in progenitor cells rather than SCs.

2.2.3 Sphere Formation Assays

Many normal SCs such as neural, hematopoietic, and mammary SCs, when maintained under special culture conditions, can form three-dimensional spheres, which are like mini-organs that can differentiate into multiple cell types. Putative CSCs identified in brain and prostate tumors as well as in melanoma also have the ability to form anchorage-independent spheres [24, 33, 34]. The advantage of using sphere-forming assays to enrich for CSC is its initial independence of specific markers. The disadvantages include the empirical nature of finding culture conditions suitable for sphere formation and the necessity of finding ways later to identify and purify the real CSCs from the spheres.

2.2.4 Label-Retaining Properties

Mammary SCs and normal keratinocyte SCs in interfollicular epidermis and hair follicle bulges are quiescent and can be identified with a pulse label with the thymidine analog bromodeoxyuridine (BrdU) or H2B-GFP followed by a long-term "chase" (i.e., removal of the label). Fast proliferating progenitor cells dilute out the BrdU label after several cell divisions whereas the slow-dividing SCs retain BrdU and are thus identified as "label-retaining cells (LRCs)" by either immunohistochemistry or flow cytometry analysis [13, 35]. Interestingly, the LRCs in human breast tumors coexpress mammary epithelial SC markers and seem to have certain SC properties [36]. Human PCa [37] and nasophar-yngeal carcinomas [38] also possess slow-cycling LRCs. The main challenge of this approach is that the LRCs have to be purified out live to show they indeed represent slow-cycling CSCs, which generally is difficult to do without a suitable genetic-tracking system. Furthermore, recent studies in HSCs suggest that not all LRCs may represent SCs [39]. On the other hand, the authors in this latter study [39] failed to show whether all the cells had been labeled with BrdU when the chase period began, as a very recent study shows that the H2B-GFP strategy labels a higher percentage of cells than using BrdU and that the label-retaining ovarian surface epithelial cells indeed possess certain SC properties [40].

2.2.5 Clonal Assay

The study in primary human keratinocytes has revealed cellular heterogeneity with respect to their ability to form a clone related to different cell sizes – small cells could form clones but large cells would undergo terminal differentiation [41]. Further work has shown that three different types of clones possess different proliferative capacities [42]. The holoclone contains tightly packed small cells with greatest replicative capacity. In contrast, the paraclone is a loosely packed clone of large cells with a short replicative life span. The third type of clone, the meroclone, contains a mixture of cells of different prolifera-tive potential and is a transitional stage between the holoclone and the para-clone [42].

Similar to primary keratinocytes, several head and neck cancer-derived cells can also form three different types of clone in culture [43]. More importantly, the holoclones but not paraclones highly express some stem cell-associated molecules, suggesting that holoclones might contain self-renewing stem-like cells [24, 43]. Our work, in several long-cultured cell lines of prostate, breast, and other cancer cells, confirmed that only a small fraction of cells can form holoclone in culture [24]. Our subsequent study in PC3 cells has revealed that holoclones are enriched for potential CSCs that can initiate serially transplan-table tumors [44].

2.3 CSC Niche

Normal SCs are found to harbor in a specialized microenvironment called the stem cell "niche", which contains capillaries, vascular endothelial cells, peri-cytes, and the fibrous proteins of the extracellular matrix. Other stromal cells, immune cells, and nerves may also be present in the niche [45]. Stimuli from the niche as well as signals from SCs themselves and from outside of niche, together, establish a regulatory network to balance between SC self-renewal and differ-entiation [46]. Under physiological conditions, the niche provides a tight con-trol over proliferation, typically maintaining cells in G0 and/or balancing proliferation and apoptosis such that the SC population remains at a constant size [13, 47, 48]. Recent investigations in HSCs have uncovered two distinct niches, an osteoblast niche and a vascular niche [49, 50]. Osteoblasts lining the endosteal surface of the bone may function as the "quiescent or dormant niche", whereas the endothelial cells lining the bone marrow (BM) and spleen sinusoids may comprise the "activated or vascular niche" that regulates HSC expansion and differentiation.

There has been some controversy over whether or not CSCs actually require specific niches. A recent study indicates that specialized microenvironments of BM (i.e., periendosteal region) seem to be required for the homing and engraftment of not only normal HSCs but also leukemic SCs [51]. CD133$^+$ brain CSCs also seem to "live" in a vascular niche that secretes factors that promote their long-term growth and self-renewal [52]. Interestingly, CSCs themselves not only are dependent on factors produced by the vasculature to maintain self-renewal and long-term growth but also generate vascular epidermal growth factor (VEGF) and other factors to induce angiogenesis to promote vascular formation [52]. Another recent study also reveals that the CD133$^+$ glioma SCs secrete more VEGF to enhance vascular formation compared to bulk cells [53]. In this case, CSCs and angiogenesis can positively feedback each other to promote tumor development and maintenance.

Intriguingly, normal SC niches may also be involved in the metastatic process, as tumor cells disseminated from the primary tumor often migrate and seed microanatomical areas characteristically occupied by somatic SCs [46]. Disseminated CSCs might acquire responsiveness to certain secreted niche signals and thus initiate metastasis from these supportive microenvironments distant from the site of primary tumor [54]. The tumor microenvironment in a secondary organ may be considered as a "metastatic niche." It is believed that the metastatic niche either passively supports tumor development or facilitates tumor formation. It has also been hypothesized that CSCs may remain dormant until activated by "appropriate" signaling from the microenvironment [55, 56]. Taken together, the potential role of the CSC niche in controlling the CSC fate provides some support for the theory that targeting the unique aberrant microenvironment of CSCs may represent a critical aspect of effective cancer therapy.

3 Chemotherapy and Drug Resistance

Traditional chemotherapeutic strategies, on the assumption that the majority of the cells within tumor are actively proliferating, have used a variety of drugs and hormonal agents that interfere with the basic cellular machinery (e.g., DNA synthesis and replication, cell cycle, and cytoskeleton) [57]. However, because cancer cells share many properties with their normal counterparts, the serious, sometimes life-threatening, side effects that arise from toxicities to sensitive normal cells limit the efficacy of cytotoxic chemotherapy [58]. Improved understanding of the molecular alterations present in the cancer cells has enabled the development of a more cancer-specific "targeted therapy" for some types of cancer [57]. Such therapeutics aim at selectively targeting proliferating cancer cells and leaving normal cells untouched, thereby reducing the common side effects. Nevertheless, all therapeutics, either targeted or non-targeted, are designed to ablate proliferating cancer cells [58], which may lead to the possibility of tumor recurrence or drug resistance due to the presence of quiescent cells or slow-dividing cells in the tumor.

Since chemotherapy became one of the main therapeutic strategies in cancer treatment, resistance has often followed. A number of studies indicate that there are three major mechanisms of drug resistance in cells: first, decreased uptake of water-soluble drugs such as folate antagonists, nucleoside analogs, and cisplatin, which require transporters to enter cells; second, various changes in cells that affect the capacity of cytotoxic drugs to kill cells, including alterations in cell cycle, increased repair of DNA damage, reduced apoptosis, and altered metabolism of drugs; and third, increased energy-dependent efflux of hydrophobic drugs that can easily enter the cells by diffusion through the plasma membrane [59]. Of these mechanisms, the one that is most commonly encountered is the increased efflux of a broad class of hydrophobic cytotoxic drugs, mediated by energy-dependent transporters, known as ATP-binding cassette (ABC) transporters, which includes seven subfamilies labeled A–G [60–62].

Interestingly, resistance occurs not only to traditional chemotherapeutic drugs but also to targeted therapeutics such as gefitinib (epidermal growth factor receptor or EGFR inhibitor), imatinib (an inhibitor of translocated BCR-ABL kinase in chronic myelogenous leukemia), and tamoxifen (targeting the estrogen receptor or ER in breast cancer) [63–65].

How do cancer cells acquire resistance to chemotherapy? Are there cells in the tumor, e.g., quiescent or slow-dividing cells that are naturally resistant to chemotherapy? Or the proliferating cells targeted by anti-cancer drugs acquire genetic changes to be resistant? The CSC hypothesis may bring us new insight on these important questions related to drug resistance.

4 CSCs in Chemoresistance and Radioresistance

Based on the CSC hypothesis, CSCs may be naturally resistant to therapeutic agents. First, most chemodrugs target proliferating cells while CSCs are thought to be generally quiescent; therefore, CSCs will be mostly spared of drugs. Solid experimental data in support of this contention are yet to be provided. Second, the putative CSC niche may protect CSCs from damage during therapeutic treatment. Third, the ABC transporters that pump out drugs are preferentially expressed in CSCs, as described above for the SP cells. Many studies have shown that the SP phenotype is mediated by MDR proteins and that the SP tumor cells confer high drug efflux capacity [66–68]. A small population of stem-like cells in small-cell lung carcinoma has also showed coexpression of CD44 and multidrug resistance protein, MDR1, suggesting that CSCs may be drug-resistant [69]. Furthermore, one recent study indicates that melanoma cells positive for ABCB5 are much more tumorigenic than the corresponding ABCB5$^-$ cells and that ABCB5 actually mediates drug resistance in melanoma, suggesting that the ABCB5$^+$ cells may represent melanoma stem cells [70]. Fourth, chemodrugs often exert their effects by eliciting cancer cell apoptosis, and overexpression of anti-apoptotic molecules such as Bcl-2 has been observed in some CSC populations [71]. Indeed, prospectively purified CSCs from human colon cancer specimen are more resistant to apoptosis than bulk cells [72]. Fifth, SCs are also thought to be more resistant to DNA-damaging agents than differentiated cells because of their ability to undergo asynchronous DNA synthesis and the enhanced capacity for DNA repair. During asynchronous DNA synthesis, the parental "immortal" DNA strand always segregates with the new SC rather than with the differentiating progeny, thus helping to protect the SC population from DNA damage [73–75]. Similarly, CSCs seem to be more resistant to DNA-damaging agents [76, 77].

Several lines of evidence indicate that CSCs may be intrinsically drug-resistant. For example, putative CSCs are found to contribute to cisplatin resistance in a Brca1/p53 mutant mouse mammary tumor model [78]. In glioblastoma, the CD133$^+$ CSCs demonstrate significant resistance to chemotherapeutic agents including teozolomide, carboplatin, paclitaxel, and etoposide in vitro [79]. In breast cancer xenografts, after several cycles of administering anti-cancer drugs to mice, the percentage of CD44$^+$CD24$^-$ CSC population increases significantly. Furthermore, these cells exhibit much higher clonogenic and tumorigenic capacity than the parental cells [38]. Importantly, breast CSCs are enriched in breast cancer patients after administering chemotherapy [38].

Besides being "naturally" resistant to therapeutics, some CSCs may also acquire further resistance through accumulating mutations following exposure, producing a population of multidrug-resistant tumor cells that can be found in many cancer patients with recurrent diseases [80].

5 Novel Cancer Therapies by Targeting CSCs and Their Microenvironment

One of the major questions raised by CSC hypothesis is whether or not current therapies are in fact targeting the right cells. As discussed above, it has been speculated that CSCs have the ability to avoid or resist current cancer therapies, although this has yet to be definitively proven in the clinical setting. In addition, CSCs may play an important role in tumor metastasis and dormancy. So, the idea that cancers could be effectively treated by selectively targeting CSCs and their microenvironmental niche, which contributes to self-renewal of these cells, has attracted tremendous clinical interest [81].

5.1 CSC-Targeted Therapy

As molecular mediators of therapeutic resistance in CSCs gradually become established, developing clinically useful inhibitors to target these pathways will be correspondingly prioritized.

5.1.1 Anti-ABC Transporters

A connection between CSCs and drug resistance is thought to exist due to the expression of ABC transporters. Inhibition of ABC transporter activity should hinder CSC drug resistance and make CSCs more sensitive to chemotherapeutics. A number of inhibitors targeting ABCB1 including verapamil, cyclosporine, PSC833, and VX710 have been identified [80, 82]. However, negative results have been observed in clinical trials of these drugs possibly because other transporters, particularly ABCG2, also need to be efficiently inhibited to achieve a significant effect in the clinic. At present, tariquidar, effective against ABCB1 and ABCG2, is being tested, but some phase III clinical trials were terminated early owing to an increased incidence of adverse effects [83].

Selective downregulation of MDR genes in cancer cells is an emerging approach in therapeutics. Technologies that enable the targeted regulation of genes, including antisense oligonucleotides, hammerhead ribozymes, and short-interfering RNA, have produced mixed results. However, sufficient downregulation of MDR genes such as MDR1 has proved difficult to attain and the safe delivery of constructs to cancer cells in vivo remains a challenges [59]. Interestingly, recent studies have revealed the possibility of using the agents targeting the EGFR, Hedgehog, Wnt/β-catenin, and/or Notch cascades to inhibit the ABC multidrug efflux transporters and/or eliminate the CSCs [84–90]. For instance, in the cyclopamine treatment for $CD44^+$ PC3 metastatic prostate cancer cells, a decrease of the expression levels of MDR1/ABCB1 and BCRP/ABCG2 was observed, suggesting that Hedgehog signaling activity may contribute to MDR expression in these cancer cells [89].

Since cancers rely on several mechanisms to escape drugs, ABC transporter inhibitors will have to be combined with other strategies to achieve efficient elimination of CSCs in vivo.

5.1.2 Inhibiting DNA Repair Capacity

CSCs may efficiently repair their DNA to escape from DNA damage, raising the possibility that inhibiting DNA repair capacity of CSCs could be an effective strategy to sensitize CSC to current therapy. Recent studies in human glioblastomas have shown that checkpoint kinase 1 (Chk1) and checkpoint kinase 2 (Chk2) play a key role in $CD133^+$ glioma stem cell survival to radiation by efficiently repairing damaged DNA; consequently, inhibition of Chk1/Chk2 kinases renders these CSCs less resistant to radiation [77]. These observations suggest that selective suppression of DNA repair mechanisms may help overcome radioresistance of CSCs.

5.1.3 Promoting Apoptosis

Although tumor cell death is controlled by several mechanisms, one of the dominant mechanisms involves mitochondria [91]. It is thus rational to target the mitochondria for therapeutic purposes due to its critical role in the regulation of apoptosis. One potential target is the mitochondrial permeability transition pore (MPTP), the most significant component of which appears to be the peripheral benzodiazepine receptor known as the translocator protein [92]. Various ligands for the translocator protein have shown both anti-proliferative and pro-apoptotic activity or may act as chemo-sensitizers via modulation of MPTP [93–95].

In addition to mitochondria, other prosurvival signaling pathways such as nuclear factor kappa B (NFκB) and BCL-2 family proteins may also become targets for cancer therapy as CSCs generally have higher activities or expressions of these pathways.

5.1.4 Sensitizing Dormant CSCs to Anti-proliferative Agents

Many types of cancer can persist as "minimal residual disease," and putative metastasis SCs can remain dormant for years, but are re-activated by as-yet unknown mechanisms, often leading to rapid disease progression [96]. One possible strategy to sensitize dormant CSCs to anti-proliferative agents would be to promote their cell-cycle entry using cytokines known to activate normal SCs. For example, imatinib treatment of chronic myelogenous leukemia (CML) CSCs intermittently activated with granulocyte-colony stimulating factor (G-CSF) in vitro resulted in an enhanced efficacy of CML–CSC elimination compared with treatment using imatinib alone [97].

However, to utilize this strategy in the clinic, new markers have to be developed to determine whether a patient has dormant disseminated disease. At present, most of the markers inform about the recurrence of the disease (e.g., uPAR, ErbB2) rather than the state of tumor cell dormancy [98]. To achieve this goal it will be important to enhance collaborations between basic research and clinical labs to test the markers of dormancy identified in experimental models in samples from bone marrow, lymph nodes, and circulating tumor cells (CTCs) [98]. These will be important for staging of cancer and for developing novel therapeutic targets.

5.1.5 Inducing CSCs into Dormancy

Therapies aimed at inducing dormancy may help overcome conventional drug resistance that is based on the ability of drugs to induce cell killing. Thus, reprogramming cancer cells into a growth arrest would allow converting the disease that would be otherwise untreatable, into a chronic asymptomatic condition. Combination of mitogenic signaling inhibitors (e.g., MEK, MET,

EGFR, IGFR inhibitors) with activators of stress pathways (e.g., p38, JNK) may induce reprogramming of tumor cells into dormancy [99].

5.1.6 Promoting Differentiation of CSCs

The tumorigenic potential of CSCs generally correlates with their capacity to undergo long-term self-renewal [46]. Self-renewal activity is inversely correlated to differentiation, raising the possibility that enforced differentiation of CSCs could be an effective strategy to decrease or eliminate CSCs activity. This type of therapeutic strategy has been used to treat hematological malignancies such as leukemia, where the cancer-initiating cells and the cellular differentiation hierarchy are well characterized [100, 101]. The first differentiation agent successful in the clinic was all-trans-retinoic acid (ATRA) in the treatment of acute promyelocytic leukemia (APL). This strategy has recently been reported in human glioblastoma, where it was shown that bone morphogenetic proteins (BMPs) promote the differentiation of not only normal neural progenitors, but also of CD133$^+$ glioma SCs toward a more mature astrocyte fate [102]. These findings should lead to renewed interest in devising therapies that promote the differentiation of cancer (stem) cells.

Although differentiation therapy does not kill cancer cells, it does have the potential to restrain their self-renewal capacity and perhaps increase the efficacy of conventional therapies, which are often most effective on differentiated cells. Furthermore, differentiation agents often have less toxicity than conventional chemotherapies [103, 104].

5.2 CSC Niche-Targeted Therapy

In light of the central role of niche in maintaining quiescence and self-renewal of CSCs, strategies for reduction of the SC population must take into account the importance of targeting niche.

HSCs need hypoxic niche to protect them from oxidative stress because reactive oxygen species induce p38-MAPK-mediated proliferation leading to HSC exhaustion [105]. Some CSCs may also be concealed in hypoxic microenvironments, which are common in solid tumors. Given that hypoxia seems to be important in maintaining CSCs, this provides an opportunity for tumor-selective therapy. Hypoxia-inducible factor 1 (HIF-1) is stabilized under hypoxic conditions and promotes survival of cancer cells in hypoxic niches, so several strategies to inactivate HIF-1 are currently under investigation at the preclinical level [106, 107].

Other niches comprising reticular and endothelial cells known to secrete factors that promote self-renewal and survival have been found in close association with the vasculature [108]. Since the niche is dependent on the presence of an efficient blood supply, one therapeutic strategy would be to target the niche endothelium. Clinical use of anti-angiogenic agents has accelerated in recent years, with more than 40 agents currently in clinical trials for various types of cancers [109]. Anti-VEGF monoclonal antibody, bevacizumab, has shown promise as part of a combination therapy regimen in several advanced cancers, including colon cancer [110] and glioblastoma [111]. Moreover, several agents that were originally developed to block EGFR (erlotinib, cetuximab, and vandetanib) have recently been shown to have an inhibitory effect on angiogenesis by blocking VEGFR or by inhibiting pro-angiogenic protein secretion [109].

Furthermore, several lines of evidence have revealed the potential benefit of targeting the tumor-specific vascular precursor cells including the circulating VEGFR-2^+ endothelial progenitor cells (EPCs) and VEGFR-1^+ pleural mesothelial cells (PMC), which may be recruited to the activated stromal compartment in the primary and secondary neoplasms, for preventing and/or counteracting the neovascularization process associated with tumor development [112–115]. More particularly, it has been shown that the use of BM-derived EPCs engineered to express an anti-angiogenic gene product, a soluble truncated form of VEGFR-2, may impair tumor growth in vivo [115].

There are several theories regarding the clinical mechanisms of anti-angiogenic drug benefit. One possibility is that anti-angiogenics simply destroy the vascular structure of the tumor, promoting profound tumor hypoxia and nutrient deprivation. Alternatively, anti-angiogenics may transiently normalize the tumor vasculature increasing oxygen and drug delivery [116]. In addition, it seems that some cancers may express VEGF receptors as well, raising the possibility that anti-VEGF therapies actually have direct anti-tumor effects.

Cell adhesion molecule CD44 is expressed on both normal and leukemic SCs and mediates adhesive interactions with the endosteal BM niche by binding to various ligands [117]. Therefore, it is possible to separate the leukemic SCs from its microenvironment by anti-CD44 therapy. In support, monoclonal antibody ligation of the CD44 effectively eliminated AML SCs derived from some patients [118]. Also, treatment of prostate and breast cancer cell lines with an siRNA against CD44 can decrease cancer cell adhesion to BM endothelial cells [119].

It is well known that signaling molecules such as Hedgehog, Wnt, BMP, fibroblast growth factor (FGF), and Notch-1 play important roles in niche control of cell fate determination [120], making it possible to develop novel cancer therapeutics by targeting these signaling pathways. Some studies have shown that the Hedgehog and Notch-1 signaling activities can be attenuated via Hedgehog inhibitor cyclopamine and Notch-1 inhibitor GSI, respectively [86, 121].

5.3 Combination Therapy Strategy

A few considerations make combination therapy necessary in clinic. First, due to inherent genomic instability, differentiated cancer cells may acquire SC phenotypes, and also possibly acquire resistance to therapeutics. Thus, eradication of the tumor will likely be achieved only by successful targeting of all cancer cells. Furthermore, most of CSC- or niche-targeted therapies aim at sensitizing CSCs to current therapy or inhibiting CSC activity including anti-apoptosis and chemoresistance to cytotoxic drugs, not killing CSCs directly. Finally, the fact the tumor cells survive anti-tumor therapeutics via variegated mechanisms suggests that single targeting therapy would not effectively eradicate the disease.

In one word, in order to eliminate CSCs and cure cancer, it seems reasonable that combining traditional therapy with one or several agents that sensitize CSCs or target CSC niche would be a good approach to rationally advance the treatment of tumors. For example, depletion of blood vessels by anti-VEGF therapy could cause a dramatic reduction in the number of medulloblastoma SCs, but this regimen had little effect on the proliferation and survival of non-CSC tumor progenitors. The combination of anti-angiogenic drugs and conventional therapies could be highly cooperative [122].

6 Conclusions and Future Directions

Cancer recurrence and metastasis are major challenges of cancer therapy. Tumor dormancy may be one of the major reasons of cancer relapse and metastasis, and due to resistance, a subset of cancer cells that survives therapy may become the origin of cancer recurrence. The revived CSC hypothesis provides us new insight on understanding cancer cell resistance to therapeutics, especially to chemotherapy. CSCs are defined as a minor population of cancer cells that possesses the capacity to self-renew and to cause the heterogeneous lineages of cancer cells that comprise the tumor. Several experimental strategies such as utilizing specific markers, SP analysis, clonal and clonogenic assays, and LRC tracking can be utilized to identify or enrich for putative CSCs. Some evidence suggests that CSCs might play key role in cancer metastasis and dormancy. Like normal SCs, CSCs might be endowed with higher intrinsic capability to escape chemotherapy through their relative quiescence, ABC transporter expression, dysregulation in apoptotic signaling and increased prosurvival mechanisms, and their capacity for DNA repair. CSC niche is the specific microenvironment in which CSCs grow. It provides critical factors for the long-term survival and self-renewal of CSCs. Because CSCs are supposed to contribute to tumor development and metastasis as well as relapse after traditional therapies, it is of a great clinical potential that novel therapeutic strategies selectively target CSCs and their microenvironmental niche.

Many clinical trials of drugs targeting bulk cancer cells or CSCs and their niches, although exciting and effective in preclinical trials, have not yielded positive results in patients. There are two possible reasons to explain this discrepancy. First, the preclinical models may be inappropriate. Numerous agents have shown very promising activity in animal models but have minimal clinical activity. One of the main reasons for this failure is the use of inappropriate mouse models for preclinical assays which are not CSC-based mouse models. So, the development of strategies to target CSCs and their niches will require new approaches for the preclinical evaluation of their efficacy [58]. In addition, drugs targeting CSCs also possibly affect normal SCs, with which CSCs share many properties. Because we use much of the knowledge gained about normal SCs to design new strategies against CSCs, most of these ideas center around attacking the stem-like properties of CSCs, and normal SCs may also be targeted in the process [54]. For example, blocking ABC transporters, such as ABCG2 and ABCB1, may make CSCs more sensitive to chemotherapy, but may also cause the body's normal SCs to become sensitive to drugs and die prematurely. So, more work is needed with regard to delineating the similarities and differences between normal SCs and CSCs in order to identify possible therapeutic strategies that would effectively and specifically eradicate CSCs while leaving normal SCs unharmed.

Acknowledgment We thank all current and past Tang lab members for their support and helpful discussions. We apologize to those colleagues whose original work could not be cited in this chapter due to space constraint. This work was supported in part by grants from NIH (R01-AG023374, R01-ES015888, and R21-ES015893-01A1), American Cancer Society (RSG MGO-105961), Department of Defense (W81XWH-07-1-0616 & W81XWH-08-1-0472), Prostate Cancer Foundation, and Elsa Pardee Foundation (D.G.T) and by two Center Grants (CCSG-5 P30 CA166672 and ES07784). JQ was supported by a post-doctoral fellowship from DOD and HY was supported by a fellowship grant from the Chinese Ministry of Education.

References

1. Luzzi KJ, MacDonald IC, Schmidt EE et al. (1998) Multistep nature of metastatic inefficiency: dormancy of solitary cells after successful extravasation and limited survival of early micrometastases. Am J Pathol 153: 865–873
2. Spillane JB, Henderson MA (2007) Cancer stem cells: a review. ANZ J Surg 77: 464–468
3. Li F, Tiede B, Massague J et al. (2007) Beyond tumorigenesis: cancer stem cells in metastasis. Cell Res 17: 3–14
4. Vaidya JS (2007) An alternative model of cancer cell growth and metastasis. Int J Surg 5: 73–75
5. Kucia M, Ratajczak MZ (2006) Stem cells as a two edged sword – from regeneration to tumor formation. J Physiol Pharmacol 57(Suppl 7): 5–16
6. Allan AL, Vantyghem SA, Tuck AB et al. (2006) Tumor dormancy and cancer stem cells: implications for the biology and treatment of breast cancer metastasis. Breast Dis 26: 87–98
7. Holmgren L, O'Reilly MS, Folkman J (1995) Dormancy of micrometastases: balanced proliferation and apoptosis in the presence of angiogenesis suppression. Nat Med 1: 149–153
8. Chambers AF, Groom AC, MacDonald IC (2002) Dissemination and growth of cancer cells in metastatic sites. Nat Rev Cancer 2: 563–572
9. Luzzi KJ, MacDonald I, Schmidt EE et al. (1998) Multistep nature of metastatic inefficiency: dormancy of solitary cells after successful extravasation and limited survival of early micrometastases. Am J Pathol 153: 865–873
10. Raff M (2003) Adult stem cell plasticity: fact or artifact? Annu Rev Cell Dev Biol 19: 1–22
11. Passegue E, Wagers AJ (2006) Regulating quiescence: new insights into hematopoietic stem cell biology. Dev Cell 10: 415–417

12. Horsley V, Aliprantis AO, Polak L et al. (2008) NFATc1 balances quiescence and proliferation of skin stem cells. Cell 132: 299–310

13. Tumbar T, Guasch G, Greco V et al. (2004) Defining the epithelial stem cell niche in skin. Science 303: 359–363

14. Morrison SJ, Spradling AC (2008) Stem cells and niches: mechanisms that promote stem cell maintenance throughout life. Cell 132: 598–611

15. Bruce WR, Van Der Gaag H (1963) A quantitative assay for the number of murine lymphoma cells capable of proliferation in vivo. Nature 199: 79–80

16. Becker AJ, Mc CE, Till JE (1963) Cytological demonstration of the clonal nature of spleen colonies derived from transplanted mouse marrow cells. Nature 197: 452–454

17. Buick RN, Till JE, McCulloch EA (1977) Colony assay for proliferative blast cells circulating in myeloblastic leukaemia. Lancet 1: 862–863

18. Raftopoulou M (2006) Cancer stem cells: the needle in the haystack. http://www.nature.com/milestones/milecancer/full/milecancer06.html

19. Lapidot T, Sirard C, Vormoor J et al. (1994) A cell initiating human acute myeloid leukaemia after transplantation into SCID mice. Nature 367: 645–648

20. Clarke MF, Dick JE, Dirks PB et al. (2006) Cancer stem cells–perspectives on current status and future directions: AACR Workshop on cancer stem cells. Cancer Res 66: 9339–9344

21. Joseph NM, Mosher JT, Buchstaller J et al. (2008) The loss of Nf1 transiently promotes self-renewal but not tumorigenesis by neural crest stem cells. Cancer Cell 13: 129–140

22. Zheng H, Chang L, Patel N et al. (2008) Induction of abnormal proliferation by non-myelinating schwann cells triggers neurofibroma formation. Cancer Cell 13: 117–128

23. Kim CF, Dirks PB (2008) Cancer and stem cell biology: how tightly intertwined? Cell Stem Cell 3: 147–150

24. Tang DG, Patrawala L, Calhoun T et al. (2007) Prostate cancer stem/progenitor cells: identification, characterization, and implications. Mol Carcinog 46: 1–14

25. Pardal R, Clarke MF, Morrison SJ (2003) Applying the principles of stem-cell biology to cancer. Nat Rev Cancer 3: 895–902

26. Mazurier F, Gan OI, McKenzie JL et al. (2004) Lentivector-mediated clonal tracking reveals intrinsic heterogeneity in the human hematopoietic stem cell compartment and culture-induced stem cell impairment. Blood 103: 545–552

27. Barker N, van Es JH, Kuipers J et al. (2007) Identification of stem cells in small intestine and colon by marker gene Lgr5. Nature 449: 1003–1007

28. Patrawala L, Calhoun T, Schneider-Broussard R et al. (2005) Side population is enriched in tumorigenic, stem-like cancer cells, whereas ABCG2+ and ABCG2– cancer cells are similarly tumorigenic. Cancer Res 65: 6207–6219

29. Clarke RB, Spence K, Anderson E et al. (2005) A putative human breast stem cell population is enriched for steroid receptor-positive cells. Dev Biol 277: 443–456

30. Kondo T, Setoguchi T, Taga T (2004) Persistence of a small subpopulation of cancer stem-like cells in the C6 glioma cell line. Proc Natl Acad Sci USA 101: 781–786

31. Hadnagy A, Gaboury L, Beaulieu R et al. (2006) SP analysis may be used to identify cancer stem cell populations. Exp Cell Res 312: 3701–3710

32. Ho MM, Ng AV, Lam S et al. (2007) Side population in human lung cancer cell lines and tumors is enriched with stem-like cancer cells. Cancer Res 67: 4827–4833

33. Fang D, Nguyen TK, Leishear K et al. (2005) A tumorigenic subpopulation with stem cell properties in melanomas. Cancer Res 65: 9328–9337

34. Singh SK, Hawkins C, Clarke ID et al. (2004) Identification of human brain tumour initiating cells. Nature 432: 396–401

35. Fuchs E, Tumbar T, Guasch G (2004) Socializing with the neighbors: stem cells and their niche. Cell 116: 769–778

36. Clarke RB, Anderson E, Howell A et al. (2003) Regulation of human breast epithelial stem cells. Cell Prolif 36(Suppl 1): 45–58

37. Patrawala L, Calhoun T, Schneider-Broussard R et al. (2006) Highly purified CD44+ prostate cancer cells from xenograft human tumors are enriched in tumorigenic and metastatic progenitor cells. Oncogene 25: 1696–1708

38. Yu F, Yao H, Zhu P et al. (2007) let-7 regulates self renewal and tumorigenicity of breast cancer cells. Cell 131: 1109–1123

39. Kiel MJ, He S, Ashkenazi R et al. (2007) Haematopoietic stem cells do not asymmetrically segregate chromosomes or retain BrdU. Nature 449: 238–242

40. Szotek PP, Chang HL, Brennand K et al. (2008) Normal ovarian surface epithelial label-retaining cells exhibit stem/progenitor cell characteristics. Proc Natl Acad Sci USA 105: 12469–12473

41. Barrandon Y, Green H (1985) Cell size as a determinant of the clone-forming ability of human keratinocytes. Proc Natl Acad Sci USA 82: 5390–5394

42. Barrandon Y, Green H (1987) Three clonal types of keratinocyte with different capacities for multiplication. Proc Natl Acad Sci USA 84: 2302–2306

43. Locke M, Heywood M, Fawell S et al. (2005) Retention of intrinsic stem cell hierarchies in carcinoma-derived cell lines. Cancer Res 65: 8944–8950

44. Li H, Chen X, Calhoun-Davis T et al. (2008) PC3 human prostate carcinoma cell holoclones contain self-renewing tumor-initiating cells. Cancer Res 68: 1820–1825

45. Baguley BC (2006) Tumor stem cell niches: a new functional framework for the action of anticancer drugs. Recent Patents Anticancer Drug Discov 1: 121–127

46. Trumpp A, Wiestler OD (2008) Mechanisms of Disease: cancer stem cells – targeting the evil twin. Nat Clin Pract Oncol 5: 337–347

47. Arai F, Hirao A, Ohmura M et al. (2004) Tie2/angiopoietin-1 signaling regulates hematopoietic stem cell quiescence in the bone marrow niche. Cell 118: 149–161

48. Zhang J, Niu C, Ye L et al. (2003) Identification of the haematopoietic stem cell niche and control of the niche size. Nature 425: 836–841

49. Kaplan RN, Psaila B, Lyden D (2007) Niche-to-niche migration of bone-marrow-derived cells. Trends Mol Med 13: 72–81

50. Li L, Xie T (2005) Stem cell niche: structure and function. Annu Rev Cell Dev Biol 21: 605–631

51. Sipkins DA, Wei X, Wu J et al. (2005) In vivo imaging of specialized bone marrow endothelial microdomains for tumour engraftment. Nature 435: 969–973

52. Calabrese C, Poppleton H, Kocak M et al. (2007) A perivascular niche for brain tumor stem cells. Cancer Cell 11: 69–82

53. Bao S, Wu Q, Sathornsumetee S et al. (2006) Stem cell-like glioma cells promote tumor angiogenesis through vascular endothelial growth factor. Cancer Res 66: 7843–7848

54. Croker AK, Allan AL (2008) Cancer stem cells: implications for the progression and treatment of metastatic disease. J Cell Mol Med 12: 374–390

55. Li L, Neaves WB (2006) Normal stem cells and cancer stem cells: the niche matters. Cancer Res 66: 4553–4557

56. Wicha MS, Liu S, Dontu G (2006) Cancer stem cells: an old idea – a paradigm shift. Cancer Res 66: 1883–1890; discussion 1895–1886

57. Raguz S, Yague E (2008) Resistance to chemotherapy: new treatments and novel insights into an old problem. Br J Cancer 99: 387–391

58. Sanchez-Garcia I, Vicente-Duenas C, Cobaleda C (2007) The theoretical basis of cancer-stem-cell-based therapeutics of cancer: can it be put into practice? Bioessays 29: 1269–1280

59. Szakacs G, Paterson JK, Ludwig JA et al. (2006) Targeting multidrug resistance in cancer. Nat Rev Drug Discov 5: 219–234

60. Chapuy B, Koch R, Radunski U et al. (2008) Intracellular ABC transporter A3 confers multidrug resistance in leukemia cells by lysosomal drug sequestration. Leukemia 22: 1576–1586

61. Coelho AC, Messier N, Ouellette M et al. (2007) Role of the ABC transporter PRP1 (ABCC7) in pentamidine resistance in Leishmania amastigotes. Antimicrob Agents Chemother 51: 3030–3032

62. de Jonge-Peeters SD, Kuipers F, de Vries EG et al. (2007) ABC transporter expression in hematopoietic stem cells and the role in AML drug resistance. Crit Rev Oncol Hematol 62: 214–226

63. Engelman JA, Zejnullahu K, Mitsudomi T et al. (2007) MET amplification leads to gefitinib resistance in lung cancer by activating ERBB3 signaling. Science 316: 1039–1043

64. Weisberg E, Manley PW, Cowan-Jacob SW et al. (2007) Second generation inhibitors of BCR-ABL for the treatment of imatinib-resistant chronic myeloid leukaemia. Nat Rev Cancer 7: 345–356

65. Ali S, Coombes RC (2002) Endocrine-responsive breast cancer and strategies for combating resistance. Nat Rev Cancer 2: 101–112

66. Hu C, Li H, Li J et al. (2008) Analysis of ABCG2 expression and side population identifies intrinsic drug efflux in the HCC cell line MHCC-97L and its modulation by Akt signaling. Carcinogenesis Sept. 26 Epub ahead of print

67. Loebinger MR, Giangreco A, Groot KR et al. (2008) Squamous cell cancers contain a side population of stem-like cells that are made chemosensitive by ABC transporter blockade. Br J Cancer 98: 380–387

68. Zhou S, Schuetz JD, Bunting KD et al. (2001) The ABC transporter Bcrp1/ABCG2 is expressed in a wide variety of stem cells and is a molecular determinant of the side-population phenotype. Nat Med 7: 1028–1034

69. Gutova M, Najbauer J, Gevorgyan A et al. (2007) Identification of uPAR-positive chemoresistant cells in small cell lung cancer. PLoS ONE 2: e243

70. Frank NY, Margaryan A, Huang Y et al. (2005) ABCB5-mediated doxorubicin transport and chemoresistance in human malignant melanoma. Cancer Res 65: 4320–4333

71. Wang S, Yang D, Lippman ME (2003) Targeting Bcl-2 and Bcl-XL with nonpeptidic small-molecule antagonists. Semin Oncol 30: 133–142

72. Todaro M, Alea MP, Di Stefano AB et al. (2007) Colon cancer stem cells dictate tumor growth and resist cell death by production of interleukin-4. Cell Stem Cell 1: 389–402

73. Cairns J (2002) Somatic stem cells and the kinetics of mutagenesis and carcinogenesis. Proc Natl Acad Sci USA 99: 10567–10570

74. Potten CS, Owen G, Booth D (2002) Intestinal stem cells protect their genome by selective segregation of template DNA strands. J Cell Sci 115: 2381–2388

75. Park Y, Gerson SL (2005) DNA repair defects in stem cell function and aging. Annu Rev Med 56: 495–508

76. Phillips TM, McBride WH, Pajonk F (2006) The response of CD24(-/low)/CD44 + breast cancer-initiating cells to radiation. J Natl Cancer Inst 98: 1777–1785

77. Bao S, Wu Q, McLendon RE et al. (2006) Glioma stem cells promote radioresistance by preferential activation of the DNA damage response. Nature 444: 756–760

78. Shafee N, Smith CR, Wei S et al. (2008) Cancer stem cells contribute to cisplatin resistance in Brca1/p53-mediated mouse mammary tumors. Cancer Res 68: 3243–3250

79. Liu G, Yuan X, Zeng Z et al. (2006) Analysis of gene expression and chemoresistance of CD133 + cancer stem cells in glioblastoma. Mol Cancer 5: 67

80. Dean M, Fojo T, Bates S (2005) Tumour stem cells and drug resistance. Nat Rev Cancer 5: 275–284

81. Shipitsin M, Polyak K (2008) The cancer stem cell hypothesis: in search of definitions, markers, and relevance. Lab Invest 88: 459–463

82. Modok S, Mellor HR, Callaghan R (2006) Modulation of multidrug resistance efflux pump activity to overcome chemoresistance in cancer. Curr Opin Pharmacol 6: 350–354,

83. Pusztai L, Wagner P, Ibrahim N et al. (2005) Phase II study of tariquidar, a selective P-glycoprotein inhibitor, in patients with chemotherapy-resistant, advanced breast carcinoma. Cancer 104: 682–691

84. Wang J, Guo LP, Chen LZ et al. (2007) Identification of cancer stem cell-like side population cells in human nasopharyngeal carcinoma cell line. Cancer Res 67: 3716–3724

85. Chen JS, Pardo FS, Wang-Rodriguez J et al. (2006) EGFR regulates the side population in head and neck squamous cell carcinoma. Laryngoscope 116: 401–406
86. Karhadkar SS, Bova GS, Abdallah N et al. (2004) Hedgehog signalling in prostate regeneration, neoplasia and metastasis. Nature 431: 707–712
87. Fan X, Matsui W, Khaki L et al. (2006) Notch pathway inhibition depletes stem-like cells and blocks engraftment in embryonal brain tumors. Cancer Res 66: 7445–7452
88. Peacock CD, Wang Q, Gesell GS et al. (2007) Hedgehog signaling maintains a tumor stem cell compartment in multiple myeloma. Proc Natl Acad Sci USA 104: 4048–4053
89. Sims-Mourtada J, Izzo JG, Ajani J et al. (2007) Sonic Hedgehog promotes multiple drug resistance by regulation of drug transport. Oncogene 26: 5674–5679
90. Clement V, Sanchez P, de Tribolet N et al. (2007) HEDGEHOG-GLI1 signaling regulates human glioma growth, cancer stem cell self-renewal, and tumorigenicity. Curr Biol 17: 165–172
91. Finkel E (2001) The mitochondrion: is it central to apoptosis? Science 292: 624–626
92. Papadopoulos V, Baraldi M, Guilarte TR et al. (2006) Translocator protein (18 kDa): new nomenclature for the peripheral-type benzodiazepine receptor based on its structure and molecular function. Trends Pharmacol Sci 27: 402–409
93. Papadopoulos K (2006) Targeting the Bcl-2 family in cancer therapy. Semin Oncol 33: 449–456
94. Chelli B, Lena A, Vanacore R et al. (2004) Peripheral benzodiazepine receptor ligands: mitochondrial transmembrane potential depolarization and apoptosis induction in rat C6 glioma cells. Biochem Pharmacol 68: 125–134
95. Chelli B, Rossi L, Da Pozzo E et al. (2005) PIGA (N,N-Di-n-butyl-5-chloro-2-(4-chlorophenyl)indol-3-ylglyoxylamide), a new mitochondrial benzodiazepine-receptor ligand, induces apoptosis in C6 glioma cells. Chembiochem 6: 1082–1088
96. Aguirre-Ghiso JA (2007) Models, mechanisms and clinical evidence for cancer dormancy. Nat Rev Cancer 7: 834–846
97. Jorgensen HG, Copland M, Allan EK et al. (2006) Intermittent exposure of primitive quiescent chronic myeloid leukemia cells to granulocyte-colony stimulating factor in vitro promotes their elimination by imatinib mesylate. Clin Cancer Res 12: 626–633
98. Aguirre-Ghiso JA (2006) The problem of cancer dormancy: understanding the basic mechanisms and identifying therapeutic opportunities. Cell Cycle 5: 1740–1743
99. Ranganathan AC, Adam AP, Aguirre-Ghiso JA (2006) Opposing roles of mitogenic and stress signaling pathways in the induction of cancer dormancy. Cell Cycle 5: 1799–1807
100. Hope KJ, Jin L, Dick JE (2004) Acute myeloid leukemia originates from a hierarchy of leukemic stem cell classes that differ in self-renewal capacity. Nat Immunol 5: 738–743
101. Lo Coco F, Nervi C, Avvisati G et al. (1998) Acute promyelocytic leukemia: a curable disease. Leukemia 12: 1866–1880
102. Piccirillo SG, Reynolds BA, Zanetti N et al. (2006) Bone morphogenetic proteins inhibit the tumorigenic potential of human brain tumour-initiating cells. Nature 444: 761–765
103. Leszczyniecka M, Roberts T, Dent P et al. (2001) Differentiation therapy of human cancer: basic science and clinical applications. Pharmacol Ther 90: 105–156
104. Sell S (2006) Cancer stem cells and differentiation therapy. Tumour Biol 27: 59–70
105. Ito K, Hirao A, Arai F et al. (2006) Reactive oxygen species act through p38 MAPK to limit the lifespan of hematopoietic stem cells. Nat Med 12: 446–451
106. Liu Y, Liu R, Mao SC et al. (2008) Molecular-targeted antitumor agents. 19. Furospongolide from a marine *Lendenfeldia* sp. sponge inhibits hypoxia-inducible factor-1 activation in breast tumor cells. J Nat Prod Nov. 7 Epub ahead of print
107. Greenberger LM, Horak ID, Filpula D et al. (2008) A RNA antagonist of hypoxia-inducible factor-1{alpha}, EZN-2968, inhibits tumor cell growth. Mol Cancer Ther 7:3598–3608
108. Kiel MJ, Yilmaz OH, Iwashita T et al. (2005) SLAM family receptors distinguish hematopoietic stem and progenitor cells and reveal endothelial niches for stem cells. Cell 121: 1109–1121

109. Folkman J (2007) Angiogenesis: an organizing principle for drug discovery? Nat Rev Drug Discov 6: 273–286
110. Hurwitz H, Fehrenbacher L, Novotny W et al. (2004) Bevacizumab plus irinotecan, fluorouracil, and leucovorin for metastatic colorectal cancer. N Engl J Med 350: 2335–2342
111. Vredenburgh JJ, Desjardins A, Herndon JE et al. (2007) Phase II trial of bevacizumab and irinotecan in recurrent malignant glioma. Clin Cancer Res 13: 1253–1259
112. Kopp HG, Ramos CA, Rafii S (2006) Contribution of endothelial progenitors and proangiogenic hematopoietic cells to vascularization of tumor and ischemic tissue. Curr Opin Hematol 13: 175–181
113. Moreira IS, Fernandes PA, Ramos MJ (2007) Vascular endothelial growth factor (VEGF) inhibition – a critical review. Anticancer Agents Med Chem 7: 223–245
114. Lyden D, Hattori K, Dias S et al. (2001) Impaired recruitment of bone-marrow-derived endothelial and hematopoietic precursor cells blocks tumor angiogenesis and growth. Nat Med 7: 1194–1201
115. Davidoff AM, Ng CY, Brown P et al. (2001) Bone marrow-derived cells contribute to tumor neovasculature and, when modified to express an angiogenesis inhibitor, can restrict tumor growth in mice. Clin Cancer Res 7: 2870–2879
116. Jain RK (2005) Normalization of tumor vasculature: an emerging concept in antiangiogenic therapy. Science 307: 58–62
117. Wilson A, Trumpp A (2006) Bone-marrow haematopoietic-stem-cell niches. Nat Rev Immunol 6: 93–106
118. Jin L, Hope KJ, Zhai Q et al. (2006) Targeting of CD44 eradicates human acute myeloid leukemic stem cells. Nat Med 12: 1167–1174,
119. Draffin JE, McFarlane S, Hill A et al. (2004) CD44 potentiates the adherence of metastatic prostate and breast cancer cells to bone marrow endothelial cells. Cancer Res 64: 5702–5711
120. Sneddon JB, Werb Z (2007) Location, location, location: the cancer stem cell niche. Cell Stem Cell 1: 607–611
121. Weijzen S, Rizzo P, Braid M et al. (2002) Activation of Notch-1 signaling maintains the neoplastic phenotype in human Ras-transformed cells. Nat Med 8: 979–986
122. Tozer GM, Kanthou C, Baguley BC (2005) Disrupting tumour blood vessels. Nat Rev Cancer, 5: 423–435

Image-Guided Photodynamic Cancer Therapy

Zheng-Rong Lu and Anagha Vaidya

1 Introduction

Photodynamic therapy is a therapeutic modality with a long history. It has been historically known in ancient India and China for the treatment of skin disorders. In Western medicine, the first experimental evidence of photodynamic therapy was reported by Raab et al. who observed the lethality of acridine dyes to paramecium in the presence of light [1]. The photodynamic effect was further demonstrated by Tappeiner and colleagues who reported killing of basal cell carcinoma using eosin and light illumination [2]. More recently, Dougherty et al. developed a hematoporphyrin derivative, which was shown to kill cancer cells in vitro and mammary tumors in mouse models in vivo [3]. Photodynamic therapy has evolved as an effective therapeutic modality for cancer treatment. In 1995, the FDA approved photodynamic therapy using Photofrin for the treatment of advanced esophageal cancer. Recent developments in biomedical imaging provide new opportunities for photodynamic therapy. Modern imaging technologies can accurately detect and diagnose malignant tumors at an early stage and can effectively assess tumor response to cancer photodynamic therapy. Combining photodynamic therapy with imaging can provide image guidance for accurate laser irradiation of tumor and timely assessment of therapeutic efficacy of photodynamic therapy. Image-guided photodynamic therapy is a new, minimally invasive cancer treatment modality that can further improve the efficacy of photodynamic therapy.

2 Photodynamic Therapy

Photodynamic therapy (PDT) involves the administration of a photosensitizer and activation of the photosensitizer with light irradiation in the tumor tissue, resulting in cancer cell death. Photodynamic therapy causes cell death through

Z.-R. Lu (✉)
Department of Pharmaceutics and Pharmaceutical Chemistry, University of Utah,
Salt Lake City, UT 84108, USA
e-mail: zhengrong.lu@utah.edu

Y. Lu, R.I. Mahato (eds.), *Pharmaceutical Perspectives of Cancer Therapeutics*,
DOI 10.1007/978-1-4419-0131-6_18, © Springer Science+Business Media, LLC 2009

two different mechanisms. When a photosensitizer accumulated in target cells is activated with laser light of a specific wavelength based on its absorbance, it absorbs photons and becomes photochemically excited. The excited photosensitizer then transfers the energy to molecular oxygen to generate singlet oxygen ($^1O_2$) and superoxide (O_2^-), which cause cell damage and cell death [4, 5]. The second mechanism involves energy transfer from the excited photosensitizer to cellular biomolecules, including DNA and RNA, catalyzing photochemical reactions of the biomolecules, such as 2 + 2 cycloaddition reactions in the nucleic acids, resulting in cytotoxicity.

In general, photosensitizers have conjugate structures that absorb light with a long wavelength (>600 nm). These compounds are preferred because a longer wavelength, e.g., red light, has minimal tissue interaction and offers better tissue penetration than a shorter wavelength. Photosensitizers are derivatives of porphyrins, chlorins, and cyanins. Photofrin (Porfimer Sodium), a hematoporphyrin derivative, was the first photosensitizer clinically approved for the treatment of advanced esophageal cancer, early non-small-cell lung cancer, advanced lung cancer, head and neck cancer, and intraepithelial neoplasia [6, 7]. Several other photosensitizers, including *meta*-tetrahydrophenylchlorin (mTHPC, Foscan®) [8, 9], benzoporphyrin derivative monoacid ring A (BPD-MA, Visudyne®) [10, 11], 5-aminolevulinic acid (ALA, Levulan®) [12,13], and methyl aminolevulinate (MLA, Metvix) [14], have also been approved for clinical applications. Figure 1 shows the chemical structures of some of the clinically approved photosensitizers. Both ALA and MLA are the precursors for in vivo synthesis of porphyrins and they can be converted to active forms of photosensitizers after in vivo administration.

Activation of photosensitizers with light is crucial in producing the photodynamic effect. Photosensitizers do not have any therapeutic efficacy without light activation. Light of the wavelength corresponding to the maximal absorption of the photosensitizers is required to produce optimal irradiation and generation of cytotoxic species. Laser light of longer wavelength has better penetration in tissues due to reduced interaction with surrounding tissues and is preferred for photodynamic therapy. The application of light is mainly expressed in terms of fluence rate, which is defined as the radiant energy per second across a sectional area (W/cm^2), and fluence, which is defined as the total energy input across a sectional area (J/cm^2). Light dose applied to the tumor tissue must be over a minimum threshold to enable tissue penetration for the maximal therapeutic effect. At the same time, a very high light dose may lead to thermal toxicity to normal tissues beyond the target tissue. Fractionated light dosing, several low doses instead of one high dose, has been observed to produce more efficacious therapy in tumors [15, 16, 17]. Although the lower fluence rate required longer treatment times, they showed lower toxic side effects when compared to higher fluence rates [18].

Photodynamic therapy causes cell death via necrosis and activation of signaling pathways that elicit apoptotic and/or autophagic response [19, 20]. Irradiation of cells in the presence of a photosensitizer leads to damage of cell

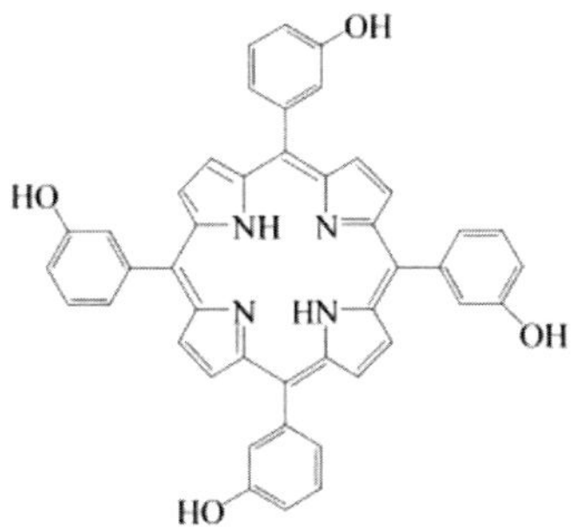

m-Tetrahydroxyphenylchlorin
(mTHPC)

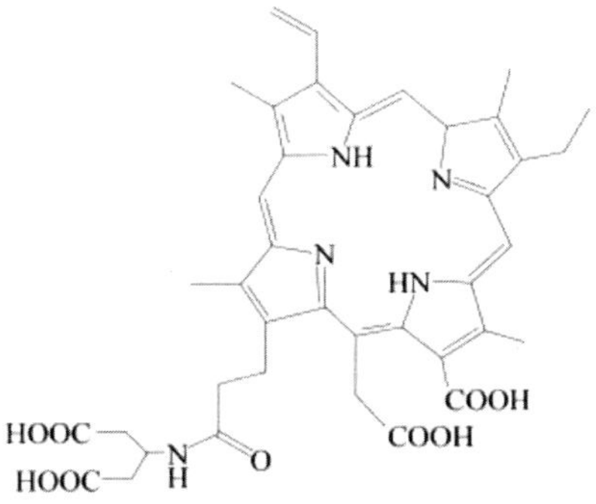

Mono-L-aspartylchlorin e$_6$ (MACE)

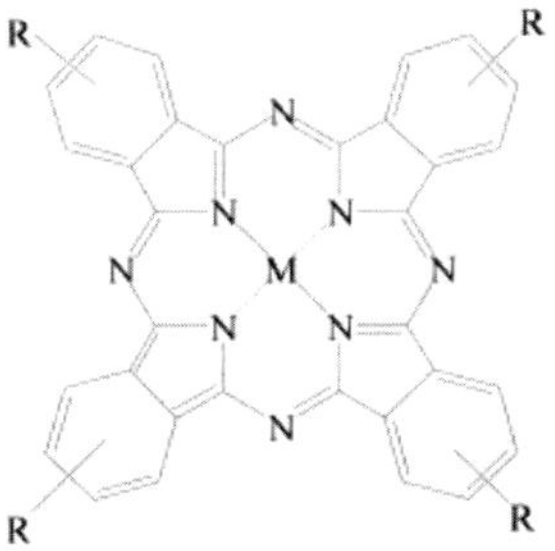

Phthalocyanine

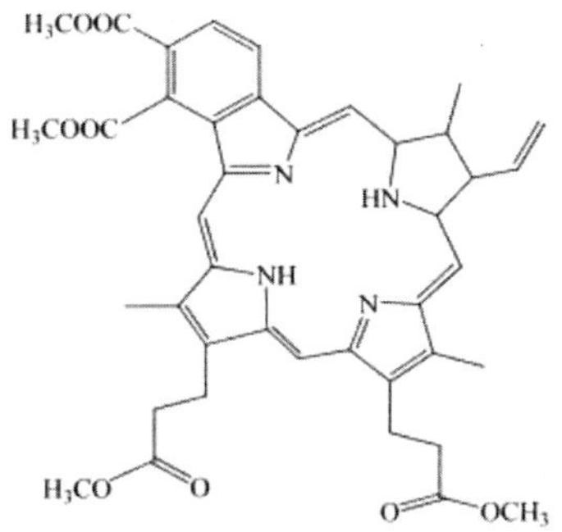

Benzophorphyrin derivative
monoacid ring A (BPD-MA)

Fig. 1 Chemical structures of some of the second-generation photosensitizers

membranes/internal structures and causes release of stress signals, ultimately triggering apoptosis or necrosis. Necrosis is a form of traumatic cell death associated with acute cell injury, while apoptosis is programmed cell death, occurring naturally in the body. Several photosensitizers are known to activate caspases, the apoptotic proteins, in the mitochondria to induce apoptosis in photodynamic therapy. Photofrin is known to elicit both apoptosis and necrosis in tumor cells in photodynamic therapy [21]. Necrosis can be caused by damage to cell membrane and disruption of cellular function [22]. Autophagy, or cellular self-digestion, is a cellular pathway involved in protein and organelle degradation and represents the response of the cell to starvation [23]. Initial autophagic response followed by apoptosis has been observed for mouse leukemia cells in response to photodynamic therapy using hypericin, which is known to target the endoplasmic reticulum [24]. Double membrane encased autophagosomal vesicles have also been observed by electron microscopy in photodynamically treated MCF-7 cells receiving phthalocyanine photosensitizer [25]. The cell-kill effects depend on the structure and composition of the photosensitizer, its uptake into the cells, and subcellular localization and it is difficult to segregate these mechanisms.

Photodynamic therapy causes vascular damage at the tissue level, which results in tumor regression as an indirect effect. The production of reactive oxygen species upon irradiation of the photosensitizer has been shown to damage the endothelium when the photosensitizer localizes in the tumor microvasculature [26]. Tumor vasculature subjected to photodynamic therapy is associated with release of thromboxane, histamine, and von Hildebrand factor [27, 28], which cause vasoconstriction, vasodilation, aggregation of blood cells, blood flow stasis, hypoxia, and cell death [29, 30]. Studies have shown that the efficacy of photodynamic therapy is determined to a large extent by the degree of damage to tumor microvasculature [31, 32]. This is corroborated by the fact that the efficacy of photodynamic therapy can be augmented by co-administration of antiangiogenic therapy [33, 34]. Targeting photosensitizers specifically on tumor stroma increases the efficacy of photodynamic therapy [35, 36].

Photodynamic therapy can also induce tumor immune response, resulting in better therapeutic efficacy. Immunity in response to photodynamic therapy is elicited by several mechanisms. Photoxidative damage triggers several cell signal transduction pathways [3, 37], causing expression of stress proteins [38,39]. It activates the nuclear factor AP-1, resulting in cytokines like IL-16, IL-10, and tumor necrosis factor-α [40, 41]. Immune response is considered more significant in long-term cancer management rather than in short-term tumor cell-kill effect.

Photodynamic therapy is well tolerated with minimal accumulative toxicity in patients as compared to chemotherapy and radiation therapy. It is minimally invasive and highly specific and does not cause scarring after the treatment. However, clinical application of photodynamic therapy is still limited to treat superficial lesions because it requires accurate light irradiation. Another challenge for effective photodynamic therapy is the specific delivery of the photosensitizer into cancer cells. Current photosensitizers do not have good specificity to cancer cells. Recent development in drug delivery and biomedical imaging allows efficient delivery of photosensitizers into tumor tissues and accurate location of non-superficial lesions for effective photodynamic therapy.

3 Bifunctional Polymer Conjugates

The conjugation of therapeutics to water-soluble biomedical polymers increases the aqueous solubility of hydrophobic drugs and reduces systemic toxicity [42, 43]. The polymer drug conjugates can preferentially accumulate in solid tumor tissues due to the hyperpermeability of tumor blood vessels or the so-called "enhanced permeability and retention (EPR) effect" [44, 45]. Polymer drug conjugates can also downregulate or overcome multiple drug resistance [46, 47]. Because of these unique properties, polymer drug conjugates exhibit much higher therapeutic efficacy than free drugs. Currently, several polymer drug conjugates are used in clinical cancer treatment, and more are in the pipeline for clinical development [48–50]. The conjugation of photosensitizers to biocompatible water-soluble polymers reduces their dark toxicity and accumulation in the skin and increases their accumulation in solid tumor tissues, resulting in high anticancer efficacy with PDT [51]. For example, conjugation of photosensitizer mesochlorin e_6 into HPMA copolymers resulted in a maximum tumor uptake of 5.5% of the total administered dose (TAD) of the photosensitizer in a mice tumor model, while the maximum tumor uptake of free mesochlorin e_6 was less than 0.5% of TAD [51, 52]. Consequently, higher anticancer efficacy with photodynamic therapy was observed with the polymeric conjugates.

Imaging probes or contrast agents can be readily incorporated into polymer conjugates to allow non-invasive tracking of the conjugates and accurate tumor detection with biomedical imaging modalities to guide photodynamic therapy for cancer treatment, particularly for the treatment of non-superficial lesions. Magnetic resonance imaging (MRI) is a non-invasive clinical imaging modality. It provides high-resolution images of soft tissues and is effective for cancer detection. Paramagnetic substances are often used as MRI contrast agents to increase image contrast between tumor tissue and surrounding normal tissue for accurate cancer detection and diagnosis. Covalent conjugation of an MRI contrast agent to the polymer photosensitizer conjugate provides bifunctional polymer conjugates. The bifunctional conjugates will allow real-time and non-invasive visualization of the biodistribution of the conjugates with MRI, accurate localization of non-superficial tumor, and the determination of the exact timing of site-directed irradiation of tumors, leading to better therapeutic efficacy.

Poly-(L-glutamic acid), PGA, is a biocompatible drug carrier and has a large number of functional side chains suitable for preparation of bifunctional conjugates. A bifunctional conjugate, PGA-(Gd-DO3A)-mesochlorin e_6 (Mce_6) conjugate, was prepared for contrast-enhanced MRI-guided photodynamic therapy [53]. Gd-DO3A is a macrocyclic MRI contrast agent with high in vivo stability, and mesochlorin e_6 is a photosensitizer. Figure 2A shows the structure of the bifunctional conjugate. Mce_6 and Gd-DO3A contents in the conjugate were 0.078 and 0.62 mmol/g-polymer, respectively. A relatively large number of Gd-DO3A chelates were conjugated because MRI has a relatively low sensitivity to visualize the contrast agents. T_1 relaxivity of the conjugate was 8.46 $mM^{-1} s^{-1}$ per complexed Gd(III) ion at 3 T. Relaxivity of an MRI contrast agent is a measurement of the ability of the agent to generate signal enhancement in contrast-enhanced MRI [54]. Usually, polymer conjugates of MRI contrast agents have higher relaxivities than corresponding free contrast agents.

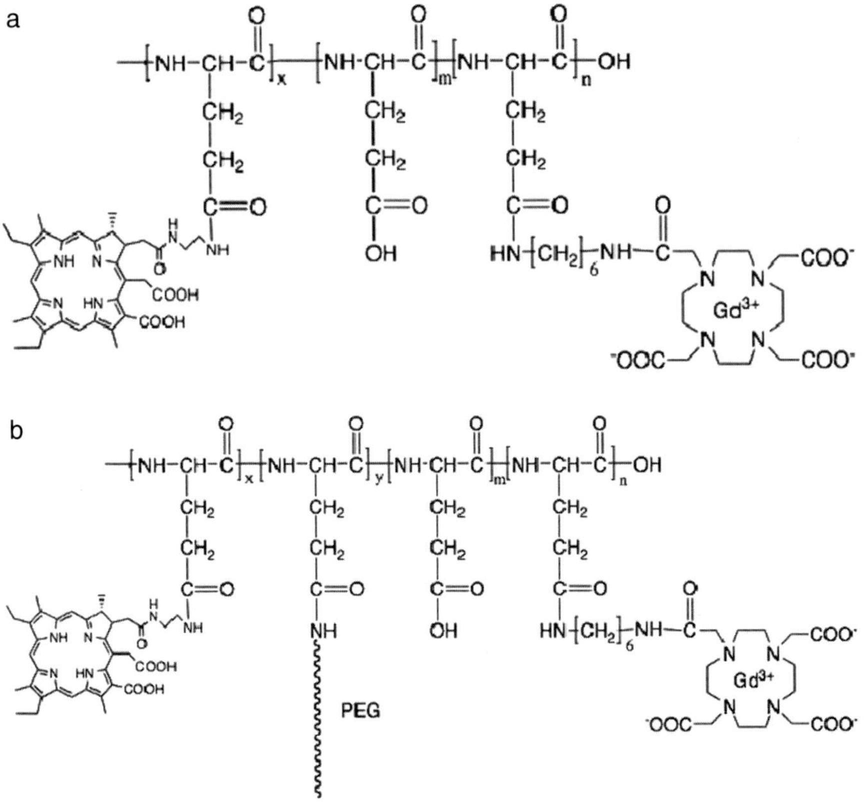

Fig. 2 Chemical structures of a bifunctional poly(L-glutamic acid)-(Gd-DO3A)-mesochlorin e$_6$ conjugate (**A**) and its pegylated bifunctional conjugate (**B**)

The bifunctional polymer conjugates can be readily modified to optimize their pharmacokinetic properties to achieve better tumor-targeting efficiency and better therapeutic outcome. The modification of bifunctional polymer conjugates with poly(ethylene glycol) (PEG) has a potential to modify the pharmacokinetics of the bifunctional conjugate by reducing non-specific tissue interaction, increasing blood circulation, and improving tumor-targeting efficiency. The conjugate of poly(L-glutamic acid) meso-chlorin e$_6$ and Gd-DO3A was modified with PEG of 2000 Da to optimize the pharmacokinetics and to improve the therapeutic efficacy of the bifunctional conjugates [55]. The structure of the PEGylated bifunctional conjugate, PEG-PGA-(Gd-DO3A)-Mce$_6$, is shown in Fig. 2B. The physical parameters of the conjugates and the control conjugate, PGA-(Gd-DO3A), are listed in Table 1. Although the conjugates were prepared from the same poly(L-glutamic acid), they had different apparent molecular weights due to the changes in their hydrodynamic volumes after various chemical

Table 1 Physical parameters of thepolymer conjugates

Polymers	Mn (kDa)	Mw (kDa)	PDI	Gd (mmol/g)	Mce_6 (mg/g)	Relaxivity $(mM^{-1} s^{-1})$
PGA-(Gd-DO3A)	25	39	1.5	0.8	–	7.9
PGA-(Gd-DO3A)-Mce_6	34	49	1.4	0.62	50	8.46
PEG-PGA-(Gd-DO3A)-Mce_6	22	35	1.6	0.43	70	4.5

modifications. The PEGylated conjugate had lower T_1 relaxivity than the non-PEGylated conjugates because PEG reduced the water exchange rate of Gd chelates.

4 Non-invasive Imaging of Pharmacokinetics of Polymer Conjugates

The pharmacokinetics and biodistribution of polymer drug conjugates are traditionally investigated by sacrificing a large number of experimental animals at various time points. Biomedical imaging allows non-invasive evaluation of the real-time pharmacokinetics and whole body distribution of polymer conjugates in the same group of animals in preclinical development. Several clinical imaging modalities, including magnetic resonance imaging (MRI), positron emission tomography (PET), computed tomography (CT), single photon emission computed tomography (SPECT), and ultrasound, can be used for non-invasive pharmacokinetic studies, including guiding cancer therapies. Among these imaging modalities, contrast-enhanced MRI produces excellent anatomic images with high spatial resolution [56].

MRI is a non-invasive clinical imaging modality. MRI provides three-dimensional images of biological structures with high spatial resolution. MR image contrast is created based on the differences in proton densities and the longitudinal or transverse relaxation rates ($1/T_1$ or $1/T_2$) of protons in the body. Paramagnetic metal chelates (e.g., Gd(III) and Mn(II) complexes) [54, 57] can alter the relaxation rates of water protons and are used as MRI contrast agents. The most commonly used clinical MRI contrast agents are stable Gd(III) chelates, including Gd-DTPA [58], Gd-(DTPA-BMA) [59], Gd-DOTA [60], and Gd-(HP-DO3A) [61]. These agents increase water proton T_1 relaxation rate and MRI signal intensity in tissues with high concentrations of the contrast agents, creating image contrast enhancement with surrounding tissues. Contrast-enhanced MRI is routinely used in cancer imaging. Polymer conjugates can be readily labeled with the paramagnetic chelates for non-invasive visualization of the in vivo properties, including biodistribution and pharmacokinetics, of the polymer conjugates.

MR signal intensity indirectly reflects the concentration of the conjugates in the organs or tissues. In T_1-weighted MR images, bright signal indicates high concentration of the paramagnetically labeled conjugates with similar relaxivities [62]. Figure 3A shows three-dimensional T_1-weighted coronal MR images of tumor-bearing mice before and at various time points after the injection of the PHPMA-GFLG-(Gd-DO3A) with an average molecular weight of 121 kDa at a dose of 0.03 mmol-Gd/kg [63]. These dynamic MR images of the same mouse clearly showed the blood pharmacokinetics of the conjugate. Strong blood signal was observed at the initial period after injection and the signal then gradually faded away. The MR images revealed that the high molecular weight polymer conjugate had relatively prolonged blood circulation. The prolonged blood circulation was shown for the conjugates with higher molecular weights. The conjugate was still visible in the blood 72 h post-injection. Prolonged blood circulation of the conjugate might result in high accumulation in tumor tissue due to EPR effect.

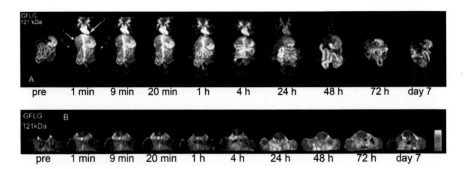

Fig. 3 (**A**) Three-dimensional MIP MR images of a mouse bearing MDA-MB-231 human breast carcinoma xenografts injected with a PHPMA-GlyPheLeuGly-1,2-ethylenediamine-(Gd-DO3A) conjugate with a molecular weight of 121 kDa before contrast and at various time points after intravenous injection of the conjugates at a dose of 0.03 mmol-Gd/kg. *Arrows* indicate the liver (*1*), heart (*2*), and tumor tissue (*3*). (**B**) Color-coded 2D axial spin-echo T_1-weighted MR images of a mouse injected with the conjugate before contrast and at various time points after the injection

MRI also revealed the dynamic and heterogeneous distribution of the labeled conjugate in tumor tissue. Figure 3B shows the color-coded contrast enhancement in tumor tissues. Significant contrast enhancement was first observed at tumor periphery after the initial injection of the conjugate and then gradually in the tumor interstitium, indicating that distribution of the polymer conjugate started at the tumor periphery and gradually diffused in the inner tumor tissue. Significant contrast enhancement was shown in tumor tissue for at least 3 days after the injection, indicating the prolonged presence of the conjugate in tumor tissue. Contrast-enhanced MRI provides non-invasive, continuous, and detailed evaluation on the biodistribution of polymer conjugates, while conventional pharmacokinetics only provides average distribution data.

The real-time pharmacokinetics and biodistribution of PEG-PGA-(Gd-DO3A)-Mce$_6$, PGA-(Gd-DO3A)-Mce$_6$, and PGA-(Gd-DO3A) were non-invasively evaluated by contrast-enhanced MRI [55]. Figure 4 shows the three-dimensional MR images of mice bearing MDA-MB-231 human breast carcinoma xenografts before and at various time points after intra-venous injection of the polymer conjugates at the same Gd(III) equivalent dose (0.05 mmol-Gd/kg). The MR images clearly revealed the structural effects of the conjugates on blood pharmacokinetics and liver distribution of the conjugates. The unPEGylated conjugates, particularly PGA-(Gd-DO3A)-Mce$_6$, showed strong enhancement in the liver, indicating high liver accumulation. PEGylated bifunctional conjugate showed much less liver enhancement, suggesting that pegylation of the conjugate significantly reduced non-specific liver accumulation of bifunctional conjugate. As a result, strong and prolonged enhancement was shown in the vasculature of

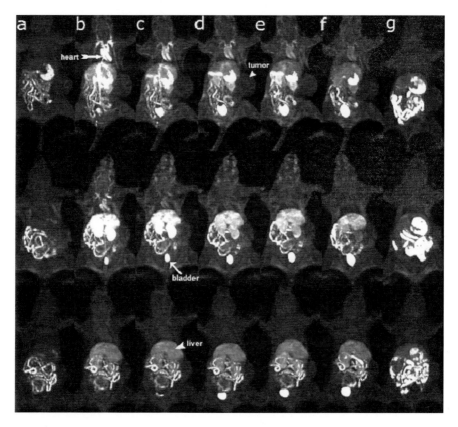

Fig. 4 Three-dimensional MIP images (coronal view) of mice before (*a*) and at 2 min (*b*), 5 min (*c*), 15 min (*d*), 30 min (*e*), 2 h (*f*), and 18 h (*g*) after intravenous injection of 0.05 mmol-Gd/kg PEG-PGA-(Gd-DO3A)-Mce$_6$ (*top panel*), PGA-(Gd-DO3A)-Mce$_6$ (*middle panel*), and PGA-(Gd-DO3A) (*bottom panel*)

the mice injected with the PEGylated conjugate, indicating prolonged blood circulation of the PEGylated conjugate. The MR images also showed that all of the conjugates could be readily excreted via renal filtration and accumulated in the urinary bladder.

Figure 5 shows axial T_1-weighted 2D spin-echo images of tumor tissues of the mice before and at various time points after intravenous injection of the conjugates [55]. Heterogeneous tumor contrast enhancement is shown in the tumor tissue, indicating heterogeneous tumor distribution of the conjugates. It appears that the PEGylated conjugate resulted in more significant tumor enhancement.

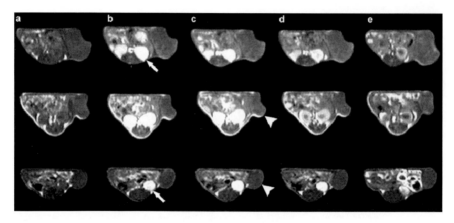

Fig. 5 Two-dimensional axial images of tumor in mice before (*a*) and at 2 min (*b*), 30 min (*c*), 2 h (*d*), and 18 h (*e*) after intravenous injection of 0.05 mmol-Gd/kg PEG-PGA-(Gd-DO3A)-Mce$_6$ (*top panel*), PGA-(Gd-DO3A)-Mce$_6$ (*middle panel*), and PGA-(Gd-DO3A) (*bottom panel*). *Arrow* points to kidneys and *arrowhead* points to tumor

Quantitative analysis of MR signal intensities provides semi-quantitative estimation of dynamic biodistribution of the conjugates in the blood, liver, and tumor. Figure 6 shows the dynamic changes of the signal-to-noise ratio (SNR) in the blood, liver, and tumor [55]. Large SNR generally indicates high concentration of Gd-DO3A-labeled conjugates, but such correlation is not linear. Nonetheless, semi-quantitative analysis clearly shows the pharmacokinetic property of the conjugates in different tissues. The bifunctional conjugate and PGA-(GD-DO3A) had similar pharmacokinetics in the blood, liver, and tumor. PGA-(Gd-DO3A)-Mce$_6$ had relatively short blood circulation and high liver uptake possibly due to the hydrophobic interaction of mesochlorin e$_6$ with the reticuloendothelial system. The modification of PGA-(Gd-DO3A)-Mce$_6$ with mPEG of 2 kDa significantly reduced the non-specific liver uptake of the photosensitizer conjugate at the same Gd(III) dose. The PEGylated conjugate resulted in more prolonged blood enhancement than PGA-(Gd-DO3A)-Mce$_6$ and higher tumor accumulation due to the "EPR" effect.

Fig. 6 The signal-to-noise ratio (SNR) in blood (**a**), liver (**b**), and tumor (**c**) for mice receiving 0.05 mmol-Gd/kg PEG-PGA-(Gd-DO3A)-Mce$_6$, PGA-(Gd-DO3A)-Mce$_6$, and PGA-(Gd-DO3A)

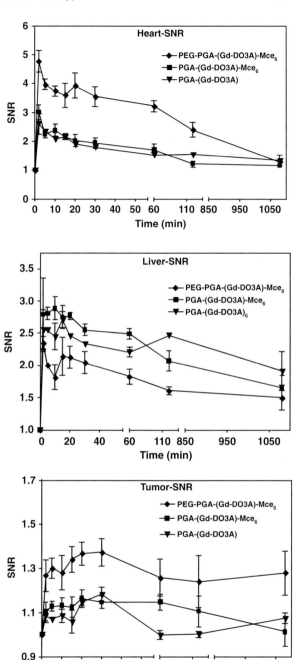

5 Cancer Treatment with Contrast-Enhanced MRI-Guided Photodynamic Therapy

The efficacy of photodynamic therapy with the bifunctional conjugates was demonstrated by irradiation of the tumor tissues with a laser of 650 nm after MR imaging [55]. Drugs containing PEGylated and non-PEGylated conjugates were injected at a dose of 6 mg-Mce$_6$/kg. PGA-(Gd-DO3A) was injected at Gd equivalent dose of 0.045 mmol/kg. Each tumor received 15 min irradiation at a dose of 180 J/cm^2, 18 and 24 h after the injection of the conjugates. Figure 7 shows the percentage of increase in tumor size after the treatments with the PEGylated, non-PEGylated, and control conjugates as compared to that before the treatments. PEG-PGA-(Gd-DO3A)-Mce$_6$ resulted in significant inhibition of tumor growth as compared to PGA-(Gd-DO3A)-Mce$_6$ and PGA-(Gd-DO3A) ($p<0.05$).

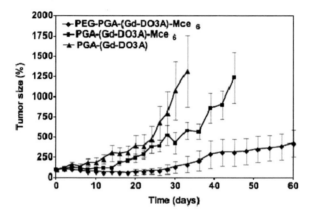

Fig. 7 Efficacy of photodynamic therapy for polymer conjugates in MDA-MB-231 xenografts-bearing nude mice. Efficacy is expressed as the percentage increase in relative tumor size for mice receiving PEG-PGA-(Gd-DO3A)-Mce$_6$ (♦), PGA-(Gd-DO3A)-Mce$_6$ (■) at a Mce$_6$ equivalent dose of 6.0 mg/kg, and PGA-(Gd-DO3A) at a dose of 0.045 mmol-Gd/kg (▲) after the tumors were irradiated at 18 and 24 h post-injection

The therapeutic efficacy of the bifunctional conjugates in photodynamic therapy correlated well with the biodistribution of the conjugates as revealed by the contrast-enhanced MRI. The PEGylated conjugate, which had high tumor accumulation with low non-specific tissue, resulted in more effective suppression of tumor growth with site-directed photodynamic therapy. In comparison, the non-PEGylated conjugate, which showed high non-specific liver accumulation and low tumor accumulation, was less effective than the PEGylated conjugate in photodynamic therapy.

The combination of contrast-enhanced MRI with photodynamic therapy based on the bifunctional conjugates can effectively localize tumor and estimate pharmacokinetics and tumor accumulation of the conjugate and provide the needed image guidance for photodynamic therapy to effectively treat non-superficial tumors. Contrast-enhanced MRI is effective to track bifunctional polymer conjugates labeled with a contrast agent, which is useful to determine the suitable timing for laser irradiation to achieve the best therapeutic outcome. High-resolution contrast-enhanced MRI images also allow accurate tumor detection. Accurate tumor localization is critical to guide laser irradiation of non-superficial tumors in photodynamic therapy. Image-guided photodynamic therapy is less invasive compared to other image-guided therapies, including image-guided thermoablation, cryoablation, laser ablation, and radiofrequency ablation, that have been used for clinical cancer treatment [64–66]. These techniques are still relatively invasive and it is very difficult to completely ablate tumor tissue without harming the normal tissue. In comparison, image-guided photodynamic therapy is a less invasive approach for specific cancer treatment.

6 Non-invasive Assessment of Tumor Response with Dynamic Contrast-Enhanced MRI

Dynamic contrast-enhanced (DCE) MRI measures the uptake kinetics of an MRI contrast agent in tumor tissue. Vascularity, the density of tumor microvessels, and tumor blood vessel permeability are important parameters for assessing response of tumor tissues to therapies. These tumor physiological properties can be evaluated from the uptake kinetics of contrast agents [67–69]. These parameters can be used to evaluate tumor response to therapies, including antiangiogenic therapy. Since macromolecules have limited extravasation in normal blood vessels and are hyperpermeable to the leaky tumor blood vasculature, DCE-MRI with macromolecular MRI contrast agents is considered to be more accurate in tumor characterization than low molecular weight contrast agents [70–73]. However, DCE-MRI with macromolecular contrast agents is limited to preclinical studies in evaluating therapeutic response because no macromolecular MRI contrast agent is available for clinical applications due to their slow excretion from the body and related safety concerns. Recently, biodegradable macromolecular MRI contrast agents based on polydisulfide Gd(III) chelates have been developed to alleviate the safety concerns and are promising for clinical development [74–77].

Tumor response to photodynamic therapy with different conjugates was non-invasively evaluated with dynamic contrast-enhanced MRI and a biodegradable macromolecular MRI contrast agent, (Gd-DTPA)-cystine copolymers (GDCP) [78]. Figure 8 shows the representative dynamic change of relative signal intensity in peripheral tumor tissue over 15 min, after intravenous administration of GDCP at a dose of 0.1 mmol-Gd/kg. The tumors had different contrast uptake kinetics after treatment with different bifunctional conjugates and the control. The tumors treated with the non-therapeutic

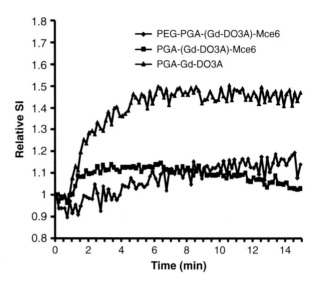

Fig. 8 Relative signal intensity plots of the DCE-MRI data showing the dynamic uptake of (Gd-DTPA)-cystine copolymers in tumor periphery of mice treated with different conjugates

control PGA-(Gd-DO3A) had rapid initial uptake kinetics because the control had no therapeutic efficacy with photodynamic therapy. Rapid and high tumor contrast uptake kinetics indicates high tumor vascular permeability and tumor viability. The non-PEGylated conjugate had intermediate therapeutic efficacy and the tumors treated with the conjugate had slower and lower uptake than those treated with the control. Low tumor contrast uptake kinetics indicates low tumor vascular permeability to the macromolecular contrast agent, indicating good tumor response to the therapy. The tumors treated with the PEGylated conjugate had much slower growth after the treatment and showed much slower uptake kinetics than the tumors treated with both PGA-(Gd-DO3A)-Mce$_6$ and PGA-(Gd-DO3A). The result suggested that the PEGylated conjugate was more effective in tumor treatment with photodynamic therapy.

The tumor uptake kinetics measured by DCE-MRI correlates well with the tumor growth curves in Fig. 7. PEG-PGA-(Gd-DO3A)-Mce$_6$ conjugate resulted in significant antitumor efficacy with photodynamic therapy. As a result, tumor microvessel density and vascular permeability significantly decreased. DCE-MRI with the biodegradable macromolecular MRI contrast agent was effective for non-invasive assessment of the tumor vascular permeability. As compared to the traditional surgery-based biopsy, DCE-MRI can provide timely and non-invasive assessment of the efficacy of photodynamic therapy with the bifunctional conjugates. DCE-MRI with the biodegradable macromolecular contrast agents is advantageous for the characterization of tumor vascularity because the agents can selectively permeate through the hyperpermeable microvasculature of tumor tissues without extravasating through normal endothelium [79].

7 Concluding Remarks

The advance of imaging technology not only improves cancer detection and diagnosis, but also provides new opportunities for development of new therapeutics and cancer treatment modalities. The combination of contrast-enhanced MRI with photodynamic therapy can provide accurate localization of non-superficial tumors and image guidance for laser irradiation of tumors. Paramagnetically labeled bifunctional conjugates are a critical component for image-guided photodynamic therapy, which provides an effective platform for the combination of contrast-enhanced MRI with photodynamic therapy. The hyperpermeability of tumor vasculature or the EPR effect of solid tumor allows preferential accumulation of bifunctional polymer conjugates in tumor tissues, which results in tumor enhancement in MRI for accurate detection and localization of non-superficial tumor. In practical application, MRI can also guide the insertion of an optical fiber to the detected non-superficial tumor for effective photodynamic therapy. Therapeutic efficacy of the image-guided photodynamic therapy can be effectively and non-invasively evaluated with dynamic contrast-enhanced MRI with a biodegradable macromolecular MRI contrast agent. Image-guided photodynamic therapy is a promising modality in personalized medicine, which provides effective tumor detection and treatment and rapid and non-invasive assessment of therapeutic efficacy.

References

1. Raab O et al. Ueber die Wirkung fluoreszierenden Stoffe auf infusorien. *Z Biol* 1900; 39: 524–526.
2. von Tappeneimer H, Jesionek A. (1903) Therapeutische versuche mit fluorescierenden stoffen. *Munch Med Wochenschr* 1903; 47: 2042–2047.
3. Dougherty TJ, Gomer CJ, et al. Photodynamic therapy. *J Natl Cancer Inst* 1998; 90: 889–905.
4. Phillips D. Chemical mechanisms in photodynamic therapy. *Progr React Kinet* 1997; 22: 175–300.
5. Oschner M. Photophysical and photobiological processes in photodynamic therapy of tumors. J Photochem Photobiol B 1997; 39: 1–18.
6. Dougherty TJ, Potter WR, Weishaupt KR. The structure of the active component of hematoporphyrin derivative. *Prog Clin Biol Res* 1984; 170: 301–314.
7. Busch TM, Hahn SM. Hypoxia and Photofrin uptake in the intraperitoneal carcinomatosis and sarcomatosis of photodynamic therapy patients. *Clin Cancer Res* 2004; 10: 4630–4638.
8. Cramers P, Ruevekamp M, Oppelaar H, Dalesio O, Baas P, Stewart FA. Foscan uptake and tissue distribution in relation to photodynamic efficacy. *Br J Cancer* 2003; 88: 283–290.
9. Hopper C, Kubler A, Lewis H, Tan IB, Putnam G. mTHPC-mediated photodynamic therapy for early oral squamous cell carcinoma. *Int J Cancer* 2004; 111: 138–146.
10. Momma T, Hamblin MR, Wu HC, Hasan T. Photodynamic therapy of orthotopic prostate cancer with benzoporphyrin derivative: local control and distant metastasis. *Cancer Res* 1998; 58: 5425–5431.

11. Keam SJ, Scott LJ, Curran MP. Verteporfin: a review of its use in the management of subfoveal choroidal neovascularisation. *Drugs* 2003; 63: 2521–2554.

12. Peng Q, Warloe T, Berg K, Moan J, Kongshaug M, Giercksky KE, Nesland JM. 5-Aminolevulinic acid-based photodynamic therapy. Clinical research and future challenges. *Cancer* 1997; 79: 2282–2308.

13. Gupta AK, Ryder JE. Photodynamic therapy and topical aminolevulinic acid: an overview. *Am J Clin Dermatol* 2003; 4: 699–708.

14. Siddiqui MA, Perry CM, Scott LJ. Topical methyl aminolevulinate. *Am J Clin Dermatol* 2004; 5: 127–137.

15. Foster TH, Gao L. Dosimetry in photodynamic therapy: oxygen and the critical importance of capillary density. *Radiat Res* 1992; 130: 379–383.

16. Coutier S, Bezdetnaya LN, Foster TH, Parache RM, Guilleminn F. Effect of irradiation fluence rate on the efficacy of photodynamic therapy and tumor oxygenation in meta-tetra (hydroxyphenyl) chlorin (mTHPC)-sensitized HT29 xenografts in nude mice. *Radiat Res* 2002; 158: 339–345.

17. Muller S, Walt H, Dobler-Girziunaite D, Fiedler D, Haller U. Enhanced photodynamic effects using fractionated laser light. *J Photochem Photobiol B. Biol* 1998; 42: 67–70.

18. Sitnik TM, Henderson BW. The effect of fluence rate on tumor and normal tissue responses to photodynamic therapy. *Photochem Photobiol* 1998; 67: 462–466.

19. Kessel D, Reiners Jr JJ. Apoptosis and autophagy after mitochondrial or endoplasmic reticulum photodamage. *Photochem Photobiol* 2004; 83: 1024.

20. Chen Y, Gibson SB. Is mitochondrial generation of reactive oxygen species a trigger for autophagy? Autophagy 2008; 4: 246–248.

21. Dellinger M. Apoptosis or necrosis following Photofrin photosensitization: influence of the incubation protocol. Photochem Photobiol 1996; 64: 183–187.

22. Hampton JA, Selman SH. Mechanisms of cell killing in photodynamic therapy using a novel in vivo drug/in vitro light culture system. *Photochem Photobiol* 1992; 56: 235–243.

23. Mizhushima N, Levine B, Cuervo AM, Klionsky DJ. Autophagy fights disease through cellular self-digestion. *Nature* 2008; 45: 1069–1075.

24. Kessel D, Arroyo AS. Apoptotic and autophagic responses to Bcl-2 inhibition and photodamage. *Photochem Photobiol* 2007; 6: 1290–1295.

25. Xue LY, Chiu SM, Azizuddin K, Joseph S, Olenick NL. The death of human cancer cells following photodynamic therapy: apoptosis competence is necessary for Bcl-2 protection but not for induction of autophagy. *Photochem Photobiol* 2007; 83: 1016–1023.

26. Fingar VH. Vascular effects of photodynamic therapy. *J Clin Laser Med Surg* 1996; 14: 323–328.

27. Reed MW, Weiman TJ, Doak KW, Peitsch CG, Schuschke DA. The microvascular effects of photodynamic therapy: evidence for a possible role of cyclooxygenase products. *Photochem Photobiol* 1989; 50: 419–423.

28. Kerdel FA, Soter NA, Lim HW. In vivo mediator release and degranulation of mast cells in hematoporphyrin derivative-induced phototoxicity in mice. *J Invest Dermatol* 1987; 88: 277–280.

29. Selman SH, Keck RW, Klauning JE, Kriemer-Birnbaum M, Goldblatt PJ, Britton SL. Acute blood flow changes in transplantable FANFT-induced urothelial tumors treated with hematoporphyrin derivative and light. *Surg Forum* 1983; 34: 676–678.

30. Fingar VH, Weiman TJ, Wiehle SA, Cerrito PB. The role of microvascular damage in photodynamic therapy: the effect of treatment on vessel constriction, permeability, and leukocyte adhesion. *Cancer Res* 1992; 52: 4914–4921.

31. Krammer B. Vascular effects of photodynamic therapy. *Anticancer Res* 2001; 21: 4271–4277.

32. Fingar VH, Taber SW, Haydon PS, Harrison LT, Kempf SL, Wieman TJ. Vascular damage after photodynamic therapy of solid tumors: a view and comparison of effect in pre-clinical and clinical models at the University of Louisville. *In Vivo 2000;* 14: 93–100.

33. Jiang F, Zhang X et al. Combination therapy with antiangiogenic treatment and photodynamic therapy for the nude mouse bearing U87 glioblastoma. *Photochem Photobiol* 2008; 84: 128–137.

34. Kaiser PK. Verteporfin photodynamic therapy and anti-angiogenic drugs: potential for combination therapy in exudative age-related macular degeneration. *Curr Med Res Opin* 2007; 23: 477–487.

35. Trachtenberg J, Bogaads A et al. Vascular targeted photodynamic therapy with palladium-bacteriopheophorbide photosensitizer for recurrent prostate cancer following definitive radiation therapy: assessment of safety and treatment response. *J Urol* 2007; 178: 1974–1979.

36. Solban N, Rizvi I, Hasan T. Targeted photodynamic therapy. Lasers Med Surg 2006; 38: 522–531.

37. Gomer CJ, Luna M et al. Cellular targets and molecular responses associated with photodynamic therapy. *J Clin Laser Med Surg* 1996; 14: 315–321.

38. Ryter SW, Gomer CJ. Nuclear factor kappa B binding activity in mouse L1210 cells following photofrin II-mediated photosensitization. *Photochem Photobiol* 1993; 58: 753–756.

39. Kick G, Messer G, Goetz A, Plewig G. Photodynamic therapy induces expression of interleukin 6 by activation of AP-1 but not NF-kappa B DNA binding. *Cancer Res* 1995; 55: 2373–2379.

40. Gollnick SO, Liu X, Owczarczak B, Musser DA, Henderson BW. Altered expression of interleukin 6 and interleukin 10 as a result of photodynamic therapy in vivo. *Cancer Res* 1997; 57: 3904–3909.

41. Anderson C, Hrabovsky S et al. Elmets. Phthalocyanine photodynamic therapy: disparate effects of pharmacologic inhibitors on cutaneous photosensitivity and on tumor regression. *Photochem Photobiol* 1997; 65: 895–901.

42. Kopecek J, Kopeckova P, Minko T, Lu Z. HPMA copolymer-anticancer drug conjugates: design, activity, and mechanism of action. *Eur J Pharm Biopharm* 2000; 50: 61–81.

43. Lu ZR, Shiah JG, Sakuma S, Kopeckova P, Kopecek J. Design of novel bioconjugates for targeted drug delivery. *J Control Release* 2002; 78: 165–173.

44. Gerlowski LE, Jain RK. Microvascular permeability of normal and neoplastic tissues. *Microvasc Res* 1986; 31: 288–305.

45. Maeda H, Sawa T, Konno T. Mechanism of tumor-targeted delivery of macromolecular drugs, including the EPR effect in solid tumor and clinical overview of the prototype polymeric drug SMANCS. *J Control Release* 2001; 74: 47–61.

46. Minko T, Kopeckova P, Kopecek J. Chronic exposure to HPMA copolymer-bound adriamycin does not induce multidrug resistance in a human ovarian carcinoma cell line. *J Control Release* 1999; 59: 133–148.

47. Minko T, Kopeckova P, Pozharov V, Kopecek J. HPMA copolymer bound adriamycin overcomes MDR1 gene encoded resistance in a human ovarian carcinoma cell line. *J Control Release* 1998; 54: 223–233.

48. Abe S, Otsuki M. Styrene maleic acid neocarzinostatin treatment for hepatocellular carcinoma. *Curr Med Chem Anti-Canc Agents* 2002; 715–726.

49. Brewerton LJ, Fung E, Snyder FF. Polyethylene glycol-conjugated adenosine phosphorylase: development of alternative enzyme therapy for adenosine deaminase deficiency. *Biochim Biophys Acta* 2003; 1637: 171–177.

50. Gianasi E, Wasil M, Evagorou EG, Keddle A, Wilson G, Duncan R. HPMA copolymer platinates as novel antitumour agents: in vitro properties, pharmacokinetics and anti-tumour activity in vivo. *Eur J Cancer* 1999; 35: 994–1002.

51. Lu ZR, Kopeckova P, Kopecek J. Polymerizable Fab' antibody fragments for targeting of anticancer drugs. *Nat Biotechnol* 1999; 17: 1101–4.

52. Lu ZR, Shiah JG, Kopeckova P, Kopecek J. Polymerizable Fab' antibody fragments targeted photodynamic cancer therapy in nude mice. *STP Pharm Sci* 2003; 13: 69–75.

53. Vaidya A, Sun Y, Ke T, Jeong EK, Lu ZR. Contrast enhanced MRI-guided photodynamic therapy for site-specific cancer treatment. *Magn Reson Med* 2006; 56: 761–7.
54. Caravan P, Ellison JJ, McMurry TJ, Lauffer RB. Gadolinium (III) chelates as MRI contrast agents: Structure, dynamics, and applications. *Chem Rev* 1999; 99: 2293–2352.
55. Vaidya A, Sun Y, Feng Y, Emerson L, Jeong EK, Lu ZR. Contrast-enhanced MRI-guided photodynamic cancer therapy with a pegylated bifunctional polymer conjugate. *Pharm Res* 2008; 25: 2002–2011.
56. Liang ZP, Lauterbur PC. *Principles of Magnetic Resonance Imaging: A Signal Processing Perspective*. New York: IEEE Inc. 2000.
57. Lauffer RB. Paramagnetic metal complexes as water proton relaxation agents for NMR imaging: theory and design. *Chem Rev* 1987; 87: 901–927.
58. Weinmann HJ, Brasch RC, Press WR, Wesbey GE. Characteristics of gadolinium-DTPA complex: A potential NMR contrast agent. *AJR* 1984; 142: 619–624.
59. Hayne L, Maravilla K, Cohen W, Gerlach R. Gd-DTPA-BMA, a new nonionic MR contrast agent: preliminary clinical results and comparison with Magnevist. *Radiology* 1989; 173: 537–540.
60. Magerstadt M, Gansow OA, Brechbiel MW, Colcher D, Baltzer L, Knop RH, Girton ME, Naegele M. Gd(DOTA): an alternative to Gd(DTPA) as a T1,2 relaxation agent for NMR imaging or spectroscopy. *Magn Reson Med* 1986; 3: 808–812.
61. Tweedle MF. The ProHance story: the making of a novel MRI contrast agent. *Eur Radiol* 1997; 7: 225–30.
62. Zheng J, Liu J, Dunne M, Jaffray DA, Allen C. In Vivo Performance of a liposomal vascular contrast agent for CT and MR-based image guidance applications. *Pharm Res* 2007; 24: 1193–1121.
63. Wang Y, Ye F, Jeong EK, Sun Y, Parker DL, Lu ZR. Noninvasive visualization of pharmacokinetics, biodistribution and tumor targeting of poly[N-(2-hydroxypropyl)methacrylamide] in mice using contrast enhanced MRI. *Pharm Res* 2007; 24: 1208–1216.
64. Kacher DF, Jolesz FA. MR imaging–guided breast ablative therapy. *Radiol Clin North Am* 2004; 42: 947–962.
65. Mortele KJ, Tuncali K, Cantisani V, Shankar S, vanSonnenberg E, Tempany C, Silverman SG. MRI-guided abdominal intervention. *Abdom Imaging* 2003; 28: 756–774.
66. Nurko J, Edwards MJ. Image-guided breast surgery. *Am J Surg* 2005; 190: 221–227.
67. Choyke PL, Dwyer AJ, Knopp MV. Functional tumor imaging with dynamic contrast-enhanced magnetic resonance imaging. *J Magn Reson Imaging* 2003; 17: 509–520.
68. Leach MO, Brindle KM, Evelhoch JL et al. The assessment of antiangiogenic and antivascular therapies in early-stage clinical trials using magnetic resonance imaging: issues and recommendations. *Br J Cancer* 2005; 92: 1599–1610.
69. Jordan BF, Runquist M, Raghunand N et al. The thioredoxin-1 inhibitor 1-methylpropyl 2-imidazolyl disulfide (PX-12) decreases vascular permeability in tumor xenografts monitored by dynamic contrast enhanced magnetic resonance imaging. *Clin Cancer Res* 2005; 11: 529–536.
70. Daldrup H, Shames DM, Wendland M et al. Correlation of dynamic contrast-enhanced MR imaging with histologic tumor grade: comparison of macromolecular and small-molecular contrast media. *AJR Am J Roentgenol* 1998; 171: 941–949.
71. Marzola P, Degrassi A, Calderan L et al. In vivo assessment of antiangiogenic activity of SU6668 in an experimental colon carcinoma model. *Clin Cancer Res* 2004; 10: 739–750.
72. Stephen RM, Gillies RJ. Promise and progress for functional and molecular imaging of response to targeted therapies. *Pharm Res* 2007; 24: 1172–1185.
73. Preda A, Novikov V, Möglich M et al. MRI monitoring of Avastin antiangiogenesis therapy using B22956/1, a new blood pool contrast agent, in an experimental model of human cancer. *J Magn Reson Imaging* 2004; 20: 865–873.

74. Cheng HL, Wallis C, Shou Z, Farhat WA. Quantifying angiogenesis in VEGF-enhanced tissue-engineered bladder constructs by dynamic contrast-enhanced MRI using contrast agents of different molecular weights. *J Magn Reson Imaging* 2007; 25: 137–145.

75. Lu ZR, Mohs AM, Zong Y, Feng Y. Polydisulfide Gd(III) chelates as biodegradable macromolecular magnetic resonance imaging contrast agents. *Intl J Nanomed* 2006; 1: 31–40.

76. Nguyen TD, Spincemaille P, Vaidya A, Prince MR, Lu ZR, Wang Y. Biodegradable intravascular (Gd-DTPA)-cystamine copolymer for contrast-enhanced steady-state free precession magnetic resonance angiography: comparison with MS-325 in a swine model. *Mol Pharm* 2006; 3: 558–565.

77. Mohs A, Nguyen T, Lu ZR et al. Pegylation of Gd-DTPA Cystine Copolymers improves pharmacokinetics and tissue retention for magnetic resonance angiography. *Magn Reson Med* 2007; 58: 110–118.

78. Feng Y, Jeong EK, Mohs A, Emerson L, Lu ZR. Characterization of tumor angiogenesis with dynamic contrast enhanced magnetic resonance imaging and biodegradable macro-molecular contrast agents in mice. *Magn Reson Med* 2008; 60: 1347–1352.

79. Stephen RM, Gillies RJ. Promise and progress for functional and molecular imaging of response to targeted therapies. *Pharm Res* 2007; 24:1172–1185.

Functional Imaging of Multidrug Resistance and Its Applications

Célia M.F. Gomes

1 Introduction

The emergence of multidrug resistance (MDR) is a major obstacle to the success of antineoplastic therapies [1]. The classical mechanism underlying MDR is the overexpression of energy-dependent transmembrane proteins behaving as drug efflux pumps. Three main proteins stand out in this family, P-glycoprotein (Pgp), multidrug resistance-associated protein-1 (MRP1), and breast cancer-related protein (BCRP). Each of these transporters has the ability to confer resistance to a broad spectrum of hydrophobic chemotherapeutic agents as a result of enhanced drug efflux [2]. These pumps, in particular Pgp, have been found in several highly resistant solid and hematological tumors and are associated with a poor prognosis [3–6]. Strategies to circumvent MDR include the co-administration of modulators, compounds that inhibit the functional activity of MDR-related transporters, and the use of cytotoxic agents that bypass the efflux mechanism [7]. Information on the functional expression of MDR-related transporters has the ability to provide a rational basis for developing potentially effective therapies that can be used in patients who are likely to be poor responders to standard chemotherapy and therefore have a poor prognosis under these circumstances.

Molecular imaging techniques using radiolabeled probes provide a minimally invasive approach for the functional assessment of MDR in cancer patients. A number of radiopharmaceuticals suitable for single-photon emission tomography (SPECT) and positron emission tomography (PET) have been developed and characterized as transport substrates of MDR transporters. Functional evaluation of MDR using imaging probes that mimic the antineoplastic agents can thus potentially be used to predict chemotherapy response and give information for the inclusion of modulators in therapeutic protocols. The most common imaging probes are the clinically approved ^{99m}Tc-labeled

C.M.F. Gomes (✉)
Institute of Biophysics/Biomathematics, IBILI – Faculty of Medicine,
University of Coimbra, Portugal
e-mail: cgomes@ibili.uc.pt

Y. Lu, R.I. Mahato (eds.), *Pharmaceutical Perspectives of Cancer Therapeutics*,
DOI 10.1007/978-1-4419-0131-6_19, © Springer Science+Business Media, LLC 2009

cationic lipophilic complexes, Sestamibi and Tetrofosmin. Their usefulness in detecting the MDR phenotype has been demonstrated in several clinical studies in different malignancies [8–10]. PET-based imaging probes including radiolabeled chemotherapeutic drugs (e.g., colchicine, daunorubicin) and modulators (verapamil) are currently undergoing investigational clinical studies and have yielded promising results [11].

A standardized SPECT/PET imaging methodology could provide very useful information in the clinical setting by determining the individual tumor susceptibility to chemotherapy at the time of diagnosis and even following chemotherapy. This knowledge could serve as a critical tool for optimizing chemotherapeutic protocols on a patient-specific basis. This chapter outlines the scientific basis of the molecular imaging probes available for functional assessment of MDR and presents examples of their application in pre-clinical and clinical studies.

2 ABC Transporters and Drug Resistance

The ability of tumor cells to develop cross-resistance to a broad range of cytotoxic agents, a trait known as multidrug resistance (MDR), limits the effectiveness of chemotherapy and is responsible for the treatment failure in several malignancies [1]. Nowadays, the emergence of MDR constitutes the major obstacle to the successful management of cancer patients. The classical mechanism underlying the MDR phenotype involves the overexpression of ATP-dependent efflux transmembrane proteins that actively remove the cytotoxic compounds preventing their intracellular accumulation at toxic levels [2]. Active drug efflux is mediated by several members of the ATP-binding cassette (ABC) superfamily of membrane transporters that share most of their sequences and present a high degree of structural homology [12]. P-glycoprotein (Pgp), the product of the human MDR1 gene, was the first ABC transporter identified and the most widely studied [13]. This protein was found to be expressed in several resistant tumor cell lines and confers resistance to a variety of structurally unrelated compounds including anthracyclines (doxorubicin, daunorubicin, epirubicin), epipodophyllotoxins (etoposide, teniposide), vinca alkaloids (vinblastine, vincristine, vindesine, vinorelbine), taxanes (docetaxel, paclitaxel), camptothecins (irinotecan, SN-38, topotecan) and others (colchicine, mitoxantrone, actinomycin D, bisantrene) [14]. Most of these drugs have distinct chemical structures and act on a variety of cellular targets, but share the property of being hydrophobic. For several years, Pgp was the only ABC transporter associated with the MDR phenotype. Subsequently other transporters were identified and recognized as energy-dependent drug efflux transporters, such as the multidrug resistance-associated protein-1 (MRP1) and the breast cancer resistance protein (BCRP) [15,16]. The chemotherapeutic substrates of these proteins are summarized in Table 1. MRP1 was cloned from a doxorubicin-resistant small-cell lung cancer cell line (H69AR) that did

Table 1 Anticancer drugs substrates of Pgp, MRP1 and BCRP

	Pgp	MRP1	BCRP
Anthracyclines	Doxorubicin, daunorubicin, epirubicin, mitoxantrone	Doxorubicin, daunorubicin, epirubicin	Doxorubicin, daunorubicin, epirubicin, mitoxantrone
Topoisomerase inhibitors	Etoposide, teniposide	Etoposide	Etoposide, topotecan, irinotecan, SN-38
Vinca alkaloids	Vincristine, vinblastine, vindesine, vinorelbine	Vincristine, vinblastine	
Taxanes	Paclitaxel, docetaxel		
Antitumor antibiotics	Actinomycin D, mitomycin C	Actinomycin D	
Antimetabolites	Cytarabine	Methotrexate	Methotrexate
Anthracenes	Bisantrene		Bisantrene
Flavonoids			Flavopiridol
Others	Colchicine		

not express Pgp [15] and is a member of the branch C of the ABC superfamily that comprises nine additional MRP1 homologues as described elsewhere [17]. The drug resistance profile caused by MRP1 is similar to that of Pgp and includes anthracyclines, vinca alkaloids, epipodophyllotoxins, camptothecins, and methotrexate but not taxanes and mitoxantrone [18,19]. Despite these similarities, MRP1 and Pgp have distinct substrates and differ on their transport mechanism. The substrates of Pgp are neutral or mildly positive lipophilic compounds, whereas MRP1 has high affinity for lipophilic anions such as heavy metal oxyanions (arsenite and antimony) that are transported as complexes of glutathione (GSH), sulfate, or glucuronate [18,20]. Moreover, the transport of some unmodified drugs such as anthracyclines or vinca alkaloids by MRP1 requires free GSH as a co-transporter or a co-factor [21].

The characterization of a mitoxantrone-resistant breast cancer cell line that displayed an efflux-based MDR phenotype without expression of Pgp or MRP1 led to the discovery of BCRP. This transporter, also known as mitoxantrone resistance protein (MXR) or placenta-specific ABC transporter (ABCP), is a half-transporter acting as a homo- or heterodimer to form an active transporter [22]. The substrate specificity of BCRP overlaps somewhat with that of Pgp and MRP1, suggesting a similar role in the pharmacokinetic of chemotherapeutic drugs. In fact, the overexpression of BCRP in tumor cells confers resistance to mitoxantrone, topotecan, SN38, flavopiridol, doxorubicin, bisantrene, etoposide, and methotrexate [16].

It is possible that other members of the ABC superfamily are involved in drug resistance. During the past few years, eight MRP1 homologues (MRP2, MRP3, MRP4, MRP5, MRP6, MRP7, MRP8, and MRP9), the bile salt export protein (BSEP), first reported as a *sister* of Pgp (S-Pgp), and the transporter associated with the antigen processing (TAP) have been shown to confer resistance to certain drugs comprising the MDR phenotype and are considered as potential mediators of drug resistance [12,23–25]. Nevertheless the clinical significance of their expression in tumor samples has not been clearly demonstrated [26,27].

2.1 Clinical Relevance

The clinical relevance of ABC transporter's overexpression in the effective treatment of cancer has been difficult to estimate. Despite the wealth of information regarding the transport mechanisms and substrate specificity of ABC transporters, translation of this knowledge from the bench to the bedside has been difficult to establish [6,26,28]. Most of the clinical studies performed so far are focused mainly on Pgp. A strong correlation between high levels of Pgp expression and poor clinical outcome has been reported in several malignancies including breast cancer, acute myeloid leukemia, osteosarcoma, ovarian cancer, lung cancer, and neuroblastoma [3–5,29–31]. Other studies, however, have failed to demonstrate such correlations and the prognostic significance of Pgp expression in therapy response remains controversial [32–34]. One of the reasons for the inconsistency in published data appears to be related with methodological issues, especially with analytical methods. In fact, there are currently no universally accepted guidelines for analytical methods or clinical validation [2]. Differences in study design and analytical methods with respect to tissue collecting and molecular targets (mRNA or protein) and the absence of standardized criteria to score the results have limited the ability to compare results from different institutions [26]. Moreover, the heterogeneity in patients groups in terms of patient number, initial or relapse samples, and differences in treatment protocols have also prevented the drawing of reliable conclusions.

2.2 Therapeutic Strategies to Overcome Drug Resistance

Reversal of MDR by non-toxic agents that block the activity of ABC transporters has been an important target for cancer therapy. Most attention has been given to inhibition of Pgp as it plays a major role in drug resistance. Since the early 1980s, a large number of compounds of diverse structure have been identified as inhibitors of Pgp and other ABC transporters [35]. These agents also referred to as MDR modulators or reversing agents were classified into three generations according to their characteristics and chronology. The first generation of modulators was not specifically developed for MDR inhibition and includes drugs with pharmacological activity such as calcium channel blockers (verapamil), calmodulin antagonists (trifluoperazine), steroid agents (progesterone, tamoxifen), and immunosuppressive drugs (cyclosporine A) [36]. The high doses required to achieve effective serum concentrations, due to their low affinity for ABC transporters, have resulted in unacceptable high toxicity limiting their application in cancer patients [37]. The second generation of modulators designed to reduce the side effects of the first-generation agents has a better pharmacological profile. They are congeners of the first-generation agents but without some of the negative pharmacological effects. Examples include PSC833 and dexverapamil derivatives of cyclosporine D and verapamil, respectively. Although less toxic, the second-generation modulators still retain some characteristics that limit their clinical usefulness due to unpredictable pharmacokinetic interactions [7]. Many anticancer agents are metabolized by cytochrome P450 3A4 isoenzyme and so are the second-generation modulators [38]. The competition of the two drugs for cytochrome P450 3A4 leads to an increase in the plasmatic concentrations of anticancer drug increasing their adverse effects. Since the pharmacokinetic interactions between modulators and cytotoxic agents are unpredictable, reducing the dose of the cytotoxic agent may result in under-dosing [38,39]. Moreover, these modulators are substrates of other ABC transporters that have a physiological role in regulating the permeability of the central nervous system, testis, and placenta to protect these systems from being exposed to xenobiotics. Their inhibition could decrease the ability of normal tissues to protect themselves from the adverse effects of anticancer drugs [40]. Recently, a new generation of Pgp modulators has been developed to specifically target Pgp based on structure–activity relationship data [37]. This third generation of modulators offers significant improvements as they are efficient at nanomolar concentrations and are not metabolized by cytochrome P450 3A4 [38]. Several compounds (tariquidar, zozuquidar, biricodar) are currently undergoing clinical trials. Data from phase I/II studies showed minimal pharmacokinetic interactions with anticancer agents, such as paclitaxel, vinorelbine, or doxorubicin, docetaxel and some of them are ongoing phase III clinical trials [41–43]. However, first reports showed either miscellaneous or negative results not meeting criteria for a study expansion [44–46]. Nevertheless the approach in which conventional chemotherapeutic agents are combined with MDR modulators is still considered valid and the search for a fourth generation of MDR modulators is ongoing [7].

A novel strategy to overcome MDR based on down-regulation of ABC transporters and enzymes involved in drug resistance has been developed. Recent advances in antisense oligonucleotide technologies have led to the development of short hairpin RNA interference (shRNA) against MDR1 mRNA. A complete reversal of Pgp-mediated drug resistance to doxorubicin, colchicine, and taxol was achieved in doxorubicin-resistant K562 cells stably expressing shRNA [47]. Ablation of Pgp in cells stably transduced with retroviral-mediated shRNA was documented by western blot and functionally confirmed by increased sensitivity of MDR1-transfected cells toward vincristine, paclitaxel, and doxorubicin [48]. In the same study, Pichler et al. used shRNA targeting a MDR1-*firefly luciferase* construct stably transfected in the liver of mice to follow in vivo by bioluminescence imaging, the downregulation of MDR1 expression [48]. Gene silencing approaches seem to have a great potential in the treatment of drug resistance tumors. The main obstacle to the development of shRNA-based therapeutic approaches is related with the delivery of the plasmid/vector to the target cells, especially in solid tumors, where delivery could be hampered by inadequate vascularization and microenvironmental factors. Moreover, due to the physiological expression of MDR1 gene in several normal epithelial and endothelial cells, it will be important to restrict delivery of shRNA to Pgp-expressing tumor cells.

2.3 Detection of ABC Transporters in Tumors

MDR-related transporters can be measured at mRNA level by reverse transcriptase polymerase chain reaction (RT-PCR) or at protein level by immunohistochemistry with monoclonal antibodies. Presently, the poor sensitivity and the lack of specificity of many commonly used antibodies along with difficulties associated with sample preparation, mostly related with contamination by normal tissue and data analysis, are impeditive for the achievement of reliable results [49,50]. The mRNA copy genes detected by RT-PCR do not always reflect the protein expression levels and the detection of MDR-related transporters at both gene and protein levels cannot predict their functional activity. Specific mutations as well as the phosphorylation status of the proteins can affect their functionality [14]. Flow cytometry assays using fluorescent markers have been developed to assess the functional activity of MDR-related proteins following administration of specific MDR inhibitors. The intracellular accumulation of Pgp substrates such as rhodamine 123, daunorubicin, Calcein-AM, or Hoechst 33342 is measured in the presence and in the absence of a Pgp-specific inhibitor [51,52]. Increases in the intracellular levels of fluorescence after exposure to a specific inhibitor reveal the presence of an active efflux pump. The functional flow cytometry as well as RT-PCR and immunohistochemistry are performed ex vivo, which implies to perform a tumor biopsy and sample processing. If this is not a significant obstacle for hematological malignancies, the same is not valid for solid tumors, which require more laborious procedures for sample collection and tissue purification.

2.4 Functional Assays Using Radiolabeled Molecules

The emergence of molecular imaging techniques using radiolabeled probes as surrogate markers of chemotherapeutic agents provides an alternative approach for functional assessment of MDR in cancer patients. Over the last decade, advances in medical imaging modalities together with the development of novel-specific imaging probes extended the traditional role of imaging in cancer from detection and staging of disease to tracking specific molecular pathways in cells or tissue function. A number of radiopharmaceuticals suitable for single-photon emission tomography (SPECT) and positron emission tomography (PET) have been developed and characterized as transport substrates of MDR transporters. Studies performed in cellular models of resistance have shown that cells exhibiting the MDR phenotype accumulate smaller amounts of radiopharmaceuticals in comparison with the sensitive counterparts, a feature that is correlated with the functionality of MDR-related proteins. Moreover, after addition of MDR modulators a considerable increase in both uptake and retention of radiotracers in resistant cells is observed, which is consistent with the blockade of MDR transporters. Such evidence suggests that functional imaging with radiotracers might be able to predict the development of resistance to chemotherapy mediated by ABC transporters. In addition, this approach provides an important tool to evaluate in vivo the efficacy of MDR modulators as an alternative to the ex vivo assays, in which the serum taken from patients receiving a modulator is assayed for its ability to reverse MDR in a Pgp-expressing cell line. The ability to obtain in vivo and non-invasively information at functional level of MDR-related transporters, using probes mimicking the antineoplastic agents is of great practical benefit for patients and offers a possibility of determining the individual tumor susceptibility to chemotherapy. This previous knowledge could serve as a critical tool for optimizing chemotherapeutic protocols on a patient-specific basis.

The following sections of this chapter are focused on the potentialities of SPECT and PET for imaging drug resistance mechanisms mediated by the expression of ABC transporters in cancer. Initially, we will introduce the radiopharmaceuticals available for SPECT imaging, highlighting some of results obtained from clinical and pre-clinical studies. Second, an overview over the advances in PET radiopharmaceuticals that are becoming available for studying MDR will be presented.

3 Functional Imaging of MDR

3.1 SPECT Imaging Agents

3.1.1 [^{99m}Tc]Sestamibi

Several gamma-emitting compounds have been synthesized, validated, and characterized as sensitive probes for Pgp and MRP1 functional activity. Most of these compounds are cationic and modestly hydrophobic similar to the chemotherapeutic agents in the MDR phenotype. The radiopharmaceutical hexakis(2-methoxy-isobutyl-isonitrile)technetium-99m commonly known as [^{99m}Tc]Sestamibi or [^{99m}Tc]MIBI (Cardiolite®) was the first imaging agent recognized as transport substrate of Pgp and the most widely used in clinical and pre-clinical studies for functional evaluation of MDR [53].

[^{99m}Tc]MIBI belongs to the class of ^{99m}Tc-labeled cationic and lipophilic compounds originally developed and clinically approved for myocardial perfusion studies. Subsequently, it has been used as a tumor-seeking agent in several malignancies [54,55]. This complex crosses the cell membranes by passive diffusion in response to the physiologically negative transmembrane potential and accumulates reversibly within the mitochondria using the electrical gradient generated by the high negative inner mitochondrial transmembrane potential [56,57].

The difference in the transmembrane potential, of the mitochondria, between normal epithelial and carcinoma cells is at least 60 mV more negative in the latter due to the higher metabolic requirements of tumor cells [58]. According to the Nernst equation, this difference would lead to a 10-fold increase in the cellular uptake of lipophilic cations [59]. This is the principle for the superior accumulation of [^{99m}Tc]MIBI in tumor cells when compared to the epithelial or connective surrounding tissues.

However, although cellular uptake of [^{99m}Tc]MIBI is driven by the plasma and mitochondrial membrane potentials, the overall accumulation of the tracer is inversely proportional to the expression levels of Pgp in tumor cells. The earlier observations that intracellular accumulation of [^{99m}Tc]MIBI varied widely among tumor cell lines [60] prompted several groups to explore the role of Pgp in transport kinetics of [^{99m}Tc]MIBI in tumor cells. Several studies performed in tumor cell lines exhibiting the MDR phenotype, either by selection with cytotoxic agents or by transfection with the MDR recombinant transporters, generally showed a reduced net uptake of [^{99m}Tc]MIBI, a feature that is closely related with the outward transport activity of Pgp.

Based on this principle, Pgp-overexpressing tumors can be detected in scintigraphic images by their low uptake ("cold" spot) and rapid washout rate from the tumor lesion, whereas drug-sensitive tumors translate into a higher uptake ("hot" spot) with a slow washout rate of the radiotracer [61]. Numerous in vitro and in vivo studies, pre-clinical and clinical, have been performed in order to appraise the usefulness of [^{99m}Tc]MIBI imaging to identify Pgp-expressing tumors on a functional basis.

After observing that [^{99m}Tc]MIBI accumulates in tumor cells in reverse ranking order of their Pgp expression levels, Piwnica-Worms et al. developed an animal model of human carcinoma for in vivo assessment of Pgp activity using [^{99m}Tc]MIBI [53]. The animal model was established by subcutaneous inoculation of human sensitive carcinoma cells KB-3-1 and its drug-resistant counterpart KB-8-5 in opposite flanks. Previous in vitro studies have shown that KB-8-5 cells overexpress Pgp are 3.2-fold resistant to adriamycin when compared to parental KB-3-1 cells [62]. A relative resistance of 2–2.5 for KB-8-5 tumors was documented by growth tumor analysis after treatment with adriamycin, further supporting the maintenance of the MDR phenotype after the inoculation of the cells in mice. The analysis of scintigraphic images 60 min after injection of [^{99m}Tc]MIBI showed a lower accumulation of [^{99m}Tc]MIBI in Pgp-expressing tumors compared to the parental tumors implanted in the opposite flank [53]. The imaging results were confirmed with quantitative biodistribution analysis of the radiotracer in tumors. In Pgp-enriched tumors (KB-8-5), the [^{99m}Tc]MIBI accumulation was 35±4% lower than in parental sensitive tumors. Similar results were observed by Barbarics et al. [63] in an animal model of human breast cancer. The MDA 435 breast carcinoma cell line and its paclitaxel-resistant derivatives, MDA/T0.1 (200-fold resistant) and MDA/T0.3 (300-fold resistant), were grown as xenografts in athymic mice to characterize the effects of chemotherapeutic agents in tumor growth. The MDA 435 parental cell line accumulated the highest percentage of the [^{99m}Tc]MIBI injected dose per gram of tissue. Compared with the parental xenografts, the resistant xenografts took up approximately 35–50% less [^{99m}Tc]MIBI. After treating the animals with the Pgp-inhibitor PSC833, the accumulation of [^{99m}Tc]MIBI in resistant tumors increased to the same levels found in parental MDA 435 xenografts. Nevertheless, the amount of PSC833 required to attain an amount of [^{99m}Tc]MIBI in MDA/T0.3 xenografts equivalent to those in MDA 435 xenografts was greater (100 mg/Kg) than that required for the MDA/T0.1 xenografts (50 mg/Kg), further indicating that PSC833 modulates Pgp activity in a dose-dependent manner.

In a rat model with a doxorubicin-resistant and drug-sensitive rat breast adenocarcinomas xenografts, Ballinger et al. observed that [^{99m}Tc]MIBI was washed out from resistant tumor with a 3-fold higher efflux rate when compared with sensitive tumors, demonstrating that functional Pgp mediates the outward transport of [^{99m}Tc]MIBI, reducing its cellular accumulation [64].

In an attempt to determine the predictive value of [^{99m}Tc]MIBI imaging, Muzzammil et al. compared the kinetic profiles of [^{99m}Tc]MIBI and doxorubicin in three variants of the human breast carcinoma cell line MCF7: sensitive MCF7/WT, doxorubicin-selected MCF7/AdrR, and MDR1-gene-transfected MCF7/BC19 cells [65]. The effects of potent second-generation Pgp modulators GG918 and PSC833 were studied regarding the accumulation of both agents and the sensitivity of the cells to doxorubicin. Cellular accumulation of [^{99m}Tc]MIBI and mean fluorescence of doxorubicin were assessed over 60 min with and without modulators. The time course of the accumulation of [^{99m}Tc]MIBI and doxorubicin differed significantly among the three cell lines under control situation, as depicted in Fig 1. The two resistant sublines,

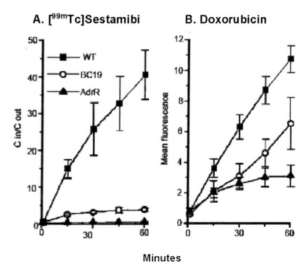

Fig. 1 Time-course accumulation of [^{99m}Tc]MIBI (**A**) and doxorubicin (**B**) in MCF7/WT, MCF7/BC19, and MCF7/AdrR cells (reprinted with permission from Macmillan Publishers, Ltd, Ref. [65])

MCF7/AdrR and MCF7/BC19, showed a deficit in both [^{99m}Tc]MIBI and doxorubicin accumulations, when compared with the wild-type cells, indicating that both drugs are transport substrates of Pgp. However, the differences in uptake between sensitive and resistant cells were greater for [^{99m}Tc]MIBI than for doxorubicin, suggesting that other cell factors may affect differently the uptake and retention of these drugs.

The MDR modulators, GG918 and PSC833, reversed the accumulation deficits of [^{99m}Tc]MIBI and doxorubicin in the MDR1-gene-transfected MCF7/BC19 cells to the MCF7/WT levels. For MCF7/AdrR cells, reversal of accumulation deficit was complete for doxorubicin but only partial for [^{99m}Tc]MIBI, suggesting that other cell factors present in MCF7/AdrR cells affect [^{99m}Tc]MIBI uptake more than doxorubicin. The resistant variant MCF7/AdrR was established through long-term exposure to doxorubicin. During drug selection, it is possible that changes in membrane, cytosolic and nuclear proteins, metabolic function, mitochondrial density, or membrane potential charge that affect uptake and retention of [^{99m}Tc]MIBI might occur, that are not reversed by Pgp modulators [53,66,67]. Supporting evidence for this explanation was the complete restoring of drug accumulation in MDR1-gene-transfected MCF7/BC19 cells, whose resistance mechanism was solely mediated by Pgp expression. Both Pgp inhibitors were effective in restoring doxorubicin and [^{99m}Tc]MIBI accumulation to the levels found in MCF7/WT cells. Moreover, PSC833 and GG918 enhanced the cytotoxic effects of doxorubicin in the two resistant cell lines. Even so, the MCF7/AdrR remained 2- to 5-fold more resistant when compared to MCF7/BC19 cells, despite the equal levels of doxorubicin fluorescence. In conclusion, both [^{99m}Tc]MIBI accumulation and doxorubicin flow cytometry techniques were able to detect Pgp-mediated MDR and its modulation, clearly distinguishing sensitive from resistant cell lines. Although [^{99m}Tc]MIBI and doxorubicin share the property of being substrates of Pgp, having similar affinity for Pgp-transport function, the radioisotope method appears to offer a better predictive value [65].

In vitro experiments demonstrated that reduced cellular uptake of [^{99m}Tc]MIBI is also related with overexpression of MRP1. Utsunomiya et al. studied the uptake and efflux kinetics of [^{99m}Tc]MIBI in a nasopharyngeal carcinoma cell line (CNE-1) [68]. Western blot and RT-PCR analysis indicated that these cells express moderate levels of both MRP1 and MRP2 but not Pgp. The maximal accumulation [^{99m}Tc]MIBI, calculated as the ratio of radioactivity concentration inside the cell to that found in the supernatant (C_{in}/C_{out}), was 6.3 and increased significantly after inhibition with verapamil and CsA when compared with control. The efflux rate of [^{99m}Tc]MIBI diminished significantly after addition of verapamil or CsA that are both not selective for Pgp and exert inhibitor effects on MRP1 activity. Additionally, PSC833 and GG918 did not elicit significant alterations on the efflux rate [^{99m}Tc]MIBI due to their specificity for Pgp.

The GSH-dependent transport of certain drugs and organic anions by MRP1 led several authors to investigate the role of GSH on the transport of

[^{99m}Tc]MIBI in MRP1-overexpressing cell lines. Prior to perform the radio-tracer kinetic studies, cells were pre-treated with buthionine sulfoximine (BSO) to reduce the intracellular content of GSH. BSO selectively inhibits γ-glutamyl-cysteine synthetase (γ-GCS), the rate-limiting step in the synthesis of GSH [20,21]. The treatment with BSO increased the uptake and retention of [^{99m}Tc]MIBI in four grade IV glioma cell lines, suggesting that transport of cationic radiotracers are carried out, in part, through the MRP1/GSH system [69]. These results were in agreement with those of Vergote [70] and Hendrikse [71] which showed that incubation with BSO induced a higher retention of [^{99m}Tc]MIBI in cells with enhanced expression of MRP1 but not in Pgp-over-expressing cells. This feature can be useful to discriminate between Pgp and MRP1 drug resistance mechanisms, as Pgp activity does not require GSH, and to evaluate the efficacy of GSH-depleting agents as well. GSH is a ubiquitous intracellular tri-peptide that plays a central role in cellular defense against toxic environmental agents and drugs [72]. Elevated levels of GSH have been impli-cated in cellular resistance to a wide range of cytotoxic drugs, in particular alkylating agents and platinum-containing compounds [73]. Modulation of cellular GSH homeostasis represents a potential strategy to sensitize tumor cells to cytotoxic drugs, an approach that could be of particular interest in MRP1 overexpressing tumor cells [20]. Experiments with MRP1-transfected cells showed that depletion of GSH results in a complete reversal of resistance to vinca alkaloids and anthracyclines [74], suggesting that changes in the intracel-lular levels of GSH have a marked effect on MRP1-mediated drug efflux for at least some of the drugs to which it conferred resistance.

Our group studied the chemosensitivity of four human osteosarcoma cell lines (Saos-2, 143B, MNNG/HOS, and U-2OS) to the main cytostatics used in the current protocols (doxorubicin, cisplatin, and methotrexate). Our purpose was to determine whether there was a relationship between drug resistance, gene expression, and functional activity of MDR-related transporters [75]. None of the cell lines were previously exposed to drugs and therefore not selected for drug resistance. We found that chemosensitivity of osteosarcoma cell lines to doxorubicin was strongly dependent on mRNA MDR1 gene expression and could be circumvented by adding a Pgp inhibitor (cyclosporine A). The radio-tracer's kinetic parameters extracted from the uptake and efflux curves corre-lated with MDR1 expression levels, hence predicting resistance to doxorubicin. Moreover, addition of cyclosporin A at the same concentration as in drug reversal studies, increased significantly the radiotracer uptake and reduces the efflux rate in resistant cells, confirming for the active role of Pgp in the mechanism of resistance to doxorubicin (Fig. 2).

These observations prompted our group to investigate the ability of [^{99m}Tc]MIBI imaging for in vivo identification of Pgp-mediated drug resistance. For that purpose, an orthotopic animal model of osteosarcoma was established by intratibial inoculation of osteosarcoma cell lines in nude mice [76]. Doxor-ubicin sensitive (143B) and resistant (MNNG/HOS) cell lines were stably transfected with the firefly luciferase to monitor the local tumor growth by

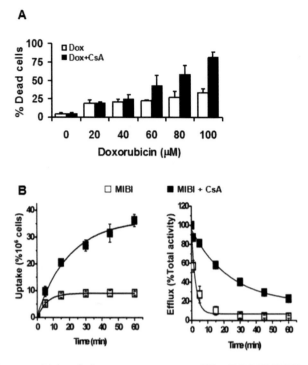

Fig. 2 (**A**) Chemosensitivity of a human osteosarcoma cell line (MNNG/HOS) to doxorubicin and reversal of drug resistance. Cells were treated for 24 h with doxorubicin at indicated concentrations with and without 5 μM CsA. The percentage of dead cells was analyzed by flow cytometry. The MNNG/HOS cell line showed a high resistance to doxorubicin, with a low and invariable percentage of dead cells. After incubation with CsA, at non-toxic concentration, the percentage of dead cells increased linearly in dose-dependent manner. (**B**) Effects of CsA on uptake and efflux kinetics of [^{99m}Tc]MIBI in MNNG/HOS cells. The same dose of CsA as in drug reversal study caused a 4-fold increase in the steady-state accumulation of [^{99m}Tc]MIBI and enhanced significantly the intracellular retention of the radiotracer as demonstrated by the slower efflux rate as compared with the control. The mRNA analysis of MDR-related genes has revealed that the MDR1 gene is up-regulated in the MNNG/HOS cell line

bioluminescence imaging. The formation of osteolytic lesions, typical of human osteosarcoma, was monitored by conventional radiography. After primary tumor growth, the animals were imaged with [^{99m}Tc]MIBI during 60 min. The kinetic parameters obtained from imaging analysis clearly discriminated sensitive from resistant tumors. Cellular accumulation of [^{99m}Tc]MIBI calculated in both early (5 min) and delayed (60 min) images was significantly higher ($p<0.05$) in 143B-sensitive tumors compared with that in MNNG-HOS-resistant tumors. A faster washout rate of [^{99m}Tc]MIBI was equally observed in MNNG-HOS-resistant tumors as demonstrated by the shorter washout half-times and higher percentage washout rate in MNNG/HOS-resistant tumors ($t_{1/2} = 87.3 \pm 15.7$ min; %WR $= 37.5 \pm 4.0$) when compared with those in 143B-sensitive tumors ($t_{1/2} = 161.0 \pm 47.4$ min; %WR $= 24.6 \pm 7.5$ %).

The treatment of animals with the Pgp-inhibitor PSC833 increased significantly the washout half-times of [^{99m}Tc]MIBI in MNNG/HOS-resistant tumors
($t_{1/2}$ = 173.0±24.5 min) to values comparable to those in 143B-sensitive tumors in
control situation. However, no significant increase was observed in [^{99m}Tc]MIBI
uptake in MNNG/HOS tumors, indicating that the uptake-related parameter is
not a consistent index to evaluate the inhibitor efficacy of PSC833 [76]. Figure 3
illustrates a representative bioluminescent image of a mouse inoculated with
osteosarcoma cells carrying a luciferase reporter gene into the right tibia and
the early and delayed scintigraphic images acquired in the absence and in the
presence of PSC833. The formation of osteolytic lesions, typical of osteosarcoma,
was detected radiographically 3–4 weeks after the inoculation of tumor cells.

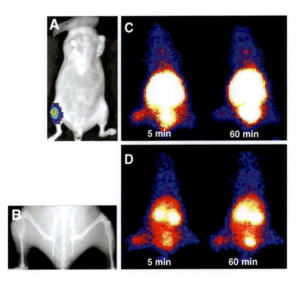

Fig. 3 (**A**) Bioluminescent image of nude mouse 4 weeks after intratibial inoculation of osteosarcoma cells carrying a luciferase reporter gene. (**B**) Radiograph taken at 4 weeks shows the
formation of osteolytic lesions in the corresponding region. [^{99m}Tc]MIBI images acquired at
early (5 min) and delayed times (60 min) in the absence (**C**) and after treatment with PSC833
(**D**). The treatment with 50 mg/kg PSC833 increased both the uptake and the retention of
[^{99m}Tc]MIBI in the tumor region

The results obtained in vivo were largely consistent with those observed in
vitro and suggest that Pgp expression is determinant on the chemosensitivity of
tumor cells to doxorubicin, an important cytostatic used in the treatment of
osteosarcoma, and can be detected non-invasively by [^{99m}Tc]MIBI imaging.
According to these results, the uptake parameter is not so robust as the wash-
out-related parameters to evaluate the functional activity of Pgp expressed in
tumors, since [^{99m}Tc]MIBI is not target specific and its uptake is markedly

influenced by several factors rather than simply Pgp activity. The enhanced washout of [^{99m}Tc]MIBI appears to be a more reliable index of Pgp activity and a better predictor of drug resistance, since it reflects the Pgp-mediated outward transport.

Inefficient blood supply, advanced cell necrosis, hypoxia, and the overexpression of the anti-apoptotic protein Bcl-2 may significantly reduce the uptake of [^{99m}Tc]MIBI in tumor lesions [77]. An adequate blood supply is a prerequisite for the effective delivery of [^{99m}Tc]MIBI to the tumoral mass. Mankoff et al. studied the influence of tumor blood supply using ^{15}O-water PET imaging on [^{99m}Tc]MIBI uptake in 37 patients with locally advanced breast carcinoma and found a significant positive correlation between early uptake and blood flow [78]. For instance, tumors containing necrotic areas accompanied by an inefficient blood supply and the occurrence of hypoxic cells can change the kinetics of [^{99m}Tc]MIBI, decreasing its intracellular accumulation, which can provide false-positive results regarding Pgp expression in tumor cells. In the absence of factors limiting the free diffusion of [^{99m}Tc]MIBI from blood to tumor cells, the early [^{99m}Tc]MIBI uptake reflects the density and the functional status of mitochondria namely the permeability of mitochondrial membrane and the preservation of the membrane potential [79]. During the early stages of drug-induced apoptosis there is an increase in the permeability of the outer mitochondrial membrane under the control of the Bcl-2 protein family resulting in mitochondrial dysfunction and dissipation of mitochondrial potentials. Bcl-2 is an anti-apoptotic protein located in the outer mitochondrial membrane that prevents cells from entering the apoptotic process. The overexpression of Bcl-2 in tumor cells prevents the permeabilization of mitochondrial membrane and the release of cytochrome c and other soluble proteins triggered by death signals protecting tumor cells from drug-induced apoptosis. This effect also impairs the trafficking of lipophilic cations across the mitochondrial membrane, reducing its accumulation within mitochondria. This evidence was further observed by Del Vecchio et al. in breast cancer patients [80]. They found that tumors who failed to accumulate [^{99m}Tc]MIBI have a low apoptotic index and a marked overexpression on Bcl-2. This relationship was further observed in vitro in breast cancer cell lines stably transfected with the human Bcl-2 gene [81]. All clones overexpressing Bcl-2 showed a dramatic reduction, up to 97% of [^{99m}Tc]MIBI accumulation as compared with wild-type and mock-transfected cells. Furthermore, after treatment with staurosporine, a potent inducer of apoptosis, [^{99m}Tc]MIBI uptake was partially restored in Bcl-2 overexpressing cells. Levels of Bcl-2 in transfected clones, as determined by immunohistochemistry, were elevated and in the range measured in tumors who failed to accumulate [^{99m}Tc]MIBI. Conversely, tumors with high in vivo uptake of [^{99m}Tc]MIBI showed only barely detectable levels of Bcl-2 (Fig. 4).

The biological information provided by an absent or a reduced accumulation of [^{99m}Tc]MIBI in early images may be related to different cellular processes and should be carefully interpreted. The lack of [^{99m}Tc]MIBI uptake

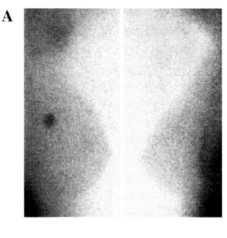

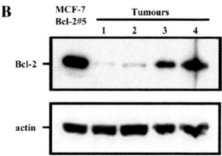

Fig. 4 (**A**) Lateral view scintimammograms obtained 10 min after i.v. injection of 740 MBq of [^{99m}Tc]MIBI in two patients with untreated breast carcinoma. On the *left*, high focal [^{99m}Tc]MIBI uptake was observed in a 2 cm ductal carcinoma (tumor 2) of the upper external quadrant of the right breast. On the *right*, no [^{99m}Tc]MIBI uptake was observed in a 3 cm ductolobular carcinoma (tumor 3) of the upper external quadrant of the left breast. (**B**) Bcl-2 levels determined by western blot analysis in breast carcinomas obtained from patients who had previously undergone [^{99m}Tc]MIBI scan as described above. Two tumors (nos. 1 and 2) had high focal ^{99m}Tc-MIBI uptake in vivo and the other two (nos. 3 and 4) showed no ^{99m}Tc-MIBI uptake on scintigraphic images. Tumors with high in vivo [^{99m}Tc]MIBI uptake (nos. 1 and 2) showed only barely detectable levels of Bcl-2 protein, whereas the two tumors with no tracer uptake on scintigraphic images (nos. 3 and 4) showed high levels of Bcl-2 protein comparable to those found in the Bcl-2 overexpressing clone MCF-7 (reprinted by permission from Springer Science + Business Media, Ref. [81])

in malignant lesions can be indicative of a non-permeable mitochondrial membrane to [^{99m}Tc]MIBI due to high expression levels of Bcl-2 or can be related with the presence of Pgp or other efflux pumps. Although both conditions constitute a drug resistance mechanism and help tumor cells to evade chemotherapy, it is important to discriminate between them in order to define the suitable approach for circumventing drug resistance.

Clinical Studies with [^{99m}Tc]MIBI

The clinical relevance of [^{99m}Tc]MIBI imaging in predicting chemotherapy response has been investigated in diverse malignancies including breast cancer, lung tumors, osteosarcoma, lymphomas, and hepatocelular carcinoma. In general, [^{99m}Tc]MIBI kinetic parameters extracted from image analysis are correlated with the expression levels of Pgp and/or MRP1, detected at gene or protein level in the tumor specimen, and with tumor response to chemotherapy.

A significant number of studies were conducted in breast cancer patients, since [^{99m}Tc]MIBI scintimammography is currently used as an auxiliary method in the diagnosis of breast cancer. A review of the published literature revealed that 41% of patients with breast cancers express Pgp at presentation, with increased levels after chemotherapy [82]. Moreover, the expression of Pgp, especially when detected following therapy, correlates with a worst prognosis in both adjuvant and neoadjuvant chemotherapies, being considered a potential biomarker of drug resistance [4,82]. The first clinical studies planned to determine whether [^{99m}Tc]MIBI imaging could detect in vivo the presence of Pgp in breast tumors examined the relationship between [^{99m}Tc]MIBI uptake and the expression of Pgp assessed by immunohistochemistry. Kostakoglu et al. observed an inverse correlation between the tumor-to-background (T/B) ratios of [^{99m}Tc]MIBI and the density of Pgp expression in tumor tissues [83]. The values for the T/B ratios were significantly lower for those tumors expressing Pgp at high levels than those with scattered and no Pgp expression ($p<0.01$ and $p<0.001$, respectively). In a prospective study, Kao et al. evaluated the relationship between the degree of accumulation of [^{99m}Tc]MIBI and Pgp or MRP1 expression in 48 patients with infiltrating ductal breast cancer [84]. The tumors with positive expression of Pgp and MRP1 showed the lowest T/B ratios (1.13 ± 0.10), whereas the tumors with negative expression Pgp and MRP1 had the highest T/B ratios (2.17 ± 0.14). A significant negative correlation has been observed between net uptake of [^{99m}Tc]MIBI and Pgp expression levels in tumor lesions; however, it was not proven any time dependence on this relationship.

Del Vecchio et al. performed a radiotracer kinetic analysis over 4 hours following injection of [^{99m}Tc]MIBI in 30 untreated breast carcinoma patients [85]. The results showed a statistically positive correlation between radiotracer efflux rate and Pgp expression levels. The efflux rate of [^{99m}Tc]MIBI in Pgp-overexpressing tumors was 2.7-fold greater than that of tumors expressing Pgp at levels comparable to benign breast lesions. A threshold value corresponding to a half-clearance of 204 min was established to discriminate Pgp-overexpressing tumors from those with basal expression levels, with 80% sensitivity and 90% specificity. Based on these findings, the authors concluded that the efflux rate constants of [^{99m}Tc]MIBI reflect the functional activity of Pgp and could be used to predict chemotherapy response of breast cancer patients. This hypothesis was further investigated in other studies. Ciarmiello et al. analyzed whether tumor clearance of [^{99m}Tc]MIBI may be predictive of therapeutic response to neoadjuvant chemotherapy in patients with locally advanced breast cancer [86].

Tumors with a prolonged retention of [^{99m}Tc]MIBI exhibited a favorable response to chemotherapy. In opposite, a rapid clearance of [^{99m}Tc]MIBI was significantly associated with a lack of tumor response to neoadjuvante chemotherapy as demonstrated by the presence of residual tumor in surgical specimens. Sciuto et al. reported similar results in a prospective study with 30 patients with locally advanced breast cancer undergoing neoadjuvant chemotherapy [8]. On this study, the washout rate of [^{99m}Tc]MIBI was calculated using the T/B ratios in early (10 min) and delayed (4 h) images as follows: $(T/B_{10\ min} - T/B_{4\ h})/T/B_{10\ min} \times 100$ (%). A cut-off of 45% was considered statistically discriminative between good and poor responders. Twelve of 30 patients who responded favorably to chemotherapy had a washout rate less than or equal to 45%. Conversely, the remaining 18 patients that have failed to respond to chemotherapy had a washout rate superior to 45%.

In a retrospective study including 46 patients with locally advanced or metastatic breast cancer, Takamura et al. evaluated the significance of [^{99m}Tc]MIBI uptake in early and delayed images in predicting tumor response to chemotherapy with epirubicin and cyclophosphamide or docetaxel [87]. Before starting chemotherapy, the patients underwent a [^{99m}Tc]MIBI SPECT study. The parameters extracted from SPECT images were the tumor-to-normal tissue ratios (T/N) of [^{99m}Tc]MIBI uptake at 10 min (early phase) and at 180 min (delayed phase) and the retention index (RI) was calculated as follows: $RI = (T/N(d))/(T/N(e))$. After chemotherapy, tumor response was determined by clinical examination.

Both early T/N(e) and delayed T/N(d) uptake ratios were significantly higher for patients who responded to chemotherapy than for non-responders. The diagnostic accuracy of the T/N(d) in predicting chemotherapy response using the arbitrary cut-off value of 3.0 was 89.1% with a positive and a negative predictive value of 81.0 and 96.0%, respectively. Although significant, the relationship between T/N(e) ratio and response to chemotherapy was less pronounced probably because the early phase of [^{99m}Tc]MIBI uptake is affected by other factors than the expression of Pgp, such as the blood flow to the tumor. Representative [^{99m}Tc]MIBI studies are shown in Fig. 5. The tumor retention index (RI) was not statistically different between responders and non-responders who seem to be attributable, at least in part, to the finding that RI was calculated using the T/N(e) ratio that is influenced by other factors than Pgp.

The expression levels of Pgp, determined by immunohistochemistry in tumor specimens prior to treatment, was significantly higher in lesions with low T/B(d) ratios when compared with those with high values, indicating that [^{99m}Tc]MIBI extrusion is accelerated in Pgp-expressing tumors. Moreover, the higher expression of Pgp was found in non-responders (Fig. 6). The results from this study suggest that the T/B ratio of [^{99m}Tc]MIBI at delayed times is useful to predict response to chemotherapy and for in vivo evaluation of Pgp expression status in patients with locally advanced or recurrent breast carcinoma.

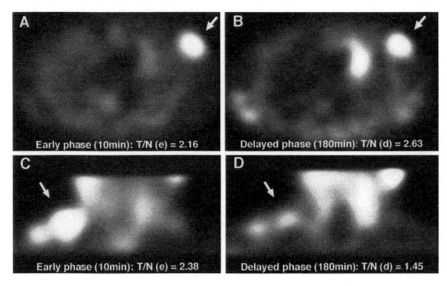

Fig. 5 Representative [^{99m}Tc]MIBI SPECT scintimammograms obtained at 10 min (early phase) and 180 min (delayed phase) after i.v. injection of [^{99m}Tc]MIBI responder (**A and B**) and non-responder (**C and D**) patients (reprinted with permission of Wiley-Liss, Inc., a subsidiary of John Wiley & Sons, Inc., Ref. [87])

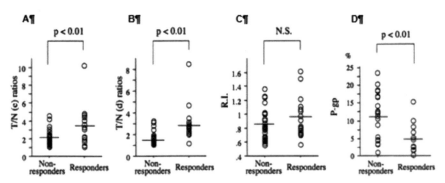

Fig. 6 Relation between chemotherapeutic response and T/N(e) ratios (**A**), T/N(d) ratios (**B**), retention index (RI) (**C**), and Pgp expression levels (**D**) in breast carcinoma patients. N.S.: not significant (reprinted with permission of Wiley-Liss, Inc., a subsidiary of John Wiley & Sons, Inc., Ref. [87])

Lung tumors represent another malignancy in which the expression of MDR-related transporters is associated with a poor prognosis [88–90]. Several studies have been published on the prognostic value of [^{99m}Tc]MIBI imaging in predicting chemotherapy response and its relationship with Pgp and/or MRP1 expression. Analysis of tumor retention and washout rates of [^{99m}Tc]MIBI by comparing early and delayed SPECT and planar images have been performed and correlated with the expression levels of Pgp and MRP1. The relation of those parameters with therapy response was also analyzed in some studies.

In a prospective study with a total of 46 patients with lung tumors, Kostakoglu et al. correlated the accumulation and washout rate of [^{99m}Tc]MIBI with the levels of Pgp expression determined by immunohistochemistry in paraffin sections [91]. All patients underwent early (30 min) and delayed (3 h) [^{99m}Tc]MIBI imaging and bronchoscopic biopsy before initiation of chemo- or radiotherapy. They found a significant inverse correlation ($p = 0.001$) between the T/B ratios and the density of Pgp expression, whereas no appreciable correlation ($p = 0.414$) was observed between the [^{99m}Tc]MIBI washout rate and the Pgp expression levels. Current data strongly suggest that, although the reduced ability for the tumors to accumulate [^{99m}Tc]MIBI correlates well with the increased levels of Pgp expression, tumor washout rates of [^{99m}Tc]MIBI do not correlate with the density of Pgp in tumor tissues. Bom et al. observed similar results in 25 patients with SCLC [92]. In this study, they calculated the T/B ratios at 1 and 4 h after injection of [^{99m}Tc]MIBI and the percent retention as follows: $\%R = (T/B_{4h})/(T/B_{1h}) \times 100$. The results were correlated with tumor response to chemotherapy evaluated according to follow-up CT and grouped as complete remission, partial remission, and no remission. The T/B ratios of patients with complete and partial remission were significantly higher compared with patients with no remission. However, the percent retention of radiotracer between 1 and 4 h did not differ significantly among the three groups. Assuming that Pgp acts as an active drug efflux pump mediating drug-outward transport, one would expect a close connection between Pgp expression and enhanced washout rate of Pgp substrates from the tumor. In both studies, they were unable to detect an active efflux mechanism associated with the considerable reduction in [^{99m}Tc]MIBI accumulation in Pgp-positive samples. This could be accepted if Pgp acts as a "flippase" transporting drugs from the inner leaflet of the lipid bilayer to the outer or to the external medium preventing drugs to accumulate within the cell. In this context, %W-O rates are not supposed to be affected dramatically by Pgp. Another explanation for the lack of correlation between [^{99m}Tc]MIBI retention and Pgp expression could be related with the time points used to derive the washout rates. In these studies, they measured the percent of change in tumor activity between 30 or 60 min and 4 h following injection of radiotracer. Probably 30 min is too late to be considered as a reference time, since active efflux occurs rapidly and might take place immediately following injection.

Zhou et al. in a study including 34 patients with histologically confirmed lung cancer underwent [^{99m}Tc]MIBI SPECT followed by surgery [93]. The early and delayed SPECT images were acquired at 15 and 180 min, respectively, after injection of [^{99m}Tc]MIBI. Sample tumors were analyzed by immunohistochemistry and RT-PCR for expression of Pgp and MRP1. The delayed uptake (at 180 min) and the efflux rate of [^{99m}Tc]MIBI (between 15 and 180 min) correlates significantly with the expression levels of Pgp. Such correlations were not observed in relation to the early tumor uptake, which suggests that early uptake is more affected by blood flow.

Neither the early and delayed uptakes nor the washout rate of [^{99m}Tc]MIBI was correlated with the MRP1 expression levels in tumor lesions. The ability of Pgp and MRP1 to wash out [^{99m}Tc]MIBI from tumor cells has been reported to be similar, in spite of their different transport mechanisms. The GSH dependence of MRP1-mediated transport might be the basis for this discrepancy. The intracellular levels of GSH and glutathione-S-transferase (GST, the enzyme that catalyzes the GSH conjugation reaction) are essential for the transport function of MRP1. GSH levels have been shown to be elevated in a number of different human cancer tissues including bone marrow, breast, colon, and lungs [94]. Therefore, the role of MRP1 in promoting drug resistance should not be dissociated from the GSH/GST intracellular levels. The same is applicable for the measurements of MRP1 activity with [^{99m}Tc]MIBI, since both uptake and efflux of [^{99m}Tc]MIBI depend on the GSH content in MRP1 overexpressing cells as demonstrated in several in vitro studies.

In another study, Akgun et al. correlated the uptake of [^{99m}Tc]MIBI and its retention in delayed images with response to multiagent chemotherapy in 40 SCLC patients [30]. The authors also investigated if there was any relationship between the survival time and the [^{99m}Tc]MIBI kinetic parameters at the time of diagnosis. Of the 40 patients, 29 were classified as good responders (complete or partial remission) and 11 as non-responders (stable disease or progressive disease). Following i.v. administration of [^{99m}Tc]MIBI, SPECT imaging at 30 min (early) and 2 h (delayed) was performed. Regions of interest were placed over the tumors and contralateral normal lung tissue on one transverse section. Uptake ratios between lesions and contralateral normal lung were obtained from early images (early ratio; ER) as well as delayed images (delayed ratio; DR). The retention index (RI%) was measured as RI% = [(DR-ER)/ER]×100. [^{99m}Tc]MIBI tumor uptake parameters were compared with chemotherapeutic response and survival time. The RI of [^{99m}Tc]MIBI in good responders was significantly higher than that in poor responders ($p < 0.05$). On the other hand, there was no significant difference between the two groups with respect to uptake in both early (30 min) and delayed (2 h) times. The patient survival time varied from 1 to 70 months with a mean survival time of 12.9 ± 13.4 months. There were no significant differences between the survival time of patients with respect to early or delayed uptake of [^{99m}Tc]MIBI. A cut-off value of 3.85% for RI provided a satisfactory discrimination between patients according to the survival time. Patients with a RI higher than 3.85% had a longer survival time (12 months) than those with lower RI (8 months), $p < 0.05$. The authors concluded that the retention index of [^{99m}Tc]MIBI, between 30 min and 2 h, could accurately predict the chemotherapy response in patients with SCLC and may be helpful in predicting survival in this pathology.

To date, a few reports have been published on the prognostic value of [^{99m}Tc]MIBI imaging in predicting chemotherapy response in osteosarcoma, the most common primary malignant bone tumor in children and adolescents. The survival rate among patients with osteosarcoma is not encouraging despite the advances in treatments including multiagent chemotherapy regimens in combination with surgery. Systemic relapses are observed in 25–50% of patients without metastases at diagnosis, mostly related to poor response to chemotherapy [95–97]. Among the different prognostic factors identified so far, the overexpression of Pgp is frequently associated with drug resistance, tumor recurrence, and poor outcome [5,98,99]. Other studies have failed to confirm this relationship and the role of Pgp as a prognostic marker remains controversial [34,100]. The results obtained from imaging studies with [^{99m}Tc]MIBI in relation to Pgp expression were equally contradictory.

Burak et al. analyzed the role of [^{99m}Tc]MIBI scintigraphy for functional imaging of the MDR phenotype in patients with musculoskeletal sarcomas [101]. They compared the uptake and the washout kinetics of [^{99m}Tc]MIBI with Pgp expression levels and tumor response to neoadjuvant chemotherapy. The tumor-to-background ratios of [^{99m}Tc]MIBI calculated either in early (10 min) or in delayed (60 min) images did not differ significantly between patients with high and low expression of Pgp. Conversely, the washout rate of [^{99m}Tc]MIBI, calculated between 10 and 60 min, was correlated with the degree of Pgp expression and was higher in patients with higher levels of Pgp than in those with a low Pgp score. According to the authors, the early images may not be sufficient to evaluate the expression of Pgp in bone and soft-tissue sarcomas, and a delayed imaging acquisition is recommended to determine the washout rate of [^{99m}Tc]MIBI. The optimal time for delayed imaging varies widely between studies. Most reports favor acquisition of the late images at least 2 h post-injection. In this study, 1 h late imaging was enough to identify differences in the washout rate of [^{99m}Tc]MIBI between patients with high and low expression of Pgp. After neoadjuvant therapy, tumor response was assessed by determining the percentage of necrosis and stratified into good responders ($\geq$90% necrosis) and no responders (<90% necrosis). Neither the expression of Pgp nor the washout rate of [^{99m}Tc]MIBI correlates significantly with the level of tumor necrosis. The absence of a relationship between the Pgp expression and the degree of necrosis is not unexpected since the multiagent chemotherapy regimens include doxorubicin, which is a Pgp substrate but also cisplatin and methotrexate that act independently of Pgp. Additionally, although the classical MDR phenotype in musculoskeletal sarcomas has been associated to Pgp, the expression of other ABC transporters, such as MRP1, should not be excluded. MRP1 confers resistance to a large drug spectrum and, as already mentioned, [^{99m}Tc]MIBI is a substrate for both Pgp and MRP1. A representative case of a patient with osteosarcoma located in the right distal femur is presented in Fig. 7. The T/B ratio derived from early (10 min) and delayed images (60 min) was 4.89 and 4.29, respectively, corresponding to a percentage washout rate of 12%. After neoadjuvant therapy, tumor regressed completely and the patient was classified as a good responder. The scintigraphy performed after treatment showed no [^{99m}Tc]MIBI uptake at the primary lesion. Surprisingly, the immunostaining of Pgp in tumor specimen was very strong, disaccording from the scintigraphic data and therapeutic response. The uncoupling between the Pgp expression and the level of its action could be the basis for this discordance. The suboptimal functional capacity of the Pgp efflux

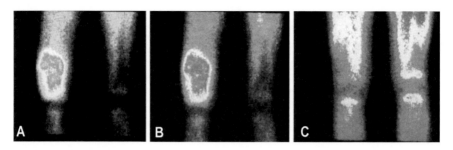

Fig. 7 A 13-years-old boy with osteosarcoma located in the right distal femur. Both early (**A**) and delayed (**B**) images acquired at 10 and 60 min, respectively, showed intense uptake of [^{99m}Tc]MIBI in the tumor lesion. The percent washout rate at 60 min was of 12%. After neoadjuvant chemotherapy, there was no [^{99m}Tc]MIBI uptake at the primary lesion site (**C**). The percent necrosis of the resection material was 99% and the patient showed complete response to chemotherapy (reprinted by permission from Springer Science + Business Media, Ref. [101])

pump due to low levels of the ATP content could generate conflicting results. To avoid false-positive results, the immunohistochemical detection of Pgp should be complemented with a functional assay.

The same group, in an independent study, investigated the role of MRP1 in drug resistance in osteosarcoma and evaluated the capability of functional imaging with [^{99m}Tc]MIBI for recognizing MRP1 expression [10]. They also examined whether kinetic parameters would help to distinguish between Pgp and MRP1 expressions. Fifteen of 24 osteosarcoma samples (62.5%) showed high levels of MRP1, 13 showed strong Pgp expression (54.2%) and 10 (41.2%) showed co-expression of both proteins (MRP1 and Pgp). Again a significant correlation between the T/B ratios and the expression of either MRP1 or Pgp was not observed. The early or delayed T/B ratios of patients with high expression of these proteins were not significantly different from those with low expression. The washout rate of [^{99m}Tc]MIBI was significantly correlated with the expression levels of MRP1, being higher in patients with high expression of MRP1 ($30.1\pm8.6\%$) than in those with low expression ($20.0\pm7.7\%$, $p=0.007$). A cut-off of 22% was defined to distinguish between cases with fast and slow [^{99m}Tc]MIBI clearance. The histological response to multiagent chemotherapy based on analysis of necrosis percentage was significantly correlated with the MRP1 immunostaining and with the washout rate of [^{99m}Tc]MIBI. The comparative analysis of [^{99m}Tc]MIBI washout rate between patients with co-expression of MRP1 and Pgp and patients with high expression of either Pgp or MRP1 showed that it is not possible to distinguish between MRP1 and Pgp expression in osteosarcoma, suggesting that [^{99m}Tc]MIBI should be actively pumped out by Pgp and MRP1 with similar efficiency. Although MRP1 differs from Pgp with respect to substrate characteristics and transport mechanisms, there is a considerable overlapping in their substrate specificity. Therefore, the overexpression of MRP1 in Pgp-negative tumors should be explored as an alternative mechanism of resistance.

Contrary to the above analysis, Gorlick et al. reported a lack of correlation of [^{99m}Tc]MIBI kinetics with both histological response to neoadjuvant chemotherapy and measurements of Pgp expression in patients with high-grade osteosarcoma [102]. A large variability was observed in the biological half-lives of [^{99m}Tc]MIBI ranging between 1.4 and 52.5 h in the cohort of patients imaged. Although the mean biological half-lives of [^{99m}Tc]MIBI has been higher in tumors without Pgp expression (13.2 h) compared with those expressing Pgp (4.4 h), the relationship was not statistically significant ($p = 0.19$). The same was observed in relation with Huvos grade. Tumors with a favorable extension of necrosis following induction chemotherapy had a mean biological half-life of 13.7 h, whereas tumor with less necrosis had a mean biological half-life of 8.1 h. The extent of necrosis was not correlated with the expression levels of Pgp measured either by immunohistochemistry or by quantitative RT-PCR, suggesting that Pgp could not serve as a prognostic factor in osteosarcoma. A concern raised by this study was also the lack of correlation between the two measurements of Pgp expression assessed by quantitative RT-PCR and immunohistochemistry ($p = 0.33$) suggesting that special attention should be paid for the methodology used when assessing Pgp expression. In this study, the authors did not consider the expression of MRP1 instead of Pgp in these lesions, which could explain some conflicting results.

A few studies have been focused on the role of [^{99m}Tc]MIBI planar scintigraphy in predicting chemotherapy response in hematological diseases. A preliminary report by Liang et al. in a group of 25 patients with malignant lymphoma showed that the mean early T/B ratio of 15 patients with good response (3.3 ± 0.6) was significantly higher than that of the 10 patients with poor response (1.2 ± 0.1) [103]. All the 15 patients with good response had negative Pgp expression. Among the 10 patients who presented a poor response to chemotherapy and had negative [^{99m}Tc]MIBI scan, only 6 were Pgp-positive. The negative [^{99m}Tc]MIBI scan in the four cases with negative Pgp expression may also be related with the MRP1 expression, an aspect that was not analyzed in this study. The differences observed in response to chemotherapy were not correlated with other prognostic factors such as tumor type, tumor stage, or patients' age. Therefore, early [^{99m}Tc]MIBI scan appears to predict more accurately, compared with other prognostic factors, chemotherapy response in patients with malignant lymphoma.

Ak et al. analyzed the relationship between the [^{99m}Tc]MIBI uptake and the expression levels of Pgp in 26 patients with newly diagnosed leukemia [104]. The patients underwent a [^{99m}Tc]MIBI whole-body planar imaging prior to chemotherapy. Planar images of pelvis and thorax were acquired 20 min post-injection of [^{99m}Tc]MIBI. The T/B ratio in bone marrow was compared with the Pgp expression in blast cells from bone marrow aspiration samples determined by flow cytometry. The results of [^{99m}Tc]MIBI imaging were concordant with the Pgp expression levels found in blast cells. The bone marrow uptake of [^{99m}Tc]MIBI was significantly ($p < 0.001$) higher in Pgp-negative patients than in those with Pgp-positive blast cells. Such observations indicate that in vivo functional imaging of bone marrow with [^{99m}Tc]MIBI could provide functional valuable information regarding Pgp activity in untreated patients with leukemia.

3.1.2 [^{99m}Tc]Tetrofosmin

[^{99m}Tc]Tetrofosmin is another lipophilic cationic compound proposed for functional imaging of MDR. It is a diphosphine complex of ^{99m}Tc also developed and approved for clinical use in myocardial perfusion studies. The cellular accumulation and retention of [^{99m}Tc]Tetrofosmin is similar to that of [^{99m}Tc]MIBI involving passive diffusion through the cell membrane in response to the negative transmembrane potential and sequestration in mitochondria. The similarity with [^{99m}Tc]MIBI prompted researchers to investigate whether [^{99m}Tc]Tetrofosmin could provide information on the functional activity of MDR-related transporters. The transport kinetics of [^{99m}Tc]Tetrofosmin has been characterized in mammalian cell lines expressing different levels of ABC transporters. Studies from Ballinger et al. in a rat breast carcinoma wild-type cell line, MatB/wt, and its doxorubicin-selected variant expressing Pgp, MatB/AdrR, demonstrated that wild-type cells accumulate 16-fold more [^{99m}Tc]Tetrofosmin than the resistant variant MatB/AdrR [105]. Furthermore, addition of PSC833 1 μM increased nine times the cellular uptake of [^{99m}Tc]Tetrofosmin in resistant MatB/AdrR cells without significant changes in parental MatB/wt cells. Similar results were observed in human breast carcinoma MCF7/wt and MCF7/AdrR cell line pair [105].

A comparative study of transport kinetics between [^{99m}Tc]MIBI and [^{99m}Tc]Tetrofosmin in drug-sensitive cells and its resistant counterparts demonstrated that functional activity of Pgp can be detected with equal sensitivity with both radiotracers. The steady-state accumulation of [^{99m}Tc]Tetrofosmin in a human epidermoid carcinoma cell line KB 3-1 (59.4±3.0 fmol/mg protein) and its colchicine-resistant derivative KB 8-5 (1.9±0.06 fmol/mg protein) were approximately half of the values obtained for [^{99m}Tc]MIBI in the same cells (104.6±4.1 and 2.85±0.1 fmol/mg protein, respectively). Nevertheless the ratio of cell accumulation (KB 3-1/KB 8-5) for [^{99m}Tc]Tetrofosmin (43.7) was similar to that obtained for [^{99m}Tc]MIBI (37.4), suggesting that both tracers could detect Pgp expression with the same efficacy. The lower cellular accumulation of [^{99m}Tc]Tetrofosmin compared with [^{99m}Tc]MIBI was systematically reported in independent studies with different resistant cell lines [68,75], a fact that is probability related with the individual characteristics of each radiotracer. In fact, despite having similar characteristics, these tracers are not identical. [^{99m}Tc]Tetrofosmin is less sensitive than [^{99m}Tc]MIBI to the electric transmembrane potentials generated in living cells. Moreover, whereas [^{99m}Tc]MIBI accumulates preferentially in mitochondria, [^{99m}Tc]Tetrofosmin remains in cytoplasm and only a small part is sequestered in mitochondria.

Several studies performed in a battery of cell lines expressing MRP1 but not Pgp clearly demonstrated that [^{99m}Tc]Tetrofosmin is also a substrate of MRP1.

Overall, cell lines overexpressing MRP1 showed a deficit in the cellular accumulation of [^{99m}Tc]Tetrofosmin, compared with their sensitive counterparts, and enhancement of radiotracer net content was observed upon addition of modulators of MRP1 transport activity such as verapamil, cyclosporin A, or probenecid [68,106]. Addition of Pgp-specific modulators (PSC833, GF120918, LY335979) did not alter the accumulation of [^{99m}Tc]Tetrofosmin in MRP1-overexpressing cells.

As observed for [^{99m}Tc]MIBI, the transport of [^{99m}Tc]Tetrofosmin by MRP1 can be modulated through depletion of GSH. Several groups observed an increase in the intracellular accumulation of [^{99m}Tc]Tetrofosmin in MRP1-overexpressing cell lines after depletion of GSH with BSO treatment [68,106,107]. These results indicate that net cell accumulation of [^{99m}Tc]Tetrofosmin is functionally affected by MRP1, which is, in turn, dependent on cellular levels of GSH.

Clinical Studies with [^{99m}Tc]Tetrofosmin

The clinical usefulness of [^{99m}Tc]Tetrofosmin scintigraphy for in vivo prediction of MDR has been demonstrated in some malignancies. The tumor uptake and washout indexes of [^{99m}Tc]Tetrofosmin have proved to be useful in detecting Pgp/MRP1 expression in tumor lesions and predicting chemotherapy response. In a study of 30 patients with infiltrating ductal breast cancer, Sun et al. suggested that [^{99m}Tc]Tetrofosmin is as capable as [^{99m}Tc]MIBI in detecting Pgp expression [108]. The tumor-to-background ratio in 12 patients with positive expression of Pgp was 1.20 ± 0.12, significantly lower ($p<0.05$) than that in 18 Pgp-negative patients (1.94 ± 0.30). [^{99m}Tc]Tetrofosmin has proved to be useful in predicting chemotherapy response in patients with lung cancer. Thirty patients with untreated lung carcinoma underwent a [^{99m}Tc]Tetrofosmin SPECT before starting chemotherapy. The scans were acquired at 10 and 120 min after injection of [^{99m}Tc]Tetrofosmin. The retention index of [^{99m}Tc]Tetrofosmin between 10 and 120 min was predictive of tumor response to chemotherapy. Fourteen of the 18 patients with high retention ($>15\%$) exhibited a favorable response to chemotherapy, whereas all the 12 tumors with a [^{99m}Tc]Tetrofosmin retention lower than 15% did not respond to chemotherapy [109]. Shiau et al. evaluated the prognostic value of [^{99m}Tc]Tetrofosmin in predicting chemotherapy response to paclitaxel in 20 patients with advanced non-small-cell lung cancer [110]. The response to chemotherapy was evaluated by clinical and radiological methods in the third month after completion of the treatment. The T/B ratio, in early and delayed images of patients with good response, was significantly higher than in patients with poor response. The immunohistochemical analysis of Pgp identified high levels of Pgp in biopsy specimens of poor responders. Such observations emphasize the ability of [^{99m}Tc]Tetrofosmin chest imaging in predicting tumor response to paclitaxel. Kao and colleagues evaluated the correlation of [^{99m}Tc]Tetrofosmin uptake with Pgp and/or MRP1 expression in small-cell lung cancer [111], malignant lymphoma [112], and parathyroid adenoma [113]. All studies revealed that tumor uptake of [^{99m}Tc]Tetrofosmin depends essentially on Pgp and/or MRP1 expression in tumor cells and therefore could be used to identify those patients that are most likely to fail chemotherapy. Yapar et al. demonstrated the ability of [^{99m}Tc]Tetrofosmin scintigraphy for detecting Pgp expression in patients with malignant bone and soft-tissue tumors [114]. The percentage washout rate of the tracer, calculated between 15 and 90 min, was correlated with the degree of Pgp expression and was higher in lesions with higher levels of Pgp (31.81±6.72%) than in those with a low Pgp score (21.0±3.49%). A cut-off value of 24.5% provided a good discrimination between lesions with and without Pgp expression with a sensitivity of 87.5% and a specificity of 100%. On the other hand, [^{99m}Tc]Tetrofosmin uptake was not correlated with Pgp expression, suggesting that Pgp is not the major factor interfering with the uptake of [^{99m}Tc]Tetrofosmin in these lesions [114]. The inability of [^{99m}Tc]Tetrofosmin uptake in detecting Pgp expression in malignant musculoskeletal tumors had already been reported in a previous study [115]. The tumor-to-background ratio of [^{99m}Tc]Tetrofosmin in tumor lesions expressing Pgp (3.01±1.48) was not statistically different from those not expressing Pgp (4.27±2.90).

3.2 PET Imaging Agents

A number of PET-based radiopharmaceuticals have been actively developed to probe the functional activity of Pgp in tumors. These tracers were developed through the incorporation of short-lived positron emitters, such as carbon-11 (^{11}C; $t_{1/2}$ = 20.3 min) or fluorine-18 (^{18}F, $t_{1/2}$ = 110 min), into organic molecules characterized as substrates or modulators of Pgp. Radiolabeling with ^{11}C has the advantage of not altering the biochemical and pharmacological properties of the compounds, as it can replace any C atom present in the molecule, but its use is restricted to centers with a cyclotron that can produce the nuclide. Fluorine-18 has a longer half-life and can be transported from the production facility to nearby centers. In some cases, fluorine-containing compounds, such as 5-fluouracil, can be labeled isotopically but ^{18}F is by far more commonly used to replace a hydrogen atom on a prospective tracer as it shares a similar van der Waal's radius with H and produces very little physicochemical effects on the labeled molecules.

3.2.1 ^{11}C-Labeled Compounds

The first ^{11}C-labeled compound synthesized for functional imaging of MDR was the anthracycline daunorubicin (DNR) which is a well-known substrate of Pgp. In vitro experiments with human ovarian carcinoma cell lines showed a 16-fold higher accumulation of [^{11}C]DNR in sensitive cells (A2780) as compared with the resistant Pgp-overexpressing counterpart (A2780AD) [116]. After treatment with verapamil, the accumulation of [^{11}C]DNR in Pgp-overexpressing cells increased to the levels found in sensitive cells further demonstrating the influence of Pgp on transport kinetics of [^{11}C]DNR. The ability of [^{11}C]DNR, in tracer dosages, to distinguish sensitive from resistant tumors was equally observed in tumor-bearing rats with a PET camera [117]. For these studies rats were inoculated with a Pgp-negative small-cell lung carcinoma cell line (GLC4) and its MDR1-gene-transfected Pgp subline (GLC4/Pgp) in opposite flanks. One hour after injection, the content of [11C]DNR in GLC4 tumors was 159±28% higher than that in GLC4/Pgp tumors. After modulation with cyclosporin A, the accumulation of [11C]DNR in GLC4/Pgp tumors increased to the levels observed in the GLC4 tumors due to blockade of Pgp efflux activity expressed in these tumors. Despite the promising results in identifying Pgp-expressing tumors, [11C]DNR has not been yet tested in clinical trials as a PET imaging tracer. The dose-dependent pharmacokinetics of DNR observed in humans [118] together with difficulties with the radiosynthesis of [11C]DNR, specially the low radiochemical yield, have limited further development of this tracer for human studies [119].

Another 11C-radiolabeled candidate for PET imaging of MDR was the calcium blocker channel antagonist verapamil. Besides its specific pharmacological activity on calcium channels, verapamil is simultaneously a modulator and a substrate of Pgp, competing with cytostatic drugs for the drug efflux pump. [11C] verapamil was initially evaluated as a Pgp probe in human ovarian carcinoma cell lines. Initial studies showed a higher accumulation of [11C] verapamil (4–5 times) in sensitive cells when compared with Pgp-expressing cells suggesting that [11C] verapamil could be a potential PET imaging tracer of Pgp in tumors. Hendrikse et al. investigated the pharmacokinetics of [11C] verapamil with PET in solid tumors and in the blood–brain barrier (BBB) [117,120]. For this study, a tumor-bearing rat model was developed. The animals were bilaterally inoculated with a Pgp-overexpressing human small-cell carcinoma (GLC4/Pgp) and its Pgp-negative counterpart (GLC4) to guaranteed equal systemic pharmacokinetics. The reversal effects of cyclosporin A on tumor pharmacokinetics of [11C] verapamil were also evaluated. The maximum uptake of [11C] verapamil in both tumors was reached within 5 min following injection. The radiotracer uptake in GLC4/Pgp tumors, expressed as percentage of injected dose per milliliter of tumor, was 23% lower than in the wild-type tumors. When the animals were treated with 50 mg/kg cyclosporin A, the content of [11C]verapamil in GLC4/Pgp tumors increased to the levels achieved in the GLC4 tumors due to blockade of Pgp-mediated efflux. Figure 8 shows a representative PET

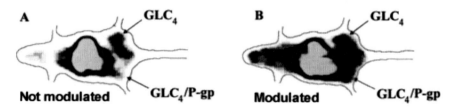

Fig. 8 Representative images from a PET study with [11C]verapamil in a male rat bearing bilateral xenografts in the absence of modulator (**A**) and after treatment with cyclosporin A (**B**) (reprinted by permission from the American Association for Cancer Research, Ref. [117]

study in a male rat bearing bilateral xenografts in the absence of modulator (A) and after treatment with cyclosporin A (B).

[[11C]verapamil is also useful to measure the functional activity of Pgp in the blood–brain barrier (BBB). In the rat brain, the levels of [[11C]verapamil increased 350% after modulation with cyclosporine A, demonstrating the usefulness of [[11C]verapamil for in vivo visualizing Pgp function and its reversal [117]. This effect is illustrated in Fig. 8. Pgp is abundantly expressed in the BBB to protect the brain against potentially toxic exogenous compounds [121]. This important role of Pgp in the BBB was observed earlier in mdr1a(-/-) Pgp-knockout mice [122,123]. Brain levels of verapamil, digoxin, and cyclosporin A were found to be increased in Pgp-knockout mice compared with mdr1a(+ / +) wild-type mice. Furthermore, the brain levels of digoxin in wild-type mice increased after blockade of Pgp with PSC833. In this way, concentrations of clinically relevant drugs acting on the central nervous system (CNS) and in solid tumors could be visualized and quantified in vivo with a non-invasive imaging technique such as PET.

A PET imaging study in healthy volunteers showed that Pgp activity in the human BBB could be measured with [[11C]verapamil. The increase observed in ^{11}C-radioactivity in the brain, after treatment with cyclosporin A, was consistent with the inhibition of Pgp in the human BBB (Fig. 9) [124]. This has implications in terms of potential drug–drug interactions at the BBB with drugs that can inhibit Pgp at therapeutic concentrations. Such applications

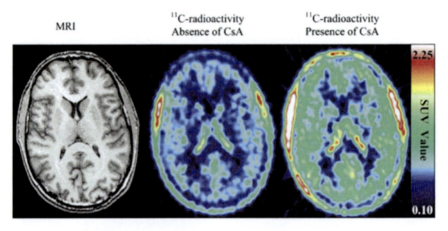

Fig. 9 Positron emission tomography images of a normal human brain after 11C-verapamil administration in the absence or presence of cyclosporine (CsA) indicate increased regional uptake (*green* to *red* areas) of ^{11}C-radioactivity in the brain in the presence of CsA. Images represent standardized uptake values (SUV) summed over a period of 5–25 min, which provide an index of regional radioactivity uptake normalized to the administered dose and weight of the subject. MRI, magnetic resonance image (reprinted by permission from Macmillan Publishers Lda, Ref. [124])

could be useful to determine the role of Pgp polymorphisms in the CNS distribution of drugs that are Pgp substrates.

The cytostatic agent colchicine, a naturally occurring alkaloid was labeled with ^{11}C and evaluated as a potential agent for MDR imaging with PET. The feasibility of using colchicine as a probe for MDR came from whole-body quantitative autoradiography studies using colchicine labeled with ^{14}C. The biodistribution studies in mice xenografted with Pgp-positive and Pgp-negative human neutoblastomas demonstrated a 2-fold higher accumulation of [^{14}C]colchicine in sensitive tumors when compared with resistant tumors [125]. In a subsequent study, the same group evaluated the ability of ^{11}C-labeled colchicine as a PET imaging agent for MDR in nude rats xenografted with sensitive human neuroblastoma cell line BE (2)-C and associated resistant strains. One hour post-injection, PET scans showed a 2-fold difference in the accumulation of [^{11}C]colchicine between sensitive and resistant tumors [126]. Colchicine is electroneutral, and contrary to [^{99m}Tc]MIBI and [^{99m}Tc]Tetrofosmin, its cellular uptake is not affected by membrane potential variations. Therefore, [^{11}C]colchicine could serve as a good predictor of resistance to electroneutral cytostatic agents such as paclitaxel and some steroid hormones. Nevertheless, the detoxification of colchicine via the bile, as demonstrated by the relatively high uptake in liver and intestine from biodistribution studies [127], makes the radiolabeled colchicine only useful in tumors away from the abdominal cavity.

3.2.2 ^{18}F-Labeled Compounds

^{18}F-labeled drugs benefit from the longer half-life of the nuclide (110 min), thus allowing us to monitor the kinetics of the modulation process and also the dynamics of the tracer in the body for longer periods when compared with ^{11}C-labeled compounds.

Paclitaxel belongs to a class of anticancer drugs (taxanes) that inhibits cellular proliferation through the stabilization of tubulin and is widely used in the treatment of patients with solid tumors. The response to treatment and the severity of adverse drug reactions vary substantially between individuals, being the expression of Pgp and its genetic variants one of the most important factors responsible for these differences. To determine the taxane biodistribution non-invasively, a synthetic scheme to make [^{18}F]fluoropaclitaxel ([^{18}F]FPAC) was developed. Previous studies have shown that paclitaxel can be fluorinated without inducing substantial alterations of its pharmacological properties [128]. The biodistribution of [^{18}F]FPAC was studied in mice with and without human breast cancer tumor xenografts in a small-animal-dedicated PET and closely followed that of the parental drug when compared with [^{1}H]paclitaxel. Paclitaxel is a neutral compound and unlike [^{99m}Tc]Sestamibi and [^{99m}Tc]Tetrofosmin does not require any electric gradient for intracellular retention. In addition, paclitaxel is not a substrate for MRP1, which makes [^{18}F]FPAC a specific probe for Pgp.

Hsueh et al. evaluated the potential of [^{18}F]FPAC to predict chemotherapy response of tumors to paclitaxel in mice bearing human breast cancer xenografts using a small-animal-dedicated PET [129]. PET images were acquired 30 min after [^{18}F]FPAC injection. Tumor uptake was expressed as standardized uptake value (mSUV) units. After imaging, the animals were treated intraperitoneally with a single dose of paclitaxel. The rate of change in tumor volume after treatment was compared with the magnitude of [^{18}F]FPAC uptake. In general, the animals with low [^{18}F]FPAC uptake demonstrated tumor progression after treatment, whereas those with high [^{18}F]FPAC uptake tended to regress. Considering any increase in tumor volume as an indicator of chemoresistance to paclitaxel, the image criterion, indexed by [^{18}F]FPAC uptake, had an overall accuracy of 82%, a sensitivity of 100%, and a specificity of 73% to identify chemoresistant tumors. To verify if the chemoresistance was related with a limited availability of the drug due to hepatic modulation, they compared the tracer accumulation in the liver with tumor uptake as well as therapeutic response. No significant correlation between tumor uptake and liver uptake of [^{18}F]FPAC or tumor response was observed, thus confirming that liver uptake cannot account for decreased tumor uptake and resistance to paclitaxel [129]. These results suggest that lower levels of [^{18}F]FPAC in tumors are related with Pgp activity and tend to be associated with higher risk of resistance to paclitaxel and tumor progression.

Another group studied in vivo the biodistribution of [^{18}F]FPAC in three non-human primates at baseline and after administration of a third-generation MDR modulator (XR9576) [130]. The potential of [^{18}F]FPAC as a MDR probe was estimated from the changes observed in [^{18}F]FPAC content in organs normally expressing Pgp following administration of XR9576. The baseline biodistribution showed high [^{18}F]FPAC accumulation in the hepatobiliary system and bowel, which is explained by the normal excretion route of paclitaxel. After modulation with XR9576, an increase was observed in the retention of [^{18}F]FPAC in the liver and in the lungs and a small increase in the efflux rate of the tracer in the kidneys. The changes in [^{18}F]FPAC uptake after modulation were considered related with alterations in the functional activity of Pgp since these tissues are rich in Pgp. These data provide strong evidence that biodistribution of [^{18}F]FPAC is similar to that of paclitaxel, as both are substrates of Pgp [131].

In a recent publication, Kurdziel et al. reported the results from [^{18}F]FPAC PET imaging studies in a mouse model, normal volunteers, and breast cancer patients [132]. The mouse model was established by the subcutaneous injection of human epithelial KB 3-1 (drug-sensitive) and KB 8-5 (drug-resistant) cell lines into the shoulders and hind legs. Due to the small size of the tumors and interference from background activity, the micro-PET images of [^{18}F]FPAC were difficult to appreciate (Fig. 10). Nevertheless, a drug-sensitive-to-drug-resistant tumor ratio of 1.35 was measured. The micro-PET imaging of surgical leg excised tumors showed significant differences in [^{18}F]FPAC uptake between

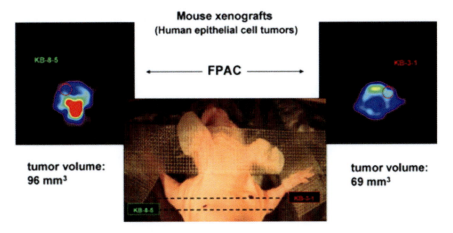

Fig. 10 Xenografts were established by subcutaneously injecting 5×10^5 cells into the right (KB 3-1; drug sensitive) and left (KB 8-5; drug resistant) shoulders of adult female nude mice. Micro-PET (Concorde micro-PET R4) imaging was performed 7 days postinoculation. While the overall FPAC uptake is low, slightly more FPAC can be seen in the drug-sensitive tumor. The drug-sensitive-to-drug-resistant tumor ratio was 1.35. Micro-PET imaging of surgically excised tumors (90 min, i.v., post-FPAC injection) showed a sensitive-to-resistant uptake ratio of 3.2 (reprinted by permission from Elsevier, Ref. [132])

drug-sensitive and drug-resistant tumors with an uptake ratio of 3.2 (Fig. 10). These results are similar to the ones reported above by Hsueh et al. in the human breast cancer mouse xenograft model.

The pilot study in normal volunteers and breast cancer patients with [^{18}F]FPAC was approved by the Virginia Commonwealth University Institutional Review Board, who developed an automated method for ^{18}F-fluorination of paclitaxel [133]. The biodistribution of [^{18}F]FPAC in normal volunteers was similar to that observed in the previous study in primates with lower background activity in chest, breast, and brain. The extensive hepatic clearance and subsequent excretion into the bowel can compromise the diagnostic value of [^{18}F]FPAC imaging in abdominal tumors.

The results from the pilot study with breast cancer patients were promising although the number of patients studied was limited. The [^{18}F]FPAC uptake in primary lesions of patients who responded to chemotherapy were not too high (SUV approx. 0.85) but remained constant over time. On the other side, patients with no significant uptake of [^{18}F]FPAC showed only a partial response to chemotherapy [132]. These findings provide evidence that [^{18}F]FPAC uptake can predict response to paclitaxel in breast cancer patients and may be useful as a clinical tool to select patients who might benefit from the addition of a Pgp modulator. The prior identification of patients who will not respond to a specific treatment can avoid the cost and morbidity associated with an ineffective chemotherapy regimen. However, further studies are needed, with a larger patient base to evaluate the reproducibility of [^{18}F]FPAC PET imaging and its impact on the management of breast cancer patients.

The synthetic pirimidine, 5-fluouracil (5-FU), is used in the treatment of a variety of epithelial tumors including, colorectal, breast cancer, ovarian, head, and neck cancers. 5-FU enters tumor cells by a facilitated nucleobase transporter and is converted into active metabolites (5′-fluoro-2′-deoxyuridine) by a complex metabolic pathway that interferes with both DNA and RNA syntheses. Of particular interest is the conversion of 5-FU to 5′-fluoro-2′-deoxyuridine (5-FUdR) and subsequent phosphorylation by thymidine kinase to the active metabolite 5′-fluoro-2′-DUMP (5-FdUMP). Unfortunately, the response rate of patients receiving 5-FU-based chemotherapy is relatively poor, varying between 10 and 30%. To further evaluate, 5-FU labeled with ^{18}F (5-^{18}FU) has been used in PET studies to understand the factors behind this strong interindividual variability. As 5-^{18}FU is biochemically identical to 5-FU, PET has been used for quantitative pharmacokinetic measurements of 5-^{18}FU in human and animal models.

Several groups tried to correlate the 5-^{18}FU uptake with the response to therapy in a variety of animal models. In a previous study, Shani and Wolf examined the 5-^{18}FU uptake in mice bearing 5-FU sensitive and resistant L-1210 lymphocytic leukemia tumors in opposite flanks [134]. Two hours after injection, the tumor-to-blood ratio of 5-^{18}FU was 1.9 in sensitive tumors and 0.96 in resistant tumors. This difference was even greater 12 h post-injection with values of 20.69 and 4.04 for sensitive and resistant tumors, respectively. These results support the hypothesis that tumor response is associated with high 5-^{18}FU uptake in a delayed phase. Wolf et al. demonstrated that early uptake values (20 min) of 5-FU reflect the influx of the drug, whereas the uptake at delayed times (120 min) represents the trapped non-metabolized 5-FU. This was confirmed with nuclear magnetic resonance spectroscopy (MRS) studies in patients. Fluorine-19 MRS allows differentiation between 5-FU and its inactive metabolites, such as α-fluoro-β-alanine without significant antitumor activity. The double examinations performed with PET and ^{19}F-labeled magnetic MRS indicated that 5-^{18}FU accumulation in metastases reflects the non-metabolized trapped 5-^{18}FU [135].

The first studies in cancer patients with 5-^{18}FU were carried out in Heidelberg. Moehler et al. investigated the predictive value of 5-^{18}FU PET for clinical response and survival of treated patients with unresectable colorectal liver metastases [136]. The standard chemotherapeutic agent of metastatic colorectal carcinoma is 5-FU, as a single agent or in combination with others. The patients were submitted to a 5-^{18}FU PET study prior to 5-FU-based chemotherapy. A semiquantitative approach of 5-^{18}FU based on the calculation of the standardized uptake value (SUV) normalized to the injected dose and body weight was performed. CT studies preceded the first chemotherapeutic cycle and were repeated within every 3–4 months after treatment. Tumor response was evaluated based on the volumetric data of metastases according to the World Health Organization guidelines. Metastases were identified in cross-sections of 5-^{18}FU PET scans. Visual inspection of images showed low trapping of

5-[18]FU in tumor regions compared with the surrounding liver tissue and a large divergence within 5-[18]FU distribution pattern for different metastases. The mean SUV in the liver metastases 120 min post-injection was approximately one-third of the mean SUV in the normal liver parenchyma and varied from 0.9 to 4.3. The patients with 5-[18]FU SUVs exceeding 2.8 had a stable disease for longer than 12 months and survival of longer than 21 months, whereas patients with 5-[18]FU SUVs lower than 1.2 showed evidences of progressive disease and had a worst survival of less than 12 months [136]. These results were in accordance with those obtained by Dimitrakopoulou-Strauss et al. [137] in a parallel study of 12 colorectal carcinoma patients. They also observed a highly variable trapping of 5-[18]FU even for multiple metastases in the same patients, and only metastases with 5-[18]FU uptake exceeding 3.0 SUV responded to chemotherapy. A significant correlation of 0.86 ($p<0.001$) was found between 5-[18]FU uptake before chemotherapy and the growth rate of the lesions after treatment as determined by CT. These preliminary results highlight the potential of PET for identifying patients who are most likely to respond to 5-FU therapy.

Several mechanisms are thought to be responsible for resistance to 5-FU. Recently, members of the subfamily ABCC of the ATP-binding cassette superfamily, including the MRP5 and MRP8, were shown to confer drug resistance to 5-FU and certain fluoropyrimidines [23,25,138]. These transporters mediated the ATP-dependent transport of 5-FU and the monophosphorylated metabolites 5-FdUMP and 5-FUMP. The accumulation of [3H]5-FU was significantly reduced by 2-fold in both stably and transient MRP5-transfected HEK cells when compared with their respective HEK-vector cells, suggesting an active role of MRP5 in the resistance to 5-FU. Furthermore, a potent transport inhibitor of MRP5 (NPPB) was shown to sensitize MRP5-transfected cells to 5-FU cytotoxicity [25]. These studies suggest that potent MDR inhibitors may be useful in reversing drug resistance to 5-FU. However, further studies are needed to explore whether MRP/ABCC transporters confer resistance to 5-FU in clinical samples. PET imaging using 5-[18]FU is a valuable tool that can be employed to clarify this point.

3.2.3 ^{67}Ga/^{68}Ga-Radiopharmaceuticals

A novel gallium(III) complex of the selected Schiff-base ligand (Ga-[3-ethoxy-ENBDMPI])[+] was synthesized and evaluated as a potential probe to assess Pgp activity. This compound is a non-metabolized cationic hydrophobic complex that can be labeled either with the single-photon emitter [67]Ga ($t_{1/2}$ = 78 h) or with the positron emitter [68]Ga ($t_{1/2}$ = 68 min) thus having potential applications in both SPECT and PET for the functional imaging of Pgp.

Cell tracer transport experiments performed in drug-sensitive KB3-1 cells and KB8-5 cells expressing modest levels of Pgp demonstrated the high sensitivity of the ^{67}Ga-complex in detecting the outward transport activity of Pgp [139]. The KB3-1-to-KB8-5 uptake ratio was 104 and the washout rate of ^{67}Ga-complex in KB8-5 cells (k = 0.20 min[-1]) was 10-fold faster when compared with that of KB3-1 cells ($k = 0.02$ min^{-1}). The residual uptake in control KB-3-1 cells after membrane depolarization with high concentrations of K$^+$/valinomicin demonstrated the membrane potential dependence of the ^{67}Ga-complex uptake and is indicative of the low non-specific membrane absorption. Further validation of ^{67}Ga-complex as a substrate of Pgp was provided by monitoring tracer accumulation in the presence of known Pgp inhibitors (LY335979, PSC833, and cyclosporin A). In KB8-5 cells a reversible effect proportional to the rank order potency of the tested inhibitors was observed.

To further evaluate the potential utility of the $^{67/68}$Ga-complex as an in vivo marker of Pgp-mediated transport activity, the complexes were injected in wild-type and mdr1a/1b (-/-) knockout mice to study the drug transport across the BBB. As previously mentioned, Pgp is expressed in the luminal surfaces of brain endothelial cells preventing the entry of amphipathic compounds into the central nervous system. Therefore, the mdr1a/1b (-/-) knockout mice offer an interesting model to evaluate the applicability of radiotracers for in vivo transport activity of Pgp. At 5 min after injection, the brain uptake of ^{67}Ga-complex in Pgp-knockout mice was 10-fold higher compared with that in the wild-type mice. As the cerebral blood flow did not differ significantly between the wild-type and the knockout mice, differences on initial brain uptake and retention of ^{67}Ga-complex were not attributed to changes in cerebral perfusion.

The potential utility of ^{68}Ga-complex as a PET radiotracer was evaluated in mice with micro-PET [139]. Five minutes after tail vein injection of the ^{68}Ga-complex, a greater net uptake in the brain of knockout mice was detected when compared with that of the wild-type mice, what is consistent with the biodistribution data obtained with the ^{67}Ga-complex. Although the $^{67/68}$Ga-complex has been recognized as a transport substrate of Pgp, the authors are cautiously optimistic regarding its applicability in SPECT and PET imaging for in vivo assessment of Pgp activity. Issues related with radiation dosimetry and radiolabeling require additional experimentation.

4 Conclusions

In this chapter, we have reviewed the potential of SPECT and PET imaging modalities for studying in vivo and non-invasively the classical mechanism of MDR in cancer. The feasibility of the clinically approved ^{99m}Tc-complexes, especially [^{99m}Tc]MIBI, for identifying drug-resistant tumors was demonstrated in numerous clinical studies in several different malignancies. A number of significant correlations were found between radiotracer kinetic parameters and Pgp and/or MRP1 expression in many cancers. Some reports also demonstrated the potential of functional imaging to predict tumor response to a particular chemotherapeutic regimen. Despite the evidences that the MDR phenotype can be assessed through a molecular imaging technique, this approach is not yet to be integrated into the clinical practice. The primary reason for this is the lack of general consensus concerning the relative prognostic value of Pgp expression as uncertain and sometimes contradictory results have been reported. Nevertheless, the majority of these studies was single institution and enrolled a limited number of patients making it difficult to draw reliable conclusions about the predictive value of Pgp or MRP1 expression. Multi-institutional studies involving a reasonable numbers of patients and meta-analysis are required to reach more reliable conclusions on the role of functional imaging in predicting chemotherapy response. An important step toward the clinical application of functional imaging of MDR is the standardization and optimization of the image acquisition protocols. The appropriate time after radiotracer injection for planar or tomographic image acquisition as well as the post-processing of the images is crucial to identify a reliable index predictive of Pgp and/or MRP1 functional activity. Presently there is no consensus regarding the imaging biomarker that better predicts the functional activity of MDR-related transporters and the overall predictive value of these studies has not been validated to warrant changes in treatment protocols.

In addition to its potential for recognizing non-invasively the MDR phenotype in cancer patients, molecular imaging techniques can also be a powerful tool in evaluating the efficacy of MDR modulators. Examples of both in vitro and in vivo assays, using cellular and animal models, respectively, illustrated the potential utility of molecular imaging probes to assess the effects of different reversing agents on the inhibition of MDR transporters. Although no compound is currently in clinical use, several agents are in the process of clinical trials and a new generation of modulators is currently being developed. The application of imaging-based biomarkers of MDR transporters, in pre-clinical models, even in early development stages of promising modulators is of particular interest in translational research, since it provides valuable data that can be used to accelerate clinical studies. For approved agents, such as verapamil and cyclosporin A, imaging probes could be applied in the clinical setting as a biomarker for assessing the efficacy of modulators in the activity of MDR transporters in tumors. This information is extremely relevant for identifying those patients that would benefit from pre- or co-administration of modulators in their therapeutic protocols.

The clinical application of PET-based imaging probes for assessing MDR is gaining increasing attention. Several chemotherapeutic agents labeled with ^{11}C or ^{18}F were characterized as MDR substrates. Although showing promising results, some of these agents suffer from complex in vivo pharmacokinetics, mediated in part by the rapid metabolism of the radiolabeled compound, and others from modest radiochemical yields, which have limited their usefulness in clinical studies. In the near future, we expect to have new PET imaging-based biomarkers molecularly targeted for MDR-related transporters with potentially clinical utility. This will be a step toward the quantitative measurement of functional activity of MDR-related transporters, in vivo and non-invasively as a valuable tool to circumvent multidrug resistance in the clinical management of cancer patients.

References

1. Gottesman MM. Mechanisms of cancer drug resistance. *Annu Rev Med* 2002; **53**:615–627.
2. Gottesman MM, Fojo T and Bates SE. Multidrug resistance in cancer: role of ATP-dependent transporters. *Nat Rev Cancer* 2002; **2**:48–58.
3. Han K, Kahng J, Kim M, Lim J, Kim Y, Cho B et al. Expression of functional markers in acute nonlymphoblastic leukemia. *Acta Haematol* 2000; **104**:174–180.
4. Clarke R, Leonessa F and Trock B. Multidrug resistance/P-glycoprotein and breast cancer: review and meta-analysis. *Semin Oncol* 2005; **32**:S9–S15.
5. Serra M, Pasello M, Manara MC, Scotlandi K, Ferrari S, Bertoni F et al. May P-glycoprotein status be used to stratify high-grade osteosarcoma patients? Results from the Italian/Scandinavian Sarcoma Group 1 treatment protocol. *Int J Oncol* 2006; **29**:1459–1468.
6. Leonard GD, Fojo T and Bates SE. The role of ABC transporters in clinical practice. *Oncologist* 2003; **8**:411–424.
7. Pauwels EK, Erba P, Mariani G and Gomes CM. Multidrug resistance in cancer: Its mechanism and its modulation. *Drug News Perspect* 2007; **20**:371–377.
8. Sciuto R, Pasqualoni R, Bergomi S, Petrilli G, Vici P, Belli F et al. Prognostic value of (99m)Tc-sestamibi washout in predicting response of locally advanced breast cancer to neoadjuvant chemotherapy. *J Nucl Med* 2002; **43**:745–751.
9. Zhou J, Higashi K, Ueda Y, Kodama Y, Guo D, Jisaki F et al. Expression of multidrug resistance protein and messenger RNA correlate with (99m)Tc-MIBI imaging in patients with lung cancer. *J Nucl Med* 2001; **42**:1476–1483.
10. Burak Z, Moretti J, Ersoy O, Sanli U, Kantar M, Tamgac F et al. 99mTc-MIBI imaging as a predictor of therapy response in osteosarcoma compared with multidrug resistance – associated protein and P-glycoprotein expression. *J Nucl Med* 2003; **44**:1394–1401.
11. West CM, Jones T and Price P. The potential of positron-emission tomography to study anticancer-drug resistance. *Nat Rev Cancer* 2004; **4**:457–469.
12. Borst P and Elferink RO. Mammalian ABC transporters in health and disease. *Annu Rev Biochem* 2002; **71**:537–592.
13. Juliano RL and Ling V. A surface glycoprotein modulating drug permeability in Chinese hamster ovary cell mutants. *Biochim Biophys Acta* 1976; **455**:152–162.
14. Ambudkar SV, Kimchi-Sarfaty C, Sauna ZE and Gottesman MM. P-glycoprotein: from genomics to mechanism. *Oncogene* 2003; **22**:7468–7485.
15. Cole SP, Bhardwaj G, Gerlach JH, Mackie JE, Grant CE, Almquist KC et al. Over-expression of a transporter gene in a multidrug-resistant human lung cancer cell line. *Science* 1992; **258**:1650–1654.
16. Doyle LA and Ross DD. Multidrug resistance mediated by the breast cancer resistance protein BCRP (ABCG2). *Oncogene* 2003; **22**:7340–7358.
17. Kruh GD and Belinsky MG. The MRP family of drug efflux pumps. *Oncogene* 2003; **22**:7537–7552.
18. Cole SP, Sparks KE, Fraser K, Loe DW, Grant CE, Wilson GM et al. Pharmacological characterization of multidrug resistant MRP-transfected human tumor cells. *Cancer Res* 1994; **54**:5902–5910.
19. Zaman GJ, Flens MJ, van Leusden MR, de Haas M, Mulder HS, Lankelma J et al. The human multidrug resistance-associated protein MRP is a plasma membrane drug-efflux pump. *Proc Natl Acad Sci USA* 1994; **91**:8822–8826.
20. Rappa G, Lorico A, Flavell RA and Sartorelli AC. Evidence that the multidrug resistance protein (MRP) functions as a co-transporter of glutathione and natural product toxins. *Cancer Res* 1997; **57**:5232–5237.
21. Hipfner DR, Deeley RG and Cole SP. Structural, mechanistic and clinical aspects of MRP1. *Biochim Biophys Acta* 1999; **1461**:359–376.

22. Doyle LA, Yang W, Abruzzo LV, Krogmann T, Gao Y, Rishi AK et al. A multidrug resistance transporter from human MCF-7 breast cancer cells. *Proc Natl Acad Sci USA* 1998; **95**:15665–15670.
23. Oguri T, Bessho Y, Achiwa H, Ozasa H, Maeno K, Maeda H et al. MRP8/ABCC11 directly confers resistance to 5-fluorouracil. *Mol Cancer Ther* 2007; **6**:122–127.
24. Haimeur A, Conseil G, Deeley RG and Cole SP. The MRP-related and BCRP/ABCG2 multidrug resistance proteins: biology, substrate specificity and regulation. *Curr Drug Metabol* 2004; **5**:21–53.
25. Pratt S, Shepard RL, Kandasamy RA, Johnston PA, Perry W, III and Dantzig AH. The multidrug resistance protein 5 (ABCC5) confers resistance to 5-fluorouracil and transports its monophosphorylated metabolites. *Mol Cancer Ther* 2005; **4**:855–863.
26. Szakacs G, Paterson JK, Ludwig JA, Booth-Genthe C and Gottesman MM. Targeting multidrug resistance in cancer. *Nat Rev Drug Discov* 2006; **5**:219–234.
27. Leonard GD, Polgar O and Bates SE. ABC transporters and inhibitors: new targets, new agents. *Curr Opin Invest Drugs* 2002; **3**:1652–1659.
28. Sheps JA and Ling V. Preface: the concept and consequences of multidrug resistance. *Pflugers Arch* 2007; **453**:545–553.
29. Yeh JJ, Hsu NY, Hsu WH, Tsai CH, Lin CC and Liang JA. Comparison of chemotherapy response with P-glycoprotein, multidrug resistance-related protein-1, and lung resistance-related protein expression in untreated small cell lung cancer. *Lung* 2005; **183**:177–183.
30. Akgun A, Cok G, Karapolat I, Goksel T and Burak Z. Tc-99m MIBI SPECT in prediction of prognosis in patients with small cell lung cancer. *Ann Nucl Med* 2006; **20**:269–275.
31. Yakirevich E, Sabo E, Naroditsky I, Sova Y, Lavie O and Resnick MB. Multidrug resistance-related phenotype and apoptosis-related protein expression in ovarian serous carcinomas. *Gynecol Oncol* 2006; **100**:152–159.
32. Schneider J, Gonzalez-Roces S, Pollan M, Lucas R, Tejerina A, Martin M et al. Expression of LRP and MDR1 in locally advanced breast cancer predicts axillary node invasion at the time of rescue mastectomy after induction chemotherapy. *Breast Cancer Res* 2001; **3**:183–191.
33. Yeh JJ, Hsu WH, Wang JJ, Ho ST and Kao A. Predicting chemotherapy response to paclitaxel-based therapy in advanced non-small-cell lung cancer with P-glycoprotein expression. *Respiration* 2003; **70**:32–35.
34. Wunder JS, Bull SB, Aneliunas V, Lee PD, Davis AM, Beauchamp CP et al. MDR1 gene expression and outcome in osteosarcoma: a prospective, multicenter study. *J Clin Oncol* 2000; **18**:2685–2694.
35. Ford JM and Hait WN. Pharmacologic circumvention of multidrug resistance. *Cytotechnology* 1993; **12**:171–212.
36. Ford JM and Hait WN. Pharmacology of drugs that alter multidrug resistance in cancer. *Pharmacol Rev* 1990; **42**:155–199.
37. Krishna R and Mayer LD. Multidrug resistance (MDR) in cancer. Mechanisms, reversal using modulators of MDR and the role of MDR modulators in influencing the pharmacokinetics of anticancer drugs. *Eur J Pharm Sci* 2000; **11**:265–283.
38. Thomas H and Coley HM. Overcoming multidrug resistance in cancer: an update on the clinical strategy of inhibiting p-glycoprotein. *Cancer Control* 2003; **10**:159–165.
39. Ozben T. Mechanisms and strategies to overcome multiple drug resistance in cancer. *FEBS Lett* 2006; **580**:2903–2909.
40. Liscovitch M and Lavie Y. Cancer multidrug resistance: a review of recent drug discovery research. *IDrugs* 2002; **5**:349–355.
41. Le LH, Moore MJ, Siu LL, Oza AM, MacLean M, Fisher B et al. Phase I study of the multidrug resistance inhibitor zosuquidar administered in combination with vinorelbine in patients with advanced solid tumours. *Cancer Chemother Pharmacol* 2005; **56**:154–160.
42. Sandler A, Gordon M, De Alwis DP, Pouliquen I, Green L, Marder P et al. A Phase I trial of a potent P-glycoprotein inhibitor, zosuquidar trihydrochloride (LY335979),

administered intravenously in combination with doxorubicin in patients with advanced malignancy. *Clin Cancer Res* 2004; **10**:3265–3272.

43. Fracasso PM, Goldstein LJ, De Alwis DP, Rader JS, Arquette MA, Goodner SA et al. Phase I study of docetaxel in combination with the P-glycoprotein inhibitor, zosuquidar, in resistant malignancies. *Clin Cancer Res* 2004; **10**:7220–7228.

44. Pusztai L, Wagner P, Ibrahim N, Rivera E, Theriault R, Booser D et al. Phase II study of tariquidar, a selective P-glycoprotein inhibitor, in patients with chemotherapy-resistant, advanced breast carcinoma. *Cancer* 2005; **104**:682–691.

45. Seiden MV, Swenerton KD, Matulonis U, Campos S, Rose P, Batist G et al. A phase II study of the MDR inhibitor biricodar (INCEL, VX-710) and paclitaxel in women with advanced ovarian cancer refractory to paclitaxel therapy. *Gynecol Oncol* 2002; **86**:302–310.

46. Gandhi L, Harding MW, Neubauer M, Langer CJ, Moore M, Ross HJ et al. A phase II study of the safety and efficacy of the multidrug resistance inhibitor VX-710 combined with doxorubicin and vincristine in patients with recurrent small cell lung cancer. *Cancer* 2007; **109**:924–932.

47. Yague E, Higgins CF and Raguz S. Complete reversal of multidrug resistance by stable expression of small interfering RNAs targeting MDR1. *Gene Ther* 2004; **11**:1170–1174.

48. Pichler A, Zelcer N, Prior JL, Kuil AJ and Piwnica-Worms D. In vivo RNA interference-mediated ablation of MDR1 P-glycoprotein. *Clin Cancer Res* 2005; **11**:4487–4494.

49. Rao VV, Anthony DC and Piwnica-Worms D. MDR1 gene-specific monoclonal antibody C494 cross-reacts with pyruvate carboxylase. *Cancer Res* 1994; **54**:1536–1541.

50. Thiebaut F, Tsuruo T, Hamada H, Gottesman MM, Pastan I and Willingham MC. Immunohistochemical localization in normal tissues of different epitopes in the multidrug transport protein P170: evidence for localization in brain capillaries and crossreactivity of one antibody with a muscle protein. *J Histochem Cytochem* 1989; **37**:159–164.

51. Efferth T, Lohrke H and Volm M. Reciprocal correlation between expression of P-glycoprotein and accumulation of rhodamine 123 in human tumors. *Anticancer Res* 1989; **9**:1633–1637.

52. Legrand O, Simonin G, Perrot JY, Zittoun R and Marie JP. Both Pgp and MRP1 activities using calcein-AM contribute to drug resistance in AML. *Adv Exp Med Biol* 1999; **457**:161–175.

53. Piwnica-Worms D, Chiu ML, Budding M, Kronauge JF, Kramer RA and Croop JM. Functional imaging of multidrug-resistant P-glycoprotein with an organo technetium complex. *Cancer Res* 1993; **53**:977–984.

54. Pauwels EKJ, McCready VR, Stoot JHMB and van Deurzen DFP. The mechanism accumulation of tumour-localising radiopharmaceuticals. *Eur J Nucl Med* 1998; **25**:277–305.

55. Maffioli L, Steens J, Pauwels E and Bombardieri E. Applications of 99mTc-sestamibi in oncology. *Tumori* 1996; **82**:12–21.

56. Piwnica-Worms D, Kronauge JF and Chiu ML. Uptake and retention of hexakis (2-methoxyisobutyl isonitrile) technetium(I) in cultured chick myocardial cells. Mitochondrial and plasma membrane potential dependence. *Circulation* 1990; **82**:1826–1838.

57. Chiu ML, Kronauge JF and Piwnica-Worms D. Effect of mitochondrial and plasma membrane potentials on accumulation of hexakis (2-methoxyisobutylisonitrile) technetium(I) in cultured mouse fibroblasts. *J Nucl Med* 1990; **31**:1646–1653.

58. Modica-Napolitano JS and Aprille JR. Basis for the selective cytotoxicity of rhodamine 123. *Cancer Res* 1987; **47**:4361–4365.

59. Modica-Napolitano JS and Aprille JR. Delocalized lipophilic cations selectively target the mitochondria of carcinoma cells. *Adv Drug Deliv Rev* 2001; **49**:63–70.

60. Delmon-Moingeon L, Piwnica-Worms D, Van den Abbeele AD, Holman BL, Davison A and Jones AG. Uptake of the cation hexakis(2-methoxyisobutyisonitrile)-technetium-99m by human carcinoma cell lines in vitro. *Cancer Res* 1990; **1**:2198–2202.

61. Sharma V, Luker GD and Piwnica-Worms D. Molecular imaging of gene expression and protein function in vivo with PET and SPECT. *J Magn Reson Imaging* 2002; **16**:336–351.
62. Shen DW, Fojo A, Chin JE, Roninson IB, Richert N, Pastan I et al. Human multidrug-resistant cell lines: increased mdr1 expression can precede gene amplification. *Science* 1986; **232**:643–645.
63. Barbarics E, Kronauge JF, Cohen D, Davison A, Jones AG and Croop JM. Characterization of P-glycoprotein transport and inhibition in vivo. *Cancer Res* 1998; **58**:276–282.
64. Ballinger JR, Muzzammil T and Moore MJ. Technetium-99m-furifosmin as an agent for functional imaging of multidrug resistance in tumours. *J Nucl Med* 1997; **38**:1915–1919.
65. Muzzammil T, Moore MJ, Hedley D and Ballinger JR. Comparison of (99m)Tc-sestamibi and doxorubicin to monitor inhibition of P-glycoprotein function. *Br J Cancer* 2001; **84**:367–373.
66. Sommers CL, Byers SW, Thompson EW, Torri JA and Gelmann EP. Differentiation state and invasiveness of human breast cancer cell lines. *Breast Cancer Res Treat* 1994; **31**:325–335.
67. Bradley G, Juranka PF and Ling V. Mechanism of multidrug resistance. *Biochim Biophys Acta* 1988; **948**:87–128.
68. Utsunomiya K, Ballinger JR, Piquette-Miller M, Rauth AM, Tang W, Su Z-F et al. Comparison of the accumulation and efflux kinetics of technetium-99m sestamibi and technetium-99m tetrofosmin in an MRP-expressing tumour cell line. *Eur J Nucl Med* 2000; **27**:1786–1792.
69. Perek N, Prevot N, Koumanov F, Frere D, Sabido O, Beauchesne P et al. Involvement of the glutathione S-conjugate compounds and the MRP protein in Tc-99m-tetrofosmin and Tc-99m-sestamibi uptake in glioma cell lines. *Nucl Med Biol* 2000; **27**:299–307.
70. Vergote J, Moretti J, de Vries EGE and Garnier-Suillerot A. Comparison of the kinetics of active efflux of 99mTc-MIBI in cells with P-glycoprotein-mediated and multidrug- resistance protein-associated multidrug-resistance phenotypes. *Eur J Biochem* 1998; **252**:140–146.
71. Hendrikse NH, Franssen EJF, van der Graaf WTA, Meijer C, Piers DA, Vaalburg W et al. 99m-Sestamibi is a substrate for P-glycoprotein and the multidrug resistance-associated protein. *Br J Cancer* 1998; **77**:353–358.
72. O'Brien ML and Tew KD. Glutathione and related enzymes in multidrug resistance. *Eur J Cancer* 1996; **32A**:967–978.
73. Cole SP and Deeley RG. Transport of glutathione and glutathione conjugates by MRP1. *Trends Pharmacol Sci* 2006; **27**:438–446.
74. Zaman GJ, Lankelma J, van Tellingen O, Beijnen J, Dekker H, Paulusma C et al. Role of glutathione in the export of compounds from cells by the multidrug-resistance-associated protein. *Proc Natl Acad Sci USA* 1995; **92**:7690–7694.
75. Gomes CMF, Paassen H, Romeo S, Welling MM, Feitsma RIJ, Abrunhosa AJ et al. Multidrug resistance mediated by ABC-transporters in osteosarcoma cell lines assessed by mRNA analysis and functional radiotracer studies. *Nucl Med Biol* 2006; **33**:831–840.
76. Gomes CM, Welling M, Que I, Henriquez NV, van der PG, Romeo S et al. Functional imaging of multidrug resistance in an orthotopic model of osteosarcoma using (99m)Tc-sestamibi. *Eur J Nucl Med Mol Imaging* 2007; **34**:1793–1803.
77. Moretti JL, Hauet N, Caglar M, Rebillard O and Burak Z. To use MIBI or not to use MIBI? That is the question when assessing tumour cells. *Eur J Nucl Med Mol Imaging* 2005; **32**:836–842.
78. Mankoff DA, Dunnwald LK, Gralow JR, Ellis GK, Schubert EK, Charlop AW et al. [Tc-99m]-sestamibi uptake and washout in locally advanced breast cancer are correlated with tumor blood flow. *Nucl Med Biol* 2002; **29**:719–727.
79. Del Vecchio S and Salvatore M. 99mTc-MIBI in the evaluation of breast cancer biology. *Eur J Nucl Med Mol Imaging* 2004; **31(Suppl 1)**:S88–S96.
80. Del Vecchio S, Zannetti A, Ciarmiello A, Aloj L, Caraco C, Fonti R et al. Dynamic coupling of 99mTc-MIBI efflux and apoptotic pathway activation in untreated breast cancer patients. *Eur J Nucl Med Mol Imaging* 2002; **29**:809–814.

81. Aloj L, Zannetti A, Caraco C, Del Vecchio S and Salvatore M. Bcl-2 overexpression prevents 99mTc-MIBI uptake in breast cancer cell lines. *Eur J Nucl Med Mol Imaging* 2004; **31**:521–527.
82. Trock BJ, Leonessa F and Clarke R. Multidrug resistance in breast cancer: a meta-analysis of MDR1/gp170 expression and its possible functional significance. *J Natl Cancer Inst* 1997; **89**:917–931.
83. Kostakoglu L, Elahi N, Kiratli P, Ruacan S, Sayek I, Baltati E et al. Clinical validation of the influence of P-glycoprotein and technetium-99m-sestamibi uptake in malignant tumors. *J Nucl Med* 1997; **38**:1003–1008.
84. Kao CH, Tsai SC, Liu TJ, Ho YJ, Wang JJ, Ho ST et al. P-Glycoprotein and multidrug resistance-related protein expressions in relation to technetium-99m methoxyisobutylisonitrile scintimammography findings. *Cancer Res* 2001; **61**:1412–1414.
85. Del Vecchio S, Ciarmiello A, Potena MI, Carriero MV, Mainolfi C, Botti G et al. In vivo detection of multidrug-resistant (MDR1) phenotype by technetium-99m sestamibi scan in untreated breast cancer patients. *Eur J Nucl Med* 1997; **24**:150–159.
86. Ciarmiello A, Del Vecchio S, Silvestro P, Potena MI, Carriero MV, Thomas R et al. Tumor clearance of technetium 99m-sestamibi as a predictor of response to neoadjuvant chemotherapy for locally advanced breast cancer. *J Clin Oncol* 1998; **16**:1677–1683.
87. Takamura Y, Miyoshi Y, Taguchi T and Noguchi S. Prediction of chemotherapeutic response by Technetium 99m – MIBI scintigraphy in breast carcinoma patients. *Cancer* 2001; **92**:232–239.
88. Oka M, Fukuda M, Sakamoto A, Takatani H, Fukuda M, Soda H et al. The clinical role of MDR1 gene expression in human lung cancer. *Anticancer Res* 1997; **17**:721–724.
89. Savaraj N, Wu CJ, Xu R, Lampidis T, Lai S, Donnelly E et al. Multidrug-resistant gene expression in small-cell lung cancer. *Am J Clin Oncol* 1997; **20**:398–403.
90. Young LC, Campling BG, Voskoglou-Nomikos T, Cole SP, Deeley RG and Gerlach JH. Expression of multidrug resistance protein-related genes in lung cancer: correlation with drug response. *Clin Cancer Res* 1999; **5**:673–680.
91. Kostakoglu L, Kiratli P, Ruacan S, Hayran M, Emri S, Ergun EL et al. Association of tumor washout rates and accumulation of technetium-99m-MIBI with expression og P-glycoprotein in lung cancer. *J Nucl Med* 1998; **39**:228–234.
92. Bom HS, Kim YC, Song HC, Min JJ, Kim JY and Park KO. Technetium-99m-MIBI uptake in small cell lung cancer 13. *J Nucl Med* 1998; **39**:91–94.
93. Zhou J, Higashi K, Ueda Y, Kodama Y, Guo D, Jisaki F et al. Expression of multidrug resistance protein and messenger RNA correlate with 99mTc-MIBI imaging in patients with lung cancer. *J Nucl Med* 2001; **42**:1476–1483.
94. Balendiran GK, Dabur R and Fraser D. The role of glutathione in cancer. *Cell Biochem Funct* 2004; **22**:343–352.
95. Meyers PA, Heller G, Healey J, Huvos A, Lane J, Marcove R et al. Chemotherapy for nonmetastatic osteogenic sarcoma: the Memorial Sloan-Kettering experience. *J Clin Oncol* 1992; **10**:5–15.
96. Provisor AJ, Ettinger LJ, Nachman JB, Krailo MD, Makley JT, Yunis EJ et al. Treatment of nonmetastatic osteosarcoma of the extremity with preoperative and postoperative chemotherapy: a report from the Children's Cancer Group. *J Clin Oncol* 1997; **15**:76–84.
97. Bielack SS, Kempf-Bielack B, Delling G, Exner GU, Flege S, Helmke K et al. Prognostic factors in high-grade osteosarcoma of the extremities or trunk: an analysis of 1,702 patients treated on neoadjuvant cooperative osteosarcoma study group protocols. *J Clin Oncol* 2002; **20**:776–790.
98. Baldini N, Scotlandi K, Barbantibrodano G, Manara MC, Maurici D, Bacci G et al. Expression of P-glycoprotein in high-grade osteosarcomas in relation to clinical outcome. *NE J Med* 1995; **333**:1380–1385.

99. Pakos EE and Ioannidis JP. The association of P-glycoprotein with response to che-motherapy and clinical outcome in patients with osteosarcoma. A meta-analysis. *Cancer* 2003; **98**:581–589.

100. Shnyder SD, Hayes AJ, Pringle J and Archer CW. P-glycoprotein and metallothionein expression and resistance to chemotherapy in osteosarcoma. *Br J Cancer* 1998; **78**:757–759.

101. Burak Z, Ersoy O, Moretti JL, Erinc R, Ozcan Z, Dirlik A et al. The role of 99mTc-MIBI scintigraphy in the assessment of MDR1 overexpression in patients with musculoskele-tal sarcomas: comparison with therapy response. *Eur J Nucl Med* 2001; **28**:1341–1350.

102. Gorlick R, Liao AC, Antonescu C, Huvos AG, Healey JH, Sowers R et al. Lack of correlation of functional scintigraphy with (99m)technetium-methoxyisobutylisonitrile with histological necrosis following induction chemotherapy or measures of P-glyco-protein expression in high-grade osteosarcoma. *Clin Cancer Res* 2001; **7**:3065–3070.

103. Liang JA, Shiau YC, Yang SN, Lin FJ, Lin CC, Kao A et al. Using technetium-99m-tetrofosmin scan to predict chemotherapy response of malignant lymphomas, compared with P-glycoprotein and multidrug resistance related protein expression. *Oncol Rep* 2002; **9**:307–312.

104. Ak I, Aslan V, Vardareli E and Gulbas Z. Assessment of the P-glycoprotein expression by 99mTc-MIBI bone marrow imaging in patients with untreated leukaemia. *Nucl Med Commun* 2003; **24**:397–402.

105. Ballinger JR, Bannerman J, Boxen I, Firby P, Hartman NG and Moore MJ. Techne-tium-99m-Tetrofosmin as a substrate for P-glycoprotein: in vitro studies in multidrug-resistant breast tumor cells. *J Nucl Med* 1996; **37**:1578–1582.

106. Chen WS, Luker KE, Dahlheimer JL, Pica CM, Luker GD and Piwnica-Worms D. Effects of MDR1 and MDR3 P-glycoproteins, MRP1, and BCRP/MXR/ABCP on the transport of Tc-99m-Tetrofosmin. *Biochem Pharmacol* 2000; **60**:413–426.

107. Perek N, Koumanov F, Denoyer D, Boudard D and Dubois F. Modulation of the multidrug resistance of glioma by glutathione levels depletion–interaction with Tc-99 M-Sestamibi and Tc-99 M-Tetrofosmin. *Cancer Biother Radiopharm* 2002; **17**:291–302.

108. Sun SS, Hsieh JF, Tsai SC, Ho YJ and Kao CH. Technetium-99m tetrofosmin mam-moscintigraphy findings related to the expression of P-glycoprotein mediated multidrug resistance. *Anticancer Res* 2000; **20**:1467–1470.

109. Fukumoto M, Yoshida D, Hayase N, Kurohara A, Akagi N and Yoshida S. Scinti-graphic prediction of resistance to radiation and chemotherapy in patients with lung carcinoma: technetium 99m-tetrofosmin and thallium-201 dual single photon emission computed tomography study. *Cancer* 1999; **86**:1470–1479.

110. Shiau YC, Tsai SC, Wang JJ, Ho YJ, Ho ST and Kao CH. Technetium-99m tetrofosmin chest imaging related to p-glycoprotein expression for predicting the response with paclitaxel-based chemotherapy for non-small cell lung cancer. *Lung* 2001; **179**:197–207.

111. Shiau YC, Tsai SC, Wang JJ, Ho YJ, Ho ST and Kao CH. To predict chemotherapy response using technetium-99m tetrofosmin and compare with p-glycoprotein and multidrug resistance related protein-1 expression in patients with untreated small cell lung cancer. *Cancer Lett* 2001; **169**:181–188.

112. Shiau YC, Tsai SC, Wang JJ, Ho YJ, Ho ST and Kao CH. Predicting chemotherapy response and comparing with P-glycoprotein expression using technetium-99m tetro-fosmin scan in untreated malignant lymphomas. *Cancer Lett* 2001; **170**:139–146.

113. Shiau YC, Tsay SC, Wang JJ, Ho ST and Kao A. Detecting parathyroid adenoma using technetium-99m tetrofosmin: comparison with P-glycoprotein and multidrug resistance related protein expression - a preliminary report. *Nucl Med Biol* 2002; **29**:339–344.

114. Yapar Z, Kibar M, Yapar AF, Uguz A, Ozbarlas S and Gonlusen G. The value of Tc-99m-tetrofosmin scintigraphy in the assessment of P-glycoprotein in patients with malignant bone and soft-tissue tumors. *Ann Nucl Med* 2003; **17**:443–449.

115. Yapar Z, Kibar M, Ozbarlas S, Yapar AF, Uguz A, Zorludemir S et al. 99mTc-tetrofosmin scintigraphy in musculoskeletal tumours: the relationship between P-glyco-protein expression and tetrofosmin uptake in malignant lesions. *Nucl Med Commun* 2002; **23**:991–1000.

116. Elsinga PH, Franssen EJ, Hendrikse NH, Fluks L, Weemaes AM, van der Graaf WT et al. Carbon-11-labeled daunorubicin and verapamil for probing P-glycoprotein in tumors with PET. *J Nucl Med* 1996; **37**:1571–1575.

117. Hendrikse NH, de Vries EG, Eriks-Fluks L, van der Graaf WT, Hospers GA, Willemsen AT et al. A new in vivo method to study P-glycoprotein transport in tumors and the blood-brain barrier. *Cancer Res* 1999; **59**:2411–2416.

118. Speth PA, van Hoesel QG and Haanen C. Clinical pharmacokinetics of doxorubicin. *Clin Pharmacokinet* 1988; **15**:15–31.

119. Brady F, Luthra SK, Brown GD, Osman S, Aboagye E, Saleem A et al. Radiolabelled tracers and anticancer drugs for assessment of therapeutic efficacy using PET. *Curr Pharm Des* 2001; **7**:1863–1892.

120. Hendrikse NH and Vaalburg W. Dynamics of multidrug resistance: P-glycoprotein analyses with positron emission tomography. *Methods* 2002; **27**:228–233.

121. Ambudkar SV, Dey S, Hrycyna CA, Ramachandra M, Pastan I and Gottesman MM. Biochemical, cellular, and pharmacological aspects of the multidrug transporter. *Annu Rev Pharmacol Toxicol* 1999; **39**:361–398.

122. Schinkel AH, Wagenaar E, van Deemter L, Mol CA and Borst P. Absence of the mdr1a P-Glycoprotein in mice affects tissue distribution and pharmacokinetics of dexametha-sone, digoxin, and cyclosporin A. *J Clin Invest* 1995; **96**:1698–1705.

123. Hendrikse NH, Schinkel AH, de Vries EG, Fluks E, van der Graaf WT, Willemsen AT et al. Complete in vivo reversal of P-glycoprotein pump function in the blood-brain barrier visualized with positron emission tomography. *Br J Pharmacol* 1998; **124**:1413–1418.

124. Sasongko L, Link JM, Muzi M, Mankoff DA, Yang X, Collier AC et al. Imaging P-glycoprotein transport activity at the human blood-brain barrier with positron emission tomography. *Clin Pharmacol Ther* 2005; **77**:503–514.

125. Mehta BM, Levchenko A, Rosa E, Kim SW, Winnick S, Zhang JJ et al. Evaluation of carbon-14-colchicine biodistribution with whole-body quantitative autoradiography in colchicine-sensitive and -resistant xenografts. *J Nucl Med* 1996; **37**:312–314.

126. Levchenko A, Mehta BM, Lee JB, Humm JL, Augensen F, Squire O et al. Evaluation of 11C-colchicine for PET imaging of multiple drug resistance. *J Nucl Med* 2000; **41**:493–501.

127. Hunter AL and Klaassen CD. Biliary excretion of colchicine. *J Pharmacol Exp Ther* 1975; **192**:605–617.

128. Gangloff A, Hsueh WA, Kesner AL, Kiesewetter DO, Pio BS, Pegram MD et al. Estimation of paclitaxel biodistribution and uptake in human-derived xenografts in vivo with (18)F-fluoropaclitaxel. *J Nucl Med* 2005; **46**:1866–1871.

129. Hsueh WA, Kesner AL, Gangloff A, Pegram MD, Beryt M, Czernin J et al. Predicting chemotherapy response to paclitaxel with 18F-Fluoropaclitaxel and PET. *J Nucl Med* 2006; **47**:1995–1999.

130. Kurdziel KA, Kiesewetter DO, Carson RE, Eckelman WC and Herscovitch P. Biodis-tribution, radiation dose estimates, and in vivo Pgp modulation studies of 18F-paclitaxel in nonhuman primates. *J Nucl Med* 2003; **44**:1330–1339.

131. Kurdziel KA, Kiesewetter DO, Carson RE, Eckelman WC and Herscovitch P. Biodis-tribution, radiation dose estimates, and in vivo Pgp modulation studies of 18F-paclitaxel in nonhuman primates. *J Nucl Med* 2003; **44**:1330–1339.

132. Kurdziel KA, Kalen JD, Hirsch JI, Wilson JD, Agarwal R, Barrett D et al. Imaging multidrug resistance with 4-[18F]fluoropaclitaxel. *Nucl Med Biol* 2007; **34**:823–831.

133. Kalen JD, Hirsch JI, Kurdziel KA, Eckelman WC and Kiesewetter DO. Automated synthesis of 18F analogue of paclitaxel (PAC): [18F]Paclitaxel (FPAC). *Appl Radiat Isot* 2007; **65**:696–700.

134. Shani J and Wolf W. A model for prediction of chemotherapy response to 5-fluorouracil based on the differential distribution of 5-[18F]fluorouracil in sensitive versus resistant lymphocytic leukemia in mice. *Cancer Res* 1977; **37**:2306–2308.

135. Wolf W, Presant CA, Servis KL, el Tahtawy A, Albright MJ, Barker PB et al. Tumor trapping of 5-fluorouracil: in vivo 19F NMR spectroscopic pharmacokinetics in tumor-bearing humans and rabbits. *Proc Natl Acad Sci USA* 1990; **87**:492–496.

136. Moehler M, Dimitrakopoulou-Strauss A, Gutzler F, Raeth U, Strauss LG and Stremmel W. 18F-labeled fluorouracil positron emission tomography and the prognoses of colorectal carcinoma patients with metastases to the liver treated with 5-fluorouracil. *Cancer* 1998; **83**:245–253.

137. Dimitrakopoulou-Strauss A, Strauss LG, Schlag P, Hohenberger P, Mohler M, Oberdorfer F et al. Fluorine-18-fluorouracil to predict therapy response in liver metastases from colorectal carcinoma. *J Nucl Med* 1998; **39**:1197–1202.

138. Guo Y, Kotova E, Chen ZS, Lee K, Hopper-Borge E, Belinsky MG et al. MRP8, ATP-binding cassette C11 (ABCC11), is a cyclic nucleotide efflux pump and a resistance factor for fluoropyrimidines 2',3'-dideoxycytidine and 9'-(2'-phosphonylmethoxyethyl)adenine. *J Biol Chem* 2003; **278**:29509–29514.

139. Sharma V, Prior JL, Belinsky MG, Kruh GD and Piwnica-Worms D. Characterization of a 67 Ga/68 Ga radiopharmaceutical for SPECT and PET of MDR1 P-glycoprotein transport activity in vivo: validation in multidrug-resistant tumors and at the blood-brain barrier. *J Nucl Med* 2005; **46**:354–364.

Gene Expression Microarrays in Cancer Research

Jian Yan and Weikuan Gu

1 Introduction

The advent of microarray technology has enabled scientists to simultaneously investigate the expression of thousands of genes. This technology has been widely used in cancer research to better characterize cancer behaviors at mRNA level and to obtain new insights into various stages of carcinogenesis. A microarray-based experiment generally involves three major components: microarray manufacturing, sample processing, and data analysis, with the goals of identifying differential genes, expression signatures, modules, or networks associated with given pathological changes (Fig. 1). In this chapter, we will introduce the outline of DNA microarray technology and some basic issues related to gene expression microarray-based experiments. The state of the art of cancer gene expression studies regarding tumor development, molecular classification, outcome, and therapeutic response prediction will be addressed. We will also consider the current challenges in data analysis and interpretation of genomics studies. Moreover, we will discuss the emerging concept of cancer systems biology and novel signature-based drug discovery strategies, which are very important for the development of individualized cancer medicine.

2 A DNA Microarray Technology Overview

Since its introduction in 1995 [1, 2], microarray technology has greatly transformed molecular biology for more than a decade. The key difference between the microarray technology and traditional approaches to measuring gene expression, such as northern blot [3] and reverse transcription polymerase chain reaction (RT-PCR), is the tremendous number of genes that can be monitored on a single array, allowing generally the simultaneous profiling of

W. Gu (✉)
Department of Orthopaedic Surgery, University of Tennessee Health Science Center, Memphis, TN 38163, USA
e-mail: wgu@utmem.edu

Y. Lu, R.I. Mahato (eds.), *Pharmaceutical Perspectives of Cancer Therapeutics*, DOI 10.1007/978-1-4419-0131-6_20, © Springer Science+Business Media, LLC 2009

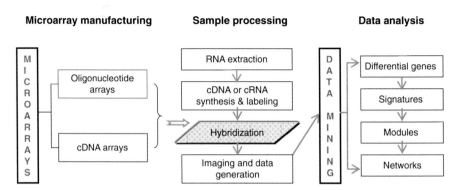

Fig. 1 A flowchart of DNA microarray experiments. A DNA microarray-based experiment consists of three major components, including microarray manufacturing, sample processing, and data analysis. Technically, various types of microarray platforms can be divided into two categories, oligonucleotide arrays and cDNA arrays. To compare global difference in gene expression between two samples, total RNAs or mRNAs are extracted, which are subject to cDNA or cRNA synthesis and labeling. The labeled samples are then hybridized to DNA microarrays to generate raw expression profiling data. Upon data mining, differential genes, expression signatures, changed modules, and networks are identified

tens of thousands of genes. This approach has deeply modified our way of performing biomedical research by switching from a gene-by-gene approach to global or genome-wide systemic studies. From its initial success as a tool for transcript-level analyses, microarray technology has spread into many areas, such as genotyping, methylation profiling, comparative genomic hybridization (CGH), and chromatin immunoprecipitation [4]. To many, the term microarray is equivalent to transcriptional profiling, which is our focus in this chapter.

2.1 Oligonucleotide Array Dominant Technology Platforms

By definition, a DNA microarray is a piece of glass, plastic, or silicon chip on which single-stranded pieces of DNA spots, called probes, are affixed in a microscopic array. These probes are used to hybridize a cDNA or cRNA sample, called target, under high-stringency conditions. Although all DNA microarrays have similar basic principles, the available technical options differ widely between platforms [5]. Two of the most important differences are the length of the probes and the number of dyes used for labeling. They can be divided into two categories: (1) cDNA arrays, usually using probes constructed with PCR products of up to a few thousand base pairs and (2) oligonucleotide arrays, using either short (25–30 mer) or long oligonucleotide (50–80 mer) probes. The probes can be either contact spotted, ink-jet deposited, or directly synthesized on the substrate. Each of these approaches has its own requirements in terms of experimental design, the amount of RNA needed, and data acquisition.

2.1.1 cDNA Arrays

In cDNA microarrays, both the probes and the targets are cDNAs. Fluorescent dyes commonly used for target cDNA labeling include green (Cy3) dye, which has a fluorescence emission wavelength of 570 nm, and red (Cy5) dye, which has a fluorescence emission wavelength of 670 nm. The two Cy-labeled cDNA samples are mixed in equal proportions and hybridized to a single microarray that is then imaged in a microarray scanner to measure fluorescence of the two fluorophores after excitation with a laser beam of a defined wavelength. The ratio of the red and green fluorescence intensities for each spot is indicative of the relative abundance of the corresponding DNA probe in the two nucleic acid target samples.

The cDNA arrays are an open-system approach, in which no sequence information is necessary before fabricating the arrays. The PCR products from cDNA banks can be synthesized using universal primers. The large size of the PCR product is also helpful in enabling stringent hybridization conditions and lowering cross-hybridization of unrelated genes, although closely related gene families will still be able to anneal to some extent. However, the preparation and the analysis of a large number of probe cDNAs are laborious and time consuming [6].

2.1.2 Oligonucleotide Arrays

In oligonucleotide microarrays, the probes are shorter sequences designed to match parts of the sequence of known or predicted open reading frames. The size of oligonucleotides used for making arrays can be short (such as 25-mer probes produced by Affymetrix) or long (such as 50-mer probes produced by Illumina). The dyes used for target labeling may be streptavidin–Alexa Fluor®647, streptavidin–phycoerythrin, Cy3 and Cy5, streptavidin–Cy3, or digoxygenin. Most of oligonucleotide arrays are detected using only one dye, called one-color or one-channel assays. Short oligonucleotide arrays were developed by Affymetrix using photolithographic methods [1]. They have been commercially available for more than 10 years and obtained wide acceptance in academic community. Up to now, they are the most commonly used oligonucleotide microarrays. Although this method is very efficient at producing thousands or millions of identical arrays, it is somewhat inconvenient and expensive for the fabrication of new arrays with added or different gene content.

To address this issue and improve work efficiency, many methods of making long oligonucleotide arrays have been developed with robotic printing or in situ synthesis. The completion of numerous genomic sequences and increased efficiency of production have combined to make the use of long oligonucleotide arrays for gene expression studies a highly attractive alternative to short oligonucleotide or cDNA arrays. Their major advantages over the others include the following: (1) the longer length probes enable more specificity in hybridization than shorter length probe arrays; (2) compared with cDNA arrays, it is much

easier to deposit the same concentration of cDNA per spot with oligonucleotides, and no denaturation step is needed for hybridization; and (3) it is more
flexible for adjusting array probe contents compared with photolithographic
methods or cDNA arrays [6].

2.2 Reliability and Reproducibility Issues in DNA Microarray Assays

Systematically searching for determinants of a phenotype using gene expression
profiling requires reasonable reproducibility, accuracy, and sensitivity in the
technology employed. However, the publication of studies with dissimilar or
totally contradictory results, obtained using different microarray platforms to
analyze identical RNA samples [7], has raised concerns about the reliability and
consistency, and hence potential application of microarray technology in the
clinical and regulatory settings. To address these concerns, the MicroArray
Quality Control (MAQC) project was initiated and led by FDA scientists
involving 137 participants from 51 organizations. In this project, gene expression levels were measured from two high-quality, distinct RNA samples in four
titration pools on seven major microarray platforms, including Applied
Biosystems, Affymetrix, Agilent Technologies, GE Healthcare, Illumina,
Eppendorf, and the National Cancer Institute (NCI) system, in addition to
three alternative expression methodologies. Each microarray platform was
deployed at three independent test sites and five replicates were assayed at
each site. The results indicate that microarray results were generally repeatable
within a test site, reproducible between test sites and comparable across platforms, even though each microarray platform has made different trade-offs
with respect to repeatability, sensitivity, specificity, and ratio compression. So
the technical performance of microarrays as assessed in the MAQC project
supports their continued use for gene expression profiling in basic and applied
research and may lead to their use as a clinical diagnostic tool as well [8].

It is estimated that the detection limit of current microarray technology
seems to be between 1 and 10 copies of mRNA per cell. However, to some
extent, inaccurate and inconsistent microarray measurements are almost una-
voidable due to several reasons: (1) the actual relationship between probe
sequences, target concentration, and probe intensity is rather poorly understood; (2) the existence of ubiquitous splice variants for at least half of the
human genes. Covering various types of alternatively spliced exons on short
oligonucleotide-based arrays is necessary to dissect the splice variant-associated
composite signals. cDNA microarrays usually have a unique long probe with
which the abundance of several splice variants can be measured. This might
explain some of the discrepancies often observed between cDNA and short
oligonucleotide microarrays; and (3) target transcript folding and cross-
hybridization can also contribute to the variation between different probes
targeting the same region of a given transcript. It is also believed that accurate

measurements of absolute expression levels and the reliable detection of low-abundance genes are currently beyond the reach of microarray technology [9].

2.3 Experimental Design for Microarray Assays

There are three primary objectives in microarray studies: class comparison, class discovery, and class prediction [10, 11]. Class comparison studies are to determine whether the expression profiles are different between the classes and, if so, to identify the differentially expressed genes. One example of a class comparison study is the comparison of gene expression profiles of grade 1 and grade 3 breast cancer patients. Class discovery studies are to identify new subtypes of a disease. Examples of class discovery are the work of Perou et al. [12], in which several molecular subtypes of breast cancer have been identified. Class prediction studies are similar to class comparison studies in that the classes are predefined. In class prediction studies, however, the emphasis is on developing valid molecular profiles with potential clinical applications, including risk assessment, diagnostic testing, prognostic stratification, and treatment selection. Many studies include both class comparison and class prediction objectives.

Experimental design depends on the study objective, but there are a few general principles that apply to all experiments. Perhaps the major issues are making sure that there is sufficient replication and avoiding the influence of confounding factors. There are also some special considerations and issues related to the design of two-channel assays, which are described below.

2.3.1 Biological and Technical Replication

In microarray studies, there are two types of replications: biological replication and technical replication. Biological replication involves hybridizations with mRNAs from different samples, whereas technical replication refers to multiple hybridizations that involve mRNA from a single biological sample. Technical replicates mean to estimate the effects of measurement variability, which is generally much smaller than biological replicates. Moreover, most commercial microarray platforms have reached a degree of reproducibility that technical replicates are of very limited value now. So technical replicates are almost never required when the study objective is to make inferences about populations that are based on sample data. They are needed only for quality-control studies. Biological replicates enable researchers to control both measurement variability and biological differences between samples. They are required in almost all experiments involving class comparison through statistical inference [13]. A recommended minimum of biological replicates for class comparison studies is five per group.

Determining sample size is one of major statistical challenges in microarray studies [14]. Several approaches have been described and tailored to specific study designs [15, 16]. Although there is no "best" methods identified, there is consensus that power analyses should be done, that microarray-tailored newer methods should be used, and that more replicates generally provide greater statistical power [13].

2.3.2 Sample Pooling

In microarray experiments, pooling refers to the study design in which RNAs collected from several individuals are combined in a pooled sample before hybridization. Labeling and hybridization are then performed on the composite sample. Many researchers favor this pooling design for several reasons: (1) sample size can be increased without using more microarrays to enhance the statistical power [13]; (2) enough RNAs can be obtained through pooling, as an alternative to RNA amplification, for performing microarray analysis [17, 18]; (3) biological subject-to-subject variability can be reduced to increase the power of statistical tests [18]. For class comparison studies, pooling is arguably beneficial [13, 19]. But pooling is not recommended for classification studies since it will interfere with the ability to accurately assess interindividual variation and covariation. Of note, when using pooling, one has to avoid bad or unusual individual samples and cannot simply analyze one pool per group [13].

2.3.3 Confounding Factors and Bias

Confounding refers to a problem that distorts the true relationship between a real causal factor and a disease [20]. A confounder can affect the outcome of interest but is unequally distributed among the study groups. Common confounders in cancer study include age, gender, cancer stage, tumor histology, and treatment received. In cancer expression profiling analysis, a simple attribution of differences in expression patterns between groups to the characteristics of disease state is inappropriate in the absence of data regarding these confounding factors. To minimize or ideally eliminate such factors, one needs to obtain comprehensive clinical/pathological annotation and stratify samples using known confounders [14].

Bias refers to an error of study design where study cases are handled differently. Possible sources of bias in microarray studies include the batch of reagents used, array batch, array version, operator, processing date, system update, platform, and pooling of tissues from multiple tissue banks. To reduce systematic study bias, one needs to develop strict inclusion and exclusion criteria, avoid inappropriate pooling of samples, and randomize processing of samples [14].

Ideally, a prospective study design should be pursued because it is one of the best ways for controlling confounding and reducing biases. This approach has just started to be adopted in two trials of breast cancer [21, 22].

2.3.4 Special Considerations with Two-Channel Microarrays

Based on the number of dyes used for target labeling, microarrays can also be categorized into two-channel (two dyes are used, such as Agilent 60-mer arrays and all cDNA arrays) and one-channel arrays (one dye is used, like most of oligonucleotide arrays). The use of two-channel arrays faces greater challenges in experimental design. The first thing to always keep in mind is that the intensities coming from the two channels should not be used separately in analysis; instead one should work directly with their ratios.

There are two common designs with two-channel arrays: direct comparison and reference design [23]. In direct comparison, two samples are labeled with red or green dye differently and hybridized on the same array. For the sake of normalization and use it as technical replication, one might hybridize each pair of samples twice, swapping the channels for half the assays ("dye swaps"). This design is sufficient for measuring differential gene expression between two conditions, but not for multiple condition comparison.

In reference design, a reference sample is used for conducting all the direct comparisons. The reference sample can be either a universal reference (such as those sold by Stratagene) or a pooled reference from the samples that will be assayed in the experiment. A pooled reference may provide better performance in a class comparison analysis [23]. A variant of the reference design is the blocked reference design, in which independent references are matched (relative to some relevant factor) to the conditions that one wants to compare and are cohybridized to each respectively. This type of design can be useful in time series experiments and in drug experiments [16, 24].

2.4 Data Analysis

Microarray data analysis is a new area of data analysis with its own unique challenges [25]. Based on the study purposes, this process can be subdivided into two components: primary analysis and integrated analysis. Primary analysis involves differential expression identification and classification for the three primary study objectives (i.e., class comparison, class discovery, and class prediction). Integrated analysis means to identify metasignatures, pathways and networks by integrating various sources of data.

2.4.1 Primary Data Analysis

Data Preprocessing

Primary data analysis starts with data preprocessing to control the effects of systematic error while retaining full biological variation. This process consists of image analysis, filtering, normalization and transformation. As for image analysis, a variety of freeware and commercial software packages have been developed and this remains an active area of research. For Affymetrix arrays, different algorithms have been proposed, and RMA (Robust Multichip Analysis) and its variant gcRMA are often favored by many investigators [13]. For non-Affymetrix platforms, image-processing algorithms abound and vary substantially with no clear "winner" emerging.

Filtering refers to exclusion of bad probes on the array or the whole array. Visual inspection of array images and color-coded plot images are the first tools that should be used to detect outlier probes or arrays [23]. Clustering (described below) is another common way to identify outlier array among the whole set of arrays in a study.

In terms of normalization, there are many options for investigators. For Affymetrix arrays, the quantile normalization method is believed to work better on Affymetrix data at the probe cell level [23]. This method makes the assumption that the samples hybridized to the different assays have roughly the same distribution of RNA abundance over the transcripts represented on the array. This algorithm transforms the intensities so that the bulk of the intensity distribution is the same for all assays in an experiment, typically with some differences in the distribution tails (which might reflect actual biological differences). But for non-Affymetrix arrays, it is unclear which normalization method produce better results [13].

Differentially Expressed Gene Identification

Differential expression analysis refers to finding genes that are expressed at different levels between two experimental conditions. Numerous methods have been applied to the identification of differentially expressed genes in microarray studies. The simplest, nonstatistical test method often used is the fold change method. In this method, the ratios between expression levels in two conditions are evaluated. Genes with a ratio higher than an arbitrary cutoff value are considered to be differentially expressed [26]. However, as a nonstatistical test, this approach offers no associated level of "confidence." It also does not provide any control on the number of false-positive findings.

The emerging standard approach is based on statistical significance and multiple hypothesis testing. The classical t test and other traditional test statistics perform well in the presence of a large number of replicates per condition. But microarray studies generally do not meet this requirement. Modified methods based on t or F statistics, which borrow variance information among genes, called regularized t-tests, are recommended if there are less than 10 samples per condition [27, 28]. More sophisticated multivariate testing methods, such as the widely used SAM [29], can provide greater power than the regularized t-tests while controlling false discovery rate (FDR) [30].

It should be noted that different methods produce gene lists that are strikingly different. For example, in a comparison of 10 common methods of differential expression identification, Jeffery et al. found that only 8–21% of genes were in common across all 10 selection methods [31]. They also made recommendations for choice of selection methods in different settings such as area under an ROC curve with datasets that have low levels of noise and large sample size, rank products with datasets that have low numbers of samples or high levels of noise, and empirical Bayes t-statistic with a wide range of sample sizes.

Classification

Classification refers to either identifying new classes within a dataset (class discovery) or assigning cases to a given class (class prediction) [13]. It is a very popular use of microarray experiments. In class discovery, unsupervised clustering approaches are utilized to classify the profiles into groups based on their similarity. A most commonly used unsupervised method in microarray studies is two-dimensional hierarchical cluster analysis, which graphically presents results in a tree diagram (dendrogram). Many questions regarding molecular classification of a disease, gene coexpression, data reduction, and data quality control could be addressed using unsupervised classification. Common non-hierarchical clustering methods include k-means method and self-organizing map [32]. However, most clusterings in microarray datasets are found not to be reproducible and resampling techniques are recommended to assess the reproducibility of clustering findings [13].

In class prediction, supervised approaches have been used to develop algorithms to assign objects to known categories. The goal may be diagnostic, offering a new way to distinguish similar-looking diseases, or it may be a true effort to predict clinical outcome. Most such methods include a training phase run on samples whose classes are already known, and a testing phase, in which the algorithm generalizes from the training data to predict classifications of previously unseen samples. Many supervised classification algorithms are available, such as k-nearest neighbors, nearest centroid, support vector machine (SVM), and classification trees [23]. But all are susceptible to overfitting to some degree, which refers to the case where an algorithm models the training samples too exactly, without sufficient generalization [13]. To address this problem, one must cross-validate it on testing data that are completely independent of the training data.

2.4.2 Integrated Data Analysis

Although primary analyses are useful for deciphering the complex molecular heterogeneity of biological phenomena, integrative bioinformatics approaches that leverage numerous other data sources have begun to show promise in uncovering important biology not apparent from these primary analysis methods [33]. This transition is accelerated with community efforts to standardize data and knowledge storage formats and access protocols and efforts to make the corresponding bases publicly available, most often through web-based access.

Meta-Analysis

With large public resources of microarray easily available, primarily ArrayExpress and the Gene Expression Omnibus (GEO), a new era is dawning on microarray analysis. One of the approaches concerns combining information from multiple independent but related existing microarray studies to increase the reliability and generalizability of results through meta-analysis. Meta-analysis has been widely used in clinical trials and epidemiological studies. Its applicability to microarray data was demonstrated for the first time in a prostate cancer study [34], where a summary of statistic-based method coupled with false discovery rate analysis was applied on four prostate cancer gene expression studies. A robust signature of overactive polyamine biosynthesis pathway was identified, which is consistent with the known elevation of polyamines in prostate cancer. Since then, microarray meta-analysis has been used to identify robust expression signatures, coexpressed genes, or gene networks [35].

Meta-analysis of microarray datasets shares many features with meta-analysis in other areas of health-care research. The main differences lie in the large numbers of variables involved and technical diversity of multiple platforms. Furthermore, most microarray studies are retrospective and many confounding factors may interfere with the interpretation of results. To help perform valid microarray meta-analysis, Ramasamy et al. [35] recently identified seven key issues and suggested a 30-step approach, consisting of (1) Identify suitable microarray studies; (2) Extract the data from studies; (3) Prepare the individual datasets; (4) Annotate the individual datasets; (5) Resolve the many-to-many relationship between probes and genes; (6) Combine the study-specific estimates; (7) Analyze, present, and interpret results.

Modular/Pathway Analysis

The complex functions of a living cell can be better understood in the framework of pathways and networks [36]. In microarray studies, a pathway often refers to a gene set with a given biological theme, also called "module" [37]. The hypothesis that genes in the same module are more likely to be coordinately regulated than a randomly selected gene set has been recently demonstrated using coherence indicators estimated in 96 pathways in tumor and normal samples [38].

Modular analysis integrates the primary microarray analysis results and their functional annotations based on precompiled databases of pathways derived from large-scale literature analysis or computer-assisted annotation, such as Gene Ontology [39], KEGG [40], Biocarta (http://www.biocarta.com/), and GenMAPP [41].

The power of pathway analysis was demonstrated by Mootha et al. [42]. By applying a method called gene set enrichment analysis (GSEA), they found that genes involved in oxidative phosphorylation are coordinately downregulated in diabetic muscle. This result was unexpected because in the original analysis, no individual genes showed significant deregulation in diabetic muscle. Only when examining functionally related gene sets were they able to identify the change. In another study, Yu et al. [43] identified a novel, robust, and biologically relevant, low-grade expression signature using the signature analysis (SA) algorithm [44]. This signature, TuM1, was not readily discernible by conventional clustering techniques. It is expressed in a subset of estrogen receptor (ER)-positive tumors and is significantly enriched with genes involved in apoptosis. This finding was validated in multiple independent breast cancer datasets generated using different array technologies.

Each type of modular analysis needs its own method of interpretation to maximize the information that is available. Interpretation of the results of modular analysis might be complicated by the variable quality of the functional descriptions. A major drawback of modular analysis is the large number of genes for which no biological classification exists; this might be the case for more than half of the genes represented on a microarray.

Gene Network Analysis

Although modular analysis is helpful for better interpretation of microarray data, individual modules are not enough to explain the complex functions of a living cell since biological processes usually involve interactions of more than one modules in the form of network. So it is very important to perform network analysis to make full use of various sources of data.

There are two main types of networks being pursued by microarray researchers: protein interactome network and transcriptional regulatory network. The study of interactome network requires detailed protein–protein interaction ("interactome") databases. Such repositories can be broadly classified into two types based on the ways they are created: (1) Those containing interactions supported by experimental evidence or (2) Those containing interactions derived from in silico predictions alone or mixed together with experimentally derived evidence. Many primary databases that contain literature-curated interactome information are publicly available, such as human protein reference database (HPRD), InAct, molecular interaction database (MINT), database of interacting protein (DIP), MIPS database, Alliance for cellular signaling (AfCS), biomolecular interaction network database (BIND), Reactome, and PDZBase. Several large transcription regulatory interaction databases are now also available to the public, such as TRANSFAC, TRED, VISTA Enhancer, and PreMod. It is good for modern biologists to know that many network-based analysis approaches have been implemented in ready-to-use and freely accessible databases and softwares [36].

When considering the current state of human molecular interaction maps and databases, it is important to note the limitations and pitfalls. First, because these information are largely incomplete and probably contain several errors, important modules and subnetworks may be missed by such analysis. For example, when considering networks generated from the literature, only well-studied proteins and interactions will be represented, and when considering networks generated from high-throughput yeast two-hybrid experiments, only nuclear and cytoplasmic proteins will be represented. Furthermore, protein–protein interactions are probably often context dependent (i.e., an interaction that occurs in a specific cell line or artificial system may not occur in vivo). Therefore, until these networks have matured, insights gained from their analysis must be treated as hypotheses requiring careful experimental validation.

2.5 Data Validation

There are two categories of approaches to independent confirmation of differential expression data: in silico analysis and laboratory-based analysis [45]. The in silico method compares array results in the literature and in public or private biological databases. Laboratory-based validation provides biomedical verification of microarray findings using semiquantitative reverse transcription PCR (RT-PCR), real-time RT-PCR, northern blot, or in situ hybridization. Tissue microarrays (TMAs) are an excellent approach for the validation of array data [45]. A TMA is a slide containing dozens to hundreds of predefined microscopic sections of tissue, enabling an investigator to measure DNA, mRNA, or protein expression using immunohistochemistry or in situ hybridization simultaneously in a large number of samples. A particular advantage of the method is to provide in situ information about gene and its expression. But the most significant drawbacks of this method are low sensitivity, poor quantitation, and sample selection bias.

To estimate the accuracy of a classification method, the standard strategy is via a training validation approach, in which a training set is used to identify the signature and a validation set is used to estimate the proportion of misclassifications [46].

However, there are many questions unresolved as to when and how validation should be performed as well as what the criteria under which a finding can be claimed to be validated are [13].

3 Characterization of Cancer Using Expression Signatures

Traditionally, cancer is characterized by gross visual information (size of the tumor, degree of spread, histological characteristics of the tumor) along with a limited number of biochemical assays. Although these methods do provide a way to classify tumor subgroups with distinct biology, it is obvious that these classifications are imprecise, offering little information on precise underlying molecular changes required for proper management. The feasibility of expression signatures in the characterization of cancer was first demonstrated in a landmark study on leukemia where expression signature was used to distinguish acute myeloid and acute lymphoblastic leukemias without previous knowledge of these classes [10]. So far, gene expression profiling of cancers represents the largest category of research using microarray technology and appears to be the most comprehensive approach to characterize cancer molecularly [47]. Among the cancers studied with microarrays, breast cancer is the most heavily explored, thus resulting in a great deal of functional information about it (Fig. 2). Breast cancer also represents a window that displays the contents and status of gene expression profiling studies of cancer [48].

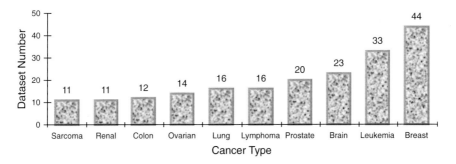

Fig. 2 Top 10 cancers studied using gene expression microarrays. Data resource: Oncomine (as of September 27, 2008) (www.oncomine.org), a large compendium of published cancer microarray data with a suite of advanced analytic tools

3.1 Tumor Individuality

The complexity of oncogenic process, involving somatic multiple mutations coupled with variability in the host's genetic constitution, produces a disease of enormous complexity. That is why Nevins et al. believe that 100 breast cancer patients may represent 100 distinct diseases [47]. The concept of each tumor as an individual was documented during the classification of breast carcinomas, because repeated samplings of the same tumor, either before and after chemotherapy or as a tumor–metastasis pair, were found to have much more similarity to each other than to any other tumor studied [49]. Furthermore, different foci in an individual may have distinct profiles and clonally related tumors in the same individual can show different expression patterns owing to divergent histories [50].

3.2 Molecular Classification of Cancer

In most human malignancies, clinical classifications are essential for prognosis assessment and cancer management. Also, they provide baseline information for unbiased comparisons in clinical research. In the last decade, traditional method-generated molecular parameters have been pursued and incorporated in cancer classifications. Molecular data may either define tumor clinical aggressiveness or represent new targets for drug development. For example, human epidermal growth factor receptor (ERBB2/HER-2) amplifications in breast cancer and epidermal growth factor receptor (EGFR) overexpression/ mutations in nonsmall cell lung cancer (NSCLC) identify a subgroup of patients with better response to trastuzumab and in some instances erlotinib, respectively [51, 52]. As a result, molecular cancer classification is critical for proper handling of cancer patients in clinical settings.

The classification of human tumors using DNA microarray technology has been an area of intense research in the last decade. For example, many studies have consistently shown that breast cancer can be molecularly classified into at least four subtypes: the basal-like subtype, the ERBB2-like subtype, and luminal-like subtypes A and B. Importantly, the newly defined molecular subgroups have distinct clinical outcomes and responses to therapy [48].

Four main histological subtypes of lung cancer are regularly distinguished by tumor morphology under the light microscope: squamous, large cell, small cell, and adenocarcinoma. In the microarray studies of lung cancer, two separate groups using different microarray platforms (Affymetrix oligonucleotide arrays and cDNA arrays) have identified similar expression signatures that accurately recapitulated these four histological subtypes [53]. Moreover, in an integrative study, Hayes et al. identified three reproducible tumor subtypes within the category of adenocarcinoma of the lung [54]. They were named bronchioid, squamoid, and magnoid to reflect their respective correlations with gene expression patterns of histologically defined bronchioalveolar carcinoma, squamous cell carcinoma, and large-cell carcinoma. Remarkably, bronchioid tumors were correlated with improved survival in early stage disease, whereas squamoid tumors were associated with better survival in advanced disease.

Identification of the primary anatomical site of tumor origin is very important for proper treatment of cancer of unknown origin. It is estimated that 4% of cancer patients present with metastatic tumors for which the origin of the primary tumor has not been determined [55]. To address this issue, Su et al. developed a multiclass molecular classification scheme based on genes whose expression was specific to tumor tissues of each anatomical site. The classifier showed 85% accuracy on test set predictions and 75% accuracy on metastasis sample predictions. Of note, an 11-gene classifier could predict the anatomical origin of up to 91% and 83% of the training and blinded tumor samples, respectively [56].

3.3 Common Transcriptional Programs for Tumor Development

A basic assumption in cancer research is that some common transcriptional programs may be shared across different types of tumors during the course of carcinogenesis, consisting of initiation, progression, and metastasis. This assumption proves to be valid by some microarray studies. For example, in a recent meta-analysis of 40 published cancer microarray datasets that represent approximately 3,700 cancer samples, Rhodes et al. meta-analyzed 36 neoplastic transformation signatures from 21 datasets (overexpressed in cancer relative to respective normal tissue), which span 12 tissue types including breast, prostate, colon, lung, liver, brain, ovary, pancreas, uterus, salivary gland, bladder, and B lymphocytes. Eventually, 183 genes were identified to be present in at least 10 of 36 signatures, 67 genes in at least 12 signatures, and 1 gene in 18 signatures. To assess the universality of the meta-signature, the top 67 genes were used to predict cancer vs. normal status in 39 analyses using a leave-one-out voting classifier. The signature was validated as a significant predictor ($P < 0.05$) in 29 of 39 analyses (from 19 of 21 datasets) [57].

In terms of cancer progression, this study meta-profiled seven "undifferentiated vs. well-differentiated" signatures spanning six cancer types. Sixty-nine genes were present in at least four of seven signatures, twenty-four genes were present in five signatures, and six genes were present in six of seven signatures, whereas zero genes were significant in five or more by chance, thus defining an undifferentiated meta-signature common to multiple types of cancer. Interestingly, a fraction of genes predominantly associated with proliferation (such as TOP2A, MCM3, CDC2, RFC4) in this meta-signature overlap with the meta-signature of neoplastic transformation, suggesting the commonality in increased proliferation in both cancer initiation and progression.

Metastasis is a fatal event that is generally regarded as a result of accumulating somatic mutation in the late phase of carcinogenesis. To elucidate the molecular nature of metastasis, Ramaswamy et al. [58] analyzed the gene expression profiles of 12 metastatic adenocarcinoma nodules of diverse origin (lung, breast, prostate, colorectal, uterus, and ovary) and compared them with the expression profiles of 64 unmatched primary adenocarcinomas representing the same spectrum of tumor types obtained from different individuals. This study identified a refined 17-gene expression signature that can distinguish primary and metastatic adenocarcinomas (Fig. 3). The enriched functional changes include overactivities of structural protein, chromosomal rearrangement, and cell communication as well as decreased activities of calmodulin binding and methylation. The generality of the expression signature was further confirmed in 279 primary solid tumors of diverse type, but not in diffuse large B-cell lymphoma, consistent with the idea that hematopoietic tumors have

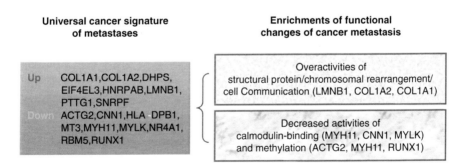

Fig. 3 A universal cancer signature of metastases. Identified by Ramaswamy et al. [58] through a microarray assay of 12 metastatic adenocarcinoma nodules of diverse origin (lung, breast, prostate, colorectal, uterus, and ovary), this 17-gene metastatic signature suggests involvement of altered functional changes of structural proteins, calmodulin binding, and methylation in cancer metastasis. The functional annotation of gene expression changes was performed using DAVID bioinformatics tools (http://david.abcc.ncifcrf.gov)

distinct mechanisms for navigating the hematologic and lymphoid compartments [58]. They found that solid tumors carrying the expression signature were
most likely to be associated with metastasis and poor clinical outcome ($P <$
0.03), suggesting the hypothesis that a gene expression program of metastasis
may already be present in the early phase of disease at the time of diagnosis.

3.4 Cancer Prognostic Prediction

In the last 5 years, gene expression profiling has been extensively used to predict
outcome of many cancer patients. Breast cancer has been a hot topic in this
field. Many disparate signatures with little overlap in their constituent genes
have been identified and validated [48]. To further validate these findings and to
find the reasons for this signature diversity, Wirapati et al. performed a largest
meta-analysis of publicly available breast cancer gene expression and clinical
data, which are composed of 2,833 breast tumors, together with a modular
analysis [59]. The performance of nine published prognostic signatures, including ONC-16, NKI-70, EMC-76, NCH-70, CON-52, p53-32, VSR, GGI-128,
and CCYC, was evaluated in this dataset collection. Using this approach, they
confirmed the presence of four stable breast cancer molecular subtypes as
originally reported by Perou and colleagues [49]. Furthermore, they validated
the equivalence of all the investigated prognostic signatures. Finally, through
modular analyses they noticed that these prognostic signatures function mostly
by identifying tumors that have high expression of proliferation genes, regardless of the subtyping based on estrogen receptor (ER) or ERBB2, suggesting
that proliferation may be the common driving force of several prognostic
signatures (Fig. 4). Importantly, this study provided a new methodological
framework applicable to other cancers for identifying consistent biological
themes behind various reported signatures.

In the case of lung cancer study, many different prognostic signatures for
survival in nonsmall cell lung cancer (NSCLC) have also been reported in the
literature [60]. To further validate the performance of these signatures, Sun
et al. conducted a large retrospective, multisite, blinded study using a total of
442 lung adenocarcinomas [60]. The results showed that several signatures
examined could accurately predict the outcome of patients. Moreover, most
signatures performed better with clinical covariates (stage, age, and sex), supporting the combined use of clinical and molecular information when building
prognostic models for early stage lung cancer.

3.5 Cancer Therapeutic Response Prediction

Our ability to treat patients based on their needs is definitely inadequate since
we do not know which therapy will be the most effective for each individual
patient. Indeed, predicting drug response is a great challenge in oncology, as
commonly used therapeutic agents are ineffective in many patients, and side

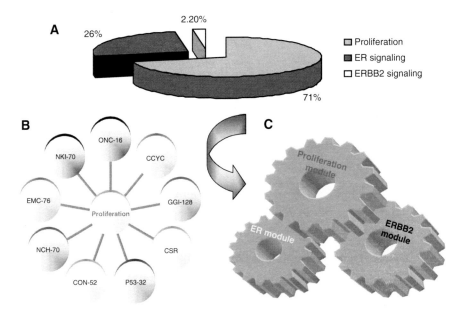

Fig. 4 Proliferation-centered gene expression changes in the prognosis of breast cancer. Based on a recent meta-analysis of gene expression profiles in breast cancer [59], most of identified gene expression changes (**A**), prognostic signatures (**B**), and altered modules (**C**) in breast cancer are related to proliferation

effects often develop. With the gene expression profiling assays, it is possible to discover correlations between a set of genes and the sensitivity or resistance of tumor cells to a given therapy toward a human cancer. Accurate prediction of patient response to drugs is a long-term goal of pharmacogenomics research as it would facilitate the individualization of patient treatment.

In an effort to find a way to predict chemotherapy sensitivity, Staunton et al. [61] conducted microarray assays using 232 cytotoxic chemotherapeutic drugs in a panel of 60 human cancer cell lines (the NCI-60). Expression profile-based classifiers of sensitivity or resistance to these compounds were generated and then evaluated on independent sets of data. About one-fourth of the classifiers performed accurately, suggesting that at least for a subset of compounds, genomic approaches to chemosensitivity prediction are feasible. These signatures have recently been further validated to be able to accurately predict clinical response in individuals treated with these drugs [62].

4 Toward Systems Biology of Cancer

Fueled mainly by the development of microarray technology, systematic study on cancer using systems biology approach has increased (Fig. 5). Systems biology represents an analytical approach to the relationships among

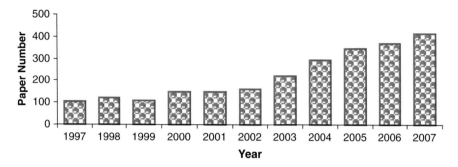

Fig. 5 Growth of research interest in cancer systems biology in the last decade. The literature search was performed using the database PubMed for the number of articles about cancer systems biology per year. Key word combination was "'systems biology" AND cancer'

components of a biological system, with the goal of understanding its emergent properties [63]. The key idea behind systems biology is that complex biological systems must be robust against environmental and genetic perturbations to be evolvable. So cancer is regarded as a highly robust disease in which the tumor eventually surpasses the host in growth [64]. To ensure the robustness of a system, four proposed mechanisms are involved: system control, fail-safe, modularity, and decoupling [64]. In the following sections, we introduce these four mechanisms using evidence obtained in cancer research, especially expression profiling studies.

4.1 System Control

System control refers to negative and positive feedbacks to attain a robust dynamic response from a regulatory network point of view. For example, the oncogene c-Myc is a key transcriptional regulator highly expressed in many cancer types. In the past decades, the molecular mechanisms by which c-Myc functions to effect tumorigenesis have been the subject of extensive research. However, the specific mechanisms by which tumorigenesis are achieved are not well understood in a perspective of traditional molecular biology. Recently, Reymann et al. [65] performed a genome-wide expression profiling analysis on lung adenocarcinomas of c-myc transgenic mice in order to elucidate the c-Myc transcriptional regulatory network. They first identified 469 upregulated genes and 8 downregulated genes in tumors. Then they analyzed the promoters of transcriptionally induced genes with respect to the binding sites of c-Myc and other transcription factors. The network analysis identified a transcriptional regulatory network, consisting of at least 17 nodes (transcription factors such as Ap2, Zf5, Zic3, and E2f) and positive and negative interactions in a hierarchical infrastructure.

4.2 Fail-Safe (Alternative)

Fail-safe, also called "alternative," is a mechanism by which a specific function is achieved through multiple means to prevent failure of robustness. It refers to having multiple heterogeneous components or modules with overlapping functions. In fact, that is all we have learnt and are puzzled in more than a decade of microarray studies: unstable gene lists with common biological themes [14]. For example, "proliferation signatures" have been observed consistently in almost all tumor microarray studies [66] and turn out to be the "core component" of various different prognostic signatures for breast cancer [59]. However, the exact gene identities that comprise these signatures often vary greatly [66]. These results suggest that the hypothesis of the existence of a universal mechanism for all individuals with a disease is not valid. Although several studies have revealed some consensus signatures as described above, these changes can explain only some basic features of tumor behavior, but not a wide variety of heterogeneity. So it is arguable that several thousands of samples are needed to make a true discovery in microarray study [67]. With this in mind, many microarray data will be easier to understand and be better interpreted.

4.3 Modularity

Modularity is a basic characteristic of complex systems. A module in a network is a set of nodes that have strong interactions and a common function. Modularity can contribute to both robustness of the whole system, by confining perturbations and damage locally to minimize the effects on, and evolution, by simply rewiring modules.

In the last two decades, using traditional strategies, cancer researchers have collected an enormous amount of information about the differences between cancer cells and their healthy counterparts, with the ultimate goal of identifying drug targets. This has, for instance, led to the identification of about 300 genes that are causally implicated in human cancer and to the discovery of the mutations in those genes [68]. Most of these genes function in signal transduction processes regulating cell growth and apoptosis [69]. It is clear that these genes work in a modular fashion. For example, compelling evidence indicate that cancer-related genes *CDK4*, *CCND1*, *Rb*, and *P16* establish a cell cycle module involved in human cancers.

Cancer involves disruptions of various cellular processes and functions due to aberrations in regulation of key proliferation and survival pathways. Some changes are common to all tumors, whereas others may be specific to certain tumors. Understanding the precise genome-wide changes in terms of modules for a given tumor has important therapeutic implications. To this end, Eran Segal et al. [37] performed an integrative analysis of 1,975 published microarrays spanning 22 tumor types. They identified 456 statistically significant modules that span various processes and functions, including metabolism, transcription, translation, degradation, cellular and neural signaling, growth, cell cycle, apoptosis, extracellular matrix, and cytoskeleton components. Then, they characterized tumors in terms of a combination of activated and deactivated modules. Some changes of modules are specific to particular types of tumor; for example, a growth-inhibitory module is specifically downregulated in acute lymphoblastic leukemias and may underlie the deregulated proliferation in these cancers. Other changes of modules are shared across a diverse set of tumors, suggestive of common tumor progression mechanisms. For example, the bone osteoblastic module was identified in a variety of tumor types.

4.4 Decoupling

Decoupling represents a preventive mechanism against damaging high-level functionalities. For example, Hsp90 not only fixes proteins that are misfolded as a result of environmental stresses but also decouples genetic variations from the phenotype using the same mechanism, therefore providing a genetic buffer against mutations. Interestingly, the most investigated tumor suppressor p53 protein also seems to be a genetic buffer [70], which may explain the unexpected survival-promoting effect of wide-type p53 in cancer cells [71]. These genetic buffers decouple the genotype from the phenotype, and they provide robustness to cope with mutation while maintaining a degree of genetic diversity.

5 Drug Discovery Through Signature Screening

Advances in genomic research in the past two decades fuelled the expectation that agents that specifically target a single disease-causing molecule—"magic bullets"—could cure cancer, diabetes, and other complex diseases. The current evidence shows that an expression signature, instead of a single disease-causing molecule, may be a reasonable target for drug development. Two approaches have been applied in this domain: signature screenings in laboratory and in silico. The framework of anticancer drug discovery through signature screening is illustrated in Fig. 6.

5.1 Signature Screening in Laboratory: Gene Expression-Based, High-Throughput Screening

Gene expression-based, high-throughput screening (GE-HTS) was developed by Stegmaier et al. to help find relevant small molecules for disease control in a library efficiently [72]. The approach starts with the identification of expression signatures for the biological states of interest ("A" vs. "B") using genome-wide

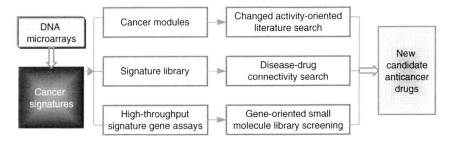

Fig. 6 Strategies for anticancer drug discovery using DNA microarrays. With signature and small-molecule libraries being available, two approaches can be applied in the screening of new candidate anticancer drugs: in laboratory and in silico. The in-laboratory method involves the identification of expression signatures and the development of high-throughput, low-cost measurement of signature genes. The in silico method means to perform literature or library search using cancer modules or signatures as targets

gene expression profiling. Next, an assay is developed for the high-throughput, low-cost measurement of the signature genes. Then, a small-molecule library is screened for compounds that induce a change from the "state A" to the "state B" signature. Using this approach, they derived a five-gene signature of leukemia differentiation and screened a library of 1,739 bioactive small molecules for compounds that induced the expression of the signature genes in a leukemia cell line. Their screening results suggested that DAPH1 (4,5-dianilinophthalimide) is a candidate acute myeloblastic leukemia (AML) differentiation-inducing agent. Although DAPH1 was previously identified as an epidermal growth factor receptor (EGFR) kinase inhibitor, it has not been developed clinically, thus precluding its evaluation with AML patients. Fortunately, they found that the Food and Drug Administration (FDA)-approved EGFR inhibitor gefitinib (Iressa) can induce myeloid differentiation in AML cell lines and primary patient-derived AML blasts at concentrations that are achievable in humans [73]. Interestingly, EGFR expression was not detected in AML cells, suggesting that gefitinib functions through a previously unrecognized EGFR-independent mechanism.

In another study, GE-HTS was used to find candidate drugs able to modulate the activity of some of the oncoproteins (including transcription factors and other previously intractable targets) that drive cancer development. The researchers used expression profiling microarrays to define a 14-gene expression signature that differentiates between Ewing sarcoma cells in which the EWS/FLI fusion protein is on and those in which it is off. They then used this signature to screen a library of about 1,000 chemicals (many already approved for other clinical uses) in a "ligation-mediated amplification assay" with a fluorescent, bead-based detection. The most active modulator of EWS/FLI activity identified by this GE-HTS approach was cytosine arabinoside (ARA-C). At levels achievable in people, this compound reduced the abundance of EWS/FLI protein and inhibited tumor growth in xenograft model of Ewing sarcoma [74].

The advantages of this method are the following: (1) GE-HTS does not require development of specialized assays for the measurement of signature genes. The gene expression signature definition, amplification, and detection are generic; and (2) a former knowledge of a target is not needed. The gene expression signature serves as a surrogate for the biological state in question. The method is thus well suited for discovery of modulators of oncogenic transcription factors in which the mutant transcription factor's transforming mechanism is not known.

5.2 Signature Screening In Silico—Connectivity Map

Gene expression signatures have been used to create the Connectivity Map for finding "connections" among small-molecule drugs, genes, and diseases [75]. In this project, expression profiles have been generated from cultured human cells treated with many small-molecule compounds (now 1309 kinds) to create a library of signatures of drug responses. This library of signatures is then used as a database that can be queried by biologists, pharmacologists, chemists, and clinical scientists in the analysis of gene expression data. In this context, the expression signature is represented as a group of gene identities, not by the actual properties of expression that are defined in the experimental setting.

The ability of the Connectivity Map database to identify new therapeutic opportunity in cancer treatment has been demonstrated in a recent study on childhood acute lymphoblastic leukemia (ALL) [76]. Glucocorticoids (GC) are critical to many biological processes and to ALL therapy. By searching the Connective Map database for profiles that coincided with a gene expression signature of GC sensitivity or resistance in ALL cells, the authors found a match target—the mTOR inhibitor rapamycin. Further experimental assays provided evidence that rapamycin could induce glucocorticoid sensitivity in lymphoid tumor cells and sensitization to apoptosis through the modulation of the antiapoptotic gene *MCL1*. These findings provide a potential path toward a new therapeutic strategy involving rapamycin and glucocorticoid.

Signature screenings in laboratory and in silico can be combined to improve the drug discovery. For example, GE-HTS was carried out for compounds capable of attenuating the aberrant androgen receptor (AR) activation seen in prostate cancer. Two of the hits were celastrol and gedunin, the molecular targets of which were unknown. To determine a potential mechanism of action, the authors treated LNCaP prostate cancer cells with gedunin, generated a expression signature, and then queried the Connectivity Map library for a match. The database returned several matches that suggested gedunin was behaving as a heat-shock protein inhibitor. Further experimentation confirmed that gedunin inhibited heat-shock protein 90 (Hsp90), a key regulator of AR, suggesting Hsp90 inhibition as a strategy for controlling AR activity in prostate cancer [77].

5.3 Module Screening In Silico—Module Map

Since tumors can be characterized as combinations of activated and suppressed functional modules in a module map [37], targeted therapies might be developed specifically for a tumor based on changed modules. This hypothesis was tested in vitro by Wong et al. [78]. With a module map for human breast cancers, they found that activation of a poor-prognosis "wound signature" is strongly associated with induction of both a mitochondria gene module and a proteasome gene module. They proposed glycolysis blockade and proteasome blockade as potential therapeutic strategies for these highly aggressive tumors accordingly. The results showed that the glycolysis inhibitor 3-bromopyruvic acid selectively killed breast cells expressing the mitochondria and wound signatures. In addition, the proteasome inhibitor bortezomib selectively killed breast cells expressing the wound signature. Thus, gene module maps may provide a new tool for rapid translation of expression signatures in human disease to targeted therapeutic strategies.

6 Future Directions and Conclusions

The advent of microarray technology has opened a new chapter of molecular cancer research. It is clear that gene expression profiling analysis has great potential for improving cancer management and for better understanding of the cancer biology. However, the future fate of microarray technology per se is being challenged by the arrival of massively parallel sequencing (MPS) technologies [79]. Also called "next-generation DNA sequencing," this technology is based on the concept of cyclic array sequencing that a dense array of DNA features is sequenced by iterative cycles of enzymatic manipulation and imaging-based data collection [80]. With this method, genomic or complementary DNA is fragmented and then ligated to common adaptors to construct template libraries through PCR. The PCR amplicons are spatially clustered either to a single location on a planar substrate or to the surface of micrometer-scale beads, which are recovered and arrayed. All array features are then manipulated with a single microliter-scale reagent volume and sequenced through imaging-based detection of fluorescent labels incorporated with each extension in parallel. The last several years have witnessed an accelerating application of this technology for a variety of goals including transcriptome profiling [80]. Hybridization-based microarrays have the advantages of a significantly lower workload and a relatively low cost. But the probe collection on a chip presents a hard constraint on its detection power. In contrast, the sequencing-based MPS approaches require more advanced instruments that are more cost- and labor intensive, but they provide in-depth analysis of gene expression profiling, allowing the potential identification of novel mRNAs [81]. It is predicted that microarray approaches may eventually become obsolete if MPS issues regarding genome assembly and annotation, cost, and ease have been worked out [82]. The present coexistence of various DNA microarray platforms and MPS technologies offers biomedical research complementary options for transcriptome profiling.

Moreover, transcriptional profiling might become less important in future because it measures a biological intermediate that is too volatile and prone to producing interfering artifacts [4]. For the identification of therapeutic targets, RNA changes need to be validated at protein level since RNA might be too far from the actual cellular effectors.

The true value of expression signatures requires a demonstration of their utility in the clinical setting. For many cancers, prognostic models based on standard clinicopathological variables already exist, and these expression signatures should demonstrate added benefit beyond the best prognostic models already in use today. Unfortunately, the performances of published signatures are much poorer than stated and the predictions are quite discordant. There is no solid evidence for favorable use of any identified expression signatures in clinic [48]. Two commercially available gene expression-based prognostic tests (MammaPrint and OncotypeDX) are currently being assessed in two large randomized clinical trials of breast cancer (TAILORx and MINDACT). In North America, TAILORx is specifically evaluating the usefulness of chemotherapy in intermediate-risk patients estimated with the Oncotype DX test. In the case of MINDACT, ongoing in the European Union, clinical validation of the prognostic test will be considered successful if the proportion of failures among patients classified as having a good prognosis by the MamaPrint test is below a predefined level. But these two trials are not primarily designed to study the clinical usefulness of the signatures [83]. It is obvious that there are many significant challenges facing investigators in the clinical validation of microarray findings, such as the complexity of biological systems, sample limitation, and variability of data mining methods [84]. Integration of expression data from primary human breast cancers with data obtained from the experimental manipulation of model systems is also a major challenge for microarray translational research [85].

Together with the rapid development of microarray technology, other important high-throughput platforms are being developed to analyze genetic and epigenetic changes in DNA, microRNA, and protein for dissecting the biological complexity of human diseases. It is a current trend to integrate various sources of information to speed up the hunting of responsible genes, modules, and networks in cancer research. For example, Gallegos Ruiz et al. [86] performed a genome-wide screening of chromosomal copy number changes with gene expression arrays in 32 radically resected tumor samples from stage I and II NSCLC patients. They identified a deletion on 14q32.2-33 as a common alteration in NSCLC (44%), which significantly influenced gene expression for Hsp90. This deletion was correlated with better overall survival ($P = 0.008$), patients whose tumors had lower Hsp90 expression also lived longer. This finding was validated in three independent sets of NSCLC patients.

Furthermore, in vitro treatment with an Hsp90 inhibitor showed potent anti-proliferative activity in NSCLC cell lines. In another study, Adler et al. used the same strategy to identify genes that may induce the transcription of the prognostic "wound response" expression signature in human breast cancer. The amplification of two genes, *MYC* and *CSN5*, appeared to be correlated with the wound response cassette. In vitro validation showed that the wound signature could be induced in MCF10A cells only when *MYC* and *CSN5* were coexpressed [87]. It is obvious that the integrative use of all these platforms should allow us to uncover genes and complex conditional interactions embedded in carcinogenesis.

In summary, microarray technology is a unique tool for cancer research. Expression profiling has become a new approach to cancer classification. Microarray studies have identified many genes and pathways potentially involved in the development of many common tumors. The emerging systems biology will improve our understanding and interpretation of complicated microarray data. We expect that expression profiling study, together with other high-throughput technologies, will eventually lead to the development of personalized and system-based approaches for optimal management of human cancer.

References

1. Lipshutz RJ et al. Using oligonucleotide probe arrays to access genetic diversity. *Biotechniques* 1995; **19**: 442–447.
2. Schena M, Shalon D, Davis RW, Brown PO. Quantitative monitoring of gene expression patterns with a complementary DNA microarray. *Science* 1995; **270**: 467–470.
3. Alwine JC, Kemp DJ, Stark GR. Method for detection of specific RNAs in agarose gels by transfer to diazobenzyloxymethyl-paper and hybridization with DNA probes. *Proc Natl Acad Sci USA* 1977; **74**: 5350–5354.
4. Hoheisel JD. Microarray technology: beyond transcript profiling and genotype analysis. *Nat Rev Genet* 2006; **7**: 200–210.
5. Hardiman G. Microarray platforms – comparisons and contrasts. *Pharmacogenomics* 2004; **5**: 487–502.
6. Barrett JC, Kawasaki ES. Microarrays: the use of oligonucleotides and cDNA for the analysis of gene expression. *Drug Discov Today* 2003; **8**: 134–141.
7. Tan PK et al. Evaluation of gene expression measurements from commercial microarray platforms. *Nucleic Acids Res* 2003; **31**: 5676–5684.
8. Shi L et al. The MicroArray Quality Control (MAQC) project shows inter- and intra-platform reproducibility of gene expression measurements. *Nat Biotechnol* 2006; **24**: 1151–1161.
9. Draghici S, Khatri P, Eklund AC, Szallasi Z. Reliability and reproducibility issues in DNA microarray measurements. *Trends Genet* 2006; **22**: 101–109.
10. Golub TR et al. Molecular classification of cancer: class discovery and class prediction by gene expression monitoring. *Science* 1999; **286**: 531–537.
11. Simon R, Radmacher MD, Dobbin K, McShane LM. Pitfalls in the use of DNA microarray data for diagnostic and prognostic classification. *J Natl Cancer Inst* 2003; **95**: 14–18.
12. Perou CM et al. Distinctive gene expression patterns in human mammary epithelial cells and breast cancers. *Proc Natl Acad Sci USA* 1999; **96**: 9212–9217.

13. Allison DB, Cui X, Page GP, Sabripour M. Microarray data analysis: from disarray to consolidation and consensus. *Nat Rev Genet* 2006; **7**: 55–65.
14. Tinker AV, Boussioutas A, Bowtell DD. The challenges of gene expression microarrays for the study of human cancer. *Cancer Cell* 2006; **9**: 333–339.
15. Dobbin K, Simon R. Sample size determination in microarray experiments for class comparison and prognostic classification. *Biostatistics* 2005; **6**: 27–38.
16. Garge NR et al. Reproducible clusters from microarray research: whither? *BMC Bioinformatics* 2005; **6(Suppl 2)**: S10.
17. Gold D et al. A comparative analysis of data generated using two different target preparation methods for hybridization to high-density oligonucleotide microarrays. *BMC Genomics* 2004; **5**: 2.
18. Churchill GA. Fundamentals of experimental design for cDNA microarrays. *Nat Genet* 2002; **32(Suppl)**: 490–495.
19. Shih JH et al. Effects of pooling mRNA in microarray class comparisons. *Bioinformatics* 2004; **20**: 3318–3325.
20. Potter JD. Epidemiology, cancer genetics and microarrays: making correct inferences, using appropriate designs. *Trends Genet* 2003; **19**: 690–695.
21. Bogaerts J et al. Gene signature evaluation as a prognostic tool: challenges in the design of the MINDACT trial. *Nat Clin Pract Oncol* 2006; **3**: 540–551.
22. Paik S. Development and clinical utility of a 21-gene recurrence score prognostic assay in patients with early breast cancer treated with tamoxifen. *Oncologist* 2007; **12**: 631–635.
23. Grant GR, Manduchi E, Stoeckert CJ, Jr. Analysis and management of microarray gene expression data. *Curr Protoc Mol Biol* 2007; **Chapter 19**: Units 19, 16.
24. Steibel JP, Rosa GJ. On reference designs for microarray experiments. *Stat Appl Genet Mol Biol* 2005; **4**: Article36.
25. Lee JK, Williams PD, Cheon S. Data mining in genomics. *Clin Lab Med* 2008; **28**: 145–166, viii.
26. DeRisi JL, Iyer VR, Brown PO. Exploring the metabolic and genetic control of gene expression on a genomic scale. *Science* 1997; **278**: 680–686.
27. Baldi P, Long AD. A Bayesian framework for the analysis of microarray expression data: regularized t -test and statistical inferences of gene changes. *Bioinformatics* 2001; **17**: 509–519.
28. Wright GW, Simon RM. A random variance model for detection of differential gene expression in small microarray experiments. *Bioinformatics* 2003; **19**: 2448–2455.
29. Tusher VG, Tibshirani R, Chu G. Significance analysis of microarrays applied to the ionizing radiation response. *Proc Natl Acad Sci USA* 2001; **98**: 5116–5121.
30. Simon R. Microarray-based expression profiling and informatics. *Curr Opin Biotechnol* 2008; **19**: 26–29.
31. Jeffery IB, Higgins DG, Culhane AC. Comparison and evaluation of methods for generating differentially expressed gene lists from microarray data. *BMC Bioinformatics* 2006; **7**: 359.
32. Slonim DK. From patterns to pathways: gene expression data analysis comes of age. *Nat Genet* 2002; **32(Suppl)**: 502–508.
33. Rhodes DR, Chinnaiyan AM. Integrative analysis of the cancer transcriptome. *Nat Genet* 2005; **37(Suppl)**: S31–37.
34. Rhodes DR et al. Meta-analysis of microarrays: interstudy validation of gene expression profiles reveals pathway dysregulation in prostate cancer. *Cancer Res* 2002; **62**: 4427–4433.
35. Ramasamy A, Mondry A, Holmes CC, Altman DG. Key issues in conducting a meta-analysis of gene expression microarray datasets. *PLoS Med* 2008; **5**: e184.
36. Han JD. Understanding biological functions through molecular networks. *Cell Res* 2008; **18**: 224–237.
37. Segal E, Friedman N, Koller D, Regev A. A module map showing conditional activity of expression modules in cancer. *Nat Genet* 2004; **36**: 1090–1098.

38. Yang HH, Hu Y, Buetow KH, Lee MP. A computational approach to measuring coherence of gene expression in pathways. *Genomics* 2004; **84**: 211–217.
39. Harris MA et al. The Gene Ontology (GO) database and informatics resource. *Nucleic Acids Res* 2004; **32**: D258–D261.
40. Kanehisa M et al. The KEGG resource for deciphering the genome. *Nucleic Acids Res* 2004; **32**: D277–D280.
41. Salomonis N et al. GenMAPP 2: new features and resources for pathway analysis. *BMC Bioinformatics* 2007; **8**: 217.
42. Mootha VK et al. PGC-1alpha-responsive genes involved in oxidative phosphorylation are coordinately downregulated in human diabetes. *Nat Genet* 2003; **34**: 267–273.
43. Yu K, Ganesan K, Miller LD, Tan P. A modular analysis of breast cancer reveals a novel low-grade molecular signature in estrogen receptor-positive tumors. *Clin Cancer Res* 2006; **12**: 3288–3296.
44. Ihmels J et al. Revealing modular organization in the yeast transcriptional network. *Nat Genet* 2002; **31**: 370–377.
45. Chuaqui RF et al. Post-analysis follow-up and validation of microarray experiments. *Nat Genet* 2002; **32(Suppl)**: 509–514.
46. Quackenbush J. Microarray analysis and tumor classification. *N Engl J Med* 2006; **354**: 2463–2472.
47. Nevins JR, Potti A. Mining gene expression profiles: expression signatures as cancer phenotypes. *Nat Rev Genet* 2007; **8**: 601–609.
48. Sotiriou C, Piccart MJ. Taking gene-expression profiling to the clinic: when will molecular signatures become relevant to patient care? *Nat Rev Cancer* 2007; **7**: 545–553.
49. Perou CM et al. Molecular portraits of human breast tumours. *Nature* 2000; **406**: 747–752.
50. Chen X et al. Gene expression patterns in human liver cancers. *Mol Biol Cell* 2002; **13**: 1929–1939.
51. Hortobagyi GN. Trastuzumab in the treatment of breast cancer. *N Engl J Med* 2005; **353**: 1734–1736.
52. Paez JG et al. EGFR mutations in lung cancer: correlation with clinical response to gefitinib therapy. *Science* 2004; **304**: 1497–1500.
53. Chung CH, Bernard PS, Perou CM. Molecular portraits and the family tree of cancer. *Nat Genet* 2002; **32(Suppl)**: 533–540.
54. Hayes DN et al. Gene expression profiling reveals reproducible human lung adenocarcinoma subtypes in multiple independent patient cohorts. *J Clin Oncol* 2006; **24**: 5079–5090.
55. Hillen HF. Unknown primary tumours. *Postgrad Med J* 2000; **76**: 690–693.
56. Su AI et al. Molecular classification of human carcinomas by use of gene expression signatures. *Cancer Res* 2001; **61**: 7388–7393.
57. Rhodes DR et al. Large-scale meta-analysis of cancer microarray data identifies common transcriptional profiles of neoplastic transformation and progression. *Proc Natl Acad Sci USA* 2004; **101**: 9309–9314.
58. Ramaswamy S, Ross KN, Lander ES, Golub TR. A molecular signature of metastasis in primary solid tumors. *Nat Genet* 2003; **33**: 49–54.
59. Wirapati P et al. Meta-analysis of gene expression profiles in breast cancer: toward a unified understanding of breast cancer subtyping and prognosis signatures. *Breast Cancer Res* 2008; **10**: R65.
60. Shedden K et al. Gene expression-based survival prediction in lung adenocarcinoma: a multi-site, blinded validation study. *Nat Med* 2008; **14**: 822–827.
61. Staunton JE et al. Chemosensitivity prediction by transcriptional profiling. *Proc Natl Acad Sci USA* 2001; **98**: 10787–10792.
62. Potti A et al. Genomic signatures to guide the use of chemotherapeutics. *Nat Med* 2006; **12**: 1294–1300.
63. Weston AD, Hood L. Systems biology, proteomics, and the future of health care: toward predictive, preventative, and personalized medicine. *J Proteome Res* 2004; **3**: 179–196.

64. Kitano H. Biological robustness. *Nat Rev Genet* 2004; **5**: 826–837.
65. Reymann S, Borlak J. Transcription profiling of lung adenocarcinomas of c-myc-transgenic mice: identification of the c-myc regulatory gene network. *BMC Syst Biol* 2008; **2**: 46.
66. Whitfield ML, George LK, Grant GD, Perou CM. Common markers of proliferation. *Nat Rev Cancer* 2006; **6**: 99–106.
67. Ioannidis JP. Microarrays and molecular research: noise discovery? *Lancet* 2005; **365**: 454–455.
68. Futreal PA et al. A census of human cancer genes. *Nat Rev Cancer* 2004; **4**: 177–183.
69. Vogelstein B, Kinzler KW. Cancer genes and the pathways they control. *Nat Med* 2004; **10**: 789–799.
70. Lahav G et al. Dynamics of the p53-Mdm2 feedback loop in individual cells. *Nat Genet* 2004; **36**: 147–150.
71. Kim E, Giese A, Deppert W. Wild-type p53 in cancer cells: When a guardian turns into a blackguard. *Biochem Pharmacol* 2009; **77** (1): 11–20.
72. Stegmaier K et al. Gene expression-based high-throughput screening(GE-HTS) and application to leukemia differentiation. *Nat Genet* 2004; **36**: 257–263.
73. Stegmaier K et al. Gefitinib induces myeloid differentiation of acute myeloid leukemia. *Blood* 2005; **106**: 2841–2848.
74. Stegmaier K et al. Signature-based small molecule screening identifies cytosine arabinoside as an EWS/FLI modulator in Ewing sarcoma. *PLoS Med* 2007; **4**: e122.
75. Lamb J. The Connectivity Map: a new tool for biomedical research. *Nat Rev Cancer* 2007; **7**: 54–60.
76. Wei G et al. Gene expression-based chemical genomics identifies rapamycin as a modulator of MCL1 and glucocorticoid resistance. *Cancer Cell* 2006; **10**: 331–342.
77. Hieronymus H et al. Gene expression signature-based chemical genomic prediction identifies a novel class of HSP90 pathway modulators. *Cancer Cell* 2006; **10**: 321–330.
78. Wong DJ et al. Revealing targeted therapy for human cancer by gene module maps. *Cancer Res* 2008; **68**: 369–378.
79. Brenner S et al. Gene expression analysis by massively parallel signature sequencing (MPSS) on microbead arrays. *Nat Biotechnol* 2000; **18**: 630–634.
80. Shendure J, Ji H. Next-generation DNA sequencing. *Nat Biotechnol* 2008; **26**: 1135–1145.
81. Liu F et al. Comparison of hybridization and sequencing-based gene expression technologies on biological replicates. *BMC Genomics* 2007; **8**: 153.
82. Coppee JY. Do DNA microarrays have their future behind them? *Microbes Infect* 2008; **10** (9): 1067–1071.
83. Koscielny S. Critical review of microarray-based prognostic tests and trials in breast cancer. *Curr Opin Obstet Gynecol* 2008; **20**: 47–50.
84. Abdullah-Sayani A, Bueno-de-Mesquita JM, van de Vijver MJ. Technology Insight: tuning into the genetic orchestra using microarrays–limitations of DNA microarrays in clinical practice. *Nat Clin Pract Oncol* 2006; **3**: 501–516.
85. Wilson CA, Dering J. Recent translational research: microarray expression profiling of breast cancer–beyond classification and prognostic markers? *Breast Cancer Res* 2004; **6**: 192–200.
86. Gallegos Ruiz MI et al. Integration of gene dosage and gene expression in non-small cell lung cancer, identification of HSP90 as potential target. *PLoS ONE* 2008; **3**: e0001722.
87. Adler AS et al. Genetic regulators of large-scale transcriptional signatures in cancer. *Nat Genet* 2006; **38**: 421–430.

Clinical Trials and Translational Applications in Cancer Therapy

Dineo Khabele and Derrick Beech

1 Introduction

Despite the gains that had been made in increasing overall survival and extending disease-free survival rates, cancer is still one of the leading causes of death in the United States [1]. There remains an urgent need for the rapid development of new cancer therapeutics. Unfortunately, only about 5% of new compounds intended for use in cancer therapy are approved for clinical use [2]. The time and enormous costs involved in conducting clinical trials are special barriers to drug development [3, 4]. Careful thought regarding each phase of investigation is critical for the successful and efficient completion and interpretation of a clinical trial and prior to widespread clinical use of a new drug. This chapter focuses on clinical trials in oncology and translational applications. The global objectives of cancer clinical trials are to evaluate promising new agents that may alleviate symptoms and/or cure the disease. As newer agents such as molecular targeted therapies are developed, questions remain as to whether current models of clinical trial design are sufficient. Nevertheless, classic design forms the basis of drug development in cancer therapy. Study objectives and endpoints are associated with specific study designs and determine the level of testing and the number of subjects required for each phase (Fig. 1) [5].

2 Classic Clinical Trial Design for New Cancer Drugs

Guidelines for clinical trials have been established by the Food and Drug Administration (FDA) [6]. The classic model of clinical trial design takes pharmaceutical compounds that have shown some promise in preclinical experimentation through several levels of testing prior to implementation in clinical practice (Fig. 1). In general, preclinical studies in vitro and in animals

D. Beech (✉)
Professor and Chair, Department of Surgery, Meharry Medical College, Nashville, TN 37208, USA
e-mail: dbeech@mmc.edu

Y. Lu, R.I. Mahato (eds.), *Pharmaceutical Perspectives of Cancer Therapeutics*, DOI 10.1007/978-1-4419-0131-6_21, © Springer Science+Business Media, LLC 2009

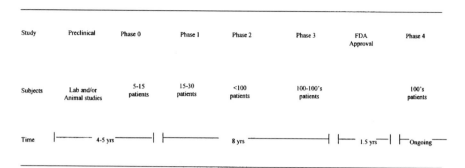

Study	Preclinical	Phase 0	Phase 1	Phase 2	Phase 3	FDA Approval	Phase 4
Subjects	Lab and/or Animal studies	5-15 patients	15-30 patients	<100 patients	100-100's patients		100's patients
Time	4-5 yrs		8 yrs			1.5 yrs	Ongoing

Fig. 1 The number of patient subjects required and the amount of time needed to complete the study

are required, in order to apply for a new Investigational New Drug (IND) application. The experimental agent is then tested for safety and efficacy in humans in phase I to phase III trials. Recent changes designed to facilitate cancer drug development and improve upon clinical trials include phase 0, and phase IV designs have been implemented by the FDA in a collaborative program with the National Cancer Institute (NCI).

2.1 Phase 0 Trials: Exploratory Studies

One method to permit early evaluation of new drugs and to more efficiently design subsequent phase I studies is to conduct phase 0 trials [7, 8]. The FDA permits investigation of new compounds with limited preliminary data through the mechanism, exploratory investigational new drug (ExpIND). The new drug can be studied concurrently with preclinical testing, in order to provide additional rationale for further human investigation. In such a trial, very low doses of the new drug are administered to a small cohort, usually 5–15 subjects, for usually less than 7 days to evaluate the mechanism of action of the agent. Pharmacokinetics and pharmacodynamics are the focus, rather than safety or efficacy. The potential efficacy is evaluated by surrogate biomarkers or specific targets of the treatment. These trials are ideal for compounds that are (1) not highly toxic, (2) have a mechanism of action, and (3) have pharmacodynamics and pharmacokinetics that can be readily evaluated. However, if the agent has been shown to be toxic in animals, if there is an unclear mechanism of action, or if there are no established pharmacodynamic assays for the drug, it is best to conduct phase I trials.

2.2 Phase I Trials: Toxicity, Pharmacokinetics, and Pharmacodynamic Studies

If phase 0 studies are not conducted, traditionally, the earliest introduction of a new agent into humans is through phase I trials [9]. Phase I studies are designed to determine pharmacologic effects, particularly dose-limiting toxicity (DLT) as well as route and timing of drug delivery by studying the pharmacokinetics and pharmacodynamics of the drug. A classic phase I trial is open to patients with different types of cancers and involves several small cohorts (about 3–5 subject per cohort) at different doses of drug. The initial cohort is treated with a dose of the drug that is typically based on a predetermined and much lower percentage of the dose that is lethal in animal studies. Study subjects are observed for toxicity, and if the drug is tolerated, with no DLT or other unacceptable side effect, another cohort is treated with a higher dose. Dose escalation continues with new cohorts of patients until the DLT is reached. Once the DLT is established in more than one patient in a cohort, then the study is halted. The dose that is one dose lower than the DLT is considered the maximal tolerable dose (MTD) and is usually recommended for further study in phase II trials.

Phase I studies are critical for development of novel agents. An example is a new histone deacetylase inhibitor (MS-275), which was tested for toxicity and pharmacologic and biological effects of three different oral dosing schedules [10]. The DLTs were hypophosphatemia and weakness observed on the weekly and twice-weekly dosing schedules – but no toxicity on the every other week schedule. Based on this study, the recommended dose for further studies was determined to be 4 mg/m^2 given weekly for 3 weeks every 28 days or 2–6 mg/m^2 given once every other week. Although not the primary intent of the study, 6 patients showed stable disease and 2 of 27 patients had partial remissions, including one patient with metastatic melanoma who remained on study for >5 years.

A key limitation to the classic phase I design is that it runs the risk of too many patients being treated at low, ineffective doses. Another constraint is that efficacy is not an endpoint of phase I trials, and a clinically meaningful benefit cannot be extrapolated from the small number of participants. Although individual responses are often observed and documented as possible surrogates of the new drug's efficacy, these results must be interpreted with caution [11]. In addition, the subjects in cancer therapeutic phase I studies are not healthy volunteers, unlike clinical trials in other medical specialties, but often heavily pretreated patients with cancers that have not responded to prior therapy. Newer approaches to phase I trials are being developed to allow for more rapid and efficient methods of determining the MTD, treating a larger number of patients at doses in the therapeutic range and reducing the toxicity of higher doses [12–14].

2.3 Phase II Trials: Response Rates and Toxicity Studies

The next level of investigation of a new cancer drug is the phase II study. Phase II trials are primarily designed to assess the efficacy of a new agent and to further evaluate its safety in larger cohorts of patients. The study design of phase II trials builds upon results from preclinical investigations and the MTD established in phase I trials. The underlying objective is to determine the drug's usefulness for future comparative studies to standard treatment. The study population is intended to be more homogenous, e.g., same disease site, unlike phase I trials which are open to a variety of tumor types.

Many phase II trials are single-arm nonrandomized studies. If there is a control arm, patients in that group receive standard of care treatment. Some of the issues with phase II trials are as follows: they (1) may expose a large number of patients to inadequate or toxic therapy; (2) take long periods of time to complete; and (3) are expensive. Most studies are designed to incorporate early stopping rules [15]. An interim analysis can be performed before the study is complete and a study stopped early, if there are no observed responses or unacceptable toxicity from the drug (a negative result) or if the responses are high and further testing in phase III trials is justified (a positive result). If the response rate is equivocal, the study is kept open for further accrual. Interim analyses and early stopping rules must be determined prior to initiating the study to limit bias in interpreting the final results.

Other strategies are being implemented to make phase II trials more efficient. One example is the multiarm multistage (MAMS) randomized trial design that allows for testing of many different agents at the same time in comparison to a single group of controls [16]. Initially, each experimental arm is compared solely to the control arm. The groups in which the experimental drugs do not show sufficient efficacy are dropped, and the remaining groups are evaluated until the primary outcomes of the study are reached. At the conclusion of the study, all arms undergo evaluation.

Phase II trials are critical for determining the utility of proceeding to additional human investigation of a new compound or testing new routes or combinations of therapy. However, the vast majority of phase II trials are negative studies that do not go to phase III trials [17]. Therefore, new paradigms of study design, particularly with novel molecularly targeted therapy, are needed to bring new compounds to clinical practice.

An example of incorporating genomic information into the design of a phase II trial is the recently published evaluation of somatic mutations in the epidermal growth factor receptor (EGFR) [18]. The authors were able to correlate specific EGFR mutations with clinical response to the EGFR inhibitor gefitinib in patients with advanced nonsmall-cell lung cancer. The authors concluded that "genotype-directed" first-line treatment with gefitnib was worthy of further study in a phase III trial. This type of study design will become more important as new molecular targets for cancer therapy are discovered.

2.4 Phase III Trials: Efficacy Studies

The gold standard test for new therapeutic agent is the randomized control clinical trial (RCT) that occurs after early phase studies have been completed. Phase III trials are large, usually multicenter studies designed to compare a new agent that showed promise in earlier phase studies to current standard treatment regimens for specific type of cancer. These RCT studies require large-enough numbers of participants to offer sufficient power to detect a statistical difference between treatment arms. Cohorts include hundreds to thousands of participants. Therefore, phase III trials require multiple institutions and sites for target accrual. The primary endpoint in phase III trials is usually progression-free survival, while secondary endpoints usually include response rate and overall survival.

An example of a multicenter, cooperative group, randomized phase III trial was the recently published comparison of intravenous paclitaxel plus cisplatin to intravenous paclitaxel plus intraperitoneal cisplatin and paclitaxel in patients with stage III ovarian cancer patients with minimal residual disease. The median duration of overall survival in the intravenous-therapy and intraperitoneal-therapy groups was 49.7 and 65.6 months, respectively [19]. Although there was a high toxicity rate, the greater than 60 months overall survival for advanced stage ovarian cancer was an important finding. This study led to new treatment guidelines for newly diagnosed, advanced stage ovarian cancers after optimal tumor debulking surgery.

2.5 Phase IV Trials: Long-Term Toxicity Studies

Once the new drug has been approved by the FDA for general clinical use, phase IV trials are conducted to assess long-term side effects. The number of subjects required for phase IV studies is usually in the thousands, and the study period is over a long period of time prospectively. Phase IV trials can be used to evaluate different doses and schedules than those initially tested in phase II and III studies. In addition, other measures such as quality of life indices and cost can be studied. Phase IV trials are difficult to conduct because of the large numbers of subjects required and the fact that they are ongoing. Phase IV studies are by necessity multicenter trials and are implemented typically through cooperative oncology groups.

3 Study Endpoints

3.1 Common Endpoints

The endpoints for phase 0 trials are pharmacokinetics, pharmacodynamics, and biomarker responses to the new drug. Phase I trials test for safety along with the pharmacokinetics and pharmacodynamics. In phase II through IV trials, common endpoints are clinical measurements of response, toxicity, time to progression or the progression-free interval, and overall survival. Several cooperative oncology groups have objective criteria to measure the severity of adverse events or serious adverse events.

3.2 Response Evaluation Criteria in Solid Tumors (RECIST)

The Response Evaluation Criteria in Solid Tumors (RECIST) criteria is the most common method of measuring responses rates for solid tumors, by physical examination and/or radiographic imaging [20]. A complete response is resolution of measurable tumors lasting at least 4 weeks. A partial response is a decrease by at least 30% in the measurable tumors with no new sites of disease. Progressive disease is at least a 20% increase in measurable disease and/or one or more new sites of disease, and stable disease defines tumors that have not met the criteria for response or progression. The overall response rate in a study is the sum of partial plus complete responses. These guidelines were designed for phase II trials to evaluate efficacy of cytotoxic drugs. However, the applicability of traditional phase II design to the study of compounds that target small molecules (e.g. tyrosine kinases) has been challenged [21]. It has been suggested that for targeted therapies, any endpoint that differentiates the treatment arm from the control can be used as a method for justifying further investigation of the new agent.

3.3 Survival

Event-free survival is measured from the time of diagnosis or treatment intervention to a defined event, typically overall survival and progression-free survival. The time to event is articulated as a median for the group or as a percentage of the group at a particular time such as the 5-year mark after diagnosis. Clearly, overall survival is a significant endpoint in cancer therapy trials. However, other cancer therapies and confounding factors such as individual co-morbidities may impact survival. Progression-free survival is often used as an endpoint in phase III trials because it more closely reflects the effects of immediate therapy. Furthermore, in studying cytostatic agents, progression-free survival may be a more appropriate endpoint.

4 Eligibility

4.1 Defining the Study Population

Defining the study population is critical in determining the immediate criteria for enrollment in a clinical trial and ultimately, if the results can be applied to the general population. The research question, hypothesis, and study design are used to identify the characteristics of participants who are eligible for the trial.

4.2 Inclusion and Exclusion Criteria

Eligible subjects are recruited based on a number of factors including particular malignant disease site, stage of disease, performance status, and underlying medical conditions. Potential study participants who are not likely to benefit or who may be at unusually high risk of adverse side effects if enrolled (e.g., renal failure) are excluded. The eligibility and exclusion criteria are typically specific to the condition and treatment under study. Inclusion and exclusion in a study should not be a matter of convenience. For example, a consecutive series of patients from a single clinic site is a sample of convenience and is inherently biased by the nature of the clinic location, patterns of referral, patient population, and other confounding factors. The process of determining the methods of subject recruitment is important in minimizing statistical bias and in the potential of generalizing the results to the population at large.

5 Statistical Considerations

5.1 Randomized Control Trials (RCTs)

In RCT studies, the method of randomization is important in reducing bias. Formal statistical models of probability are the best method of assigning subjects. It is important that the assignment to a particular study arm is made after the participant's eligibility is established and informed consent has been obtained.

A double-blind study is designed to hide which treatment is being administered from both the study participants and the treating physicians. Ideally, to eliminate as much bias as possible in a double-blind study, all personnel involved with the participant's treatment, data collection, data management, and analysis should be blinded. A single-blind study in which the study group assignment is unknown to either the study participant or the treating physician is still subject to bias. An open-label study where assignments are known to study participants, treating physicians, and study personnel is the most biased study design, and the results should be interpreted in this context. The gold standard is a double blind, RCT. However, single institution studies may be a practical initial approach for small exploratory investigations.

5.2 Sample Size, Power, and Significance

In order to calculate the number of participants required for the study or the sample size, the investigator must know the desired power, significance level, and expected magnitude of the effect to be observed. The statistical power of a clinical study is the probability of detecting a difference in the effect of the investigational drug, compared to standard treatment, if indeed a true difference exists. The complement of power $(1 - \text{power})$ is the probability of failing to find an effect when one does exist, a false negative or type II or β error. Common values for type II error are 0.2 (or 1 in 5) and 0.1 (or 1 in 10), which correspond to power of 0.8 and 0.9, respectively. The study significance level is the probability of detecting an apparent effect when none exists, and differences observed are the result of chance, a type I error. Common values for a false positive or type I α error are 0.05 (1 in 20) and 0.01 (1 in 100). Increases in type I and II errors and low power are observed with small sample size. On the other hand, if a sample size is too large, there is an increased chance of subjecting study participants to unnecessary risk, wasting resources, and prolonging the study duration. Furthermore, too large of a sample size may be statistically significant, but clinically irrelevant. Early stopping rules are determined a priori by statisticians and clinical investigators to ensure the study design takes into account the statistical considerations as well as the pathogenesis and clinical progression of individual types of cancer.

5.3 The Null Hypothesis

Comparisons are most frequently made to determine whether there is a difference between treatments, or between treatment and control, with respect to the null hypothesis (the premise that there is no difference between the two conditions) [22]. Thus, the null hypothesis is rejected if any difference is seen. Theoretically, the tests are two sided. The null hypothesis will be rejected if the observed value is greater or less than the null value (i.e., if any difference is observed). It can be argued that for practical purposes, however, a new cancer treatment is of interest only if it changes clinical practice by having a favorable effect on the patient's prognosis. Tests to determine whether a treatment changes a parameter relative to the null hypothesis that it causes no change or decreases (increases) the parameter are referred to as one sided because the null hypothesis is rejected only if the effect is in one direction. One-sided hypotheses have greater power with smaller numbers of observations but produce less information about the relation between treatments. They also are open to overgeneralization of positive results if the directionality of the test is misinterpreted. This one-sided hypothesis is in contrast to the two-sided hypothesis in which the new therapy could be worse than standard of care. Testing the two-sided hypothesis requires a much larger sample size. However, typically one is most interested in the new agent performing better than standard therapy. Thus, most studies test the null hypothesis that the response rate is less than expected and the alternative hypothesis that the response rate is greater than anticipated. The expected value is determined by statisticians.

Determining the magnitude of expected response a priori is critical. A difference of 15–20% response rate between the investigational drug and standard treatment in solid tumors can typically be achieved. A larger difference is not likely to be observed clinically but requires a smaller number of patients. If the response rate of the standard of care is close to 50%, detection of a difference from the new treatment requires more patients than if the rate is at much higher or lower extremes.

6 Ethical Considerations

6.1 The Ethical Basis for Clinical Trials

Ethical considerations must be applied from the design to the completion of a clinical trial. Clear scientific hypotheses and objectives are critical. It is difficult to justify a clinical study if it is not clinically important or relevant. There are added ethical considerations for cancer patients, many of whom have been heavily pretreated with other chemotherapy agents and many of whom are terminally ill and may not derive any direct benefit from the agent being studied, particularly in phase 0 and I trials [23]. Clinical trials are conducted under guidelines issued in the Belmont Report of 1978 that protects human subjects and follows principles of respect for persons, beneficence, and justice. Scientific conduct is also guided by ethical principles in that competent and rigorous analysis is required to prevent compromise of the results [24].

6.2 Special and Vulnerable Populations

The NCI has a policy for inclusion of women and minorities to ensure that research findings can be applicable to all those at risk of the disease. Women have historically been excluded from clinical trials. Emerging information shows that dosing and toxicity may differ in men and women [25]. In addition, recent data suggest that molecular markers may have differential implications based on gender. For example, observed polymorphisms in the EGFR have opposite effects on overall prognosis in men and women [26].

Information about ethnicity and race is also important for clinical trials. The response to chemotherapy in African-American women may be affected by the fact that the basal type "triple negative" breast cancers are more prevalent among black women [27]. Minorities in general are underrepresented in clinical trials. The reasons are complex and include lack of access to care, lack of information and awareness, and mistrust of the medical establishment [28, 29]. Furthermore, minorities are often not offered an opportunity to enroll in trials. Strategies to include minorities in clinical trials are to increase access and awareness and to offer minorities a chance to participate in trials [30]. In addition, the use of patient navigators as suggested for improving cancer care among minorities [31] may facilitate minority access and involvement in clinical trials.

Children and prisoners are considered to be vulnerable populations because of issues of potential ethical issues related to informed consent and coercion. Participation in clinical trials is permitted for vulnerable populations, but only if the risks of the trial are minimal. Finally, cancer patients in general can be considered vulnerable because many subjects are terminally ill by the time they enroll in clinical trials [23]. It is important to be aware of the potential ethical issues and similar to other vulnerable populations, minimize the risks and ensure proper informed consent.

7 Challenges and Future Prospects for Translation of Clinical Trials

In an era of exciting and promising discovery of new therapeutic agents for the treatment of cancer, it is important to make sure that clinical trials are conducted in such a way that the ultimate results have meaning for those affected by the disease. An understanding of the classic study designs of clinical trials is important in bringing new therapeutic agents from preclinical investigation to the clinic. However, as the complexity of treatment strategies increases such as with combination chemotherapy and with novel molecular targets for treatment, clinical trial design will need to adapt to such changes. More rapid methods of moving from discovery to clinical delivery will be required. At the same time, attention to including diverse populations affected by specific cancers is important for the widest applicability of the research findings. Finally, with newer and more complex treatment strategies for cancer, there may be new emphasis on endpoints other than overall survival, such as maintaining stable disease, improving quality of life, and analysis of cost.

References

1. Jemal A, Siegel R, Ward E, Hao Y, Xu J, Murray T, Thun MJ. Cancer statistics, 2008. *CA Cancer J Clin* 2008; **58**: 71–96.
2. Kola I. The state of innovation in drug development. *Clin Pharmacol Ther* 2008; **83**: 227–230.
3. DiMasi J, Grabowski HG. Economics of new oncology drug development. *J Clin Oncol* 2007; **25**: 209–216.
4. Vickers AJ, Jang K, Sargent D, Lilja H, Kattan MW. Systematic review of statistical methods used in molecular marker studies in cancer. *Cancer* 2008; **112**: 1862–1868.
5. Nottage M, Siu LL. Principles of clinical trial design. *J Clin Oncol* 2002; **20**: 42S–46S.
6. FDA, Food and Drug Administration. 2008. http://www.fda.gov/oc/gcp/.
7. Murgo AJ, Kummar S, Rubinstein L, Gutierrez M, Collins J, Kinders R, Parchment RE, et al. Designing phase 0 cancer clinical trials. *Clin Cancer Res* 2008; **14**: 3675–3682.
8. Kummar S, Kinders R, Rubinstein L, Parchment RE, Murgo AJ, Collins J, Pickeral O, et al. Compressing drug development timelines in oncology using phase '0' trials. *Nat Rev Cancer* 2007; **7**: 131–139.
9. Storer BE. Design and analysis of phase I clinical trials. *Biometrics* 1989; **45**: 925–937.
10. Gore L, Rothernberg ML, O'Bryant CL, Schultz MD, Sandler AB, Coffin D, McCoy C, et al. A phase I and pharmacokinetic study of the oral histone deacetylase inhibitor, MS-275, in patients with refractory solid tumors and lymphomas. *Clin Cancer Res*; 2008; **14**: 4517–4525.
11. Horstmann E, McCabe MS, Grochow L, Yamamoto S, Rubinstein L, Budd T, Shoemaker D, et al. Risks and benefits of phase 1 oncology trials, 1991 through 2002. *N Engl J Med* 2005; **352**: 895–904.
12. Rosa D, Harris DJ, Jayson GC. The best guess approach to phase I trial design. *J Clin Oncol* 2006; **24**: 206–208.
13. Calvert AH, Plummer R. The development of phase I cancer trial methodologies: the use of pharmacokinetic and pharmacodynamic end points sets the scene for phase 0 cancer clinical trials. *Clin Cancer Res* 2008; **14**: 3664–3669.

14. Booth CM, Calvert AH, Giaccone G, Lobbezoo MW, Seymour LK, Eisenhauer EA. Endpoints and other considerations in phase I studies of targeted anticancer therapy: recommendations from the task force on Methodology for the Development of Innovative Cancer Therapies (MDICT). *Eur J Cancer* 2008; **44**: 19–24.
15. Chen K, Shan M. Optimal and minimax three-stage designs for phase II oncology clinical trials. *Contemp Clin Trial* 2008; **29**: 32–41.
16. Parmar MK, Barthel FM, Sydes M, Langley R, Kaplan R, Eisenhauer E, Brady M, James N et al. Speeding up the evaluation of new agents in cancer. *J Natl Cancer Inst* 2008; **100**: 1204–1214.
17. Ratain MJ. Phase II oncology trials: let's be positive. *Clin Cancer Res* 2005; **11**: 5661–5662.
18. Sequist LV, Martins RG, Spigel D, Grunberg SM, Spira A, Janne PA, Joshi VA, et al. First-line gefitinib in patients with advanced non-small-cell lung cancer harboring somatic EGFR mutations. *J Clin Oncol* 2008; **26**: 2442–2449.
19. Armstrong DK, Bundy B, Wenzel L, Huang HG, Baergen R, Lele S, Copeland LJ, et al. Intraperitoneal cisplatin and paclitaxel in ovarian cancer. *N Engl J Med* 2006; **354**: 34–43.
20. Therasse P, Arbuck SG, Eisenhauer EA, Wanders J, Kaplan RS, Rubinstein L, Verweij J, et al. New guidelines to evaluate the response to treatment in solid tumors. European Organization for Research and Treatment of Cancer, National Cancer Institute of the United States, National Cancer Institute of Canada. *J Natl Cancer Inst* 2000; **92**: 205–216.
21. Ratain MJ, Eckhardt SG. Phase II studies of modern drugs directed against new targets: if you are fazed, too, then resist RECIST. *J Clin Oncol* 2004; **22**: 4442–4445.
22. Ratain MJ, Karrison TG. Testing the wrong hypothesis in phase II oncology trials: there is a better alternative. *Clin Cancer Res* 2007; **13**: 781–782.
23. Abdoler E, Taylor H, Wendler D. The ethics of phase oncology trials. *Clin Cancer Res* 2008; **14**: 3692–3697.
24. Beecher HK. Ethics and clinical research. *N Engl J Med* 1966; **274**: 1354–1360.
25. Huang RS, Kistner EO, Bleibel WK, Shukla SJ, Dolan ME. Effect of population and gender on chemotherapeutic agent-induced cytotoxicity. *Mol Cancer Ther* 2007; **6**: 31–36.
26. Press OA, Zhang W, Gordon MA, Yang D, Lurje G, Iqbal S, El-Khoueiry A, et al. Gender-related survival differences associated with EGFR polymorphisms in metastatic colon cancer. *Cancer Res* 2008; **68**: 3037–3042.
27. Morris GJ, Naidu S, Topham AK, Guiles F, Xu Y, McCue P, Schwartz GF, et al. Differences in breast carcinoma characteristics in newly diagnosed African-American and Caucasian patients: a single-institution compilation compared with the National Cancer Institute's Surveillance, Epidemiology, and End Results database. *Cancer* 2007; **110**: 876–884.
28. Khabele D. Racial and ethnic health disparities, women and cancer. *The Medscape Journal* 2005. http://cme.medscape.com/viewprogram/4412.
29. Colon-Otero G, Smallridge RC, Solberg LA Jr, Keith TD, Woodward TA, Willis FB, Dunn AN. Disparities in participation in cancer clinical trials in the United States : a symptom of a healthcare system in crisis. *Cancer* 2008; **112**: 447–454.
30. Ford JG, Howerton MW, Lai GY, Gary TL, Bolen S, Gibbons MC, Tilburt J, et al. Barriers to recruiting underrepresented populations to cancer clinical trials: a systematic review. *Cancer* 2008; **112**: 228–242.
31. Vargas RB, Ryan GW, Jackson A, Rodriguez R, Freeman HP. Characteristics of the original patient navigation programs to reduce disparities in the diagnosis and treatment of breast cancer. *Cancer* 2008; **113**: 426–433.

Index

685